Health Assessment for Nursing Practice

7TH EDITION

Susan Fickertt Wilson, PhD, RN
Emeritus Associate Professor
Harris College of Nursing and Health Sciences
Texas Christian University
Fort Worth, Texas

Jean Foret Giddens, PhD, RN, FAAN, ANEF
Dean and Professor
Yingling Endowed Chair of Nursing
School of Nursing
Virginia Commonwealth University
Richmond, Virginia

ELSEVIER

Elsevier
3251 Riverport Lane
St. Louis, Missouri 63043

HEALTH ASSESSMENT FOR NURSING PRACTICE, SEVENTH EDITION   ISBN: 978-0-323-66119-5

Previous editions copyrighted 2017, 2013, 2009, 2005, 2001, and 1996.

Library of Congress Control Number 2020941147

Executive Content Strategist: Lee Henderson
Senior Content Development Manager: Luke Held
Senior Content Development Specialist: Jennifer Wade
Publishing Services Manager: Julie Eddy
Senior Project Manager: Cindy Thoms
Design Direction: Brian Salisbury

Printed in India

Last digit is the print number: 9 8 7 6 5 4 3 2 1

To my daughter, Megan, for her continued love, patience, and support; to Craig Greenway for his role in this project, and to the faculty, colleagues, and students who have challenged me through the years.

SFW

To my husband, Jay, for his unconditional support; to my mentors and role models, for their guidance throughout my career; to my co-author, Susan Wilson, who has been a tremendous writing partner over the past 20 years and who has an intense passion for making this book as useful as possible for our students; and to nursing students, who are the future of our profession.

JFG

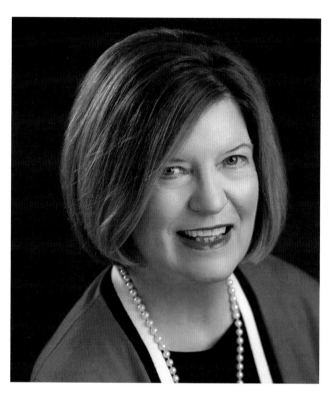

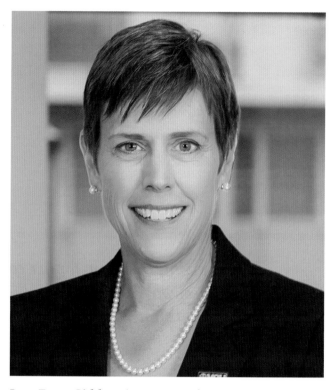

Susan Fickertt Wilson is an Emeritus Associate Professor from Harris College of Nursing and Health Sciences at Texas Christian University in Fort Worth, Texas. She now resides in North Las Vegas, Nevada. Dr. Wilson earned a Bachelor of Science in Nursing from the University of Texas Medical Branch, a Master of Nursing from the University of Washington, and a Doctor of Philosophy in Allied Health Teaching and Administration from Texas A&M University. Dr. Wilson has over 40 years of teaching experience, including 30 years teaching health assessment. Her teaching experience includes baccalaureate and master's degree programs in Texas and Alaska. Her content areas in nursing education include adult health nursing, pathophysiology, pharmacology, health assessment, curriculum development, and spirituality. This text is a synthesis of her experiences performing and teaching health assessment.

Jean Foret Giddens is Dean, Professor, and the Doris B. Yingling Endowed Chair at the School of Nursing at Virginia Commonwealth University in Richmond, Virginia. Dr. Giddens earned a Bachelor of Science in Nursing from the University of Kansas, a Master of Science in Nursing from the University of Texas at El Paso, and a Doctor of Philosophy in Education and Human Resource Studies from Colorado State University. Dr. Giddens has been involved with nursing education since 1984. Her teaching experience includes associate, baccalaureate, and master's degree programs in New Mexico, Texas, Colorado, and Virginia. Her content areas in nursing education include adult health nursing, health assessment, nursing process, curriculum development, and innovative educational strategies.

Sue K. Goebel, MS, RN, WHNP, SANE
Associate Professor of Nursing
Department of Health Sciences
Colorado Mesa University
Grand Junction, Colorado;
Women's Health Nurse Practitioner
Integrative Medicine Center
Grand Junction, Colorado
Chapter 17 and Chapter 20

Leigh Small, PhD, RN, PNP-PC
Associate Dean of Academic Programs
Michigan State University
College of Nursing
East Lansing, Michigan
Chapter 19

REVIEWERS

Laura Brennan, MS, RN
Assistant Professor and Director: Undergraduate
Pre-licensure Program
Department of Nursing and Health Sciences
Elmhurst College
Elmhurst, Illinois

Anna M. Bruch, RN, MSN
Nursing Professor
Health Professions
Illinois Valley Community College
Oglesby, Illinois

Donna Carlson, MSN, RN
Lab/Simulation Instructor, Pre-Licensure
College of Nursing and Health Care Professions
Grand Canyon University
Phoenix, Arizona

Robin Halemeyer, MSN, RN
Professor
Department of Nursing
Lewis and Clark Community College
Godfrey, Illinois

Denise E. King, MSN, RN-BC, CCM
BSN Faculty
Department of Nursing
Dominican University
River Forest, Illinois

LaDonna K. Northington, DNS, RN, BC
Professor, Assistant Dean of Undergraduate Programs
School of Nursing
University of Mississippi School of Nursing
Jackson, Mississippi

Tina Rowe, DNP, CRRN, RN
Nursing Instructor
Department of Nursing
Jefferson State Community College
Clanton, Alabama

Joella A. Tabaka, MSN, RN
Professor
Department of Nursing
Olivet Nazarene University
Oak Brook, Illinois

Mila L. Walker, Ed S, MSN, RN, BC
Clinical Assistant Professor
Science of Nursing Care
Indiana University School of Nursing
Indianapolis, Indiana

Linda M. Wines, RN, MS, CNE
Assistant Professor
Hunt School of Nursing
Gardner-Webb University
Boiling Springs, North Carolina

If a teacher is indeed wise, he does not bid you enter the house of his wisdom, but rather leads you to the threshold of your own mind.

KAHLIL GIBRAN *The Prophet*

Following this teaching we have revised this text *Health Assessment for Nursing Practice* to retain the strong features and add others. The underlying principles of the previous editions are steadfast. As with the previous editions, the seventh edition is based on the assumption that every patient—from neonate to older adult—is an interactive, complex being who is more than a collection of his or her parts. Each patient's health status depends on the interactions of physiologic, psychologic, sociocultural, and spiritual factors. These interactions occur within their physical environments (what they eat, drink, and breathe; what type of activity and work they participate in and where they live), their social environments and health beliefs (friends, family, and support systems; when and how they seek health care), and their internal environments (what they eat and drink, how they sleep, and how often they exercise).

As faculty, we are challenged with several responsibilities toward our students:

- Demonstrate caring and compassion when we interact with patients to act as role models for students.
- Help students become knowledgeable and skilled in history-taking and physical assessment.
- Model for students as well as teach them how to be objective and nonjudgmental.
- Assist students to mobilize their resources to apply health assessment knowledge and skills to patients of all ages and from a multitude of cultures and ethnic groups.

We know that students will need this content for the remainder of their professional lives. This textbook is a toolbox of information and techniques. As a wise teacher, you lead students to the threshold.

ORGANIZATION

Health Assessment for Nursing Practice is organized into four units to assist students and faculty to find their areas of interest. Unit 1, entitled Foundations for Health Assessment, provides a strong foundation for students, covering issues pertinent to nursing practice with all age-groups, such as Introduction to Health Assessment, Obtaining a Health History, Techniques and Equipment for Physical Assessment, and General Inspection and Vital Signs. Also included are chapters on Cultural Competence, Pain Assessment, Mental Health Assessment, and Nutritional Assessment.

Unit 2, entitled Health Assessment of the Adult, is organized by body system. Each chapter in this unit includes a review of Anatomy and Physiology, a Health History, an Examination section, a section on Common Problems and Conditions, and a Clinical Application and Clinical Judgment section.

The Anatomy and Physiology section is found at the beginning of the chapter because physical assessment techniques allow the student to answer the question, "How does this patient's anatomy and physiology compare with that expected for his or her age group and ethnic group?"

The Health History section instructs the student on history data to collect by providing sample questions to ask patients along with the reasons for asking those questions. The text below each question describes the variances that the student may find. Included in the Health History section are headings for Present Health Status, Past Health History, Family History, Personal and Psychosocial History, and Problem-Based History. Risk factor boxes for disorders in each body system are found within the history section to remind students to discuss these behaviors with patients to help them maintain health and reduce risk of disease. The areas of risk factor identification and health promotion are unique to this text. These areas indicate our commitment to not only teach students how to gather data from patients and examine their bodies to detect health and disease, but also to teach them how to help patients attain and maintain a higher level of health.

The Examination section begins with a table that outlines procedures performed routinely and in special circumstances as well as procedures completed by an advanced practice registered nurse. A list of the appropriate Equipment needed for these procedures is included in the table. This section guides the student sequentially in the procedures routinely performed during the physical assessment of an adult, telling what to do, how to do it, and what to expect. Photographs are provided to enhance learning. The subsequent section describes the examination procedures performed in special circumstances. The indication for performing each procedure is followed by expected and abnormal findings. The left column, Procedures With Expected Findings, details the techniques of the assessment and the expected findings, and the right column describes Abnormal Findings. Following the examination section, techniques performed by advanced practice registered nurses are described briefly. When applicable, a section on Patients With Situational Variations may include examinations of patients with limited mobility and patients with a mastectomy.

The Clinical Application and Clinical Judgment section at the end of each chapter contains a Case Study and Review Questions. Case Studies describe subjective and objective data about a patient and ask the student to use clinical reasoning skills to answer questions. Answers for the Review Questions are included in Appendix B to facilitate self-study.

Health Promotion for Evidence-Based Practice boxes outline recommendations for health promotion and reducing health risks. These special feature boxes follow the Health History section so that data are collected at the time of history taking. The Common Problems and Conditions section toward the end of each chapter has been updated. Ethnic, Cultural, and Spiritual Variations boxes throughout the body systems chapters contain racial, cultural, and religious variations the nurse should consider when assessing patients.

Unit 3, entitled Health Assessment Across the Life Span, begins with an overview of growth and development and continues with chapters on Assessment of the Infant, Child, and Adolescent; Assessment of the Pregnant Patient; and Assessment of the Older Adult. These chapters describe how to individualize the examination for patients of different ages and in pregnancy. Each chapter includes a box that lists the differences in anatomy and physiology pertinent to those patients. Health history and examination follow along with procedures and expected and abnormal findings. The Common Problems and Conditions section toward the end of each chapter has been retained in these chapters as they pertain to the patients described.

Unit 4, entitled Synthesis and Application of Health Assessment, contains Conducting a Head-to-Toe Examination, Documenting the Comprehensive Health Assessment, and Adapting Health Assessment. These chapters provide guidelines and photographs for combining the body system assessments into one comprehensive examination, for communicating the findings to other health care professionals, and for adapting the physical assessment to patients receiving medical or surgical treatment.

Appendix A provides abbreviations for selected terms.

A Glossary at the end of the book provides definitions to enhance student comprehension of key concepts and terms.

Chapters were updated and revised based on feedback from both faculty and students. Two content areas have had intentional enhancements in this edition.
- Recognizing and screening for victims of human trafficking have been added to relevant chapters such as the Health History
- Individualizing assessments for people in the lesbian, gay, bisexual, transgender, queer, and questioning (LGBTQ+) community has been added to relevant chapters such as the Health History, Assessments of the Breasts, and Reproductive System.

Consider each chapter a different type of tool from the toolbox. Collectively they provide all that students need to perform a comprehensive health assessment.

SUMMARY OF SPECIAL FEATURES

- Most chapters in Unit 2 (body system chapters) have a Concept Overview section at the beginning of the chapter. A concept relevant to that chapter is featured; interrelated concepts are also shown with an explanation of how these concepts are linked.
- Updated Health Promotion for Evidence-Based Practice boxes include recommendations for health promotion and reducing risk.
- Risk Factors boxes are found in the Health History and highlight information specific to various body systems and disorders.
- Unique and revised Clinical Judgment boxes provide a case situation and walk students through the thought process of how an experienced nurse makes decisions. The steps presented include noticing or recognizing cues, interpreting or analyzing cues and forming hypothesis, then responding or taking action, and finally reflecting on the clinical situation.
- Frequently Asked Questions boxes answer common questions students have as they are learning health assessment. These "FAQs" appear throughout Unit 2.
- Case Studies feature a clinical situation involving a health condition and the ensuing applicable health assessment involved, as well as recognition of important cues within the data. Answers to the Case Studies are provided in Appendix B to help students evaluate their learning.
- Ethnic, Cultural, and Spiritual Variations boxes anticipate the unique needs of a multicultural patient population.
- Within each of the Unit 2 chapters, a Documenting Expected Findings box provides an example of how examination data are presented in a documentation note. This box is found at the end of the Examination section.
- A Lab Guide with skills checklists accompanies this book to assist students when practicing health assessment in laboratory settings.

TEACHING AND LEARNING AIDS

The Evolve website for this book contains extensive student and instructor resources and can be accessed at http://evolve.elsevier.com/Wilson/assessment. This dynamic educational component allows students and faculty to access the most current information and resources for further study and research.

The comprehensive Evolve Instructor Resources include TEACH for Nurses, a resource that ties together every chapter resource necessary for the most effective class presentations. TEACH for Nurses incorporates objectives, key terms, nursing curriculum standards (including BSN Essentials and Concepts), student and instructor chapter resources, in-class/online case studies, and teaching strategies consisting of student activities, online activities, and discussion topics. The ExamView Test Bank has been updated and includes approximately 650 test questions. Also included is a comprehensive Image Collection, which contains hundreds of full-color images that can be imported into the PowerPoint Lecture Slides for use in classroom lectures. Audience Response Questions and Case Studies are also provided for the PowerPoint lecture slides. Evolve Instructor Resources also now include 20 Next Generation NCLEX® Exam-style case studies, including 15 single-episode cases and 5 unfolding cases to help prepare students for the NGN.

Evolve Student Resources include animations, case studies, content updates, key points, audio sounds, review questions, and video clips. Evolve Student Resources also now include 10 Next Generation NCLEX® Exam-style case studies to help students prepare for the NGN. Visit http://evolve.elsevier.com/Wilson/assessment to access these resources.

CONTENTS

Introduction to Health Assessment

Health assessment refers to a systematic method of collecting and analyzing data for the purpose of planning patient-centered care. The nurse collects health data from the patient and compares these with the ideal state of health, taking into account the patient's age; gender; culture; ethnicity; and physical, psychological, and socioeconomic status. Data about the patient's strengths, weaknesses, health problems, and deficits are identified. The nurse incorporates the patient's knowledge, motivation, support systems, coping ability, and preferences to develop a plan of care that will help the patient to maximize his or her potential.

One approach to developing a plan of care is using the American Nurses Association (ANA) *Standards of Practice.*[1] The first six standards are based on the nursing process (i.e., assessment, diagnosis, outcome identification, planning, implementation, and evaluation; Box 1.1). The first and foundational step is assessment, described as the collection of "pertinent data and information relative to the healthcare consumer's health or the situation."[1,p.53] The assessment and subsequent analysis of data are performed by nurses in all settings. Five core competencies identified by the Institute of Medicine are essential for all health care professionals to demonstrate in all areas of practice. These include: (1) provide patient-centered care, (2) work in interdisciplinary teams, (3) use evidenced-based practice, (4) apply quality improvements, and (5) use informatics.[2] These five competencies are integrated into all areas of care, including health assessment.

COMPONENTS OF HEALTH ASSESSMENT

Components of health assessment include conducting a health history, performing a physical examination, reviewing other data from the health record (as available), and documenting the findings (Fig. 1.1). These steps lead to data analysis and interpretation (discussed later in this chapter) so that a patient-centered plan of care can be developed and implemented. The amount of information collected by the nurse during a health history and the extent of the physical examination depend on the setting, the situation, the patient's needs, and the nurse's experience. Structured patient assessment formats provide an outline of elements to include in the assessment, which then enhances the quality and consistency of the data collected and the care provided by health care clinicians.[3] Many standardized formats are evidence based (meaning they are based on scientific evidence) and are used to guide comprehensive health assessments. They are also a specific or focused component of a health assessment (e.g., standardized pain scales, wound assessment scales, risk for fall assessment scales).

Health History

A health history consists of subjective data collected during an interview. This history includes information about the patient's current state of health, current medications, previous illnesses and surgeries, a family history, personal and psychosocial history, and review of systems. Patients may report feelings or experiences associated with health problems. These patient reports are called *symptoms* and are considered subjective data (Box 1.2). Subjective data acquired directly from a patient are considered *primary source data*. If data are acquired from another individual (e.g., a family member), they are referred to as *secondary source data*. More information about conducting a health history is presented in Chapter 2.

Physical Examination

A physical examination involves the collection of objective data; these data are sometimes referred to as *signs* (see Box 1.2). During a physical examination, objective data are collected using the techniques of inspection, palpation, percussion, and auscultation. In addition, the patient's height, weight, blood pressure, temperature, pulse rate, respiratory rate, and oxygen saturation are measured. Specific physical examination skills and techniques are presented in chapters throughout this textbook.

BOX 1.1 STANDARDS OF NURSING PRACTICE

Standard 1: Assessment
The registered nurse collects pertinent data and information relative to the health care consumer's health or the situation.

Standard 2: Diagnosis
The registered nurse analyzes the assessment data to determine actual or potential diagnoses, problems, or issues.

Standard 3: Outcome Identification
The registered nurse identifies expected outcomes for a plan individualized to the health care consumer or the situation.

Standard 4: Planning
The registered nurse develops a plan that prescribes strategies to attain expected, measurable outcomes.

Standard 5: Implementation
The registered nurse implements the identified plan.
5A: Coordination of Care—The registered nurse coordinates care delivery.
5B: Health Teaching and Health Promotion—The registered nurse uses strategies to promote health and a safe environment.

Standard 6: Evaluation
The registered nurse evaluates progress toward attainment of goals and outcomes.

From American Nurses Association: *Nursing: scope and standards of practice,* ed 3, Silver Spring, MD, 2015, American Nurses Association.

BOX 1.2 CLARIFICATION OF TERMS

Signs and Symptoms
- *Signs* are objective data observed, felt, heard, or measured. Examples of signs include rash, enlarged lymph nodes, and swelling of an extremity.
- *Symptoms* are subjective data perceived and reported by the patient. Examples of symptoms include pain, itching, and nausea.

Occasionally data may fall into both categories. For example, a patient may tell the nurse that he "feels sweaty"—a symptom. At the same time the nurse may observe excessive sweating, or diaphoresis—a sign.

Clinical Manifestation
Clinical manifestation is a term often used to describe the presenting signs and symptoms experienced by a patient.

plan of care and prevents the patient from having to provide the same information to another health care provider. The health record serves as the legal permanent record of the patient's health status at the time of the health care encounter. Thus it serves as a baseline for the evaluation of subsequent changes and decisions related to care. The format for documentation varies from agency to agency, although the electronic health record (EHR) is most widely used. An EHR is a digital version of personal health information maintained by health providers over time. It is used by all health care professionals involved in an individual's care and includes data from the history, physical examination, laboratory and diagnostic tests, and surgical procedures and progress notes (Fig. 1.2). Ultimately, the goal is for EHRs to integrate the documentation of care across participating health systems for any single patient.[4] The basic underlying principles of documentation require data to be recorded accurately, concisely, without bias or opinion, and at the point of care. Documentation of a comprehensive health assessment is presented in Chapter 23.

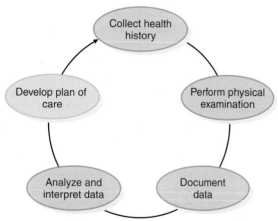

FIG. 1.1 Health history, examination, data documentation, and data analysis are antecedents to developing a plan of care.

Documentation of Data

Health assessment data are documented at the time of the health care encounter, making the information available to other health care professionals involved in the care. Complete, accurate, and descriptive documentation improves the

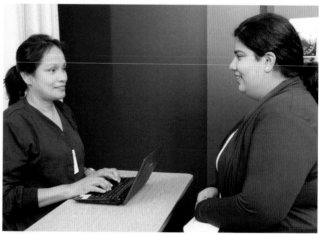

FIG. 1.2 The nurse may take notes while conducting a health assessment. (Copyright © iStock/monkeybusinessimages.)

TYPES OF HEALTH ASSESSMENTS

The amount of information gained during a health assessment depends on several factors, including the context of care and the patient needs.

Context of Care

The term *context* refers to circumstances or situations associated with an event or events. The phrase *context of care* refers to the circumstances or situations related to the health care delivery. Circumstances contributing to the context of care include the setting or environment; the physical, psychological, or socioeconomic circumstances involving patients; and the expertise of the nurse. Because of these variables, different types of assessments are performed (e.g., a comprehensive health assessment, a problem-based or focused health assessment, an episodic assessment, a shift assessment, and a screening assessment; Box 1.3). In some settings such as a hospital or a community-based primary care setting, a comprehensive history is collected and an examination is performed. In an urgent care or emergency department setting, a problem-based or focused assessment may be indicated, although additional subjective and objective data that may have a direct or indirect impact on the management of the patient are collected.

Patient Needs

The type of health assessment performed by the nurse is also driven by patient needs. The patient's age, general level of health, presenting problems, knowledge level, and support systems are among many variables that impact patient need. For example, a healthy 17-year-old male presenting to a primary care clinic for a sports physical clearly has different needs than a 78-year-old, recently widowed patient with diabetes, presenting to the same clinic with increasing fatigue.

Health Assessment Skills

This textbook presents basic health assessment skills with an overview of advanced health assessment skills. Learning every assessment skill described in this book is not realistic for the beginning student; in fact, few health professionals apply all health assessment skills. Research involving the physical assessment skills used in clinical practice has shown that nurses incorporate some skills regularly and others less frequently. In a study representing a sample of 193 nurses across multiple areas of clinical practice, respondents report performing only 30 of 124 examination skills on a routine basis; the remaining skills were performed occasionally or not performed at all.[5] Replication studies conducted by Anderson and colleagues[6] and Birks and colleagues[7] report similar findings, with a variance in only a few skills. Secrest, Norwood, and duMont[8] report that 92.5% of physical assessment skills on a 120-item survey were taught and practiced in baccalaureate nursing programs, yet only 29% of nurses in clinical practice actually perform those skills on a regular basis. A survey of baccalaureate students in one nursing program found that fewer than half of the skills taught in the physical examination course were actually used in clinical practice.[9] In yet another study, researchers reported that inspection was the predominate assessment strategy used and that 70% of health assessment skills often taught in nursing programs were never performed or learned. The biggest influencer of skills performed was shaped by the practice area.[10] In these studies, the large majority of the skills routinely performed by nurses represent inspection and auscultation involving cardiovascular and respiratory systems. These findings suggest the need to clearly differentiate the skills that are more likely to be used in practice from those that are used infrequently. Box 1.4 presents the *core* physical assessment skills identified through research. Throughout this textbook, the techniques that are frequently performed by most nurses in most settings are differentiated from the techniques that are less commonly performed by nurses or indicated only in special circumstances. Furthermore, a brief description of the assessment techniques typically performed by an advanced practice nurse (e.g., a clinical nurse specialist, nurse practitioner, or certified

---

BOX 1.3 TYPES OF HEALTH ASSESSMENT

- **Comprehensive assessment:** This involves a detailed history and physical examination performed at the onset of care in a primary care setting or on admission to a hospital or long-term care facility. The comprehensive assessment encompasses health problems experienced by the patient; health promotion, disease prevention, and assessment for problems associated with known risk factors; or assessment for age- and gender-specific health problems.

- **Problem-based/focused assessment:** This involves a history and physical examination that is limited to a specific problem or complaint (e.g., a sprained ankle). This type of assessment is commonly used in a walk-in clinic or emergency department, but it may also be applied in other outpatient settings. In addition to collecting data on a specific problem, the nurse also considers the potential impact of the patient's underlying health status.

- **Episodic/follow-up assessment:** This type of assessment is usually done when a patient is following up with a health care provider for a previously identified problem. For example, a patient treated by a health care provider for pneumonia might be asked to return for a follow-up visit after completing a prescription of antibiotics. An individual treated for an ongoing condition such as diabetes is asked to make regular visits to the clinic for episodic assessment.

- **Shift assessment:** When individuals are hospitalized, nurses conduct assessments each shift. The purpose of the shift assessment is to identify changes to a patient's condition from the baseline; thus the focus of the assessment is largely based on the condition or problem the patient is experiencing. Adapting an assessment to the hospitalized patient is discussed in Chapter 24.

- **Screening assessment/examination:** This is a short examination focused on disease detection. A screening examination may be performed in a health care provider's office (as part of a comprehensive examination) or at a health fair. Examples include blood pressure screening, glucose screening, cholesterol screening, and colorectal screening.

BOX 1.4 CORE EXAMINATION SKILLS

Skin
- Inspect skin.*
- Inspect skin lesions and wounds.*

Head, Eyes, Ears, Nose, Throat
- Inspect face.*
- Inspect oral cavity.*
- Assess hearing (based on conversation).*
- Inspect external eyes.*
- Inspect pupils and response to light and accommodation.*
- Assess visual acuity.

Chest and Lungs
- Inspect chest.*
- Evaluate breathing effort.*
- Auscultate lung sounds.*
- Palpate thoracic expansion.

Cardiovascular
- Auscultate heart sounds and apical pulse.*
- Auscultate carotid artery.
- Palpate the distal pulses.*
- Palpate and inspect the nails (capillary refill).*
- Inspect and palpate extremities for edema.*
- Palpate extremities for temperature.*
- Inspect extremities for skin color and hair growth.*

Musculoskeletal
- Inspect upper and lower extremities for size and symmetry.*
- Palpate extremities for tenderness.*
- Observe range of motion.*
- Assess muscle strength.*
- Inspect spine.
- Assess gait.*

Abdomen
- Inspect abdomen.*
- Auscultate bowel sounds; aortic vascular sounds.*
- Palpate abdomen lightly (generalized tenderness and distention).*

Neurologic
- Assess mental status and level of consciousness.*
- Evaluate speech.*
- Assess Glasgow Coma Scale.
- Assess sensation to extremities.

Genitalia
- Inspect male genitalia (penis/scrotum).*
- Inspect female genitalia.

*Indicates core assessment skill in three studies.
Data from Giddens JF: A survey of physical assessment techniques performed by RNs: lessons for nursing education, *J Nurs Educ* 46:83-87, 2007; Secrest JA, Norwood BR, Dumont PM: Physical assessment skills: a descriptive study of what is taught and what is practiced, *J Prof Nurs* 21(2):114-118, 2005; Anderson B, Nix E, Norman B, McPike H: An evidence-based approach to undergraduate physical assessment practicum course development, *Nurse Educ Pract* 14:242-246, 2014.

nurse midwife) are presented at the end of the examination section.

CLINICAL REASONING AND JUDGMENT

The outcome of a health assessment is a portrait of a patient's physical status, strengths and weaknesses, abilities, support systems, health beliefs, and activities to maintain health in addition to health problems and lack of resources for maintaining health. The nurse analyzes and interprets these data to determine the best course of action for a plan of care. To be clear, physical assessment is not to be approached as just a task to be completed. The collection of data without actively applying and integrating the information in a purposeful way does little to benefit the patient. Another critical but perhaps understated purpose of health assessment is the ongoing monitoring of the patient for subtle changes (and being aware of early signs of deteriorating status).[11] Early recognition of cues by a nurse (as collected through assessment) that indicate a change in a patient's health status is central to the early detection of a deteriorating status and initiation of appropriate interventions.[12-13]

Data Organization

After collecting and documenting data, nurses organize or cluster them so the problems appear more clearly. This may be done based on a body system format (e.g., cardiovascular, musculoskeletal, auditory, visual) or a conceptual format (e.g., gas exchange, perfusion, mobility).

Data Analysis, Interpretation, and Developing a Problem List

Data are analyzed to determine findings that are expected as well as abnormal findings. This analysis helps the nurse to identify problems experienced by patients and initiate an appropriate plan of care (see Fig. 1.1). A key component of data analysis and interpretation is the formulation of a problem list, which is a summary of health problems identified as a result of the health assessment process. The list is typically placed in order of the most important or most active problems first, followed by problems of less concern. The problem list is updated over time as the patient's condition changes or as problems resolve.

Clinical Judgment

The term *clinical judgment* is defined as "an interpretation or conclusion about a patient's needs, concerns, or health problems and/or the decision to take action (or not), use or modify standard approaches, or improvise new ones as deemed appropriate by the patient's response."[14,p 204] Although the nurse's clinical judgment depends on an accurate collection of assessment data, the interpretation of these data guides the nursing actions. According to Tanner, clinical judgment is influenced more by the nurse's experiences, knowledge, attitudes, and perspectives than the data alone.[14] In a comparison of expert and novice nurses, Hoffman and colleagues found that expert nurses collect and cluster a wider range of assessment cues in decision-making.[12] This can be illustrated in the following situation:

A 50-year-old man arrives at a walk-in medical clinic reporting a gradual onset of a cough over the course of the day that began while he was at work. He states that he takes no medications and smokes one-half pack of cigarettes a day. His vital signs and oxygen saturation are within normal limits.

- A novice nurse seeing this patient is likely to collect and document these initial data, auscultate his lungs, and inform the primary care provider that a patient with a cough and wheezing is waiting to be seen.
- An experienced nurse seeing this patient notices subtle cues (that he is anxious, his skin is somewhat pale and moist, and he is slightly restless). This nurse intuitively asks additional questions about the onset of symptoms and learns that he has felt nauseous and was exposed to chemical fumes at work. Although his vital sign data are in the "normal" range, this nurse recognizes that the respiratory rate and pulse are borderline high and the oxygen saturation is at the lower end of the expected range. This nurse suspects that the patient is becoming hypoxic and administers low-flow oxygen. The nurse informs the primary care provider that this patient is a priority for evaluation.

Both nurses in the preceding scenario noted the same initial signs and symptoms; however, the analysis and interpretation of data differ, resulting in different nursing actions. These differences can partly be explained by clinical judgment. As described by Tanner,[14] the process of clinical judgment includes four components: noticing, interpreting, responding, and reflecting. Noticing involves recognizing that a situation is or is not consistent with what nurses anticipate or expect to see based on the context of the patient situation. Tanner describes this process as a perceptual grasp of the situation. Although assessment is linked to noticing, the process of assessment in itself does not automatically lead to noticing. Noticing is based on the nurse's expectations associated with multiple variables, including clinical experience, knowledge, and the clinical context. The next step, interpreting, is a process in which the nurse uses patterns of reasoning (involving analysis and intuition) to gain an understanding of the situation. Once an understanding is gained, the nurse determines the appropriate actions and interventions to take (if any)— what Tanner refers to as responding. Reflecting is a critical component of the development of clinical judgment. Tanner differentiates reflection-*in*-action (in other words reflecting

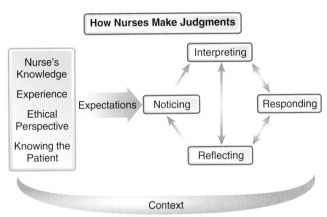

FIG. 1.3 Clinical judgment model. *Noticing* refers to the nurse's expectations and initial grasp of a situation. It triggers reasoning patterns that allow the nurse to interpret the situation and respond with interventions. *Reflection-in-action* specifically relates to evaluating outcomes of interventions, whereas *reflection-on-action* represents the contribution of an experience to a nurse's collective experiences. (From Tanner C: Thinking like a nurse: a research-based model of clinical judgment in nursing, *J Nurs Educ* 45:204-211, 2006.)

on past experiences while in the midst of another situation) from reflection-*on*-action (thinking about a situation that has occurred and developing a better understanding of what happened and the appropriateness of the patient outcomes). By reflecting, nurses use what is learned from clinical experiences for future encounters (Fig. 1.3).

More recently, the National Council of State Boards of Nursing (NCSBN) has developed a clinical judgment model (CJM) that represents an integration of the Intuitive-Humanistic Model (represented by the work of Tanner[14] described above), the Dual Process Reasoning Theory, and the Information-Processing Model.[15] According to the NCSBN CJM, clinical judgment involves a series of underlying cognitive operations that include recognizing and analyzing cues associated with a clinical problem, developing and prioritizing a hypothesis based on those cues, which leads to the ability to take action and evaluate outcomes.[15]

HEALTH PROMOTION AND HEALTH PROTECTION

An essential component of health care is the promotion of health. Health promotion begins with health assessment; thus health promotion is found throughout this textbook. Through the process of health assessment, nurses assess patients' current health status, health practices, and risk factors. Interpretation of such data allows nurses to target appropriate health promotion needs for patients. *Health promotion* is behavior motivated by the desire to increase well-being and actualize human health potential. *Health protection* is behavior motivated by the desire to actively

TABLE 1.1 LEVELS OF HEALTH PROMOTION

LEVEL OF PREVENTION	FOCUS	EXAMPLES
Primary prevention	Protection to prevent occurrence of disease	Immunizations, pollution control, nutrition, exercise
Secondary prevention	Early identification of disease before it becomes symptomatic to halt the progression of the pathologic process	Screening examinations and self-examination practices (e.g., colorectal screening, mammography, blood pressure screening)
Tertiary prevention	Minimize severity and disability from disease through appropriate therapy for chronic disease	Diabetes mellitus management Cardiac rehabilitation Hypertension management

avoid illness, detect it early, or maintain functioning within its constraints.[16]

Three levels of health promotion—primary prevention, secondary prevention, and tertiary prevention—address the promotion of health regardless of a patient's health status. Nurses are instrumental in providing education and care to help an individual meet his or her health promotion needs.

The focus of *primary prevention* is to prevent a disease from developing through the promotion of healthy lifestyles. *Secondary prevention* consists of screening efforts to promote the early detection of disease. *Tertiary prevention* is directed toward minimizing the disability from acute or chronic disease or injury and helping the patient to maximize his or her health. Table 1.1 clarifies these levels of health promotion.

CLINICAL APPLICATION AND CLINICAL JUDGMENT

See Appendix B for answers to exercises in this section.

REVIEW QUESTIONS

1. A 52-year-old male patient is admitted to the hospital with a new diagnosis of rectal cancer. Which type of assessment does the nurse conduct on his admission?
   1. A comprehensive assessment
   2. A problem-based health assessment
   3. An episodic assessment
   4. A screening assessment for colorectal cancer

2. After collecting data, the nurse begins data analysis with which activity?
   1. Documenting information from the history
   2. Organizing the data collected
   3. Reporting data to other care providers
   4. Recording data from the physical examination

3. Which situation illustrates a screening assessment?
   1. A patient visits a clinic for the first time and the nurse completes a history and physical examination.
   2. A hospital sponsors a health fair in a community to measure blood pressure and cholesterol levels.
   3. A nurse at an urgent care center checks the blood pressure, pulse, temperature, and respirations of a patient reporting leg pain.
   4. A patient with diabetes mellitus comes to the laboratory to get her blood glucose tested prior to a visit with a health care provider.

4. The nurse documents which information in the patient's history?
   1. The patient is scratching his left arm.
   2. The patient's skin feels warm.
   3. The patient reports itching of her eyes.
   4. The patient's temperature is 100°F (37.8°C).

5. Select the example given below that represents information a nurse collects from a patient during a physical examination.
   1. Shiny skin and lack of hair found on lower legs
   2. Concerned about lack of money to pay for prescriptions
   3. Complains of tingling in both feet while sleeping
   4. Family history of colon and breast cancer

CASE STUDY 1

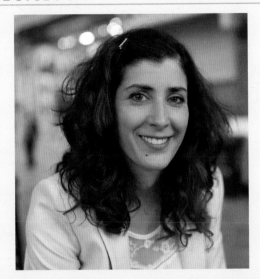

Sharon Faulkner is a 42-year-old woman being seen in a community clinic with abdominal pain. She tells the nurse the pain she is experiencing in her right upper abdomen feels like a knife and that it goes all the way to her shoulder. She is also very nauseous. She tells the nurse that she is exhausted and has not slept for three nights because the pain keeps her awake. The nurse observes dark circles under Sharon's eyes. Her vital signs are as follows: blood pressure, 132/90 mm Hg; heart rate, 104 beats/min; respiratory rate, 22 breaths/min; temperature, 101.8°F (38.8°C). A complete blood count laboratory test reveals that Sharon has an elevated white blood cell count. She lies on the examination table in a fetal position and tells the nurse that it hurts too much for her to get up and move.

1. List the subjective data described in this case study.
2. List the objective data described in this case study.

CASE STUDY 2

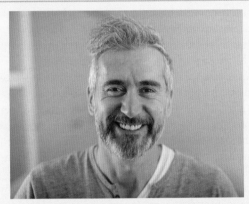

Mark Lyons is a 41-year-old man in the orthopedic unit with a complex femur fracture. Listed in the next paragraph are data collected by the nurse.

Interview Data

Mark states, "I fell off my horse while riding. The horse stepped on my leg and crushed the bone in my upper leg." He describes intense pain in his right leg and states that the pain medication helps only a little. He wants to move but cannot because of an immobilizer device. Mark says, "My butt hurts because I can't move around." He tells the nurse, "I have not had a bowel movement for 3 days, and the last time the stool looked like hard, dry rabbit turds. Normally at home I go every day." Mark has not been hungry either. He says that "the food is horrible." He also complains that he is so bored he can't stand it. "I'm used to being active; being stuck in bed is driving me crazy. Television shows aren't worth watching."

Examination Data

- *Vital signs:* blood pressure, 108/72 mm Hg; pulse, 88 beats/min; respiration, 16 breaths/min; temperature, 98.1°F (36.7°C); height, 5 ft 5 in (165 cm); weight, 135 lb (61 kg).
- *Prescribed medications:* Ibuprofen 400 mg every 4 to 6 hours; oxycodone 1 or 2 by mouth every 4 to 6 hours as needed for severe pain (i.e., pain level 8 or over on 10-point scale.). He has taken two oxycodone pills every 6 hours over the past several days for pain management.
- *Diet:* Regular diet. Has eaten, on average, 30% of meals. Fluid intake has averaged 1000 mL/day.
- *Activity:* Complete bed rest.
- *Respiratory:* Breathing even/unlabored. Lungs clear to auscultation bilaterally.
- *Cardiovascular:* All distal pulses in lower extremities palpable. Heart rate and rhythm regular. No peripheral edema.
- *Abdomen:* Slightly distended. Bowel sounds auscultated throughout abdomen.
- *Musculoskeletal:* Immobilization device to right leg. Reports sensation to foot/toes, rapid capillary refill. Other extremities: full range of motion. No pain over joints and muscles.
- *Integument:* Skin warm and dry. Pin sites for external fixation device without redness or drainage. Redness over sacrum, 2 inch in diameter. Skin intact.

The following three problems are applicable to Mark. List the data presented in this case study that support each problem. NOTE: Some data may be placed under more than one problem.

1. Pain
   a. Subjective data
   b. Objective data
2. Altered elimination (constipation)
   a. Subjective data
   b. Objective data
3. Risk for skin breakdown
   a. Subjective data
   b. Objective data

CHAPTER

2

Obtaining a Health History

evolve

http://evolve.elsevier.com/Wilson/assessment

Health assessment involves collecting data about a patient's health history followed by a physical examination. As noted in Chapter 1, the health history consists of subjective data collected during an interview involving the nurse and patient. The purpose of the health history is to obtain important information from the patient so a plan to promote health, prevent disease, resolve acute health problems, and minimize limitations related to chronic health problems can be developed. In many settings, patients are asked to complete a health history questionnaire, which typically consists of a series of yes-or-no questions pertaining to specific problems or symptoms that they may have experienced. Although a questionnaire is useful for collecting some elements of a heatlh history, it is never a substitute for an interview. Any past medical problems or symptoms reported on a questionnaire should be investigated further.

THE INTERVIEW

The health history is obtained through an interview process where the nurse facilitates discussion to collect data. Structured formats are used in many health care settings to enhance the quality and consistency of data collected.[1] During the interview, the patient's story is revealed. This perspective is a helpful reminder that each patient is unique; thus each interview reveals specific information about that individual. Information gathered includes defining health, beliefs about attaining and maintaining health, and understanding the patient's expectations for health. Such expectations are based on his or her life experiences, family and friends' experiences, and culture. Nurses also learn about patients' health concerns and the social, economic, and cultural factors that influence their health and their responses to illness. Data generated from an interview provide the foundation for personalized, safe, and effective health care for each individual. A successful patient interview includes selecting an appropriate physical setting, using a patient-centered approach, and creating a positive rapport with the patient.

The Physical Setting

Before conducting an interview, the nurse considers the physical setting, which can impact the exchange of information. Ideally, an interview is conducted in a private, quiet, comfortable room free from environmental distractions where the nurse and patient can sit face to face.

The importance of privacy, especially when discussing issues that are highly personal, cannot be overemphasized. Patients may not be willing to share sensitive information openly and honestly if they are fearful of being overheard or are in the presence of friends or family members. For example, consider the potentially compromising situation if the nurse asks a patient about drug use or sexual activity in the presence of family members. Privacy is best gained by conducting the interview in an unoccupied room. Unfortunately, the physical layout of some patient care areas makes finding a completely private place to conduct an interview difficult; thus the nurse must make every effort to allow for as much privacy as possible. If the interview occurs in an environment with multiple treatment areas or in a semiprivate hospital room, draw the curtains to provide some degree of privacy and block out visual distractions.

Patients should be physically comfortable during the interview. When possible, patients should remain in street clothes during the interview and change into a gown for the physical examination. The nurse and patient should sit at a distance from one another that provides for a comfortable flow of conversation. The patient's comfort level is partly related to personal space (i.e., the area that surrounds the person's body). The amount of space the patient needs varies and is influenced by his or her culture and previous experiences in similar situations. In addition, if possible, the room temperature should be set at a comfortable level.

Finally, the interview should be conducted in a quiet setting without distractions. Interruptions by other individuals should be avoided. Unnecessary noise should be eliminated, and unnecessary equipment should be removed from the area or turned off, if possible. With the exception of emergencies, cell phones and pagers should not be answered while conducting an interview.

A Patient-Centered Approach

The premise of patient-centered care is that patients, families, and health care providers engage in shared decision-making for all health decisions.[2-3] A central element of patient-centered care involves treating each patient as a unique individual, respecting the patient for who he or she is, and responding to needs and preferences. The nurse considers a wide range of variables (including age, culture, gender identity and expression, language and physical or emotional distress, sensory impairments, and cognitive impairment) when conducting an interview to ensure the patient's unique needs and preferences are revealed.

Age

The patient's age can influence the participation, accuracy, and completeness of data provided. Adults and adolescents are usually able to fully participate in an interview and answer questions for themselves. When obtaining a health history on a child, the nurse typically involves a parent or guardian, although an older child should be included in the process as appropriate. Older adults may have some decline in abilities with age; thus accommodations should be considered as needed.

Culture

Nurses work with patients from many different cultural backgrounds. Patient-centered care is provided when nurses accept and respect differences and identify cultural factors that may influence patients' beliefs about health and illness. The health care system places accountability for cultural competence with all heath care professionals.[4] Cultural competence, as defined by Campinha-Bacote, refers to "The ongoing process in which the health care professional continuously strives to achieve the ability and availability to work effectively within the cultural context of the patient (individual, family, community)."[5] To deliver culturally competent care, nurses must interact with each individual as a unique person who is a product of past experiences, beliefs, and values that have been learned and passed down from one generation to the next (Fig. 2.1). However, nurses remember that all individuals within a specific cultural group do not think and behave in a similar manner. They avoid stereotyping patients because of their culture or ethnicity. There may be as much diversity within a cultural group as there is across cultural groups. The nurse should ask patients about experiences that illustrate what has been of value to them and that characterize their culture. This increases the nurse's understanding and demonstrates interest in them as individuals. Further information about cultural considerations is presented in Chapter 5.

Gender Identity and Expression

The term *gender identity* represents a person's own internal sense of gender—which can include male, female, a blend of

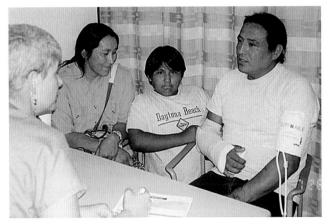

FIG. 2.1 Interact with the patient as a unique person and be sensitive to cultural diversities.

BOX 2.1 COMMON TERMS ASSOCIATED WITH GENDER IDENTITY

- Cisgender—gender identity consistent with the sex assigned at birth.
- Transgender—gender identity that does not match the sex assigned at birth; male identifies as female (transfemale) or female identifies as male (transmale).
- Nonbinary—person does not identity strictly as male or female.
- Agender—person does not identify with any gender.

both, or neither. Gender identity is formed by age three.[6] *Gender expression* refers to how an individual presents his or her gender within the context of a culture and society.[7] Nurses should be aware of these distinctions and incorporate the patient's views as part of the health history, as appropriate. Box 2.1 presents common terms associated with gender identity.

Language

As the country's population becomes progressively diverse, the number of patients who have limited English proficiency (LEP) increases. When the nurse and patient do not share a common language, a certified translator is used to gain accurate data for the health history. State and federal laws mandate the provision of interpreting services for patients with LEP; this is also an element within the accreditation guidelines for health care agencies.[8] Although using family members as translators may be tempting, this practice is discouraged because the family members may alter the meaning of what is said or describe what they think is wrong with the patient. Conducting an interview through a translator takes considerably more time than a typical interview because everything said must be repeated.

Physical or Emotional Distress

Ideally, patients are mentally alert and in no physical or emotional discomfort. Conducting an interview with a patient who is in physical or emotional distress is difficult. In such a case, limit the number and nature of questions to those that are absolutely necessary for the given situation, and save any additional questions for later.

Sensory Impairment

Some individuals may have hearing or vision impairments that may make the interview more challenging. For the hearing impaired, the nurse speaks slowly and clearly and faces the individual so he or she can see the nurse's face. Individuals with a hearing impairment may not provide complete information if unable to fully hear the questions asked. Holding the interview in a quiet room without extraneous noise is important. Individuals with visual impairments may need assistance completing written interview forms.

Cognitive Impairment

When nurses interview patients with a cognitive impairment (e.g., dementia, delirium, or psychosis), they may rely on data from a secondary source (such as a family member or caregiver) to obtain pertinent and essential information. Additional information may also be gained from a preestablished health record, if it exists. Adults with confusion or memory loss may still be involved in an interview, but nurses should keep questions simple and consult with family members to clarify data as needed. A designated health care agent (medical power of attorney) should be assigned for individuals who are unable to participate in health care decisions due to a cognitive impairment. Specific laws regarding power of attorney and advance directives vary by state.[9]

Establishing Rapport

Perhaps the most important factor for a successful interview is the ability to establish a positive rapport (or relationship) with the patient. Establishing a positive rapport leads to trust that enhances the sharing of personal information. Factors that affect the rapport include the professional behavior of the nurse and effective communication.

Professional Behavior

First impressions are powerful. A first impression is made during an initial encounter and leads to the formation of an opinion regarding the other individual. The first impression nurses make starts with their appearance, dressing, and grooming. A clean appearance, modest professional attire, and an identification badge are imperative. Nurses avoid extremes in dress and manner so appearance does not become an obstacle or a distraction to the patient's responses. Nurses should strive to convey a professional, confident, and caring demeanor. A stiff, formal attitude or being too casual or displaying a "laid-back" attitude may fail to instill confidence. Examples of professional behaviors that contribute to positive first impressions are being prompt, knocking before entering a room, introducing oneself, and being fully present to the situation.

Effective Communication

Interpersonal skills are central to effective communication. Skilled nurses conduct interviews in an efficient, calm, and unhurried manor. Nurses actively listen to patients and project a genuine interest in them and what they are saying. Patients have the need to feel understood; nurses should make every attempt to understand their point of view, communicate acceptance, and treat them with respect. Failure to do so jeopardizes the flow of information. Nonverbal behavior is also very important. Posture, gestures, eye contact, and facial expression project to patients the nurse's level of interest, acceptance, and understanding of them. Avoid reactions (e.g., startle, surprise, frowning, laughter, grimacing) based on a patient's appearance or the information shared. Also avoid focusing more on the process of recording data instead of focusing on the patient. Ideally, one should listen first and then record the data.

Phases of the Interview

The interview consists of three phases: introduction, discussion, and summary (Box 2.2). To begin the introduction phase, the nurse greets the patient and introduces himself or herself. (Fig. 2.2). This is the opportunity to make an important first impression with the patient and begin establishing

---

BOX 2.2 PHASES OF AN INTERVIEW

Introduction Phase
- Greet the patient; introduce self to patient.
- Establish purpose of the visit from patient.
- Describe the purpose and process of the interview.

Discussion Phase
- Facilitate and maintain a patient-centered discussion.
- Use various communication skills and techniques to collect data.

Summary Phase
- Summarize the data with the patient.
- Allow the patient to clarify the data.
- Create a shared understanding of the problems with the patient.
- Plan for next steps and end interview

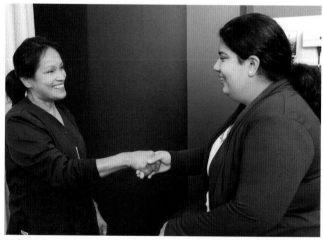

FIG. 2.2 Introduce yourself when you begin an interview. (Copyright © iStock/monkeybusinessimages.)

rapport. When patients are adults, address them by their title (e.g., Mr., Mrs., Miss, or Ms.) and surname initially. As a follow-up, ask "What is your preferred name? or "How would you like to be addressed?" Avoid using their first name unless they request it or when they are adolescents or children. If other individuals are in the room, acknowledge each person and determine his or her role and level of participation in care. During the introduction the nurse establishes the purpose of the visit and explains the purpose and process of the interview.

Next the interview moves into the discussion phase. The nurse collects the health history by gathering data about various aspects of the patient's health. Although the role of the nurse is to facilitate the direction of conversation, ideally the conversation is *patient-centered,* meaning the patient is free to share concerns, beliefs, and values in his or her own words.[10] During the discussion phase, a variety of communication skills and techniques are used to enhance the conversation and data collection.

The summary phase of the interview is the time for closure. Main points gained from the interview are summarized, and data that have implications for health promotion, disease prevention, or the resolution of their health problems are emphasized. The summary allows for clarification of data and provides validation to the patient that the nurse has an accurate understanding of his or her health issues, problems, and concerns. Finally, the nurse and patient plan for the next steps and end the interview.

FREQUENTLY ASKED QUESTIONS

What are the key points to ensure a successful interview with a patient?

- **Make a good first impression.** A professional greeting is essential to establish initial rapport. The nurse should consider his or her personal appearance and body language.
- **Be prepared.** Review the patient's medical record (if it is available) before meeting the patient. This not only helps the nurse to anticipate some of the issues that may arise, but it also lets the patient know that the nurse is interested enough to invest time prior to the first meeting.
- **Be an attentive listener throughout the interview.** The nurse must use active listening skills and be fully engaged in the conversation. (Active listening is described under Techniques that Enhance the Interview.)
- **Avoid using medical jargon.** The nurse should use lay language when asking questions, as appropriate to ensure the patient understands the information provided.

The Art of Asking Questions

The art of obtaining information from patients and listening carefully to their responses is an essential competency. Questions must be clearly spoken and understood by patients. Define words that patients may not understand and avoid the use of technical terms if possible. Slang words such as "pee" as opposed to "urinate" may be used if necessary to

describe certain conditions. Questions are adapted to a patients' developmental level, knowledge, and understanding. For example, the nurse may ask a young child where he or she hurts but would ask an adult more detailed questions such as the onset, duration, and characteristics of the pain. Patients are encouraged to be as specific as possible. For example, if the nurse asks how many glasses of water the patient drinks each day and the patient says, "Oh, a few," the nurse clarifies what the patient means by asking, "How many is a few? Three? Four? Five?" This approach yields a more specific answer and provides the patient's interpretation of "a few."

The nurse asks one question at a time and waits for the reply before asking the next question. If several questions are asked at a time, a patient may become confused about which question to answer, or the nurse may be uncertain about which question the patient is answering. For example, the nurse asks, "Have you had immunizations for tetanus, hepatitis B, and influenza?" If the patient answers "yes," it is not clear whether the patient means "yes" to all three or to one only. If something a patient says is confusing, the nurse must ask for clarification. The explanation may clear up the confusion, or it may indicate that the patient has been misinformed or there is some underlying emotional or thought-processing difficulty that impairs understanding.

The nurse is attentive to the feelings that accompany the patient's responses to some questions. These responses may signify that additional information is needed during the interview or that problems exist that need to be addressed in the future. For example, if the patient reports that her mother died of breast cancer and she begins to cry, this may indicate a future need to discuss coping or adjustment strategies with her.

Some areas of questioning (e.g., sexuality, domestic violence, human trafficking, or the use of alcohol or drugs) are more sensitive than others. What is perceived as sensitive may vary from patient to patient. When asking questions about sensitive issues, nurses explain that they need to ask personal or sensitive questions and that all nurses ask these questions of all patients. Another technique is referred to as *permission giving.* For example, the nurse could say, "Many people have experimented with drugs; have you ever used street drugs?" or "Many young people your age have questions about sex. What questions or concerns do you have?" With the permission-giving technique, the nurse communicates to the patient that it is safe to discuss such topics.

Patients may ask the nurse questions during the interview. The nurse can answer them using terms that patients understand but avoiding giving in-depth answers or providing more information than necessary. If patients ask broad questions or questions that the nurse is unprepared to answer at that time, the nurse asks for more information about the situation such as, "Tell me more about what you are thinking." This provides some direction to answer broad questions or allows the nurse to refer the patient to appropriate resources.

Types of Interview Questions

There are two categories of interview questions—open-ended and directive questions. Both types of questions are useful to incorporate into an interview.

Open-ended Questions

Begin the interview with *open-ended questions* such as, "How have you been feeling?" or "What brings you in to the clinic today?" These broadly stated questions encourage a free-flowing, open response. The aim of open-ended questions is to elicit responses that are more than one or two words. Patients may respond to this type of question by describing the onset of symptoms in their own words and at their own pace. However, the open-ended question should focus on the patient's health. A question that is too broad such as, "Tell me a little about yourself," may be too general to provide useful information. A challenge associated with open-ended questions is that some patients may be unable to focus on the specific topic of the question or take excessive time to tell their story. In these cases the nurse needs to refocus the interview. However, flexibility is necessary when using this type of question because the patient's associations may be important and the nurse must allow the patient the freedom to pursue them.

Directive Questions

To gain more precise details, nurses ask more specific, *directive questions* (also called closed-ended questions) that require only one or two words to answer or lead patients to focus on a set of thoughts. For example, the nurse may ask, "Do you become short of breath when walking a flight of stairs?" or "How many days have you been unable to eat?" Another reason for using this type of question is to give patients options when answering questions such as, "Is the pain in your stomach sharp, dull, or aching?" This type of question is valuable in collecting data, but it must be used in combination with open-ended questions because failing to allow patients to describe their health in their own words may lead to inaccurate conclusions.

Techniques That Enhance the Interview

The professional behavior exhibited by the nurse and the art of asking questions (presented previously) are fundamental for establishing the patient's trust. In addition, a number of communication techniques are used to enhance patient responses and facilitate communication during the interview.

Active Listening

Active listening involves listening with a purpose to the spoken words, as well as noticing nonverbal behaviors. This is performed by concentrating on what the patient is saying and the subtleties of the message being conveyed, together with the facial expressions and body language observed. The nurse must pay full attention to the patient's response rather than trying to predict how the patient will respond to the question or formulate the next question. When assumptions are made, the nurse may ask an illogical question; or, if the nurse is concentrating on how the next question will be worded, attention is shifted away from the information that the patient is providing.

Facilitation

Facilitation uses phrases to encourage the patient to continue talking. These include verbal responses such as, "Go on," "Uh-huh," and "Then?" and nonverbal responses such as head nodding and shifting forward in your seat with increased attention.

Clarification

Clarification is used to obtain more information about conflicting, vague, or ambiguous statements. As an example, if the patient said, "I was so angry I almost lost it," the nurse seeking clarification may respond by asking "What do you mean by 'almost lost it'?" or, as another example, if the patient said, "I just wasn't able to return to work," the nurse might ask "What do you think kept you from returning to work?"

Reflection

Reflection is a technique used to gain clarification by restating a phrase used by the patient in the form of a question. This encourages elaboration and indicates that the nurse is interested in more information. As an example:

Patient: "I got out of bed and I just didn't feel right."

Nurse: "You didn't feel right?"

Patient: "Uh huh, I was dizzy and had to sit back on the bed before I fell over."

Confrontation

Confrontation is used when inconsistencies are noted between what the patient reports and observations or other data about the patient. For example, the nurse might say, "I'm confused. You mentioned that you are following your diet and exercising three times a week, yet your weight has increased since your last visit. Can you help me to understand this?" However, the use of confrontation can be tricky. The nurse's tone of voice is important when using confrontation; use a tone that communicates confusion or misunderstanding rather than one that is accusatory and angry.

Interpretation

The nurse uses interpretation to share with the patient the conclusions drawn from data given. After hearing the conclusion, the patient can confirm, deny, or revise the interpretation. For example, "Let me share my thoughts about what you have just told me. The week you were out of the office you exercised, felt no muscle tension, felt relaxed, and slept well. I wonder if your work environment is contributing to the anxiety that you're experiencing."

Summarization

A summary condenses and orders data obtained during the interview to help clarify a sequence of events. This is useful when interviewing a patient who rambles on or does not provide sequential data.

Behaviors That Interfere With the Interview

There are a number of nurse behaviors that can disrupt the flow of an interview, interfere with the quality of data collection, and possibly impair the patient-nurse relationship. These behaviors can often be avoided by considering the interview from the patient's perspective.

Using Medical Terminology

Using medical terminology, abbreviations, or jargon not known to patients interferes with the communication process. Some examples include saying "hypertension" instead of "high blood pressure," "dysphagia" rather than "difficulty in swallowing," "CVA" rather than "stroke," or "myocardial infarction" rather than "heart attack." Using medical terminology might confuse the patients, lead them to misunderstand the question, or cause them to feel too embarrassed to ask for clarification. Such a scenario can lead to inaccurate data collection.

Expressing Value Judgments

Value judgments expressed by the nurse have no place in an interview. For example, the nurse should ask, "If you have had a mammogram, do you recall when you had the last one?" rather than saying, "You have had regular mammograms, haven't you?" The latter question forces the patient to respond in a way that is consistent with the nurse's values, or it might cause the patient to feel guilty or defensive when she must answer to the contrary.

Interrupting the Patient

Allow patients to finish sentences; do not become impatient and finish their sentences for them. The ending the nurse might add to a sentence may be different from the one that the patient would have used. Associated with interrupting is changing the subject before a patient has finished giving information about the last topic discussed. Nurses may feel pressured for time and are eager to move on to other topics, but they should allow patients the opportunity to complete their thoughts.

Being Authoritarian or Paternalistic

The nurse who uses the approach, "I know what is best for you, and you should do what I say," risks alienating the patient. Despite personal beliefs held by the nurse, a patient's health is his or her own responsibility. The patient may choose to follow or ignore the advice and teaching offered by the nurse.

Using "Why" Questions

This type of questioning can be perceived as threatening and may put patients on the defensive.[3] When patients are asked why they did something, the implication is that they must defend their choices. Instead of asking, "Why did you stop taking the antibiotics?" the nurse could say, "I noticed several doses of prescription are left in the bottle" and wait to see if the patient offers an explanation. If no explanation is forthcoming, the nurse can follow up with, "I'm curious to know whether you intended to take all the antibiotics."

Awkward Moments and Challenging Situations

Personal Questions

Patients may ask the nurse questions about his or her personal life. A brief, direct answer usually satisfies their curiosity. Sharing personal experiences that are supportive of patients may be helpful (e.g., parenting issues or stress management techniques) and may enhance the relationship with patients and increase the nurse's credibility.

Silence

When an awkward silence occurs, the nurse may feel an urge to break it with a comment or question. However, remember that patients may need the silence as a time to reflect or gather courage. Some issues can be so painful to discuss that silence is necessary and should be accepted. It may indicate that they are not ready to discuss this topic or that the approach needs to be evaluated. The nurse should become comfortable with silence; it can be useful.

Displays of Emotion

Patients may express a variety of emotions, such as sadness, fear, or anger, during an interview. Crying is a natural emotion. Saying, "Don't cry" is not a therapeutic response. A therapeutic approach is to provide tissues and let patients know that it is all right to cry by giving a response such as, "Take all the time you need to express your feelings." Postpone further questioning until the patient is ready. Crying may indicate a need that can be addressed at a later time. A compassionate response to a patient who is crying demonstrates caring and may enhance the nurse-patient relationship.

At times a patient may be angry, which can make the interview a challenge. One approach is to deal with it directly by first identifying its source. The nurse may say, "You seem angry; can you tell me what is going on?" If a patient chooses to discuss the anger, he or she may reveal whether the anger is self-directed, directed at someone else, or directed at the nurse. If the patient is angry with someone else, discuss with him or her an approach for talking with that person about the reason for the angry feelings. When patients are angry with the nurse, encourage them to discuss their feelings. Acknowledge their feelings and, if appropriate, apologize. Nurses may be able to continue working with a patient after the angry feelings have been discussed; but, if the patient would prefer to interact with another nurse, their request should be honored. Regardless of the outcome, nurses should model a healthy, appropriate approach to managing anger.

Overly Talkative Patient

Some patients are difficult to interview because they are overly talkative. They may feel a need to go into every detail of a problem or illness and become distracted as they tell their story. Some patients focus on events in the remote past with no apparent relevance to their present situation. Still others may want to discuss issues that do not relate directly to themselves, such as other people or current world events. Although each situation is unique, ideally the nurse tactfully redirects the conversation. The use of directive or closed-ended questions may help to maintain direction and flow of the conversation.

Others in the Room

Patients may be accompanied by other individuals. When this is the case, avoid making assumptions regarding the relationship among those present. Ask the others, "What is your relationship to the patient?" Or, you can ask the patient, "Who did you bring with you today?" which gives them an opportunity to introduce those who have accompanied them.

All patients should be involved with the interview to the extent that their age, mental ability, or physical ability allows. When patients are unable to answer questions for themselves, others may assist with the interview. For example, the parent or guardian of a child usually answers interview questions on behalf of a young child. Patients who are able to speak for themselves should be given an opportunity to be interviewed directly and in private if possible. If other individuals are present, the nurse should obtain the patient's permission for them to remain in the room during the interview.

Disruptive Individuals

At times, the individuals who accompany patients are disruptive to the interview. For example, sometimes a parent, spouse, or friend will answer questions for the patient. Usually these individuals are trying to be helpful, but this may also suggest a dominant personality or, worse, an abusive situation or a human trafficking situation. Such situations can adversely affect the accuracy of data collected, and the nurse must validate with the patient that the information is correct. If others persist in answering for a patient, the nurse can specifically request them to allow the patient to answer or ask them to leave until the end of the interview.

A disruptive interview may also occur when others are present and create a distraction for the patient and/or nurse. As one example, attempting to conduct an interview with a woman who is accompanied by two active young children often causes constant distractions. If children are too young to wait in the waiting room, the nurse should find developmentally appropriate activities for them while the interview is completed.

THE HEALTH HISTORY

Types of Health Histories

A health history is obtained from patients on every visit; however, the amount of data collected for a history depends largely on the setting and the purpose of the visit. A history is a component of all the types of health assessments described in Chapter 1 (Box 1.3), including a comprehensive assessment, a problem-based or problem-focused assessment, and an episodic or follow-up assessment. If the patient has a pre-established health record available, the nurse should access the record and review it before the patient visit, if possible.

The *comprehensive health history* is performed for new patients in any setting, including a hospital admission, an initial clinic visit, or home visit. A comprehensive health history requires more time than other types of histories because a complete database is being established. The admission process for many hospitals includes obtaining a comprehensive database. However, the patient's condition must be considered. For example, a critically ill patient admitted to the hospital may be unable to participate in a comprehensive interview; thus it would be inappropriate to pursue it at that time. Family members may be of assistance in providing important, essential information to the nurse for the seriously ill patient. A comprehensive health history should be conducted once the patient is stable. An example of a documented comprehensive health history for an adult is presented in Chapter 23.

The history for a *problem-based* or *problem-focused health assessment* includes data that are limited in scope to a specific problem. However, it must be detailed enough so the nurse is aware of other health-related data that may affect the current problem. For example, the history for a patient with a lacerated foot should include information about the incident and symptoms and also medications that the patient is taking currently, medication allergies, other health problems that the patient has, and immunization status. Imagine the disastrous result that could occur if this patient had a history of diabetes mellitus and a severe allergy to penicillin and this information were not discovered. A problem-focused interview is also used when a patient seeks help to address an urgent problem such as relief from asthma attack or for chest pain. Further data may be collected once the patient has been stabilized, particularly if he or she requires ongoing care.

The history associated with an *episodic* or *follow-up assessment* generally focuses on a specific problem or problems for which a patient has already received treatment. An interview for an episodic visit focuses on the changes that have taken place since the last visit, particularly with an interest in disease management and the early detection of complications or a decline in health. As an example, a patient receiving chemotherapy as a treatment for cancer makes episodic visits to monitor his or her condition.

Components of the Health History

Because the scope of a health history varies with the type of health assessment conducted, the nurse can expect variations in the format of the history. However, many components are found consistently in all health histories. A comprehensive health history includes the following components:

- Biographic data
- Reason for seeking care
- History of presenting illness
- Present health status
- Past health history
- Family history
- Personal and psychosocial history
- Review of systems

Biographic Data

Biographic data are collected at the first visit and updated as changes occur. These data begin to form a picture of the patient as a unique individual. Box 2.3 lists the data obtained.

Reason for Seeking Health Care

The reason for seeking care is a brief statement of the patient's reason for requesting the services of a health care professional and is often recorded in direct quotes. Often the reason for seeking health care is described in terms of a *chief concern* or *presenting problem*. As an example, the patient's reason for seeking health care may be recorded as "Back pain for two days." A patient may present for a routine examination or well visit and thus does not have a presenting problem. When multiple problems are verbalized, they are all listed and the patient is asked to prioritize the problems. A patient may initially be uncomfortable giving the nurse the actual reason for seeking care. When this is the case, the patient may not divulge the true reason he or she came until the end of the visit, when he or she begins to feel more comfortable. A patient who is unable to provide an address; seems unsure of current location, current date, and time; seems nervous or afraid and avoids eye contact; provides an inconsistent history; and/or is accompanied by a person who answers for the patient, may be a victim of human trafficking (Box 2.4). When these indicators are present, the nurse should talk with the patient alone. Examples of screening questions for suspected victims of human trafficking are presented in Box 2.5. Keep in mind that victims frequently feel hopeless and may not report their situation to the nurse even when given an opportunity.[11]

The patient's condition dictates how the nurse proceeds. Urgency dictates expediency. Patients with severe pain, dyspnea, or injury should not be subjected to a prolonged

---

BOX 2.3 BIOGRAPHIC DATA

- Name and preferred name
- Gender and gender identity
- Address, telephone number, and email address
- Birth date
- Birthplace (important when born in a foreign country)
- Race/ethnicity
- Religion
- Marital status
- Occupation
- Contact person
- Source of data

Note: Gender is commonly used to describe a person's sex (biologic male or female distinction) in the context of social and cultural differences. Gender identity refers to an individual's view of themselves (see Box 2.1).

BOX 2.4 RECOGNIZING VICTIMS OF HUMAN TRAFFICKING

Human trafficking is defined as a commercial sex act induced by force, fraud, or coercion or in which the person induced to perform such an act has not attained 18 years of age. Nearly 80% of victims are female and present for a variety of health reasons. Since nurses are often the first health professionals to have contact with victims, they are in a unique position to identify those at increased risk and recognize red flags that indicate the victim may need help.

- Vulnerable Individuals for Human Trafficking
  - Individuals who have experienced childhood abuse or neglect
  - Children in foster care and juvenile justice system
  - Runaway or homeless youth
  - Victims of violence
  - Lesbian, gay, bisexual, and transgender individuals
  - Racial and ethnic minorities, particularly Native Americans, Native Hawaiians, and Pacific Islanders
  - Non-English speaking, limited language skills
  - Undocumented immigrants, refugees, migrant workers
  - Individuals with low socioeconomic status
  - Uneducated individuals
  - Individuals with history of substance abuse
- Common Reasons for Seeking Health Care
  - Mental health issues (anxiety, depression, posttraumatic stress disorder [PTSD]), substance abuse)

- Physical injuries: burns, fractures
- Malnutrition
- Skin conditions
- Dental injuries and disease
- Sexually transmitted diseases (STDs); human immunodeficiency virus (HIV); acquired immunodeficiency syndrome (AIDS)
- Complications of abortion
- Gastrointestinal disorders
- Evidence of sexual violence
- Indicators or "Red Flags" of Human Trafficking:
  - Unable to provide address (victims are moved frequently)
  - Unsure of present location, current date, or time
  - Accompanied by a person who answers for the patient, interprets for the patient, or refuses to let the patient have privacy
  - Not in possession of personal identification documents or money
  - Provides an inconsistent or scripted history
  - Unwilling or hesitant to answer questions about injury or illness
  - Displays evidence of controlling or dominating relationships (excessive concerns about pleasing persons who accompany him or her)
  - Demonstrates fear or nervous behavior or avoids eye contact

National Conference of State Legislatures: Human trafficking and the health care system, *Legisbrief* 26(14), 2018; Trafficking Victims Protection Act of 2000: https://www.govinfo.gov/content/pkg/PLAW-106publ386/pdf/PLAW-106publ386.pdf; The Joint Commission: Quick Safety 42: Identifying human trafficking victims, 2018. Retrieved from: https://www.jointcommission.org/issues/article.aspx?Article=Dtpt66QSsiI%2FHRkIecK TZPAbn6jexdUPHfIBjJ%2FD8Qc%3D; Schwarz C, Unruh E, Cronin K, et al: Human trafficking identification and service provision in the medical and social service sectors, *Health Hum Rights* 18(1)181-191, 2016; Washburn J: What nurses need to know about human trafficking, *J Christ Nurs* 35(1): 18-25, 2018;

BOX 2.5 SCREENING QUESTIONS FOR VICTIMS OF HUMAN TRAFFICKING

- Where do you live, sleep, and eat?
- Are you allowed to leave the place where you are living or working? Under what circumstances?
- Has your identification or documentation been taken from you?
- Have you ever run away from home or a program? What did you do to survive during that time?
- Do you feel people are controlling you and forcing you to do things you do not want to do?
- Are you frightened by people in your everyday life or work setting?
- Have you been threatened with harm if you try to leave?
- Has anyone threatened or harmed your family?
- Can you quit your job or situation if you want to?
- Are you provided with protective equipment at work (gloves, glasses, masks, helmets)?
- Has anyone force you to do something physically or sexually that you did not feel comfortable doing?
- Do you feel your only option is to say in this situation?
- Would you know how to seek help if you needed it?
- Are you afraid to get help?

From: The Joint Commission: Quick Safety 42: Identifying human trafficking victims, 2018. Retrieved from: https://www.jointcommission.org/issues/article.aspx?Article=Dtpt66QSsiI%2FHRkIecKTZPAbn6jexdUPHfIBjJ%2FD8Qc%3D; Washburn J: What nurses need to know about human trafficking, *Journal of Christian Nursing* 35(1): 18-25, 2018.

history. Biographic data may be delayed to pursue the health concern. This approach enables the nurse to analyze the data quickly, identify the cause of the health concern, prioritize the patient's needs, and plan how to alleviate the signs or symptoms.

History of Presenting Illness and Symptom Analysis

When patients seek health care for a specific presenting illness or problem, the nurse investigates it further by conducting a *symptom analysis,* which is a systematic method of collecting data about the presenting problem. Remember, not all individuals seeking health care have a specific presenting problem (e.g., a person presenting for routine health care or wellness visit). For this reason, a symptom analysis is not always indicated. Several formats are used to conduct a symptom analysis, but the analysis should include all of the following variables: onset of symptoms, location and duration of symptoms, characteristics, aggravating factors, related symptoms, treatment, and severity of symptoms (Box 2.6).

Present Health Status

The current health status focuses on the patient's current health conditions, medications the patient is currently taking, and known allergies.

- *Current health conditions.* Examples include diabetes, hypertension, heart disease, sickle cell anemia, cancer, seizures, pulmonary disease, arthritis, and depression. Ask

BOX 2.6 MNEMONIC FOR SYMPTOM ANALYSIS: OLD CARTS

Onset: When Did the Symptom Begin?
- When and how did the symptom(s) begin?
- Did it develop suddenly or over a period of time? (Ask for the specific date, time, day of week if appropriate.)
- Where were you or what were you doing when the symptom started
- Does anyone else with whom you have been in contact have a similar symptom?

Location: Where Is the Symptom?
- Is the symptom in a specific area? If so, describe.
- Is it vague and generalized?
- Does the symptom radiate to another area?

Duration: How Long Does the Symptom Last?
- Is the symptom constant or intermittent (does it come and go)?
- If constant, does the severity of symptom change?
- If intermittent, how many times a day, week, or month does the symptom occur and for how long? How do you feel between episodes of the symptom?
- Since you first noticed the symptom, has it become worse? About the same?

Characteristics: Describe the Symptom
- How does the symptom feel or look?
- Describe the sensation: stabbing, dull, aching, throbbing, nagging, sharp, squeezing, itching.
- If applicable, describe the appearance: color, texture, composition, and odor.

Aggravating Factors: What Makes the Symptom Worse?
- Is the symptom aggravated by an activity or situation (e.g., walking, climbing stairs, eating, a particular body position)? If so, describe.
- Are there psychological or physical factors in the environment that may be contributing to the symptom (e.g., stress, smoke, chemicals)? If so, describe.

Related Symptoms: Are Other Symptoms Present?
- Have you noticed that other symptoms have occurred that you think may be related (e.g., fever, nausea, pain)? If so, describe.

Treatment: What Factors Alleviate the Symptom?
- Is the symptom relieved with change in body position, application of heat or cold, change in diet, or use of over-the-counter drugs?
- Have you tried any self-treatments or taken any medications to relieve the symptom? If so, have any of these treatments been effective?
- Have you previously sought treatment from a health care provider for this symptom?

Severity: Describe the Intensity of the Symptom
- Describe the size, extent, number, or amount.
- On a scale of 0 to 10, with 10 being most severe, how would you rate your symptom?
- Is the symptom so severe that it interrupts your activities (e.g., work, school, eating, sleeping)?

the patient how long he or she has had the condition(s) and the impact of the illness on daily activities.

- *Medications.* Inquire about prescription, over-the-counter, and herbal preparations. Include the reason for taking the medication, how long the patient has been taking it, the dose and frequency, any adverse effects, and the patient's perception of its effectiveness. In addition, ask about any home remedies used for health conditions.

- *Allergies.* Ask about allergies to foods, medications, environmental factors, and contact substances. Be sure to ask specifically about substances to which patients could be exposed in the health care setting such as latex and iodine. The nurse should explain the term *allergy* to ensure that the patient understands it. Many people do not know the difference between an adverse effect (e.g., nausea) and a true allergic reaction (e.g., a rash or difficulty in breathing). When the patient reports an allergy to a medication or substance, ask for a description of the symptoms that occurred to determine whether the reaction is an adverse effect or an allergic reaction.

Past Health History

Past health history (also known as the past medical history) is important because past conditions may have some effect on the patient's current health needs and problems. The following data categories are included:

- *Childhood illnesses:* measles, mumps, rubella, chickenpox, pertussis, *Haemophilus influenzae* infection, streptococcal throat infection, otitis media (ask if there were complications in later years such as rheumatic fever or glomerulonephritis that can occur after streptococcal throat infection)
- *Surgeries:* types, dates, outcomes
- *Hospitalizations:* illnesses, dates, outcomes
- *Accidents or injuries:* type (fractures, lacerations, loss of consciousness, burns, penetrating wounds), dates, outcomes
- *Immunizations:* tetanus, diphtheria, pertussis, mumps, measles, rubella, rotavirus, poliomyelitis, hepatitis A or B, influenza, pneumococcal pneumonia, human papillomavirus (HPV), meningococcal vaccines, and varicella. For foreign-born patients: bacille Calmette-Guérin (BCG). Immunizations are discussed further in Chapter 18.
- *Last examinations:* type (physical, dental, vision, hearing, electrocardiogram [ECG], chest radiograph, skin test for tuberculosis; for women: Papanicolaou [Pap] test, mammogram; for men: prostate examination), dates, and outcomes
- *Obstetric history:* number of pregnancies (gravidity), number of births (parity), and number of abortions/miscarriages, if applicable. If working with a pregnant patient or woman in childbearing years, further information is recorded; see Chapter 20

Family History

A history of the patient's blood relatives (biologic grandparents, parents, aunts, uncles, and siblings), spouse, and children is obtained to identify illnesses of genetic, familial, or environmental nature that may affect the patient's current

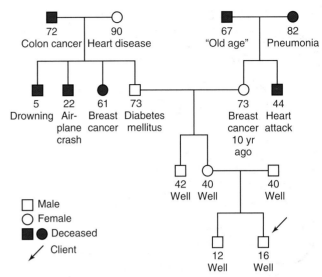

FIG. 2.3 A sample genogram identifying great-grandparents, grandparents, parents, aunts, uncles, and siblings.

or future health. As recommended in the *Essentials of Genetic and Genomic Nursing,* trace back at least three generations.[12] Specifically ask about the presence of any of the following diseases among family members: Alzheimer disease, cancer (all types), diabetes mellitus (specify type 1 or type 2), coronary artery disease (including myocardial infarction), hypertension, stroke, seizure disorders, mental illness (including depression, bipolar disorder, schizophrenia), substance abuse, endocrine diseases (specify), and kidney disease. The family history can be documented in narrative form, or it can be illustrated. A genogram is a tool consisting of a family-tree diagram depicting members within a family over several generations. This tool is useful in tracing diseases with genetic links. Symbols are used to indicate males and females and those who are alive and deceased. Include the current ages of those who are alive and the cause of and age at death of those who are deceased (Fig. 2.3).

Personal and Psychosocial History

This history explores a variety of topics, including any information that affects or reflects the patient's physical and mental health.

Personal status. Ask the patient for a general statement such as "How would you describe yourself?" or "How do you feel about yourself?" Ask about cultural/religious affiliations and practices. Ask about education; occupational history, work satisfaction, perception of having adequate time for leisure and rest, and current hobbies and interests.

Family and social relationships. Ask about general satisfaction with interpersonal relationships, including significant others, people with whom the patient lives, and the patient's role within the family. Sometimes health information about significant others, sexual partners, and roommates is relevant to the patient's health, so be sure to ask about the current state of health of these individuals. Ask about social interactions with friends, participation in social organizations (community, school, work), and participation in spiritual or religious

BOX 2.7 DOMESTIC VIOLENCE

Recognizing Domestic Violence
- *What:* Domestic violence can be either physical or emotional and occurs within the home.
- *Victims:* Women and children are victims most frequently, although men also are victims of domestic violence.
- *Perpetrators:* Most often an intimate partner or parent figure is the perpetrator.
- *Contributing factors:* Domestic violence is often associated with drug or alcohol use (or both).

Screening Questions for Domestic Violence
Ask the patient: When the patient answers "yes" to any question, ask additional questions to obtain more specific data.
- Have you been physically injured (hit, kicked, punched) by someone in your home in the last year? If so, describe.
- Many women are victims of domestic violence. Do you feel safe in your current relationship with your husband or significant other?
- Are you afraid of an individual with whom you have previously had a relationship?

groups. If interactions are limited, find out what makes the patient avoid social interaction—perhaps this is by choice, or there could be an underlying problem. Be aware of issues associated with domestic violence; make a point of screening all patients for this (Box 2.7).

Diet/nutrition. The patient should describe appetite and typical dietary intake for both food and fluids. Inquire about food preferences and dislikes, food intolerances, use of caffeine-containing beverages, dietary restrictions, and use of dietary supplements such as vitamins or protein drinks. Ask about recent changes in appetite or weight, changes in how food tastes, or problems with nutritional intake (e.g., indigestion, pain or difficulty associated with eating, heartburn, bloating, difficulty chewing or swallowing). Also ask about overeating, sporadic eating, or intentional fasting. Further information about a dietary history is presented in Chapter 8.

Functional ability. This functional assessment focuses on a person's ability to perform self-care activities such as dressing, toileting, bathing, eating, and ambulating. Functional ability also includes a person's ability to perform skills needed for independent living such as shopping, cooking, housekeeping, and managing finances. Ask the patient questions related to his or her perceived ability to complete these tasks. An assessment of functional ability is especially important for adults with physical or mental disabilities and for older adults. Further information about assessment of functional ability is presented in Chapter 21.

Mental health. Ask the patient about personal stress and the sources of stress. Common causes of stress include recent life changes such as divorce, moving, family illness, new baby, new job, and finances. Also ask about feelings of anxiety or nervousness, depression, irritability, or anger. Explore with the patient personal coping strategies for stressful situations and previous counseling or mental health care. Further information about obtaining a mental health history is presented in Chapter 7.

Tobacco, alcohol, and illicit drug use. The personal habits most detrimental to health include tobacco use, excessive intake of alcohol, and the use of illicit street drugs. Obtain specific information, including the substance used, the amount used, and the duration of the habit.

- *Tobacco:* Identify the type of tobacco used (cigarette, electronic cigarettes, cigars, pipe, chewing tobacco) and the frequency of use. For cigarette smokers, record the smoking history in *pack-years*. Pack-years refers to the number of packs smoked per day multiplied by the number of years smoked. For example, a patient who reports smoking approximately one pack a day for 25 years has a 25 pack-year smoking history. Many patients will report the number of cigarettes they smoke in a day, so knowing there are 20 cigarettes per pack is important. As an example, a person reporting smoking 5 cigarettes a day (¼ pack) for 15 years would have a 3.75 pack-year history.
- *Alcohol:* Identify the type and amount of alcohol consumed. Ask how many alcoholic drinks are consumed in a day; if not daily, then the weekly or monthly use. Ask about driving under the influence of alcohol. Screening questionnaires such as the Alcohol Use Disorders Identification Test (AUDIT) can be used to assess problem drinking and are discussed further in Chapter 7.
- *Illicit drug use:* Ask specifically about the use of marijuana, cocaine, crack cocaine, barbiturates, and amphetamines. Ask about high-risk behaviors such as sharing needles or driving under the influence of drugs.

Health promotion activities. Ask the patient which activities are regularly performed to maintain health. Ask specifically about exercise (type of exercise, frequency), stress management strategies, sleep habits, routine health examinations, and safety practices (e.g., seat belt use, wearing safety goggles, wearing helmets). Health promotion practices are assessed further in the review of systems section.

Environment. The history also includes data related to environmental health. Obtain a general statement of the patient's assessment of environmental safety or concerns. Variables to consider include potential hazards within the home (the lack of fire and smoke detectors, poor lighting, steep stairs, inadequate heat, open gas heaters, inadequate pest control, violent behaviors), hazards in the neighborhood or community (noise, water and air pollution, heavy traffic on surrounding streets, overcrowding, violence, firearms, sale/use of street drugs), and hazards associated with employment (inhalants, noise, heavy lifting, machinery, psychological stress). Also ask patients about recent travel outside the United States (when and which countries visited, length of stay).

Review of Systems

A review of systems is conducted to inquire about the past and present health of each of the patient's body systems. Conduct a symptom analysis when the patient acknowledges the presence of symptoms (see Box 2.6). If sufficient data have been collected about a body system in the present illness/present health status section, these questions are not repeated. For example, if you completed a symptom analysis on "cough" when completing the present health status, you need not repeat questions about cough in the review of systems.

Symptoms listed in the review of systems are written in medical terms. A brief definition of each term is included where necessary to facilitate patient understanding. For example, if the nurse wants to know if the patient has dyspnea, the nurse asks, "Do you become short of breath?" If the patient says, "No," the nurse documents "no dyspnea," but if the patient says, "Yes," questions from the symptom analysis are used, and the findings are documented. Therefore use medical terms for documentation and communication with other health care providers, but use only terms understood by the patient during the interview. Although some health promotion data are included in other sections of the health history, additional information is collected during the review of systems.

An outline of symptoms to ask the patient follows. This list, organized by body system or region, is not inclusive; rather, it is an example of the kinds of questions to ask. More detailed questions are presented in the chapters that follow. Remember that a comprehensive health assessment includes most of the questions; in a focused health assessment, nurses ask questions only about systems related to the reason for seeking care. In an episodic or follow-up assessment, the questions are limited to asking the patient about changes that have taken place since the last visit.

General symptoms
- Pain; general fatigue, weakness; fever; problems with sleep; unexplained changes in weight

Integumentary system (see Chapter 9)
- *Skin:* skin disease, problems, lesions (wounds, sores, growths); excessive dryness, diaphoresis (sweating), or odors; changes in temperature, texture, or pigmentation; discoloration; rashes, pruritus (itching); frequent bruising
- *Hair* (refers to all body hair, not just head and pubic area): changes in amount, texture, character, distribution; alopecia (loss of hair); itching scalp
- *Nails:* changes in texture, color, shape
- *Health promotion:* plan to limit sun exposure; use of sunscreen; skin self-examination; type and frequency of nail care

Head and neck (see Chapter 10)
- *Head:* headaches; significant trauma; vertigo (dizziness); syncope (brief lapse of consciousness)
- *Eyes:* discharge, redness, pruritus (itching); excessive tearing; ophthalmalgia (eye pain) ; changes in vision (generalized or field of vision); difficulty reading; visual disturbances such as blurred vision, photophobia (sensitivity to light), blind spots, floaters, halos around lights, diplopia (double vision), or flashing lights; use of corrective or prosthetic devices; interference with activities of daily living
- *Ears:* otalgia (ear pain); excessive cerumen (earwax); discharge; recurrent infections; changes in hearing (deceased hearing or increased sensitivity to environmental noises); tinnitus (ringing or crackling); use of prosthetic devices; change in balance; interference with activities of daily living
- *Nose, nasopharynx, and paranasal sinuses:* nasal discharge; epistaxis (nosebleed); sneezing; obstruction; sinus pain; postnasal drip; change in the ability to smell; snoring
- *Mouth and oropharynx:* sore throat; tongue or mouth lesion (abscess, sore, ulcer); bleeding gums; use of prosthetic devices (dentures, bridges); altered taste; dysphagia (difficulty swallowing); difficulty chewing; changes to the voice or hoarseness
- *Neck:* lymph node enlargement; edema (swelling) or masses in neck; pain/tenderness; neck stiffness; limitation in movement
- *Health promotion:* use of protective headgear and eyewear; protection of ears from excessively loud noise; dental hygiene practices (brushing/flossing); dental care from dentist

Breasts (see Chapter 16)
- *General:* breast pain/tenderness; edema (swelling); lumps or masses, breast dimpling; nipple discharge; changes to the nipples
- *Health promotion:* date of last mammogram (if applicable)

Respiratory system (see Chapter 11)
- *General:* cough (nonproductive or productive); hemoptysis (coughing up blood); frequent colds; dyspnea (shortness of breath); night sweats; wheezing; stridor (abnormal, high-pitched, musical sound); pain on inspiration or expiration; exposure to smoke or other respiratory irritants
- *Health promotion:* handwashing (reduction of respiratory infection); tuberculosis screening; wearing a mask for occupational or environmental respiratory irritants or hazards; annual influenza immunizations (flu shots); smoking cessation; secondhand smoke exposure

Cardiovascular system (see Chapter 12)
- *Heart:* palpitations (sensation the heart is racing or fluttering); chest pain; dyspnea (shortness of breath); orthopnea (difficulty in breathing unless sitting up); paroxysmal nocturnal dyspnea (periodic dyspnea during sleep)
- *Blood vessels:* coldness in the extremities; numbness; edema (swelling); varicose veins; intermittent claudication (leg pain with exercise that ceases with rest); rest pain (leg pain with exercise that does not cease with rest); paresthesia (abnormal sensations); changes in color of extremities
- *Health promotion:* dietary practices to limit salt and fat intake; cholesterol screening; blood pressure screening; use of support hose if work involves long periods of standing; avoidance of crossing legs at the knees; exercise/activity

Gastrointestinal system (see Chapter 13)
- *General abdominal symptoms:* abdominal pain; heartburn, nausea/vomiting; hematemesis (vomiting blood); jaundice (yellowish color to skin and sclera); ascites (increase in the size of the abdomen caused by intraperitoneal fluid accumulation)
- *Elimination:* bowel habits (frequency, appearance of stool); pain or difficulty with defecation; excessive flatus (gas), change in stools (color, consistency); problems with diarrhea or constipation; blood in stool (hematochezia); hemorrhoids; use of digestive or evacuation aids (stool softener, laxatives, enemas)
- *Health promotion:* dietary analysis (compare diet with MyPlate); use of dietary fiber supplements; colon cancer screening

Urinary system (see Chapter 13)
- *General:* characteristics of urine (color, contents, odor); hesitancy (difficulty initiating urine flow); frequency (repeated need to urinate); urgency (sudden, almost uncontrollable need to urinate); change in urinary stream; nocturia (excessive urination at night); dysuria (painful urination); flank pain (pain in back between ribs and hip bone); hematuria (blood in the urine); dribbling or incontinence (inability to control urination); polyuria (excessive excretion of urine); oliguria (decreased urination)
- *Health promotion:* plan to prevent urinary tract infections (females); Kegel exercises (performed to strengthen muscles of the pelvic floor to help prevent urine leakage)

Reproductive system (see Chapter 17)
- *Male genitalia:* presence of lesions; penis or testicular pain or masses; penile discharge; hernia
- *Female genitalia:* presence of lesions, pain, discharge, odor; menstrual history (date of onset, last menstrual period [LMP], length of cycle); amenorrhea (absent menstruation); menorrhagia (excessive menstruation); dysmenorrhea (painful menstruation); metrorrhagia (irregular menstruation); pelvic pain
- *Sexual history:* ask about current and past involvement in sexual relationships and sexual preferences; nature of sexual relationship(s) (heterosexual, homosexual, bisexual); type and frequency of sexual activity; number of sexual partners (past and present); sexual identity; satisfaction with sexual relationships; method of contraception used (if applicable); changes in sex drive; problems with infertility; exposure to sexually transmitted infections; females: dyspareunia (pain during intercourse); postcoital bleeding (bleeding after intercourse); males: impotence; premature ejaculation
- *Health promotion:* methods to prevent unwanted pregnancy; protection from sexually transmitted infections; testicular or vulvar self-examination; Papanicolaou (Pap) test (females); prostate screening (males)

Musculoskeletal system (see Chapter 14)
- *Muscles:* twitching; cramping; pain; weakness
- *Bones and joints:* joint edema (swelling); pain; erythema (redness); stiffness; deformity; crepitus (noise with joint movement); limitations in range of motion; arthritis; gout; interference with activities of daily living
- *Back:* back pain; pain down buttocks and into legs; limitations in range of motion; interference with activities of daily living
- *Health promotion:* amount and kind of exercise per week; calcium intake; osteoporosis screening

Neurologic system (see Chapter 15)
- *General:* syncope (fainting episodes); loss of consciousness; seizures (which body parts moved, incontinence, characteristics); cognitive changes; changes in memory (short term, recent, long term); disorientation (time, place, person); dysphasia (difficulty communicating)
- *Motor and Gait:* loss of coordinated movements; ataxia (inability to coordinate muscle movement; paralysis (partial versus complete inability to move); paresis (weakness); tremor; spasm; interference with activities of daily living
- *Sensory:* paresthesia (abnormal sensations; e.g., "pins and needles," tingling, numbness); pain (describe sensation and location)

AGE-RELATED VARIATIONS

This chapter discusses principles of interviewing and conducting a health history with adult patients. Nurses will find that a health history may require a different approach and focus on different information, depending on the age of the patient.

INFANTS, CHILDREN, AND ADOLESCENTS

The pediatric health history is similar to that of the adult, with the addition of questions about pregnancy, prenatal care, growth and development, and behavioral and school status, as applicable. For the young child, most data are obtained from the adult accompanying the child, but the nurse should include the child as much as appropriate for his or her age. By age 7, most children can provide a dependable report on their health status (e.g., how they are feeling, where they are hurting).[13] When obtaining a health history from an adolescent, the nurse determines whether an adult or a pediatric database and history format are more appropriate. In addition, a decision is made whether to interview the adolescent with the parent present or alone. Chapter 19 presents further information regarding conducting a health history for this age group.

PREGNANCY

A comprehensive health history is obtained at the first prenatal visit to establish baseline data. This is similar to the information presented in this chapter but with a special emphasis on data that could impact pregnancy outcomes. Prenatal visits are considered episodic visits to monitor the health of the pregnancy. See Chapter 20 for further information.

OLDER ADULTS

The primary difference in conducting a health history with an older adult from that previously described is the incorporation of various age-related questions and questions involving functional status. In addition, depending on the age of the older adult, data about childhood immunizations or developing a genogram may not be necessary. Remember that more time may be needed to conduct a comprehensive health history for an older adult because he or she may have multiple symptoms and conditions, take numerous medications, and have a long past health history. Chapter 21 presents further information regarding the health history for an older adult.

CLINICAL APPLICATION AND CLINICAL JUDGMENT

See Appendix B for answers to exercises in this section.

CASE STUDY

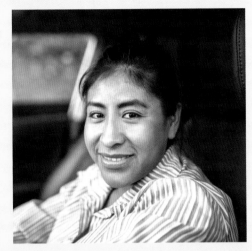

During an interview, Leotie Deschene provides the following family history. She is 37 years old, married, and in good health. Her husband is 43 and also in good health. The couple has a 12-year-old son, an 11-year-old daughter, and a 10-year-old son, all in good health. Leotie has a 42-year-old brother and three sisters who are 32, 36, and 40 years old. All of her siblings are in good health. Both of Leotie's parents are alive. Her 70-year-old father has mild emphysema and is an only child. Her mother is 66 and has hypertension. Leotie's mother has three siblings. The oldest brother (Leotie's uncle) is 74 and suffers from glaucoma. Another brother is 72 and is in good health. A sister is 69 and has osteoarthritis. All of Leotie's grandparents are deceased. Her paternal grandfather died at age 89 of prostate cancer. Her paternal grandmother died of heart failure at age 91. Leotie's maternal grandfather died at age 86 of prostate cancer; her maternal grandmother died of "old age" at age 96. Leotie does not know anything about her great-grandparents.

ACTIVITY

Draw a genogram for Leotie's family history with the information provided.

REVIEW QUESTIONS

1. The nurse is interviewing an adult Navajo woman. Which statement demonstrates cultural sensitivity and acceptance of the patient?
   1. "How often do you visit the medicine man for your health care?"
   2. "Tell me about your health care beliefs and practices."
   3. "Many Navajo people are afraid of hospitals. Are you afraid?"
   4. "Have you ever had a physical examination by a physician or a nurse practitioner?"

2. Which statement is appropriate to use when beginning an interview with a new patient?
   1. "Have you ever been a patient here before?"
   2. "Tell me a little about yourself and your family."
   3. "Did you have any difficulty finding the clinic?"
   4. "What is your purpose for coming to the clinic today?"

3. While giving a history, a patient describes several events out of order that occurred in different decades in his life. What technique does the nurse use to understand the timeline of these events?
   1. Draw conclusions about the order of events from data the patient provided.
   2. Ask the patient to elaborate about these events.
   3. State the order of events as understood and ask the patient to verify the order.
   4. Ask the patient to repeat what he said about these events in the order they occurred.

4. A patient is very talkative and shares much information that is not relevant to his history or the reason for his admission. Which action by the nurse improves data collection in this situation?
   1. Use closed-ended questions.
   2. Ask the patient to stay on the subject.
   3. Ask another nurse to complete the interview.
   4. Terminate the interview.

5. For which patient is a focused health history most appropriate?
   1. A new patient at the health clinic for an annual examination
   2. A patient at the health care provider's office for a sport physical
   3. A patient discharged 11 months ago who is being readmitted today
   4. A patient presenting to a clinic with a lacerated finger

6. A nurse is interviewing a male patient who reports he has not had a tetanus immunization in about 15 years because he had a "bad reaction" to the last tetanus immunization. What is the most appropriate response by the nurse in this case?
   1. Notify the health care provider that this immunization cannot be given.
   2. Document that the patient is allergic to the tetanus vaccine.
   3. Ask the patient to describe the "bad reaction" to the vaccine in more detail.
   4. Give the vaccine after explaining that adverse reactions are rare.

7. The patient reports having a persistent cough for the past 2 weeks and that the cough disrupts sleep and has not been helped by over-the-counter cough medicines. Which question is most appropriate for the nurse to ask next?
   1. "What do you think is causing this persistent cough?"
   2. "What other symptoms have you noticed related to this cough?"
   3. "Have you tried taking sleeping pills to help you sleep?"
   4. "Did you think this will just go away on its own?"

Techniques and Equipment for Physical Assessment

evolve
http://evolve.elsevier.com/Wilson/assessment

Conducting a physical assessment requires the use of infection control practices, assessment techniques, optimal patient positions for examination, and equipment. Safety measures are described throughout the chapter. Correct technique and proper use of equipment are essential for accurate data collection and patient safety. This chapter provides an overview of these topics. The use of techniques and equipment as related to specific body systems is discussed in subsequent chapters.

INFECTION CONTROL PRACTICES

The prevention and control of infection underlies all areas of healthcare practice. Infection rates are considered one of the patient safety indicators identified by the Agency of Healthcare Research and Quality.[1] All health care professionals, including nurses, are responsible for incorporating infection control principles. Two levels of infection control guidelines exist: standard precautions and transmission-based precautions.

Standard Precautions

Standard precautions are applied in all aspects of patient care and in all health settings.[2] These measures reduce the risk of transmitting infection from body fluids and non-intact skin. Body fluids include blood, secretions, and excretions from mucous membranes (with the exception of sweat). Even though performing a health assessment is a relatively safe activity, it has the potential for infection transmission that can occur from patient to nurse, from nurse to patient, or from patient to patient via the nurse, equipment used by the nurse, or the environment. The primary elements of standard precautions recommended by the Centers for Disease Control and Prevention (CDC)[2] include:
- Hand hygiene
- Personal protective equipment
- Respiratory hygiene/cough etiquette
- Appropriate patient placement
- Managing contaminated equipment (including sharps)
- Environmental infection control

Some of these elements are infrequently applied when conducting a health assessment, but all nurses are expected to know when and how to incorporate each element, should it be needed. These specific elements are described further in the following sections.

Hand Hygiene

The single most important action to reduce the transmission of infection is hand hygiene, an essential element of standard precautions (Fig. 3.1). The CDC estimates that, on average, providers perform hand hygiene less than half of the time they should, despite it being a very simple and effective way to prevent infection.[3] Because of ongoing poor compliance and high rates of infections transmitted by personnel in health care settings, The Joint Commission now cites noncompliance of hand hygiene as a deficiency if a surveyor observes any individual failing to perform hand hygiene in the process of direct patient care.[4]

Hand hygiene is performed before and after direct contact with a patient. This includes direct contact with a patient's intact skin, non-intact skin, mucous membranes, blood or any body fluids, or any wound dressings, as well as any objects, including medical equipment, chairs, and tables, in the patient care area.[5] Hand hygiene is also performed during the care for the same patient if the nurse is moving from a contaminated body site (such as perineal area or open wound) to a clean body site. Hand hygiene is performed also after removing gloves following patient contact, as well as before eating, and after using the bathroom. *Note: Wearing gloves is never a substitute for hand hygiene!*

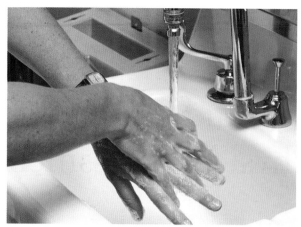

FIG. 3.1 Correct handwashing technique includes rubbing from the palms to the back of the hands with fingers interlocked.

There are two acceptable methods for cleaning hands in the health care setting: washing with soap and water or, when hands are not visibly dirty, using alcohol-based hand sanitizers.[5] Box 3.1 presents recommendations for hand hygiene techniques.

FREQUENTLY ASKED QUESTIONS

Which is a better method for performing hand hygiene: using alcohol-based hand sanitizer or washing with soap and water?

Both approaches to hand hygiene are acceptable. However, the use of alcohol-based sanitizer is the preferred method for cleaning the hands *when the hands are not visibly dirty*. Reasons for this preference are that hand sanitizer requires less time, is more effective at killing pathogens on the hands, reduces bacterial counts on the hands, causes less skin irritation compared to soap and water, and is more accessible than sinks.

From Centers for Disease Control: Hand Hygiene in Healthcare Settings: Show Me the Science, updated 2016. Retrieved from: https://www.cdc.gov/handhygiene/science/index.html.

Personal Protective Equipment

Standard precautions guidelines for infection control include personal protective equipment (PPE; e.g., gloves, masks or respirators, eye protection, face shields, and gowns) worn by health care providers.[6] Box 3.2 presents a guideline for the use of personal protective equipment. The specific PPE used depends on the specific precautions in place. Regardless of the equipment used, the sequence for putting on PPE is gown, then mask or respirator, then goggles and/or face shield, and then gloves. The sequence for removing PPE follows a reverse order—gloves, goggles/face shield, mask, and then gown—although removal of the gown and gloves at the same time is also permissible.[7] Hand hygiene is performed immediately upon removal of all PPE.

BOX 3.1 TECHNIQUES FOR PERFORMING HAND HYGIENE

Using Alcohol-Based Hand Sanitizer

- Apply a generous amount of product to hands. Use a product with at least 60% alcohol. (Most preparations used in health care settings contain between 60% and 95% ethanol or isopropanol.)
- Cover all surfaces (including fingers and back of hands). The efficacy of hand hygiene depends on the volume of product applied and the areas covered. Areas most often missed are the thumbs, fingertips, and between the fingers.
- Rub hands together until hands feel dry.

Note: The entire process should take about 20 seconds.

Washing With Soap and Water

- Wet the hands first with warm water and then apply soap product to cover the surface of the hands completely.
- Rub hands together vigorously for **at least** 15 seconds, covering all surfaces of the hands and fingers.
- Rinse the hands with warm water and dry them thoroughly with a disposable towel. Turn the faucet off using the towel.

Note: Avoid using hot water to avoid excessive drying of the skin. Some sources recommend washing for 20 seconds; either time frame is acceptable.

From Centers for Disease Control: Hand Hygiene in Healthcare Settings: Clean Hands for Healthcare Providers, 2018. Retrieved from: https://www.cdc.gov/handhygiene/providers/index.html.

Respiratory Hygiene/Cough Etiquette

These precautions apply to any patient care environment to contain respiratory secretions among patients and visitors who are symptomatic for respiratory infections.[8] Specific measures for symptomatic individuals include:

- Cover mouth/nose with a tissue when coughing or sneezing and promptly dispose of the contaminated tissues in a no-touch trash receptacle.
- Perform hand hygiene when the hands are contaminated with respiratory secretions and from contaminated objects and materials.
- When individuals in the health care setting are coughing, offer them a mask to contain respiratory secretions. This is particularly important during periods of respiratory infection outbreaks, such as the flu or coronavirus.
- A spatial separation of at least 3 feet among people in the waiting area is ideal when space and chairs are available. However, a separation of 6 feet is used when mandates for social distancing are implemented, such as when the coronavirus outbreak began in 2020.

Patient Placement

Within patient care settings, the placement of patients is another consideration of infection control practice. A patient should be placed in a single room if he or she is suspected of having a highly transmittable infection or is likely to contaminate the environment. Likewise, if the patient is known to be immunosuppressed and at risk of acquiring an infection, he or she should be placed in a single room for protection.

BOX 3.2 STANDARD PRECAUTION GUIDELINE: PERSONAL PROTECTIVE EQUIPMENT

Gloves

Gloves should be worn when contact with a patient's blood or other body fluid is possible or when handling equipment contaminated with blood or other body fluids. Gloves are worn for three primary reasons:

1. To protect the health care worker from exposure to blood-borne pathogens carried by the patient
2. To protect the patient from microorganisms on the hands of the health care worker
3. To reduce the potential of infection transmission from one patient to another patient via the hands of the health care worker

The use of gloves does not reduce the frequency or importance of hand hygiene. Hands must be washed before performing a procedure, even when gloves are worn and again immediately after removal of gloves. Gloves should be changed between procedures on the same patient to prevent cross-contamination. If a glove breaks during a procedure, it should be removed promptly and replaced with a new glove. Gloves should be discarded after all procedures; they should never be washed and reused.

Masks, Eye Protection, Face Shields

The nurse should wear a mask with eye protection or a face shield during procedures that may result in splashes or sprays of the patient's blood, body fluids, secretions, or excretions. Such equipment protects the mucous membranes of the eyes, nose, and mouth from contact, thus reducing the likelihood of pathogen transmission. Although not routinely needed for health assessment, this equipment become necessary in selective patient encounters.

Gowns

A gown should be worn during procedures to protect the health care worker's arms and other exposed skin surfaces, and to prevent the contamination of clothing with the patient's blood or other body fluids or contact with other potentially infectious material.

From Siegel JD, Healthcare Infection Control Practices Advisory Committee: *2007 Guideline for Isolation Precautions: Preventing Transmission of Infectious Agents in Healthcare Settings,* 2007. Retrieved from: https://www.cdc.gov/hai/pdfs/Isolation2007.pdf.

Contaminated Patient Care Equipment and Sharps

Another aspect of standard precautions involves the management of contaminated patient care equipment.[6] The nurse should wear gloves when touching equipment contaminated with blood or other body fluid. Multiple-use patient equipment that has been soiled with blood or other body fluids (e.g., a vaginal speculum) should not be reused until it has been adequately cleaned and reprocessed. Single-use items must be disposed of properly after patient use. The nurse must be cautious when handling contaminated sharp equipment. (Note: Gloves do not provide protection from a sharp injury such as a needle stick.) The appropriate handling of sharps includes the following principles:

- Never recap a needle after patient use.
- Never attempt to remove a needle from a disposable syringe.
- After use, place disposable syringes and needles directly into a "sharps container" (i.e., a puncture-resistant container designated for contaminated sharp items). If the sharps container is full, do not attempt to force additional sharps in the container, as this may lead to a stick injury.

The CDC and Safe Injection Practice Coalition has launched the One & Only Campaign (https://www.cdc.gov/injectionsafety/one-and-only.html) to raise awareness among patients and health care providers about safe injection practices and to eliminate infections associated with unsafe injection practices.[9]

Environmental Control

Environmental control refers to the process of decontaminating the patient care environment. This includes the routine care, cleaning, and disinfection of environmental surfaces, particularly frequently used surfaces such as examination beds, tabletops, counter surfaces, and examination lights. Specific protocols for decontamination are required within all patient care settings.

Transmission-Based Precautions

These guidelines are designed for the control of infections among patients with known or suspected infections caused by certain pathogens of epidemiologic significance. Transmission-based precautions include (1) contact precautions, (2) droplet precautions, and (3) airborne precautions. Additional information about transmission-based precautions can be found on the Centers for Disease Control and Prevention website (www.cdc.gov).

Latex Allergy

Occupational latex allergy has become a problem for many health care professionals because latex is found in gloves and many other types of medical equipment and supplies. A latex allergy is a reaction to the proteins in latex rubber. The amount of exposure required to produce a latex allergy reaction is unknown, but frequent exposure increases the risk of developing allergic symptoms.[10] An estimated 9.7% of health care workers have latex allergy, compared with 7.2% of susceptible patients and 4.3% of the general population.[11] The three types of latex reactions include (1) irritant contact dermatitis (contact dermatitis of the skin, not involving the immune system), (2) Type I reaction (an immune-based systemic reaction caused by an antigen-antibody reaction and resulting in the release of histamine), and (3) Type IV contact dermatitis (a delayed hypersensitivity involving the immune system in response to the chemicals in latex occurring 24 to 48 hours after contact). The use of nonpowdered latex gloves and nonlatex gloves has been shown to reduce the incidence of latex allergy.[12] The National Institute for Occupational Safety and Health recommendations for preventing latex allergy in nurses are summarized in Box 3.3.

Patients may also have a latex allergy; those particularly at risk are children with spina bifida and people who have had multiple medical procedures and surgeries, especially genitourinary surgery. For this reason, nurses should routinely ask

BOX 3.3 PREVENTING LATEX ALLERGY

- Use nonlatex gloves for any activities that are not likely to involve contact with infectious materials.
- If latex gloves are to be used, use a powder-free, low-allergen glove, if possible.
- Do not use oil-based hand lotions when wearing latex gloves.
- Immediately after removing latex gloves, wash the hands with mild soap and dry them thoroughly.

From National Institute for Occupational Safety and Health: *Latex allergy: a prevention guide,* NIOSH publication no. 98–113, Cincinnati, 1998, NIOSH. Retrieved from: https://www.cdc.gov/niosh/docs/98-113/.

patients about latex allergy; if it exists, they should protect patients from coming in contact with latex gloves and other medical equipment made of latex, such as urinary catheters and gastrostomy tubes.

TECHNIQUES OF PHYSICAL ASSESSMENT

Data for physical assessment are collected using four basic assessment techniques: inspection, palpation, percussion, and auscultation.

Inspection

The term *inspection* refers to data obtained by a visual examination of the body, including body movement and posture, as well as that obtained by smell. The physical examination begins with inspection, a technique used throughout the entire exam with each body system. For example, when inspecting the lungs and respiratory system, the nurse observes the shape of the chest, paying attention to breathing (noting the rate, depth, and effort of respiration) and noticing the overall color of the skin, lips, and nail beds. During inspection, the patient is draped appropriately to maintain modesty while allowing sufficient exposure for examination; adequate lighting is essential.

Inspection can be hindered when the nurse has preconceived assumptions about the patient. For this reason, thoroughly observing the patient with a critical eye is important. By concentrating on the patient without being distracted, the nurse notices potentially important data. Although inspection at first may seem like an easy assessment technique to master, practice is necessary to develop expertise.

Sometimes the use of equipment facilitates the inspection of certain body systems. For example, a penlight may be used to increase the light in a specific location (looking into a mouth, looking at a skin lesion) or to create shadows by directing light at right angles to the area being inspected—a technique referred to as *tangential lighting* (Fig. 3.2). Other instruments, such as an otoscope, an ophthalmoscope, or a vaginal speculum, are used to enhance the inspection of specific body systems or structures. Equipment used to facilitate the inspection is presented later in this chapter.

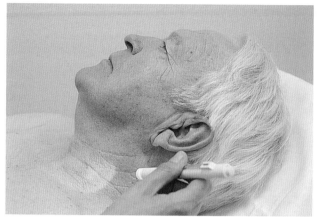

FIG. 3.2 Tangential light using a penlight to inspect jugular vein pulsations.

Palpation

Palpation involves using the hands to feel texture, size, shape, consistency, pulsation, and location of certain parts of the patient's body. It is also used to identify areas the patient reports as being tender or painful. This technique requires the nurse to move into the patient's personal space. The nurse's touch should be gentle, the hands warm, and nails short to prevent discomfort or injury to the patient. Touch has cultural significance and symbolism. Each culture has its own understanding of the uses and meanings of touch. Because of this, the nurse must tell the patient the purpose of and need for the touch (e.g., "I'm feeling for lymph nodes now") and manner and location of touch (e.g., "I'm going to press deeply on your abdomen to feel the organs"). Gloves are worn when palpating mucous membranes or any other area where contact with body fluids is possible.

The palmar surfaces of the fingers and finger pads are more sensitive to palpation than the fingertips; thus they are better for determining position, texture, size, consistency, masses, fluid, moisture, and crepitus. The ulnar surface of the hands extending to the fifth finger is the most sensitive to vibration, whereas the dorsal surface (back) of the hands is more sensitive to temperature.

Palpation using the palmar surfaces of the fingers may be light or deep and is controlled by the amount of pressure applied. Light palpation is accomplished by pressing down to a depth of approximately 1 cm and is used to assess skin, pulsations, and tenderness (Fig. 3.3A). Deep palpation is accomplished by pressing down to a depth of 4 cm with one or two hands and is used to determine size and contour of an organ (Fig. 3.3B). A bimanual palpation technique uses both hands, one anterior and one posterior, to entrap a mass or an organ (such as the uterus, kidney, or large breasts) between the fingertips to assess size and shape. Light palpation should always precede deep palpation because deep palpation may cause tenderness or disrupt fluid, which may interfere with collecting data by light palpation.

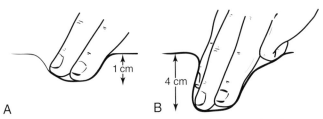

FIG. 3.3 (A) Superficial palpation. (B) Deep palpation.

Percussion

Percussion is performed to evaluate the size, borders, and consistency of internal organs; detect tenderness; and determine the extent of fluid in a body cavity. There are two percussion techniques: direct and indirect.

Direct Percussion

Direct percussion involves striking a finger or hand directly against the patient's body. The nurse may use direct percussion technique to evaluate the sinus of an adult by tapping a finger over the sinus or to elicit tenderness or pain over the kidney by striking the costovertebral angle (CVA) directly with a fist (Fig. 3.4). How and where to strike the CVA is discussed in Chapter 13.

Indirect Percussion

Indirect percussion requires the use of both hands and is performed by different methods, depending on which body area is being assessed. One method, indirect fist percussion of the kidney, involves placing the nondominant hand palm down (with fingers together) over the CVA and gently tapping the back of the hand with the fist of the dominant hand. Another method, indirect finger percussion, is performed by placing the distal aspect of the middle finger of the nondominant hand against the skin over the organ being percussed and striking the distal interphalangeal joint (between the cuticle and first joint) with the tip of the middle finger of the dominant hand. The position of the other fingers of the nondominant hand is important; they are spread apart and slightly elevated off the patient's skin so they do not dampen the vibrations (Fig. 3.5). The force of the downward snap of the striking finger comes from the rapid flexion of the wrist. The wrist must be relaxed and loose while the forearm remains stationary. Make the striking finger rebound as soon as it makes contact with the striking surface so the vibration is not muffled. Listen for the vibrations created by the percussion. The tapping produces a vibration 1.5 to 2 inches (4 to 5 cm) deep in the body tissue and subsequent sound waves. Percuss two or three times in one location before moving to another. Stronger percussion is needed for obese or very muscular patients because the thickness of tissue can impair the vibrations; the denser the tissue, the quieter the percussion tones.

Five percussion tones are described in Table 3.1. *Tympany* is normally heard over the abdomen. *Resonance* is heard over healthy lung tissue, whereas *hyperresonance* is heard in over-inflated lungs (as in emphysema). *Dullness* is heard over the

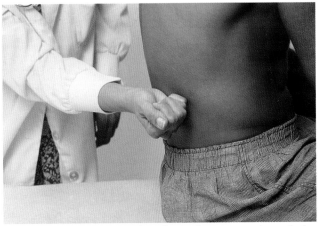

FIG. 3.4 Hand position for direct fist percussion of the kidney.

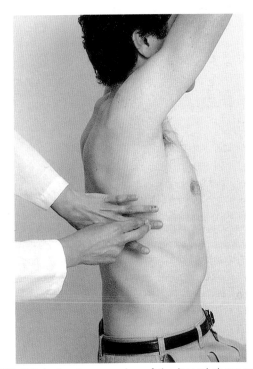

FIG. 3.5 Indirect percussion of the lateral chest wall.

liver, and *flatness* is heard over bones and muscle. Detecting sound changes is easier when moving from resonance to dullness (e.g., from the lung to the liver).

Auscultation

Auscultation involves listening to sounds within the body. Although some sounds are audible to the ear without the use of special equipment (e.g., respiratory stridor, severe wheezing, and abdominal gurgling), a stethoscope is usually used to facilitate auscultation. The stethoscope blocks out extraneous sounds that may interfere with hearing sounds produced by the heart, blood vessels, lungs, and intestines (Fig. 3.6). Listen for the sound and its characteristics: intensity, pitch, duration, and quality (Box 3.4). Concentration is required

TABLE 3.1 PERCUSSION TONES

AREA PERCUSSED	TONE	INTENSITY	PITCH	DURATION	QUALITY
Lungs	Resonant	Loud	Low	Long	Hollow
Bone and muscle	Flat	Soft	High	Short	Extremely dull
Viscera and liver borders	Dull	Medium	Medium high	Medium	Thudlike
Stomach and gas bubbles in intestines	Tympanic	Loud	High	Medium	Drumlike
Air trapped in lung (emphysema)	Hyperresonant	Very loud	Very low	Longer	Booming

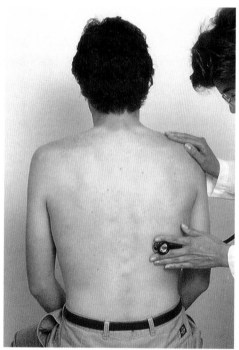

FIG. 3.6 Auscultation using a stethoscope. The diaphragm of the stethoscope is stabilized between the index and middle fingers.

BOX 3.4 CHARACTERISTICS OF SOUNDS HEARD BY AUSCULTATION

- *Intensity* is the loudness of the sound, described as soft, medium, or loud.
- *Pitch* is the frequency or number of sound waves generated per second. High-pitched sounds have high frequencies. Expected high-pitched sounds are breath sounds, whereas cardiac sounds are low pitched.
- *Duration of sound vibrations* is short, medium, or long. Layers of soft tissue dampen the duration of sound from deep organs.
- *Quality* refers to the description of the sounds (e.g., hollow, dull, crackle).

because sounds may be transitory or subtle. Closing the eyes may improve listening because it reduces distracting visual stimuli. The isolation of specific sounds such as sounds of air during inspiration or a single heart sound is referred to as *selective listening.*

Precautions should be taken to optimize the quality of auscultation findings. Auscultation is best performed in a quiet room because environmental noise can interfere with hearing the sounds. The stethoscope must be placed directly onto the skin because clothing (including a patient gown) obscures or alters sounds. Warm the head of the stethoscope before placing it on the patient. If the patient becomes cold and shivers, involuntary muscle contractions could interfere with auscultation findings. The friction of body hair rubbing against the diaphragm of the stethoscope could be mistaken for abnormal lung sounds (crackles). Bumping the stethoscope tubing while auscultating produces a loud tapping sound that obscures the underlying auscultation findings. Because the diaphragm and bell of the stethoscope are placed on the patient's skin, they must be cleaned with alcohol between patients to prevent the spread of infection.

EXAMINATION SETTING

The physical assessment is usually conducted in a health care setting. There are several characteristics of an optimal space for examination. Providing privacy is a priority, particularly during examination procedures where the patient is exposed. A private examination room provides the best level of privacy and also reduces the risk of interruptions during the examination. The examination space should have good lighting to facilitate inspection, should be quiet to facilitate hearing sounds during auscultation or percussion, and should be a warm temperature to maximize patient comfort. The examination setting should be furnished with an examination table or bed that maximizes options for patient positioning, an examination stool, and a bedside table. Finally, the equipment needed to conduct the examination should be readily available, accessible, and functional.

PATIENT POSITIONING

The patient may assume a number of positions during the examination; the positions depend on the type of examination to be performed and the condition of the patient. The sitting and supine positions are the most common. Various positions for examination are presented in Table 3.2. Draping the patient appropriately is important to provide for modesty while allowing the exposure needed for the examination. The inability to assume a particular position may be a significant finding about the patient's physical status and require the nurse to make necessary accommodations. For example, a

TABLE 3.2 POSITIONS FOR EXAMINATION

POSITION	AREAS ASSESSED	RATIONALE	LIMITATIONS
Sitting	Head and neck, back, posterior thorax and lungs, anterior thorax and lungs, breasts, axilla, heart, vital signs, and upper extremities	Sitting upright provides full expansion of lungs and better visualization of symmetry of upper body parts.	Physically weakened patient may be unable to sit. The nurse should use supine position with the head of bed elevated instead.
Supine	Head and neck, anterior thorax and lungs, breasts, axilla, heart, abdomen, extremities, pulses	This is the most normally relaxed position. It provides easy access to pulse sites.	If patient becomes short of breath easily, the nurse may need to raise the head of the bed.
Dorsal recumbent	Head and neck, anterior thorax and lungs, breasts, axilla, heart, abdomen	This position is used for abdominal assessment because it promotes relaxation of abdominal muscles.	Patients with painful disorders are more comfortable with knees flexed.
Lithotomy[a]	Female genitalia and genital tract	This position provides maximal exposure of genitalia and facilitates insertion of vaginal speculum.	Lithotomy position is embarrassing and uncomfortable; thus the nurse minimizes the time that a patient spends in it. The patient is kept well draped.
Sims	Rectum and vagina	Flexion of hip and knee improves exposure of rectal area.	Joint deformities may hinder the patient's ability to bend the hip and knee.
Prone	Musculoskeletal system	This position is used only to assess the extension of the hip joint.	This position is poorly tolerated in patients with respiratory difficulties.
Lateral recumbent	Heart	This position assists in detecting murmurs.	This position is poorly tolerated in patients with respiratory difficulties.
Knee-chest[a]	Rectum	This position provides maximal exposure of rectal area.	This position is embarrassing and uncomfortable; thus the nurse minimizes the time that the patient spends in it. The patient is kept well draped.

[a]Patients with arthritis or other joint deformities may be unable to assume this position.
From Potter PA, Perry AG: *Basic nursing: essentials for practice,* ed 6, St Louis, 2006, Mosby.

patient who is short of breath may not be able to tolerate a supine position. In this situation, the nurse should raise the head of the bed or examination table for certain aspects of the assessment (e.g., abdominal assessment).

EQUIPMENT USED DURING THE EXAMINATION

Examination equipment is used to facilitate the collection of data. Keep in mind that not all equipment presented in this chapter is used for all examinations. The type of equipment used varies, depending on the type of examination and the problem being assessed.

Thermometer

A thermometer is an instrument used to measure body temperature. Common thermometers used in health care settings are the electronic thermometer, the tympanic membrane thermometer, and the temporal artery thermometer.

The standard electronic thermometer, used for the measurement of oral, axillary, or rectal temperatures, consists of a battery-powered display unit, a thin wire cord, and a temperature-sensitive probe (Fig. 3.7A). The probe is covered with a disposable sheath before use and placed either under the tongue with the mouth closed, in the axilla with the upper arm held close to the chest, or in the rectum. The probe measures the temperature of the blood flowing near the tissue surface. The thermometer calculates and displays the temperature either in Fahrenheit or Celsius on a digital screen within 15 to 30 seconds.

The tympanic membrane thermometer (Fig. 3.7B) is an infrared radiation device that measures the temperature of blood flowing near the tympanic membrane. The device works when the temperature-sensitive probe, covered with a disposable sheath, is inserted into the patient's external auditory canal; a temperature measurement either in Fahrenheit or Celsius is displayed on the screen in less than 5 seconds.

The temporal artery thermometer (Fig. 3.7C) is an infrared radiation device that provides a temperature measurement from the temporal artery. Depress the scan button on the thermometer and slide it from one side of the patient's forehead to behind the ear. Heat emitted from the skin surface of the forehead and behind the ear is detected while scanning the temporal artery to record the temperature. The device is noninvasive and demonstrates sufficient accuracy in studies involving children between the age of 1 and 4 and among adults in a critical care setting.[13-14] A newer infrared radiation device that has become increasingly prevalent for body temperature measurement is the noncontact infrared thermometers (NCIT). This is a type of thermal radiation thermometer that uses laser technology to obtain a temperature reading. However, a recent study recommended further calibration of the NCIT is needed to ensure its accuracy.[15]

Body temperature is routinely measured using peripheral thermometers such as tympanic membrane, temporal artery, axillary, or oral. Over the past decade, a number of studies comparing the accuracy of the various devices to measure body temperature in a wide range of populations have been conducted with variable results. A meta-analysis of these studies concluded that peripheral thermometers lack accuracy and should not be used as a basis for clinical decisions.[16] Although using an electronic thermometer and infrared devices provide easy measurement of body temperature, they are generally less reliable than obtaining a core body temperature and should be used for screening.[15,17–20] The gold standard for core body temperature is that of blood in the pulmonary artery. Since this site is impractical for daily monitoring, the site that provides the most practical option is the rectal temperature.[16] However, core temperature is not measured as part of a routine physical assessment because it involves invasive approaches.

Stethoscope

A stethoscope is used to auscultate sounds within the body that are not audible with the naked ear. Although there are several types of stethoscopes (acoustic, magnetic, electronic, and stereophonic), the acoustic stethoscope is used routinely for a physical examination (Fig. 3.8A).

The acoustic stethoscope is a closed cylinder that transmits sound waves from the source through the tube to the ears. It does not magnify sounds but allows difficult-to-hear sounds to be heard more easily by blocking out extraneous noise from the room. The stethoscope consists of four components: the earpieces, the binaurals, the tubing, and the head. The earpieces, which may be hard or soft, should fit snugly and completely fill the ear canal. The binaurals are metal tubes connecting the stethoscope tubing to the earpieces. They allow the earpieces to be angled toward the nose so sound is projected toward the tympanic membrane. The tubing is usually made of a firm polyvinyl material and no longer than 12 to 18 inches (30 to 46 cm). If the tubing is longer than 18 inches (46 cm), the sounds may become distorted.

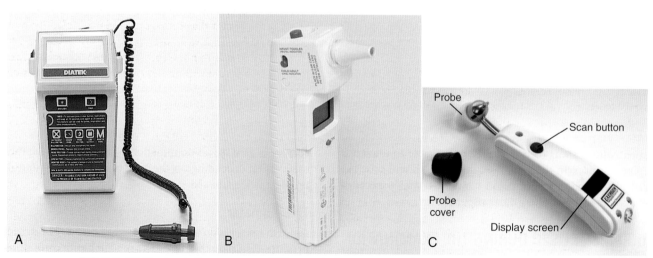

FIG. 3.7 (A) Electronic thermometer. (B) Tympanic thermometer. (C) Temporal artery thermometer. (B, From Seidel et al., 2011. C, From Bonewit-West, 2012.)

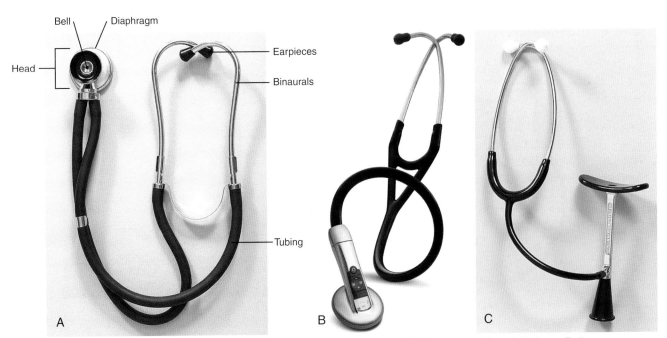

Head
Bell
Diaphragm
Earpieces
Binaurals
Tubing

A   B   C

FIG. 3.8 (A) Acoustic stethoscope. (B) Digital stethoscope. (C) Fetoscope. (A and C, From Ball et al., 2015. B, From Swarup S, Makaryus: Digital stethoscope: technology update. *Medical Devices: Evidence and Research* 11:29–36, 2018.)

The head of the stethoscope consists of two components: the diaphragm and the bell. It should be heavy enough to lie firmly on the body surface without being held. This piece is configured by a closure valve so only the diaphragm or the bell may be activated at any one time. The diaphragm consists of a flat surface with a rubber or plastic ring edge. It is used to hear *high-pitched* sounds such as breath, bowel, and normal heart sounds. Its structure screens out low-pitched sounds. The nurse holds the diaphragm firmly against the patient's skin, stabilizing it between the index and middle fingers (see Fig. 3.6). The bell of the stethoscope is constructed in a concave shape. It is used to hear soft, *low-pitched* sounds such as extra heart or vascular sounds (bruit). When using the bell, the nurse presses it lightly on the skin with just enough pressure to ensure that a complete seal exists around it. If the bell is pressed too firmly on the skin, the concave surface is filled with skin, and the bell functions as a diaphragm and inhibits sound waves. Some stethoscopes have varying head sizes that are interchangeable. When assessing an infant or a young child, the nurse uses a pediatric stethoscope, which has a small head. The diaphragm and bell should span one intercostal space of the patient's thorax.

A digital stethoscope represents a recent advancement in healthcare technology. The digital stethoscope (which attained FDA clearance in 2015)[21] converts an acoustic sound to electronic signals that can be amplified and then digitalized for transmittal to a computer and incorporation into a patient's electronic health record[22] and is especially helpful to support telehealth. Although similar in appearance to an acoustic stethoscope, the diaphragm of the acoustic stethoscope has a transducer with a microphone that allows for a recording, an electronic display, and Bluetooth capabilities (Fig. 3.8B). Although this technology may not be used for general health assessment immediately, as this technology evolves, such devices will be used in clinical practice with increasing frequency.

A special type of acoustic stethoscope known as a fetoscope (Fig. 3.8C) is used to auscultate the heart sounds of the fetus. The fetoscope has a metal attachment that rests against the nurse's head. This metal piece assists the conduction of sound so the fetal heart tones are heard more easily.

Equipment to Measure Blood Pressure

Blood pressure is usually measured indirectly (noninvasively) using a manual sphygmomanometer or an electronic automated blood pressure device. The sphygmomanometer consists of the gauge to measure the pressure (manometer), a blood pressure cuff that encloses an inflatable bladder, and a pressure bulb with a valve used to manually inflate and deflate the bladder within the cuff (Fig. 3.9A). A stethoscope is used in conjunction with the sphygmomanometer to auscultate the blood pressure.

The automated blood pressure device attaches to a blood pressure cuff (Fig. 3.9B). It operates by sensing circulating blood flow vibrations through a blood pressure cuff sensor and converting these vibrations into electric impulses. These impulses are translated to a digital readout that generally consists of the blood pressure, mean arterial pressure, and pulse rate. The device can be programmed to repeat the measurements on a scheduled basis and alarm if the measurements are outside the desired limits. This feature is especially useful for patients requiring frequent blood pressure monitoring. A stethoscope is not required when the automated device is used.

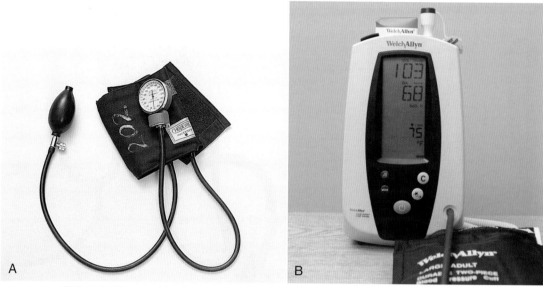

FIG. 3.9 (A) Aneroid sphygmomanometer. (B) Automated blood pressure device.

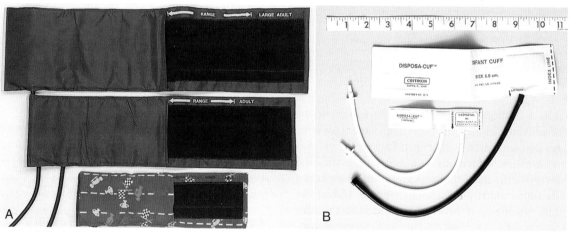

FIG. 3.10 Blood pressure cuffs in various sizes. (A) Reusable cuffs in large adult *(top)*, adult *(middle)*, and child *(bottom)* sizes. Note the range lines above the Velcro material on the right side of each cuff. (B) Disposable infant *(top)* and neonatal *(bottom)* cuffs. (B, From Seidel et al., 2011.)

Blood pressure cuffs come in a variety of sizes and are either reusable (occlusive cloth shell) or disposable (a vinyl material; Fig. 3.10). Both have a Velcro-type material on one end used to secure the cuff when it is wrapped around the arm. To obtain accurate results, the nurse must select a blood pressure cuff that is the correct size for the patient. If the cuff is too wide, it underestimates the blood pressure; if it is too narrow, it overestimates the blood pressure. Ideally the cuff width should be 40% of the circumference of the limb to be used. The bladder within the cuff should encircle at least 80% of the upper arm. Recommended cuff sizes are based on arm circumference and presented in Table 3.3. On most cuffs, range lines are indicated to assess the proper size. When a correctly sized cuff is applied, the cuff edge should lie between the range lines (see Fig. 3.10). Adult cuffs are available in two widths. The standard cuff is adequate for most adults.

If the adult is large or obese, an oversized cuff may be used. If the adult has an extremely obese arm, the nurse uses a larger cuff designed to measure the blood pressure around a thigh. There are many different sizes of cuffs for children. The width of the cuff should cover two-thirds of the child's or infant's upper arm. Correct cuff selection affects the accuracy in blood pressure measurement. Although selecting the correct cuff size may seem relatively easy, only 43% of nurses participating in a study assessing their knowledge about blood pressure measurement answered questions on the assessment of the cuff size correctly.[23] In another study, 22% of participants reported being unable to regularly obtain the correct cuff size.[24]

Wrist blood pressure monitors have emerged as another option for blood pressure monitoring; however, these devices are commonly used in home settings. Like the automated

TABLE 3.3 SIZES FOR BLOOD PRESSURE CUFFS BASED ON ARM CIRCUMFERENCE

ARM CIRCUMFERENCE (MEASURED AT MIDDLE OF ARM)	NAME AND SIZE* OF CUFF
5–7.5 cm (2–3 in)	Newborn: 4 × 8 cm (1.5 × 3.1 in)
7.5–13 cm (3–5.2 in)	Infant: 6 ×12 cm (2.4 × 4.7 in)
13–20 cm (5.2–7.9 in)	Child: 9 × 18 cm (3.5 × 7.1 in)
22–26 cm (8.8–10.4 in)	Small adult: 12 × 22 cm (4.7 × 8.6 in)
27–34 cm (10.8–13.6 in)	Adult: 16 × 30 cm (6.3 × 11.8 in)
35–44 cm (14–17.6 in)	Large adult: 16 × 36 cm (6.3 × 14.2 in)
45–52 cm (18–20.8 in)	Adult thigh: 16 × 42 cm (6.3 × 16.5 in)

*Note: Cuff measurement represents width and length.
Based on American Heart Association Recommendations (Pinkering TG, Hall JE, Appel LJ, et al.: Recommendations for blood pressure measurement in humans and experimental animals. Part 1: Blood pressure measurement in humans, *Hypertension* 45:142–161, 2005) and Welton PK, Carey RM, Aronow WS, et al: ACA/AHA/ AAPA/ABC/ACPM/AGS/APhA/ASH/ASPC/NMA/PCNA guideline for the prevention, detection, evaluation, and management of high blood pressure in adults: executive summary. *Hypertension* 71:1269–1324, 2018.

blood pressure devices mentioned previously, the wrist monitors use oscillometric technology to estimate arterial blood pressure (meaning the device detects vibration of blood in the artery and converts this into digital readings). The reliability of these devices has been questioned, and for this reason, they are not recommended by the American Heart Association.[25]

Pulse Oximeter

Oxygen saturation in arterial blood is measured using a pulse oximeter, consisting of a light-emitting diode (LED) probe connected by a cable to a monitor (Fig. 3.11). The LED emits light waves that reflect off oxygenated and deoxygenated hemoglobin molecules circulating in the blood. This reflection is used to estimate the percentage of oxygen saturation in arterial blood and a pulse rate. The sensor probe is taped or clipped to a highly vascular area—typically a digit (finger or toe) or an earlobe; for infants, a foot, the palm of a hand, or a thumb is used. Pulse oximetry is considered highly accurate in the measurement of oxygen saturation over the range of 70% to 100%, although if the probe is applied to cold fingers or toes, the accuracy may be affected.

Scales to Measure Body Weight and Height

Measurement of body height and weight is accomplished using a scale. A standing platform scale is used for older children and adults (Fig. 3.12A). The scale should be calibrated

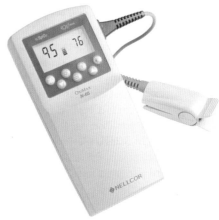

FIG. 3.11 Pulse oximeter shown with a clip and tape sensor probe. (Image used by permission from Nellcor Puritan Bennett LLC, Boulder, CO, part of Covidien.)

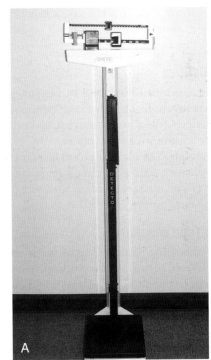

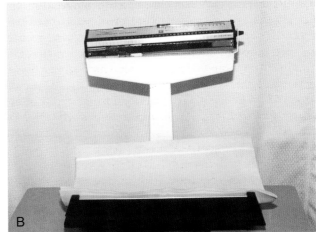

FIG. 3.12 (A) Adult platform scale. (B) Infant platform scale.

to 0 (zero) before measuring a patient's weight. The weight can be recorded in increments as small as 0.25 lb or 0.1 kg. Height is measured using the height attachment. This should be pulled up before the patient stands on the platform and then lowered until it is in firm contact with the top of the patient's head (see Fig. 4.2). Height is usually recorded in inches or centimeters for infants and in feet and inches or centimeters for children, adolescents, and adults. Measurement of height and weight using a platform scale is discussed further in Chapter 4.

Electronic scales are also used in many health care facilities. The patient steps on the scale, the weight is calculated, and a digital readout is provided (either in pounds or kilograms). Calibration of these scales occurs automatically with each use.

Infants are weighed using an infant platform scale (Fig. 3.12B). These work similarly to the adult platform scale but can measure weight in ounces or grams. The child may sit or lie on the platform while the weight is measured. Because the infant platform scale does not have a height attachment, height (length) is measured using a mat or board. This is discussed further in Chapter 4.

Skinfold Caliper

One method to estimate body fat is by measuring the thickness of subcutaneous tissue with a skinfold caliper. Different models of calipers (e.g., Lang or Herpendem) can be used to measure the thickness of subcutaneous tissue at different points on the body (Fig. 3.13). The most frequent location for thickness evaluation is the posterior aspect of the triceps. The use of calipers to measure skinfold thickness is discussed further in Chapter 8.

Ruler and Tape Measure

Obtaining an accurate measurement of size is accomplished with a ruler or tape measure. A small transparent metric ruler with markings in both millimeters and centimeters is useful for measuring lesions or other marks on the skin. A disposable paper tape measure is useful in various situations such as measuring the length of an infant, determining the circumference of an extremity, or measuring an open wound. A tape measure that has inches on one side and centimeters on the

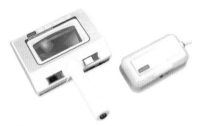

FIG. 3.14 Wood lamp. (From Pfenninger, Fowler, 2011.)

reverse side is ideal. Nurses can estimate size using their hands or fingers if they know landmark measurements (e.g., the fingertip to the distal interphalangeal joint).

Wood Lamp

The black-light effect of a Wood lamp is used to detect fungal infections of the skin or corneal abrasions of the eye. The examination room should be darkened to enhance the determination of the lesion color. Skin lesions caused by a fungal infection exhibit a fluorescent yellow-green or blue-green color when examined with a Wood lamp (Fig. 3.14). When fluorescein dye is placed in the eye, the Wood lamp can also detect scratches or abrasions of the cornea.

Magnification Device

Many nurses use a small handheld magnification device to assist with inspection. Some of these devices come with a battery-powered light source. Magnification and lighting facilitate the inspection of wounds, skin lesions, and parasites.

Penlight

The penlight provides a focused light source to facilitate inspection; thus it has many uses during a physical examination. It may be used to illuminate the inside of the mouth or nose, highlight a lesion, or evaluate pupillary constriction (see Fig. 3.2). To be effective, the penlight must have a bright light source. In addition, some penlights have a pupil-size gauge printed on the side of the light cylinder that allows the nurse to measure pupil size.

Visual Acuity Charts

A screening examination for visual acuity, color perception, and field perception is performed using visual acuity or eye charts. Several types of charts may be used, and the nurse must select a chart that is appropriate for the patient.

Distance Vision Charts

Either the Snellen or Sloan chart is used to screen for vision for English-speaking adults and children ages six and older.[26] These charts are hung on a wall at a distance of 20 feet from the patient (although some charts have been configured for use at 10 feet). The Snellen chart consists of 11 lines of letters of decreasing size (Fig. 3.15A). The letter size indicates the degree of visual acuity when read from a distance of 20 feet. The patient is tested one eye at a time. Ask the patient to read the smallest line possible. Beside each line of letters is the

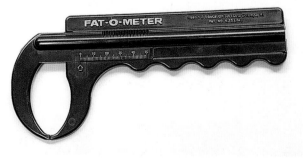

FIG. 3.13 Skinfold calipers.

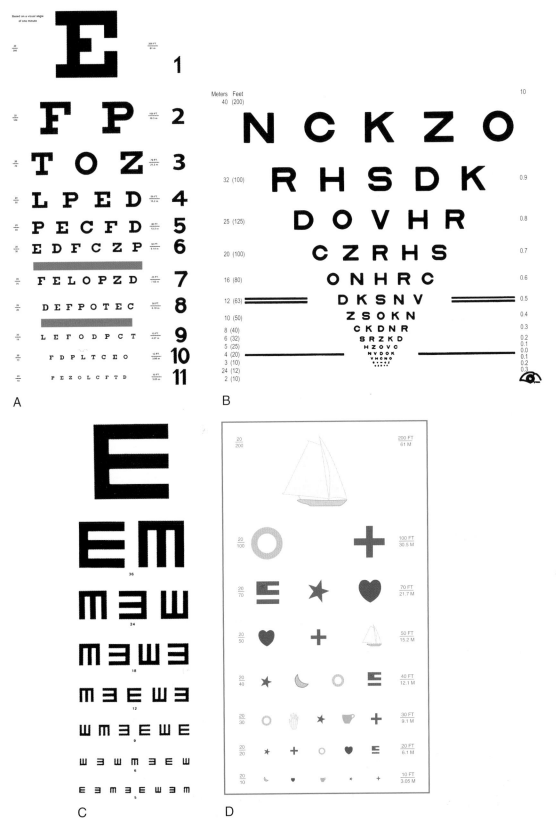

FIG. 3.15 (A) Snellen visual acuity chart. (B) Sloan chart. (C) Tumbling E chart. (D) Allen chart. (From Yoost and Crawford, 2016.)

corresponding acuity rating that should be recorded (e.g., 20/40, 20/100). The top number of the recording indicates the distance between the patient and the chart, and the bottom number indicates the distance at which a person with normal vision should be able to read that line of the chart. Ask the patient to name the colors of the horizontal lines as a screening for color perception. The top line is green, and the bottom line is red. Also ask the patient which line is longer as a screening for field perception measurement (the green line is longer).The Sloan chart consists of 5 letters to a row, and each row of letters is of decreasing size; they are scored in the same way as the Snellen chart (Fig. 3.15B).

For non–English-speaking individuals or those who cannot differentiate letters, the "Tumbling E" chart can be used (Fig. 3.15C). The nurse describes the "E" as a table with three legs and asks the patient to point in the direction that the table legs point. The scoring of the Tumbling E chart is the same as that of the Snellen chart.

Although children can use the Tumbling E chart, the HOTV or picture charts may be more appropriate for young children. The HOTV chart uses four letters, and the child is asked to identify the letters (H, O, T, or V) displayed. Picture/symbol charts (such as the Lea or Allen charts) show pictures and symbols in decreasing size. For example, the Allen chart depicts a sailboat, a flag, a star, heart, an O, and + (Fig. 3.15D). See Chapter 10 for further information regarding the assessment of visual acuity.

Near-Vision Examination

The Rosenbaum chart is used to evaluate near vision and consists of a series of numbers, Es, Xs, and Os in graduated sizes (Fig. 3.16). The patient should hold the chart 14 inches away from the face and read the smallest line possible. The nurse tests and records vision for each eye separately. Acuity

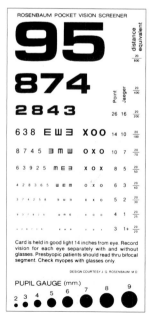

FIG. 3.16 Rosenbaum near-vision chart. (From Seidel et al., 2006.)

is located on the right side of the chart and is recorded as distance equivalents (20/20), the Jaeger equivalent (J-1+), or point equivalent (P-3). Asking the patient to read a newspaper held at 14 inches from the face is an alternate method to evaluate near vision. The patient should be able to read the newspaper without difficulty.

Ophthalmoscope

Inspection of the internal structures of the eye is accomplished using an ophthalmoscope, an instrument that consists of a series of lenses, mirrors, and light apertures. This instrument consists of a head and a handle; the handle is a power source containing batteries or connects to a wall-mounted electrical source. The head and handle fit together by a turn-and-lock system.

The head of the standard ophthalmoscope (Fig. 3.17A) consists of two movable parts: the lens selector dial and the aperture setting. The lens selector dial allows the nurse to adjust a set of lenses that control focus. The unit of strength for each lens is referred to as a *diopter.* When the lens selector dial is turned clockwise, the positive-sphere lenses (black numbers) are brought into place. The black numbers on the lens selector dial indicate increasingly positive diopter; these help the nurse focus on near objects within the patient's eye. Likewise, when the lens selector disk is turned counterclockwise, the negative-sphere lenses (red numbers) are brought into place. The red numbers indicate increasingly negative diopter and help the nurse focus on objects that are farther away within the patient's eye. The positive and negative lenses compensate for myopia or hyperopia in both the nurse's and patient's eyes and also permit focusing at different places within the patient's eye.

The aperture has several settings that permit light variations during the examination. The large light can be used for an examination of the internal eye if the patient's pupils have been dilated. The small light can be used if the patient's pupils are very small or if the pupils have not been dilated. The red-free filter actually shines a green beam of light. This filter facilitates the identification of pallor of the disc and permits the recognition of retinal hemorrhages by making the blood appear black. The slit light permits easy examination of the anterior of the eye and determination of elevation or depression of a lesion. The grid light facilitates an estimation of size, location, and pattern of a fundal lesion.

Another type of ophthalmoscope head, known as the PanOptic head, is designed to allow for a wider field of view and greater magnification, creating an improved view of the eye structures as compared with a standard ophthalmoscope head (Fig. 3.17B). The PanOptic head attaches to the same handle as the standard ophthalmoscope head. Eye examination using an ophthalmoscope is discussed further in Chapter 10.

Otoscope

Inspection of the external auditory canal and tympanic membrane is performed with an otoscope. The traditional otoscope consists of two primary components: the head and the handle. Some otoscopes also have a pneumatic attachment

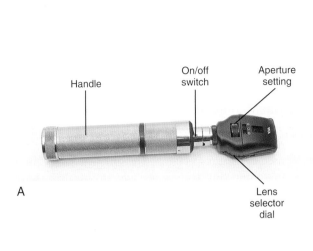

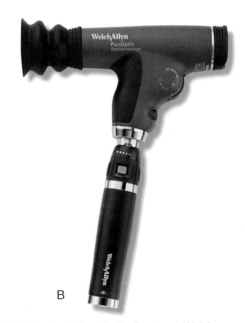

FIG. 3.17 (A) Ophthalmoscope with a standard head. (B) PanOptic head. (B, Courtesy Welch Allyn, Skaneateles Falls, NY.)

(Fig. 3.18A). The head of the otoscope consists of a magnifying lens, a light source, and a speculum that is inserted into the auditory canal. On newer models of otoscopes, such as the MacroView, an adjustable focus allows for greater magnification and field of view compared with the traditional otoscopes (Fig. 3.18B). Specula come in various sizes. Choose the largest-size speculum that fits into the patient's ear canal. The handle of the otoscope is the power source; it either contains batteries or connects to a wall-mounted electrical source. The pneumatic attachment is used to evaluate the fluctuation of the tympanic membrane. This attachment consists of a small rubber tube with a bulb attached to the head of the otoscope. When the bulb is squeezed, it produces small puffs of air against the tympanic membrane, causing the membrane to move. No fluctuation of the membrane may indicate pressure from behind the membrane. See Chapter 10 for further discussion on the use of the otoscope.

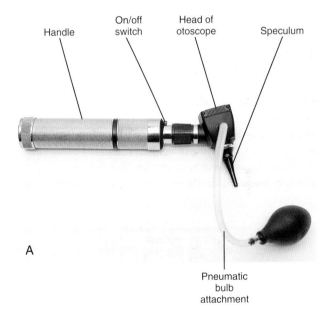

Audioscope

An audioscope is used to perform basic screening for hearing acuity. The handheld, battery-operated audioscope is inserted into the patient's external ear (Fig. 3.19) and provides a fast, simple test to detect hearing problems. It systematically and automatically creates tones at the different frequencies: 1000, 2000, 4000, and 5000 Hz. A light appears when the specific tone at a given frequency is sounded. The patient is instructed to raise an index finger when the tone is heard, which should correspond to the light seen on the audiometer. Hearing assessment is discussed further in Chapter 10.

Tuning Fork

The tuning fork has two purposes in a physical examination: auditory screening and assessment of vibratory sensation. To

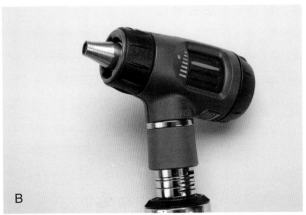

FIG. 3.18 (A) Traditional otoscope with pneumatic bulb. (B) MacroViewotoscope.

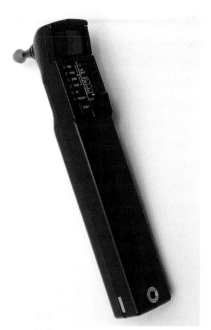

FIG. 3.19 Audioscope.

activate a tuning fork, the nurse holds it at the base with one hand and squeezes the prongs together or taps the prongs against the heel of one hand. Once a tuning fork is activated, the vibrations produce sound waves described as cycles per second or hertz (Hz).

For auditory evaluation, a high-pitched tuning fork with a frequency of 500 to 1000 Hz should be used, meaning it produces 500 to 1000 cycles per second (Fig. 3.20). A fork that vibrates in this frequency range can estimate hearing loss in the range of normal speech (300 to 3000 Hz). Inaccurate results are produced if the nurse strikes the prongs together vigorously or uses a tuning fork with a lower frequency. See Chapter 10 for further discussion on using a tuning fork to assess hearing with the Rinne and Weber tests.

For an assessment of vibratory sensation, the nurse uses a tuning fork with a pitch between 100 and 400 Hz. To activate,

the nurse holds the tuning fork at the base and sharply strikes the prongs on the heel of one hand. The vibrating tuning fork is then placed over a bone, such as the malleus (ankle bone), and the patient is asked to indicate if the vibration is felt. Patients who are unable to feel the vibration have reduced peripheral sensation. See Chapter 15 for further information on assessment using a vibratory sensation.

Nasal Speculum

The internal surfaces of the nose can be inspected using a nasal speculum to open the nares. Two instruments can be used as a nasal speculum. The simple nasal speculum is used in conjunction with a penlight to visualize the lower and middle turbinates of the nose (Fig. 3.21). The instrument is used by gently squeezing the handle of the speculum, causing the blades of the speculum to open and spread the nares, which permits the inspection of the internal nose. The second type of nasal speculum is a broad-tipped, cone-shaped device that is placed on the end of an otoscope. The nasal cavity can be inspected by using the light source and viewing lens of the otoscope.

Doppler

A Doppler is a device that amplifies sounds that are difficult to hear with an acoustic stethoscope. Ultrasonic waves are used to detect difficult-to-hear vascular sounds such as fetal heart tones or peripheral pulses (Fig. 3.22). A variety of Doppler devices are used for different applications (such as vascular Dopplers and fetal Dopplers). To use the device, the nurse applies a coupling gel to the patient's skin and slides the transducer over the skin surface until the blood flow is heard. The probe on the distal end of the Doppler amplifies the subtle changes in pitch as blood ebbs and flows through the vessels. The resulting sound heard is a swishing, pulsating sound. A volume control helps amplify the sound further. Depending on the type of Doppler used, the sound is amplified either through a microphone (allowing others in the room to hear) or through a headset where only the examiner can hear it.

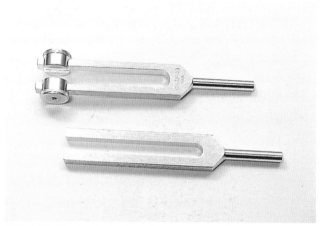

FIG. 3.20 Tuning forks for vibratory sensation *(top)* and auditory screening *(bottom)*.

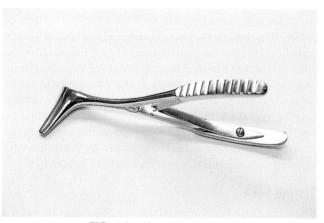

FIG. 3.21 Nasal speculum.

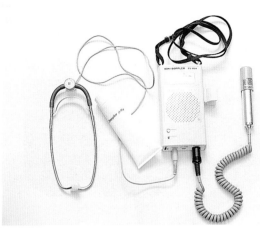

FIG. 3.22 Doppler.

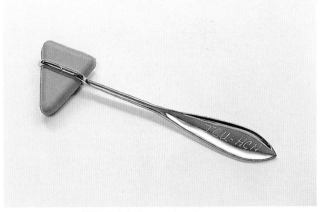

FIG. 3.24 Percussion hammer.

Goniometer

The degree of flexion or extension of a joint can be measured using a goniometer, which is a two-piece ruler joined in the middle with a protraction-type measuring device (Fig. 3.23). After the goniometer is placed over a joint, the patient extends or flexes the joint allowing the nurse to measure the degree of flexion and extension on the protractor. Goniometer use is discussed further in Chapter 14.

Percussion Hammer and Neurologic Hammer

Deep tendon reflexes are tested with a percussion (reflex) hammer. This device consists of a triangular rubber component on the end of a metal handle (Fig. 3.24). The hammer is configured so either the flat or the pointed surfaces can be used to elicit the reflex response. The flat surface is commonly used when striking a tendon directly and observing the patient response. The pointed surface may be used either to strike the tendon directly or to strike the nurse's finger, which is placed on a small tendon such as the patient's biceps tendon. A neurologic hammer can also be used to test deep tendon reflexes. It is similar to a percussion hammer, but the rubber-striking end is rounded on both sides. The technique to assess deep tendon reflexes is found in Chapter 15.

Monofilament

A monofilament is a small, flexible, wire-like device attached to a handle used to test for sensation on the lower extremities (Fig. 3.25). The wire is placed on the skin surface and then bent (the wire bends at 10 g of linear pressure). The patient should indicate when and where the monofilament is felt. Patients who are unable to feel the monofilament when it is bent have reduced peripheral sensation. Typically the monofilament is used to assess sensation to the foot in several locations, including the plantar aspect of the foot, great toe, heel, and ball of the foot. It is used only over areas with intact skin. Examination of peripheral sensation with a monofilament is discussed further in Chapter 15.

Vaginal Speculum

A vaginal speculum is used to spread the walls of the vaginal canal as part of the pelvic examination. This allows the nurse to inspect the vaginal walls and cervix and collect samples for diagnostic testing. There are three types of vaginal specula: the Graves, the Pederson, and the pediatric or virginal. All of the specula are composed of two blades and a handle and are available as either reusable metal or disposable plastic models (Fig. 3.26). The Graves speculum is available in a variety of sizes, with blades ranging from 3.5 to 5 inches in length and 0.75 to 1.25 inch in width. The bottom blade is slightly longer than the top blade. This configuration conforms to the longer posterior vaginal wall and aids visualization. The Pederson

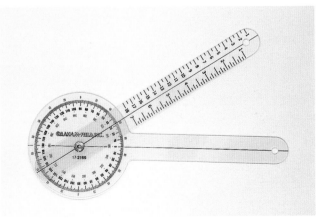

FIG. 3.23 Goniometer.

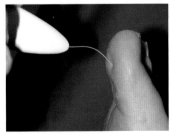

FIG. 3.25 Monofilament assessing peripheral sensation. (From Walker et al., 2014.)

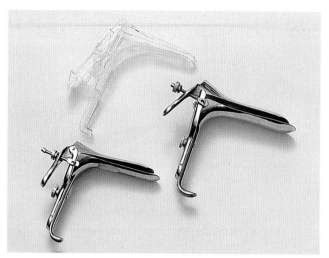

FIG. 3.26 Vaginal specula.

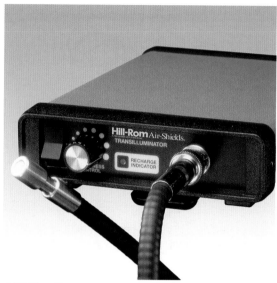

FIG. 3.27 Transilluminator. (Courtesy Draeger Medical, Telford, PA.)

speculum has blades that are as long as those of the Graves speculum, but are much narrower and flatter. The pediatric or virginal speculum is smaller in all dimensions of width and length.

Metal and plastic specula differ slightly in the ease of use and positioning. The metal speculum has two positioning devices. The top blade is hinged and has a thumb lever attached. When the thumb lever is pressed down, the distal end of the top blade rises and opens the speculum. The blade can be locked open at that point by tightening the screw on the thumb lever. The proximal end of the speculum can also be opened wider if necessary by loosening and then tightening another thumbscrew on the handle.

The bottom blade of a disposable plastic speculum is fixed to a posterior handle, and the upper blade is fixed to the anterior lever handle. When the lever is pressed, the distal end of the top blade opens; at the same time the base of the speculum widens. As the speculum opens, it goes through a series of clicking sounds until it snaps into the desired position. The patient should be forewarned about the clicking and snapping sounds. In addition, some of the plastic models have a port through which a light source can be inserted directly into the speculum. See Chapter 17 for further discussion on use of the speculum.

Transilluminator

Characteristics of tissue, fluid, and air within a specific body cavity can be differentiated using a transilluminator. It consists of a strong light source with a narrow beam at the distal section of the light (Fig. 3.27). When the examination room is darkened and the light is placed directly against the skin over a body cavity such as a sinus area, the transilluminator disseminates its light source under the surface of the skin. On the basis of the character of the glowing light tones, the nurse can determine whether the area under the surface is filled with air, fluid, or tissue.

CLINICAL APPLICATION AND CLINICAL JUDGMENT

See Appendix B for answers to exercises in this section.

REVIEW QUESTIONS

1. A nurse plans on changing a patient's wound dressing and then performing perineal care on that same patient. In following standard precautions, the nurse takes which actions immediately after completing the wound care?
   1. Documents the size and appearance of the wound and treatment as ordered
   2. Helps the patient to a supine position and drapes the patient to perform perineal care
   3. Performs hand hygiene immediately after removing the gloves
   4. Removes gloves, performs hand hygiene, and dons a new pair of gloves

2. A patient reports his right leg feels cooler than his left. What part of the hand does the nurse use to palpate his legs to assess skin temperature?
   1. The dorsal surface of both hands
   2. The ulnar surfaces of both hands
   3. The pads of the fingers of both hands
   4. The palmar surface of both hands

3. How does the nurse use a stethoscope to auscultate the chest of an adult?
   1. By pressing the bell firmly against the skin to hear heart sounds
   2. By pressing the bell lightly against the skin to hear breath sounds
   3. By pressing the diaphragm firmly against the chest to hear breath sounds
   4. By pressing the diaphragm lightly against the chest to hear heart sounds

4. A nurse is preparing to take a patient's blood pressure with a large blood pressure cuff that is 7 inches wide. The patient's upper arm circumference is 17 inches. How accurate will this patient's blood pressure be using this blood pressure cuff?
   1. Accurate, reflects the actual value
   2. Higher than the actual value
   3. Lower than the actual value
   4. Cuff size does not influence the measured value

5. A nurse is unable to palpate a pedal pulse on the patient's right leg. What action does this nurse take at this time?
   1. Use an audioscope to auscultate the pulse.
   2. Use a Doppler to auscultate the pulse.
   3. Use a stethoscope to auscultate the pulse.
   4. Use a goniometer to auscultate the pulse.

6. What equipment does a nurse use to inspect a skin lesion on the patient's arm?
   1. Wood lamp
   2. Transilluminator
   3. Skin calipers
   4. Penlight

7. A patient with Type I diabetes mellitus complains of reduced sensation in the feet. What equipment does the nurse use to gather additional data about this reduced sensation?
   1. Doppler
   2. Monofilament
   3. Percussion hammer
   4. Pulse oximeter

8. An English-speaking adult patient describes a change in his ability to see at a distance. Which equipment is used to assess this patient's visual acuity?
   1. Penlight
   2. Ophthalmoscope
   3. Snellen chart
   4. Transilluminator

4

General Inspection and Measurement of Vital Signs

evolve

http://evolve.elsevier.com/Wilson/assessment

Initial data collected at the beginning of the examination includes initial observations and measurement of vital signs. Specifically, these baseline data are collected from the patient before specific body systems are examined. The initial observations are often referred to as *general inspection*, although the terms *general survey* and *general observations* have the same meaning. Other baseline data include height, weight, and vital signs (including temperature, heart rate, respiratory rate, blood pressure, oxygen saturation, and pain assessment).

GENERAL INSPECTION

Begin the general inspection the moment you meet the patient. This involves observing physical appearance and hygiene, body structure, body movement, emotional status, disposition, and behavior (Fig. 4.1). The general inspection requires paying attention to detail and provides clues about any possible problems the patient may be experiencing. Initial impressions gained from these preliminary observations direct the nurse to further examine areas that do not initially appear normal. However, these initial impressions obtained as part of the general survey may be clarified as the nurse gains additional data during the examination, and through reflection on what was observed. In other words, the nurse avoids cognitive bias and forming premature conclusions by keeping an open mind to the presence of and meaning of additional data gained throughout the examination.

Appearance

The general appearance includes a variety of observations, including the overall state of health, age, level of consciousness, obvious sign of distress, skin, and hygiene. Consider the following things as you observe the overall appearance:
- What is the patient's overall state of health? Does the patient appear to be in good health? Does the patient

have an ill appearance? Does the patient have an obvious injury?
- Does the patient appear close to his or her stated age? Some patients appear older or younger than their stated age as a result of a number of factors such as drug and alcohol use, excessive sun exposure, chronic disease, and endocrine disorders (altered growth patterns or sexual development).
- Is the patient awake, alert, and responsive to you?
- Does the patient exhibit any obvious signs of physical distress? Is the patient short of breath, anxious, or in obvious pain?
- Notice the color and condition of the patient's skin. Are there any variations in color or is there an obvious presence of lesions?
- What is the patient's general hygiene? Is the patient clean and well groomed? Are any odors detected? Does the patient have a disheveled appearance?

Body Structure and Position

Observations involving the body structure include inspecting the stature, a general impression of the nutritional status (i.e., well nourished, cachectic, or obese), and the body symmetry (i.e., right and left sides of the body appear similar in size). Also note the patient's position or posture. Does he or she sit and stand up straight? For example, a patient with spinal deformities or back pain may have a slumped posture when standing or sitting. A patient who is having difficulty breathing may sit slightly forward, bracing the arms on his or her knees in what is referred to as the *tripod position*. A patient who is in pain may exhibit guarding or assume a *fetal position* when lying down.

Body Movement

Note how the patient moves. Does he or she walk with ease? Is the gait balanced and smooth with the symmetric

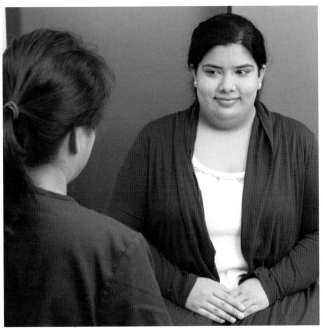

FIG. 4.1 The General inspection begins immediately on meeting the patient.

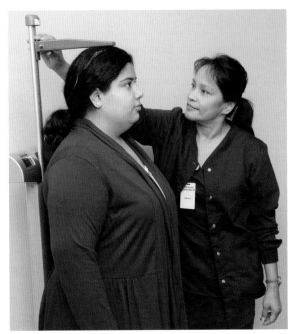

FIG. 4.2 Measurement of Height using a platform scale.

movement of all extremities? Note the use of assistive devices for ambulating such as a cane or walker. Note the ease of movement from standing to sitting and from sitting to lying. Does the patient move all the extremities? Are there obvious limitations in range of motion in any of the extremities? Does the patient seem to guard the extremities or show any evidence of pain with movement? Also observe for the presence of involuntary movements such as a tremor or tic.

Emotional Status, Disposition, and Behavior

The emotional status, disposition, and behavior are evaluated by noting alertness, the facial expressions, the tone of voice, and the affect. Does the patient maintain eye contact? Does he or she converse appropriately? Are the facial expressions and body language appropriate for the conversation? Is the clothing worn appropriate for the weather, age, and situational context? Is the behavior appropriate?

HEIGHT AND WEIGHT

The assessment of height and weight usually occurs at the onset of the physical examination.

Height

Height, a standard anthropometric measure, is gained as part of health assessment and is influenced by age, genetics, and dietary intake. As one of two primary measures of growth, height increases from birth through adulthood; adult height is attained between the age of 18 and 20. Many older adults loose height as part of the aging process. Height is usually measured using a platform scale with a height attachment. The height attachment is pulled up, and the

horizontal headpiece extended before the patient steps on the scale to avoid poking him or her as the headpiece is extended. Ask the patient to stand on the scale (without shoes); lower the attachment until the horizontal headpiece touches the top of the patient's head (Fig. 4.2). The vertical measuring scale can measure in inches or centimeters.

Weight

Another standard anthropometric measure is body weight or mass. A number of factors influence body weight including genetics, age, dietary intake, exercise, health conditions, and fluid volume. Genetics influence height and body size, including bone structure, muscle mass, and gender. Body weight is important in nutritional assessment to determine the changes in weight over time (if previous body-weight measurements are available) and in some situations to calculate medication dosage. Nutritional assessment is discussed further in Chapter 8. An unintentional change in weight can be a significant finding. For example, an increase in weight may be the first sign of fluid retention. For every liter of fluid retained (1000 mL, or approximately 1 quart), weight increases by 2.2 lb (1 kg). In addition, unexplained weight loss may be one indication of a disease process.

When measuring weight using a balance scale, ask the patient to stand in the middle of the scale platform while the large and small weights are balanced. The scale uses a counterbalance system of adding or subtracting weights in increments as small as 0.25 lb (0.1 kg) to achieve a level horizontal balance beam on the scale. Move the larger weight to the 50-lb (22.7-kg) increment less than the patient's weight. Adjust the smaller weight to balance the scale. Read the weight to the nearest 0.25 lb (0.1 kg).

VITAL SIGNS

Baseline and ongoing indicators of a patient's health status are referred to as the *vital signs* measurement. Vital signs include measurement of temperature, heart rate, respiratory rate, blood pressure, and oxygen saturation and are usually assessed at the onset of the physical examination. Assessing the presence of pain is also included with the assessment of the vital signs. Pain assessment is discussed in Chapter 6.

Temperature

Body temperature is regulated by the hypothalamus. Heat is gained through the processes of metabolism and exercise and lost through radiation, convection, conduction, and evaporation. The expected temperature ranges from 96.4°F to 99.1°F (35.8°C to 37.3°C), with an average of 98.6°F (37°C). This is the stable core temperature at which cellular metabolism is most efficient.

Temperature changes occur as a result of normal variations and activities. Diurnal variations of 1°F to 1.5°F (0.6°C to 0.9°C) occur, with the lowest temperature found early in the morning and the highest in the late afternoon and early evening. During the menstrual cycle a woman's temperature increases by 0.5°F to 1°F (0.3°C to 0.6°C) at ovulation and remains elevated until menses ceases. This elevation is caused by the secretion of progesterone. Moderate-to-vigorous exercise increases temperature.

Temperature is measured by several routes, including oral, tympanic, temporal, axillary, and rectal. Thermometers measure body temperature in Fahrenheit and Celsius.

Oral Temperature

The measurement of temperature by the oral route is done using an electronic thermometer. This provides a safe and relatively accurate measurement, although smoking or the ingestion of hot or cold liquids or food impacts on the accuracy of measurement.[1] Delay taking oral temperature readings for at least 10 minutes in such situations.

To take the temperature, cover the probe with a disposable sheath. Place the probe under the patient's tongue in the right or left posterior sublingual pocket. This area receives its blood supply from the carotid artery; thus it reflects inner core temperature indirectly. Ask the patient to keep the mouth closed while temperature is being measured. An electronic oral thermometer should remain in place until the audible signal sounds and the temperature registers on the display screen. Because the plastic sheath does not break, the assessment of temperature by the oral route with an electronic thermometer is safe for use with children of school age. An electronic thermometer with a pacifier-shaped probe is well tolerated by infants and toddlers and has been shown to be comparable in accuracy with the adjusted rectal core temperature.[2]

Temporal Artery Temperature

A temporal artery thermometer provides a measurement of the temperature of the temporal artery using infrared

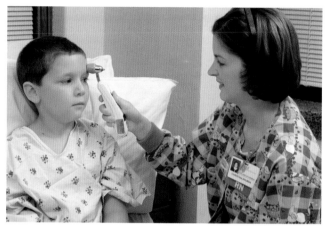

FIG. 4.3 Taking a temporal artery temperature. (From Potter et al., 2013.)

technology. Heat emitted from the surface of the skin on the forehead is detected while scanning the temporal artery to record the temperature.

To take the temperature, first place a disposable cover on the probe. Place the probe on the center of the patient's forehead, depress the scan button, and maintain contact with the skin while sliding the probe across the forehead into the hairline and behind the ear; then release the button and read the temperature measurement (Fig. 4.3). Moving the probe to the area behind the ear before reading the thermometer accounts for the evaporative cooling effect with diaphoresis. This device has shown a high level of accuracy among children and adults in critical care settings.[3,4]

Tympanic Membrane Temperature

The tympanic thermometer uses infrared technology to measure the temperature of the blood flowing near the tympanic membrane within the ear.

To take the temperature, cover the probe with a protective sheath and place inside the external ear canal with firm but gentle pressure (Fig. 4.4). Tugging the ear upward on the helix for adults (and downward on the earlobe for infants and children) should be done to help straighten the external auditory canal to ensure the accuracy of the measurement. The probe must come in contact with all sides of the ear canal. (NOTE: The probe does not extend all the way to the tympanic membrane.) The thermometer is removed after the audible signal occurs (approximately 2 to 3 seconds) and the temperature reading is displayed.

Axillary Temperature

The axilla is a common site for measuring temperature in infants and children; however, it is an infrequently used site for temperature measurement in adults. The axillary site is thought to poorly reflect core body temperature because it is not close to any major blood vessels and because the thermometer is placed between skin surfaces. Multiple studies have shown that temperature measurements at the axillary site are less accurate than in alternative sites.[5–7]

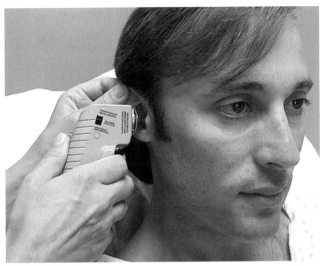

FIG. 4.4 Taking a tympanic membrane temperature. (From Harkreader, Hogan, and Thobaben, 2007.)

To take an axillary temperature, place the probe of an electronic thermometer in the middle of the axilla with the arm held against the body until the audible signal occurs and the temperature appears on the screen. Normal temperature readings from the axilla are approximately 1° below the normal temperature taken orally.

Rectal Temperature

Rectal temperature reflects core body temperature and is considered more accurate than noninvasive approaches.[3,5-9] Despite this, rectal temperature measurement is performed less frequently than tympanic, temporal, or oral measurements because it is invasive, is less comfortable, requires more time, and has an increased risk of infection transmission compared with other routes.

To take a rectal temperature, place the patient in the Sims position with the upper leg flexed. Appropriate privacy should be provided. Insert a disposable sheath over the thermometer probe and apply a water-soluble lubricant. Wearing gloves, insert the lubricated thermometer probe in the rectum 1 to 1.5 inches (2.5 to 3.8 cm) and hold it in place until the audible signal occurs and the temperature is displayed on the screen. Rectal temperature readings are approximately 1 degree higher than oral readings.

Heart Rate

Heart rate is commonly assessed indirectly by palpating a pulse. The pulse *rate* is the number of pulsations felt in 1 minute. The *rhythm* refers to the regularity of the pulsations (i.e., the time between each beat). Further discussion of heart rate and rhythm is found in Chapter 12.

To take a pulse, place your fingers over the artery and feel for the pulsations while also noticing the rhythm. Pulses are palpated using the finger pads of the index and middle fingers. Firm pressure is applied over the pulse but not so hard that the pulsation is occluded. If the pulse is difficult to locate, vary the amount of pressure and palpate the location where you expect to find it. If the rhythm is regular (time between each beat is consistent), count the number of pulsations palpated for 30 seconds and multiply by 2 or count for 15 seconds and multiply by 4. If the pulse rhythm feels irregular (time between each beat varies), note whether there is a regularity to the rhythm (e.g., a skip every fourth pulsation), which is documented as a "regular irregularity," or if the rhythm lacks regularity, which is documented as an "irregular irregularity." When rhythm irregularities are found, count the number of pulsations for 1 minute. Expected heart rates for various age groups are listed in Table 4.1. Changes in heart rate can be caused by a number of variables including physical exertion, fever, anxiety, hypotension, hormonal imbalances, and many other underlying conditions.

Although a pulse can be taken in many areas, the radial artery is most frequently used to measure heart rate because it is accessible and easily palpated. The radial pulse is found at the radial side of the forearm at the wrist (Fig. 4.5). The brachial and carotid arteries are common alternative sites to assess pulse rate. The brachial pulse is located in the groove between the biceps and triceps muscles just medial to the biceps tendon at the antecubital fossa (in the bend of the elbow) (Fig. 4.6). The carotid pulse is found by palpating along the medial edge of the sternocleidomastoid muscle in the lower third of the neck (Fig. 4.7). The heart rate can also be assessed by auscultating the heart (known as the apical pulse) and counting the heart sounds for 1 minute. To auscultate the heart, place

TABLE 4.1 NORMAL VITAL SIGNS THROUGHOUT THE LIFE SPAN

VITAL SIGN	INFANT	TODDLER	SCHOOL-AGE CHILD	ADOLESCENT	ADULT
Heart rate (beats/min)	100–160	98–140	75–118	60–100	60–100
Respiratory rate (breaths/min)	30–53	22–37	18–25	12–20	12–20
Blood pressure (mm Hg)					
• Systolic range	72–104	86–106	97–115	110–131	<120
• Diastolic range	37–56	42–63	57–76	64–83	<80

From American Heart Association: Pediatric Advanced Life Support Provider Manual, 2015 and Whelton PK, Carey RM, Aronow WS, et al: 2017 ACC/AHA/AAPA/ABC/ACPM/AGS/ APhA/ASH/ASPC/ NMA/PCNA guideline for the prevention, detection, evaluation, and management of high blood pressure in adults: executive summary: a report of the American College of Cardiology/American Heart Association Task Force on Clinical Practice Guidelines. *Hypertension* 71:1269–1324, 2018.

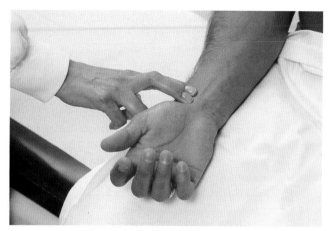

FIG. 4.5 Palpating the radial pulse.

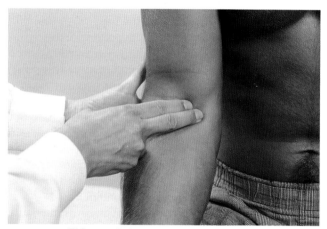

FIG. 4.6 Palpating the brachial pulse.

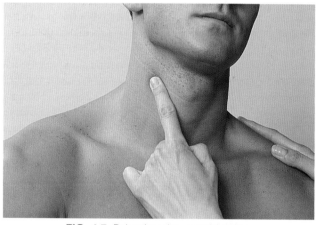

FIG. 4.7 Palpating the carotid pulse.

the bell or diaphragm of the stethoscope over the fifth intercostal space at the left midclavicular line over the mitral area. Auscultation of the heart is discussed further in Chapter 12.

Respiratory Rate

Assessment of the respiratory rate involves counting the number of times a patient completes a ventilatory cycle (inhalation and exhalation) each minute. Men usually breathe diaphragmatically, which increases the movement of the abdomen, whereas women tend to be thoracic breathers, which is noted with movement of the chest. Count the respiratory rate when patients are unaware that you are doing so; this prevents them from becoming self-conscious of the assessment and perhaps changing the breathing rate or pattern. Many nurses obtain the pulse rate and leave their fingers on the pulse site while they count the respirations so patients are unaware of when counting the pulse rate ends and counting the respiratory rate begins. Respiratory rates vary with age (see Table 4.1). Other factors that increase respiratory rate are fever, anxiety, exercise, and increased altitude. Increases in respiratory rates associated with altitude are generally noticed beginning at approximately 8000 feet for those not acclimated; the higher the altitude, the greater the effects.[10]

In addition to assessing the rate, note the rhythm, depth, and effort of breathing. Rhythm is the pattern or regularity of breathing and is described as regular or irregular. Depth is assessed by observing the excursion or movement of the chest wall. It is described as deep (full lung expansion with full exhalation), normal, or shallow. Shallow breathing (small volume of air movement in and out of lungs) may be difficult to observe. The effort that goes into breathing is also observed. Normally, breathing should be even, quiet, and effortless when patients are sitting or lying down. The assessment of respirations is discussed further in Chapter 11.

Blood Pressure

Blood pressure is the force of blood against the arterial walls and reflects the relationship between cardiac output and peripheral resistance. Cardiac output is the volume of blood ejected from the heart each minute. Peripheral resistance is the force that opposes the flow of blood through vessels. For example, when the arteries are narrow, the peripheral resistance to blood flow is high, which is reflected in an elevated blood pressure. Blood pressure depends on the velocity of the blood, intravascular blood volume, and elasticity of the vessel walls.

Blood pressure is measured in millimeters of mercury (mm Hg). *Systolic blood pressure* is the maximum pressure exerted on arteries when the ventricles contract or eject blood from the heart. By contrast, *diastolic blood pressure* represents the minimum amount of pressure exerted on the vessels; this occurs when the ventricles relax and fill with blood. Blood pressure is recorded with the systolic pressure written on top of the diastolic pressure (e.g., 122/76), but it is not a fraction. The difference between the systolic and diastolic pressure is called the *pulse pressure*, which normally ranges from 30 to 40 mm Hg. Normal blood pressure parameters are shown in Table 4.1. A series of blood pressure measurements may also be taken when the patient is in a lying, sitting, and standing position to assess for *orthostatic hypotension*. (A 20– to 30–mm Hg drop in blood pressure when the patient moves from a lying or sitting position to standing indicates orthostatic hypotension.)

Blood Pressure Measurement: Methods and Sites

Blood pressure can be measured directly or indirectly. Direct measurement is accomplished by inserting a small catheter into an artery that provides continuous blood pressure measurements and arterial waveforms. This direct measurement is done in the critical care setting when continuous monitoring is required. In all other settings, blood pressure is measured indirectly either by auscultation (also known as *manual blood pressure measurement*) using a sphygmomanometer and a stethoscope (Fig. 4.8) or an automated blood pressure device—also known as *oscillometric blood pressure measurement* (see Chapter 3).

Indirect blood pressure is typically measured using the upper arm. Measuring blood pressure on the bare upper arm has been the "gold standard" for years. Alternative sites for measurement when the upper arm is inaccessible or when a properly fitting blood pressure cuff for use on the upper arm is unavailable include the thigh, calf, ankle, wrist, and forearm. However, the reliability of blood pressure readings (compared with the upper arm) for some of these alternative sites bring to question the interchangeability of readings from different sites.[11–12]

Measurement of blood pressure—auscultation method.

The procedure for measuring blood pressure by auscultation at the upper arm is described in detail in Box 4.1, based on the most current clinical practice guideline.[13] Blood pressure can be measured with individuals in a lying position using the same positioning of the arm, cuff placement, and procedure for measurement as used when the patient is sitting.

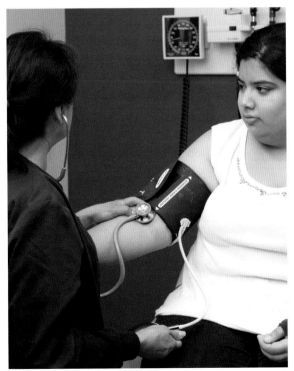

FIG. 4.8 Auscultating kortokoff sounds to measure blood pressure.

Patient Preparation
- Avoid consumption of caffeine, nicotine, or exercise for at least 30 min preceding measurement.
- Ask patient to empty the bladder, and remove clothing from the upper arm.
- Place patient in a sitting position, feet on the floor with the back supported.*
- Patient should relax and avoid talking for several minutes before blood pressure is taken.

Blood Pressure Measurement
- Position arm slightly flexed at heart level with the palm turned up.
- Palpate the brachial pulse in the antecubital space. Apply an appropriately sized blood pressure cuff (see Chapter 3) 1 inch (2.5 cm) above the site of brachial pulsation. The bladder of the cuff should be centered over the artery. The cuff should fit evenly and snugly around the arm.
- Position the sphygmomanometer at eye level no more than 3 ft (1 m) away. Close the valve on the pressure bulb clockwise until it is tight but easily releasable with one hand.
- Palpate the brachial or radial pulse with the fingertips of one hand while inflating the cuff rapidly; note the point at which you no longer feel the pulse and continue to inflate 20–30 mm Hg above this point. Slowly release the valve to deflate the cuff and note the point at which the pulse reappears; this is the palpated systolic pressure. Immediately deflate the cuff completely.
- After waiting for 30 seconds, place the stethoscope over the brachial pulse and inflate the cuff 20–30 mm Hg above the palpated systolic pressure. Release the valve and allow the cuff to deflate slowly at a rate of 2 mm Hg per second.
- Notice the pressure reading on the sphygmomanometer when the first Korotkoff sound is heard: this is the systolic pressure. Continue to deflate the cuff slowly and note the point at which the sounds disappear: this is the diastolic pressure.
- Deflate the cuff completely and remove it from the patient's arm. Record the measurement.
- This procedure may be repeated on the other arm for comparison purposes.

*Note: Measurements made with patient sitting on examination table (with legs dangling) or in lying position do not meet procedure criteria.[14]

The auscultation method requires careful listening for *Korotkoff* sounds (named for the Russian physician who first described them). Blood flows freely through the artery until the inflated cuff occludes the artery enough to interrupt blood flow and silence any sounds. As the cuff pressure is slowly released, the nurse listens for the sounds of the blood pulsating through the artery again. The initial sound is called the *first Korotkoff sound* and is characterized by a clear, rhythmic thumping corresponding to the pulse rate that gradually increases in intensity (Fig. 4.9). The pressure reading at which

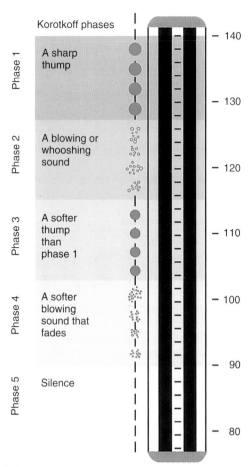

FIG. 4.9 Sounds auscultated during blood pressure measurement can be differentiated into five Korotkoff phases. In this example the blood pressure is 140/90. (From Potter et al., 2013.)

this sound is first heard indicates the systolic pressure. A swishing sound heard as the cuff continues to deflate is the *second Korotkoff sound*. The *third Korotkoff sound* is a softer thump than the first; the *fourth Korotkoff sound* is muffled and low pitched as the cuff is further deflated. The *fifth Korotkoff sound* actually marks the cessation of sound and indicates that the artery is completely open. The manometer pressure noted at the fifth Korotkoff sound is the diastolic pressure. A great deal of practice is required to differentiate all five sounds, but this differentiation is usually not necessary; in most cases only the first (systolic) and fifth (diastolic) Korotkoff sounds are recorded.

To take a blood pressure reading from the thigh, the patient should be placed in the prone or supine position. The prone position is preferred, but the supine position can be used with the patient bending the knee slightly to allow access to the popliteal artery. Wrap an adult thigh cuff (16 × 42 cm or 6.3 × 16.5 inches) around the lower third of the thigh, centering the bladder of the cuff over the popliteal artery. The measurement process similar as described for taking a blood pressure measurement in the arm (see Box 4.1). Normally the systolic blood pressure is 10 to 40 mm Hg higher in the leg

than in the arm but the diastolic pressures of arms and legs are similar.

Measurement of blood pressure—automated blood pressure monitor. The procedure for measuring blood pressure with an automated blood pressure monitor differs somewhat from the procedure presented in Box 4.1. Because the automated monitor is an electronic device, Korotkoff sounds are not auscultated. The monitor senses circulating blood flow vibrations through a sensor in the blood pressure cuff, converts the vibrations into electric impulses, and translates the impulses into a digital readout indicating systolic and diastolic pressures.

One of the concerns raised with automated blood pressure devices relates to accuracy of blood pressure obtained. Familiarity with the equipment and following manufacturer guidelines are needed to optimize accurate results. For the automated blood pressure monitor to be accurate, the cuff must fit properly and be placed correctly on the arm so the sensor is directly over the brachial artery. Even when used correctly, the accuracy of automated blood pressure devices has come into question. First, because of variability in calibration among devices, the potential for inconsistent readings occurs when multiple devices are used. Several studies comparing automated and manual approaches confirm acceptable accuracy and consistency for systolic readings; however, diastolic accuracy is less clear.[14-16] For this reason, if the blood pressure measurement using an automated device is very high or if there is any doubt about the blood pressure measurement obtained with an automated device, the blood pressure should be rechecked by auscultation as described in Box 4.1.

Physiologic Factors That Affect Blood Pressure Measurements

A number of patient-related factors can affect blood pressure and should be considered when interpreting blood pressure measurements.

- *Age:* From childhood to adulthood there is a gradual rise.
- *Gender:* After puberty, females usually have a lower blood pressure than males; however, after menopause, a woman's blood pressure may be higher than a man's.
- *Pregnancy:* During pregnancy, diastolic blood pressure may gradually drop slightly during the first two trimesters of pregnancy, but then it typically returns to the prepregnant levels by term.
- *Race:* The incidence of hypertension is twice as high in African Americans as in whites.
- *Diurnal variations:* Blood pressure is lower in the early morning and peaks later in the afternoon or early evening.
- *Emotions:* Feeling anxious, angry, or stressed may increase the blood pressure.
- *Pain:* Experiencing acute pain may increase blood pressure.
- *Personal habits:* Ingesting caffeine or smoking a cigarette within 30 minutes before measurement may increase blood pressure.
- *Weight:* Obese patients tend to have higher blood pressures than nonobese patients.

BOX 4.2 ERRORS IN UPPER ARM BLOOD PRESSURE MEASUREMENT

Errors Resulting in False-High Blood Pressure Measurement

- Allowing the patient to keep legs crossed during measurement
- Positioning the patient's arm below the level of the heart
- Using a cuff that is too narrow for the extremity
- Wrapping the cuff too loosely or unevenly
- Deflating the cuff too slowly (slower than 2–3 mm Hg per second)
- Reinflating the cuff before completely deflating it
- Failing to wait 1–2 minutes before obtaining a repeat measurement

Errors Resulting in False-Low Blood Pressure Measurement

- Positioning the patient's arm above the level of the heart
- Using a cuff that is too wide
- Not inflating the cuff enough
- Deflating the cuff too rapidly (faster than 2–3 mm Hg per second)
- Pressing the diaphragm too firmly on the brachial artery

Common Errors Associated With Blood Pressure Measurement

The accuracy of blood pressure measurement is significantly affected by the technique used. Research has found that many health care providers demonstrate incorrect technique or lack sufficient knowledge about blood pressure measurement, leading to the recommendation from the Subcommittee of Professional and Public Education of the American Heart Association to retrain all health professionals on a regular basis.[14] Incorrect technique can result in false-low or false-high measurements, potentially leading to inaccurate diagnosis or unnecessary medical care. Box 4.2 presents common errors in blood pressure measurement.

Oxygen Saturation

In many settings, measurement of oxygen saturation is included routinely with vital signs. As discussed in Chapter 3, oxygen saturation is measured by a pulse oximeter—a device that estimates the oxygen saturation of hemoglobin in the blood. The probe is usually either clipped or taped to the patient's fingertip; the toe, earlobe, and nose are alternative sites. The oxygen saturation level appears as a digital readout within 10 to 15 seconds after the oximeter is placed. Oxygen saturation levels lower than 90% are considered abnormal and require further evaluation.

Pain

Routine assessment of a patient's pain or comfort level is standard practice in all health care settings and is often assessed with vital sign measurement. The Joint Commission has specific standards that include pain screening and pain assessment.[17] An in-depth discussion of pain assessment is presented in Chapter 6.

AGE-RELATED VARIATIONS

This chapter discusses conducting a general inspection and measurement of vital signs with adult patients as a primary focus. Vital signs are assessed in individuals of all ages, but the approach and techniques used to collect the information may vary, depending on the patient's age.

INFANTS AND CHILDREN

The measurement of height (recumbent length), weight, head, and chest circumference is an important indicator of growth. These data are plotted on growth charts to assess the growth patterns of infants and children and compare their growth with infants and children of the same age and gender. Although the same general process for a general inspection and the measurement of vital signs in infants and children is followed as described previously, nurses should use the specific age-appropriate approaches and techniques presented in Chapter 19.

OLDER ADULTS

The process for measuring height, weight, and the vital signs in the older adult does not differ from what has been previously described.

CLINICAL APPLICATION AND CLINICAL JUDGMENT

See Appendix B for answers to exercises in this section.

REVIEW QUESTIONS

1. The nurse obtains vital signs on a 42-year-old man having his annual physical examination. He has no medical conditions and states that his health is excellent. The nurse uses an automated blood pressure device to measure his blood pressure, and obtains a reading of 62/40. Which action by the nurse is most appropriate?
   1. Obtain a different cuff and take the blood pressure again.
   2. Take the blood pressure again using the auscultation method.
   3. Place the patient in a supine position and take the pressure on the leg.
   4. Record the blood pressure and continue with the examination.

2. Which set of vital signs should the nurse recognize as out of the expected range?
   1. 42-year-old man: pulse, 74 beats/min; respiration, 16 breaths/min; temperature, 98.2°F (36.8°C)
   2. 11-year-old girl: pulse, 88 beats/min; respiration, 32 breaths/min; temperature, 98.0°F (36.7°C)
   3. 3-year-old boy: pulse, 130 beats/min; respiration, 34 breaths/min; temperature, 98.0°F (36.7°C)
   4. 1-month-old girl: pulse, 120 beats/min; respiration, 42 breaths/min; temperature, 98.0°F (36.7°C)

3. The nurse records the following general inspection findings on a patient: "41-year-old male in no distress; very thin, skin tone slightly jaundiced, disheveled appearance, and appears older than his stated age. Patient with flat affect and makes minimal eye contact." What additional information should be added to this general inspection?
   1. His body movement
   2. The family history
   3. The estimated size of his liver
   4. His pulse rate

4. A patient is experiencing respiratory distress. Which method of temperature measurement would be the most appropriate?
   1. Oral temperature
   2. Axillary temperature
   3. Temporal artery
   4. Rectal temperature

5. A 62-year-old patient tells the nurse that he has recently had frequent fainting spells. After palpating the radial pulse, 13 pulsations are counted in 15 seconds with a regularly irregular rhythm. What is the most appropriate action for the nurse to take at this time?
   1. Reassess the pulse rate after he walks around the room for several minutes.
   2. Reassess the pulse rate for 15 seconds using the carotid artery.
   3. Take an apical pulse for 5 full minutes, counting the number of skipped beats.
   4. Palpate the pulse for 1 minute and determine the pattern to the irregularity.

6. Which action results in the patient's blood pressure being falsely low?
   1. Deflating the cuff too rapidly
   2. Using a cuff that is too narrow
   3. Wrapping the cuff too loosely on the arm
   4. Asking the patient to cross his legs during measurement

7. A nurse notices that the patient has gained 11 lb since a visit last month. If this weight gain is due to fluid retention, how much fluid has the patient retained?
   1. 1 liter
   2. 3 liters
   3. 5 liters
   4. 11 liters

Culture Competence

Nurses provide care to individuals, families, and communities who represent a wide range of diversity. Developing cultural competence facilitates the quality of care in all areas of nursing practice, including health assessment. Nurses who provide culturally competent care demonstrate acceptance of the patient's health beliefs and are sensitive to their preferences when taking a history, conducting a physical examination, and interpreting data. The American Nurses Association (ANA) not only considers Assessment as one of six standards of practice, but also cites culturally congruent practice as a standard of professional performance.[1] Attaining cultural competence is not an end point; rather, it is a process that evolves over the nurse's career. Cultural expertise is attained as a result of intentional learning over time, together with encounters with individuals and families from a variety of cultures.

ETHNIC, CULTURAL, AND SPIRITUAL AWARENESS

Changing Demographics

The demographics of the United States have changed dramatically over the past several decades, and changes are projected to continue in the decades to come. Although population growth is expected to increase at a slower pace, dramatic changes to the make-up of the population are forecasted. According to the US Census Bureau projections, three major trends will be seen: (1) the population will be older, (2) the population will be increasingly diverse, and (3) immigration will outpace the birthrate in the United States. By 2030 (for the first time in US history), older adults (over age 65) are projected to outnumber children as the baby boomers age. Net international migration is projected to overtake natural increase in 2030. The white non-Hispanic population is projected to shrink from 199 million in 2020 to 179 million by 2060; by comparison, the white-Hispanic origin population is projected to grow from 253 to 275 million over the same time period. The two or more races population is projected to be the fastest growing over the next several decades, followed by single-race Asians and Hispanics.[2] The term *fifth minority* has been used to describe those who are multiracial,[3] with the other four minorities being Hispanic, black, Asian and Pacific Islanders, and American Indian and Alaska Native.[4]

Cultural Diversity

All people are influenced by their unique cultural beliefs and practices, and thus the changing demographics reflect people with diverse ethnic, cultural, and spiritual practices. People who have immigrated to the United States have varied levels of cultural assimilation. At one end of the continuum are those who have moved to the United States from other countries without changing many of their behaviors or beliefs. They may live in small communities inhabited by people with a common cultural heritage. At the other end of the continuum are those who moved to the United States from other countries and adopted many beliefs, values, and behaviors of American culture. Between the two ends of this continuum are people with varying cultural, ethnic, and spiritual behaviors and beliefs that represent a blending of foreign and American influences. Belief systems act as lenses through which people filter everything they view. As people interact with new individuals and new environments, their own culture may change.

Diversity refers to differences in gender, age, culture, race, ethnicity, religion, sexual orientation, physical or mental disabilities, and social and economic status. As a nurse, you have the responsibility to care for individuals who may not have the same skin color, language, health practices, beliefs, religious practices, gender identify, and values as your own. When this occurs, the goal is to meet patients where they are and to work with their beliefs and value systems to provide effective and appropriate care. Consider the following scenario:

Rosa Martinez is a 72-year-old Hispanic woman who speaks Spanish as her primary language. Conversing in broken English, she tells the nurse that she has injured her lower back and now has continuing aches and stiffness. She was unsure about seeking care but came at the urging of her daughter. Maria sought care from a curandera, who gave her an herbal formula to take orally and had made herbal poultices for her to apply to her back. Rosa tells the nurse that these remedies are working and that she is not sure whether treatment from the clinic will help her. The nurse caring for Ms. Martinez has at least three facts to consider: (1) the language barrier; (2) an alternative health care provider, Maria, the curandera, in whom Mrs. Martinez has much confidence; and (3) the use of alternative folk remedies (i.e., the herbal formulas and poultices).

Definitions

Understanding the meanings of the terms *culture, ethnicity, race, spirituality, religion, sex, gender, gender identity,* and *gender expression* is necessary for cultural assessment. *Culture* is defined as knowledge, belief, art, morals, laws, customs, and any other capabilities and habits acquired by a person as a member of society. It includes religious affiliation, language, physical size, gender, sexual orientation, age, disability, political orientation, socioeconomic status, occupational status, and geographic location, all of which influence a person's perceptions, behaviors, and evaluations.[5] *Ethnicity* refers to the characteristics that a group may share in some combination, such as a common geographic origin; race; language and dialect; religious beliefs; a shared tradition and symbols; literature, folklore, and music; food preferences; settlement and employment patterns; and an internal sense of distinctiveness (Fig. 5.1).[6] Consider the following scenario:

A nurse is obtaining a history from an older Navajo woman. After each question, there is a long silence. The patient often stares at the floor. The nurse wonders if the patient has cognitive impairment or does not understand the questions. However, in Navajo culture, silence indicates that she is paying close attention to the nurse and is a culturally appropriate behavior. As a Navajo, she values silence. A person who interrupts while someone is speaking is perceived as immature.[7]

The previous example illustrates how behaviors can be interpreted differently by two individuals from different cultural backgrounds.

Race is genetic in origin and includes physical characteristics such as the skin color, blood type, eye color, and hair color. The Human Genome Project provides evidence that all human beings are 99.9% identical in their genetic make-up. Although less than 0.1% of a difference exists among races, some differences are evident when performing health assessments.[8]

The term *spirituality* is defined as "a search for the sacred" (God, Jesus, Mohammed, the Buddha, Brahman, ultimate

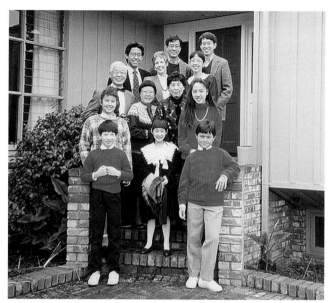

FIG. 5.1 Ethnicity indicates a common race, language, and dialect, and a shared tradition.

truth or reality).[9, p 40] A concept analysis revealed that *spirituality* is defined by four themes: as religious systems of beliefs and values; as life meaning, purpose, and connection with others; as nonreligious systems of beliefs and values; and as metaphysical or transcendental phenomena.[10] Religion may or may not be part of one's spirituality. *Religion* refers to the organized system of beliefs, rituals, and practices in which an individual participates, whereas spirituality is a broader concept. Spirituality practices may include prayer, meditation, walking in the woods, listening to music, painting, journaling, the intentional appreciation of beauty, or being present in the world with others.[11] Consider the following scenario:

Fatima Amir, a 46-year-old Arab woman who speaks both Arabic and English, is admitted for surgery. The nurse says to Ms. Amir, "I noticed you indicated your religion as Islamic. What do we need to know about your faith practices that might influence your care both now and after surgery?"

Instead of making assumptions about her faith practices, the nurse caring for Ms. Amir asks about how she practices her faith. While Islamic law requires same-gender providers for physical care, such as bathing; keeping the body covered at all times; and knocking before entering her room and waiting for permission to enter, Ms. Amir may not follow these practices.[12]

Sex refers to a person's genetic composition and its phenotypic expression. *Gender* is society's perception of a person's sex as male/man or female/woman. *Gender identity* is a person's internal sense of self as a man, woman, both, or neither. It usually develops by age 3 and remains relatively stable over a lifetime. *Gender expression* is a person's visible expression of social norms, such as mannerisms, dress, speech, or behavior conventionally regarded as masculine, feminine, both, or neither.[13] Consider the following scenario:

Patricia Collins, age 23, presents to the clinic for an annual exam. Her emotional and sexual attraction have been for women since childhood. During the sexual history, Ms. Collins reports that she has a female partner. As a follow-up question, the nurse asks, "Is there anything else you want me to add in your history?" Ms. Collins responds, "Yes, please don't talk to me about birth control; that is something I will never need."

The nurse caring for Ms. Collins has at least two facts to consider: (1) her lesbian lifestyle and (2) discussion about need for Papanicolaou (Pap) test to screen for cervical cancer.[14]

STANDARDS OF CARE

To emphasize the importance of culturally and linguistically appropriate services (CLAS) in health care, the Office of Minority Health (OMH) of the US Department of Health and Human Services issued national standards to ensure that all people entering the healthcare system receive equitable and effective treatment (Fig. 5.2). These standards provide for CLAS to help eliminate racial and ethnic health disparities and improve the health of all people living in the United States of America. The principal standard states, "Provide effective, equitable, understandable and respectful quality care and services that are responsive to diverse cultural health beliefs and practices, preferred languages, health literacy and other communication needs."[15]

The interpreter resources of the health care facility should be used when translators are needed, as opposed to a patient's family members or other hospital employees. Interpreters can not only help with language translation but also may be able to provide cultural insights that can help with care delivery. When demand is not high, some organizations use virtual interpreter services such as Skype or other web-based sources. Remember to document not only the use of a translator but also the purpose, such as obtaining a history and performing an exam. The use of translation apps on smartphones or the use of family members are not recommended as a substitution for

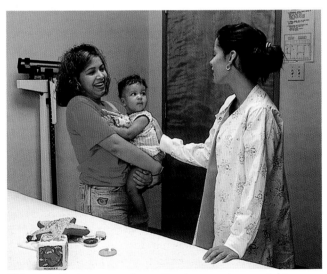

FIG. 5.2 Patients receive effective, understandable, and respectful care.

formal interpreter services. The accuracy of translation on smartphones can be poor and the vocabulary may be limited because they were designed for basic sentences such as ordering meals and getting directions when traveling. Using family members increases the risk of inaccurate translation and may violate patient confidentiality.[16]

The ANA Code of Ethics describes compassionate and respectful nursing care. In addition, one of the ANA's Standards of Practice describes Culturally Competent Care. Further, the ANA issued a position statement advocating for lesbian, gay, bisexual, transgender, queer or questioning (LGBTQ+) populations. The "+" designation is used to include other sexual and gender minorities not captured within the acronym LGBTQ. The ANA's position states, "Nurses must deliver culturally congruent, safe care and advocate for the LGBTQ+ populations."[17]

CULTURAL COMPETENCE

Performing a culturally competent patient assessment requires nurses to take several steps: (1) develop cultural competence through developing a sensitivity to differences between their own culture and that of the patient; (2) avoid stereotyping and assuming the meaning of the behavior of others; and (3) incorporate questions in the history to learn about the patient's health beliefs, health practices, spiritual/religious beliefs, and gender identity.

Develop Cultural Competence

The process of developing cultural competence involves mastering five interrelated components: cultural desire, cultural awareness, cultural knowledge, cultural skill, and cultural encounters. To start this process, nurses must be motivated or have a *cultural desire* to become competent to interact with people from different cultures. This begins when nurses give up their prejudices and biases toward people of different cultures and respect and care for them regardless of their cultural values, beliefs, or practices.[5]

Nurses begin their *cultural awareness* through an in-depth self-examination of their own cultural background. They identify their own cultural/ethnic group. Being aware of their own religious and cultural lens is important because these lens influence the way they hear and understand others.[18] Next, nurses identify their feelings gained from experiences they have had with people from different groups. Were assumptions made about people based solely on their appearance, dress, or skin color? What thoughts come to mind when patients speak with an accent or in broken English? Developing cultural awareness is enhanced by cultural humility. In a concept analysis, cultural humility was defined as a process of openness, self-awareness, being egoless, and incorporating self-reflection and critique after interacting with diverse individuals. Nurses with cultural humility are open to interactions with culturally diverse persons without assumptions or biases. They want to learn from patients about what is important to them. Also, these nurses are aware of their strengths, limitations, values, beliefs, behavior, and appearance to others. The quality of "egoless" refers to those with humble attitudes who approach others as equals. Self-reflection and critique refer to a critical process of reflecting on one's thoughts, feelings, and actions. Developing cultural humility is a *process* that is ongoing, through life-long learning and self-reflection.[19] Through reflection and self-examination some nurses may come to realize that they are harboring prejudices they were unaware of. As the desire for cultural competence increases and the awareness of the lack of this competence is realized, nurses seek additional knowledge.[5]

Gaining *cultural knowledge* begins when nurses learn about the beliefs, religions, values, traditions, and customs of other cultural groups. This information provides an insight into the differences and similarities among people. Cultural knowledge can expand to the incidence of disease and its prevalence and ethnic pharmacology.[5] While nurses learn about other cultures, they should not assume that all people from a particular culture are the same. They must use their knowledge as a foundation for learning about the beliefs, values, and customs of each patient as a unique being.

Cultural skill is demonstrated when nurses collect relevant cultural data about the patient's health problem and perform a culturally based health assessment.[5] An interpreter may be necessary to communicate with patients. During interviews, nurses should apply the art of asking questions described in Chapter 2 and implement cultural competence, as described in this chapter.

Cultural encounters provide opportunities for nurses to interact with patients from culturally diverse backgrounds (Fig 5.3). With continued application of their cultural awareness, knowledge, and skills, nurses become proficient in their assessments and modify their existing beliefs about cultural groups to prevent stereotyping.[5] A study to evaluate the cultural competence of graduating nursing students concluded that *cultural awareness*, rather than *cultural competence*, was a more realistic goal for this population.[20]

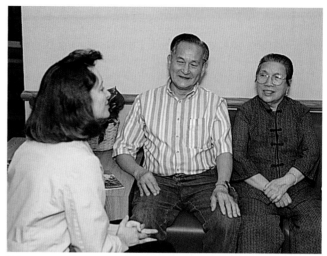

FIG. 5.3 When interviewing patients, recognize that cultural diversity exists.

Developing culture competence is a continuous process supported by the ANA's Standards of Practice. Table 5.1 shows examples of congruence between these standards and the process for developing cultural competence described previously.

Avoid Stereotyping

Nurses must show respect and acknowledge an individual's uniqueness regardless of that person's skin color, physical features, cultural heritage, sexual orientation, or spirituality. One's cultural heritage plays an important part in identifying an individual's "roots" and perhaps helps explain their attitudes, beliefs, and health practices. However, each major cultural group is composed of unique individuals and families who may have values and attitudes that differ from the cultural norm. Nurses must not assume that individuals or families who are Asian or Pacific Islanders all share culturally similar beliefs. Within the Asian or Pacific Islander

TABLE 5.1 **DEVELOPING CULTURALLY COMPONENT CARE**	
CAMPINHA-BACOTE'S COMPONENTS OF CULTURALLY COMPETENT CARE	**ANA STANDARD 8: CULTURALLY CONGRUENT CARE**
Cultural Desire: an internal motivation to develop skills interacting with people from other backgrounds.	
Cultural Awareness: a process of self-reflection of one's own culture and their reactions to people from other backgrounds.	Assess one's own beliefs, and cultural heritage.
Cultural Knowledge: a process to intentionally learn about beliefs, customs, traditions of people from other backgrounds.	Participate in lifelong learning to appreciate cultural preferences.
Cultural Skill: the ability to assess and interpret information, adapt communication style, establishing relationships.	Communicate respectfully with appropriate language and behaviors.
Cultural Encounters: the interaction with individuals from diverse cultural backgrounds.	Use knowledge of health beliefs, practices, and communications patterns when interacting with health care consumers.

Campinha-Bacote J: *The process of cultural competence in the delivery of healthcare services: A culturally competence model of care,* ed 4 Cincinnati, OH, 2003, Transcultural C.A.R.E. Associates.
American Nurses Association (ANA): Nursing scope and standards of practice, ed 3, Silver Springs, MD, 2015, Nursebooks.org.

group are Chinese, Filipino, Japanese, Asian Indian, Korean, Vietnamese, Cambodian, Thai, Bangladeshi, Burmese, Indonesian, Malayan, Laotian, Kampuchean, Pakistani, Sri Lankan, Hawaiian, Samoan, Tongon, Tahitian, Palauan, Fijian, and Northern Mariana Islanders. Each of these groups has a unique heritage and set of beliefs. Thus nurses should avoid making assumptions based on racial or ethnic backgrounds.

Likewise, individuals who identify with one religion do not necessarily have all the same beliefs or practices. For example, people can claim to be Jewish but not practice their religion in the same way or accept all of the beliefs of that faith. This variation applies to people of all faiths. Thus an assessment of each person's faith beliefs is necessary to gain an accurate understanding of that individual.

If you learn nothing else from this chapter, learn that all individuals are unique, deserving of respect and a personalized assessment of their beliefs, values, and traditions. Even people who share the same culture and background are not necessarily the same. Furthermore, they may act one way in one role but differently in another.

Apply Cultural Competence to a Health History

When conducting the health history, nurses ask patients and families about their health beliefs and practices that could reflect their cultural heritage (Fig. 5.4). They should also ask patients about spiritual beliefs and practices that are important to them. Today many people expect the health care provider will ask about their religious backgrounds. In one study about discussing spirituality with patients, 83% of subjects reported that they would like their provider to ask about their religion. Only 17% of the subjects reported never wanting to be asked about religion.[21] Nurses are *not* responsible for knowing about the health beliefs, practices, religions, and values of all cultural and racial groups. However, they are responsible for asking patients about their health beliefs, practices, religious beliefs,

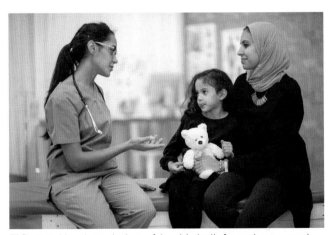

FIG. 5.4 Use knowledge of health beliefs and communication patterns when interacting with patients. (Used with permission from istockphoto.com.)

sexual orientation, attitudes, and values because this information forms the foundation for respectful, patient-centered, and holistic care. Keep in mind that a person may identify with one or more racial groups and also with one or more cultural groups, such as a religious affiliation, age group, the homeless; migrant worker; or a lesbian, gay, bisexual, or transgender individual.

Cultural assessment forms part of the personal and psychosocial history. Questions are asked to gather information about the unique beliefs, value systems, and spiritual practices of individuals of other cultures. Ask one question at a time, allow ample time for a response, use active voice, and avoid medical jargon.

To improve their cultural awareness and sensitivity, nurses should notice patients' behaviors during the initial interview for clues about preferred communication practices. For example, if patients do not make eye contact, they may be demonstrating that this is a preferred way of communicating in their culture. If patients back up as nurses approach them, they may prefer more personal space. If patients withdraw when touched by the nurse, they may view touching as prohibited or restricted. Also, look at the patient's immediate surroundings for clues about patient values and preferences. For example, look for religious symbols such as religious books (such as the Koran, Bible, or Torah) or other articles such as a cross or rosary beads. Also, notice if the patient is wearing an amulet, cross, chain, or charm on the neck, wrist, or waist. These may have special meaning to the patient, such as protection from physical and psychological illness, harm, or misfortune.[6] Such observations provide an opportunity to ask the patient about the meaning of the articles. For example, "I notice you have your rosary beads." In response, the patient may comment on the meaning to him or her.

Introductory Questions
- What name do you prefer?
- Where were you born? Which cultural practices are important to you?

Primary Language and Method of Communication
- What is your primary language?
- Which language is usually spoken in your home?
- How well do you speak, read, and write English?
- Will you need the services of a translator during the time you are in this health care facility?
- Tell me about your preferred styles communication, such as use of eye contact, touch, silence, personal space, or communicating with specific family members.
- How do you show respect for others?

Personal Beliefs About Health and Illness
- Do you believe that you have control over your health? If not, what or whom do you believe controls it?
- What are some practices or rituals that you believe will improve your health?

- Do you use or have you used any alternative healing methods, such as acupuncture, acupressure, *ayurvedic medicine*, healing touch, or herbal products? If so, how effective were these methods?
- Whom do you consult when you are ill?
- Which specific practices or rituals do you believe should be used to treat your health problem?
- Who makes the health decisions in your family?
- Which health topics do you feel uncomfortable talking about?
- Which examination procedures do you find embarrassing?

Beliefs About a Current Health Problem (Sickness)[22,23]

- What do you call this sickness?
- What do you think caused the sickness?
- Why do you think it started when it did?
- What do you think the sickness does? How does it work?
- How bad is your sickness?
- What kind of treatment do you think you should receive?
- What are the most important results you hope to receive from this treatment?
- What do you fear most about this sickness?
- What problems has your sickness caused for you?

Religious or Spiritual Influences

Box 5.1 presents a spiritual assessment tool. A study to evaluate this tool using an ethnically diverse sample concluded it was a feasible tool for clinical assessment of spirituality.[24] Box 5.2 lists barriers to assessing spiritual needs.

- If time or the situation only permits asking one question, ask, "What spiritual needs or concerns related to your health do you have at this time?"[25] How would you describe your current spiritual or religious orientation?
- In what ways is your spirituality/religion meaningful to you?
- What practices do you perform as a part of your daily religious and spiritual life (e.g., meditation, prayer, Bible reading)?
- How do your beliefs affect your health practices?
- How does your faith help you cope with illness?
- Are there any specific aspects of medical care that your religion discourages or forbids?
- Are there any religious/spiritual practices or rituals you would like to have available while you are receiving care? What part of your religion/spirituality would you like the nurses to consider as they care for you?
- What knowledge or understanding would strengthen your relationship with the nurses?[26]

Roles in the Family

- Who makes the decisions in your family?
- What is the composition of your family? How many generations or family members live in your household?

BOX 5.1 SPIRITUAL ASSESSMENT TOOL

The questions below can be remembered using the acronym FICA, meaning *faith, importance, community, apply, address.*
- What is your *faith* tradition?
- How *important* is your faith to you?
- What is your *church* or *community* of faith?
- How do your religious and spiritual beliefs *apply* to your health?
- How can we *address* your spiritual needs?

From Puchalski CH, Romer AL: Taking a spiritual history allows clinicians to understand patients. *J Palliat Med* 3:129–137, 2000.

BOX 5.2 BARRIERS TO ASSESSING SPIRITUAL NEEDS

Personal and Individual Barriers
- Nurses may view the assessment of a patient's spiritual needs as a private or family matter or a pastoral responsibility, but not their responsibility.
- Nurses may experience personal embarrassment, discomfort, or uncertainty about their own spirituality.
- Nurses may be uncomfortable when dealing with conditions and situations that frequently result in spiritual distress (e.g., suffering, grief).

Knowledge Barriers
- Nurses may lack knowledge about spirituality and the religious beliefs of others.
- Nurses may have minimal, if any, education related to spiritual assessment.

Adapted from McEwen M: Spiritual nursing care: state of the art. *Holistic Nurs Pract* 19:161–168, 2005.

Special Dietary Practices

- What is the main type of food eaten in your home?
- Are there any foods that are forbidden by your culture or foods that are a cultural requirement? If so, what are they?
- Who in your family is responsible for food preparation?
- Are there any specific beliefs about food, such as those believed to cause or cure illness? If so, what are they?

REMEMBER

The most important behaviors in cultural assessment are to be sensitive, to ask questions, to gather information specific to the individual patient, and to avoid stereotyping. Also remember to document your assessment findings so that all health care team members have data from your cultural assessment as they interact with this patient.

Regardless of the patient's race, cultural heritage, or sexual orientation, each individual is unique. Before you become involved in the detailed task of a physical assessment, first take the time to get to know the patient and his or her family.

CLINICAL APPLICATION AND CLINICAL JUDGMENT

See Appendix B for answers to exercises in this section.

REVIEW QUESTIONS

1. A school nurse notices a teen with a bandage on his arm and black fluid under the edge of the bandage. She asks the teen what happened to his arm. He replies that his mother applied axle grease to a boil. What is the nurse's most appropriate response to this teen?
   1. Tell the teen to remove the bandage and wash his arm.
   2. Remove the dressing to inspect and palpate the boil.
   3. Advise the teen to tell his mother to use antibiotic cream rather than axle grease.
   4. Suggest the teen see a health care provider to treat the boil.

2. How does a nurse begin the process of becoming culturally competent?
   1. By caring for patients from different cultures
   2. By abandoning prejudgment of others
   3. By being motivated to study other cultures
   4. By learning to speak a foreign language

3. A woman comes to the clinic with a complaint of back pain. During the history, she tells the nurse that she usually uses acupuncture for her ailments. What is the nurse's best response?
   1. "How effective was the acupuncture?"
   2. "Acupuncture is good for some problems, but not for back pain."
   3. "Why did you use acupuncture?"
   4. "Is acupuncture a common treatment in your culture?"

4. A nurse is assessing a woman whose religious beliefs do not allow blood transfusions. She has severe anemia, is very weak, and has altered mental status. What should the nurse do to provide culturally competent care to this woman?
   1. Examine his or her feelings about the role of religious beliefs in making decisions about life.
   2. Recognize that he or she cannot provide care to patients whose religious beliefs endanger their lives.
   3. Try to convince the patient to have a blood transfusion to save her own life.
   4. Determine whether the patient is competent to make her own decisions about health care.

5. A nurse at a clinic is admitting a new patient. During the assessment, she learns that this patient lives as a female but was born with male genitalia. The nurse feels uncomfortable after learning about this gender variance. What should this nurse do to provide competent care to this patient?
   1. Ask another nurse to complete the assessment of this patient.
   2. Try to subdue or hide her feelings from the patient.
   3. Discuss with the patient the reasons for living as a woman.
   4. Reflect on her own values, beliefs, feelings, and attitudes.

6. An older man who is near death has been admitted to the hospital, and his family members are at his bedside. Which question or statement should the nurse use during the admission assessment to address the spiritual needs of the patient and his family appropriately?
   1. "What is your religion? I'll make the appropriate spiritual arrangements."
   2. "Tell me what death means to people from your culture."
   3. "Are there any special needs that you and your family have at this time?"
   4. "I'll call the hospital priest so he can administer last rites."

7. A nurse admits a Hispanic woman who describes having traditional cultural beliefs. What action by the nurse demonstrates culturally competent care?
   1. Consult the hospital chaplain about how to meet her spiritual needs.
   2. Contact a *curandero* to visit her when possible.
   3. Ask her about her spiritual and cultural needs.
   4. Ask the family members what care they want for their relative.

CHAPTER

6

Pain Assessment

Pain is the most common reason people seek health care and has been described as a "significant public health problem" in the United States.[1] The assessment of pain represents a fundamental aspect of nursing care and applies to nearly all areas of nursing practice. Nurses should assess for pain as part of every patient encounter. Most health care facilities have policies and procedures that mandate an evidenced-based approach to pain assessment that includes the use of validated tools to obtain data about the patient's pain.[2] Pain assessment is performed not only as an initial assessment but also as a reassessment following pain management interventions. In 2018, The Joint Commission (TJC) released new guidelines for pain assessment and management, which include the expectation that "The hospital has defined criteria to screen,

assess, and reassess pain that are consistent with the patient's age, condition, and ability to understand."[3] Further, the American Nurses Association (ANA) recommends "ongoing reassessment with the patient of the efficacy of pain relief interventions."[4,p 6–7]

A widely accepted definition of pain recommended by the International Association for the Study of Pain (IASP) states that pain is "an unpleasant sensory and emotional experience associated with actual or potential tissue damage."[5,p 250] The definition of pain by McCaffery is that "pain is whatever the experiencing person says it is, existing wherever he says it does."[6,p.95] This definition represents the belief that one person cannot judge the perception or meaning of pain experienced by another person.

CONCEPT OVERVIEW

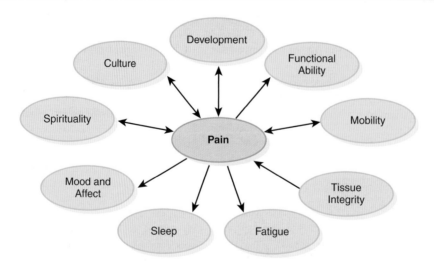

The concept for this chapter is *Pain*. Multiple concepts are associated with pain and effect its interpretation. Pain is associated with actual or potential tissue damage. A loss or

disruption of tissue integrity often results in pain, because sensory nerves react to the irritation from the local damage.[7] A person's expression and interpretation of pain varies widely, depending on his or her culture and spirituality. A person's level of development impacts both how pain is interpreted and communicated. Thus, as shown in the illustration, there are two-way arrows for spirituality, culture, development, and mobility. Pain can impair functional ability and sleep, and can lead to fatigue, particularly when sleep is interrupted. Those with severe or persistent pain may have altered mood and affect.[8] The following case provides a clinical example featuring several of these interrelated concepts.

Haim is a 41-year-old man with osteoarthritis in the hips. Osteoarthritis is associated with injury to the bone and cartilage in joints leading to pain (tissue integrity). He reports significant pain when walking and a reduction in joint mobility. He also has pain at night that interrupts his sleep, causing fatigue. Over time, his hip pain has limited his ability to do many daily activities he previously enjoyed (functional ability), resulting in depression (mood and affect) and a decreased quality of life.

ANATOMY AND PHYSIOLOGY

THE PAIN PROCESS

The physiology of pain involves a journey from the site of where the peripheral receptors are stimulated to the spinal cord, up the spinal cord to the cerebral cortex, and back down the spinal cord. The pain process begins when nociceptors respond to stimuli causing tissue damage. These nociceptors are primary sensory nerves located in tendons, muscles, subcutaneous tissue, epidermis, dermis, and skeletal muscles.

As nociceptors are stimulated, they initiate the second phase of the journey, which is to stimulate sensory peripheral nerves. These sensory nerve fibers carry pain impulses and include the large A-delta and the small C fibers shown in Fig. 6.1. The A-delta fibers are associated with a sharp, pricking, acute, or well-localized pain of short duration. The C fibers are associated with a dull, aching, throbbing, or burning sensation that is diffuse, has a slow onset, and has a relatively long duration. When these fibers are stimulated by nociceptors, they initiate an action potential that travels along peripheral nerves to the dorsal horn of the spinal cord. Located in the dorsal horn is the substantia gelatinosa, called the *gate*, which controls the stimulation of sensory tracts within the spinal cord. According to the gate theory of pain, when the gate is opened, pain impulses enter the spinal cord and ascend in the spinothalamic tract to the thalamus, resulting in the perception of pain.[9]

The third phase of the journey occurs when the thalamus receives impulses from the spinothalamic tract and sends them to the parietal lobe in the cerebral cortex and onto the limbic system. When impulses reach the parietal lobe, the patient feels the pain. Stimulation of the limbic system generates the emotional response to the pain, such as crying or anger.[9]

The pain journey ends when the body produces substances to reduce the perception of pain. As sensory nerve fibers travel through the brainstem, they stimulate descending nerves that inhibit nociceptor stimuli. These nerves travel down to the dorsal horn of the spinal cord, where they release substances such as endogenous opioids (e.g., endorphins and enkephalins) that inhibit the transmission of noxious stimuli and produce analgesia.[9] For example, endorphins and enkephalins occupy opioid receptor sites throughout the brain and spinal cord that prevent A and C nerve fibers from opening the gate (see Fig. 6.1).

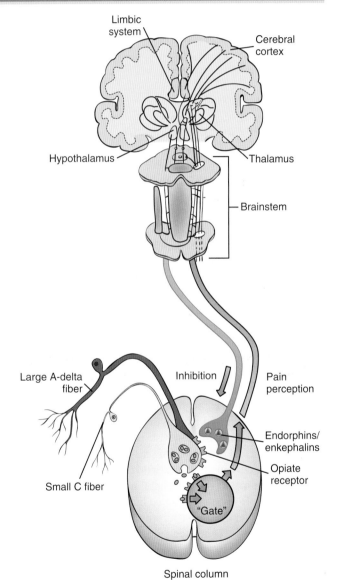

FIG. 6.1 The Journey of the pain process. **(1)** Nociceptors stimulate the free nerve endings; **(2)** nociceptor stimulation initiates action potentials along large A-Delta or small C fibers to open the gate to the substantia gelatinosa and ascend to the brain and the spinal thalamic track through the thalamus; **(3)** impulses move from the thalamus to the parietal lobe (cerebral cortex) and limbic system; and **(4)** the body produces endorphins and enkephalins to occupy the opiate receptor sites to close the gate to slow or stop the pain experience.

TYPES OF PAIN

A clear distinction among the different types of pain may not always be possible, because pain can be classified in a variety of ways. For example, it can be classified based on the duration and also by the inferred pathology.[9]

Classification by Pain Duration

Acute pain has a recent onset (less than 6 months), results from tissue damage, is usually self-limiting, and ends when the tissue heals. It is a stressor initiating a generalized stress response and may cause physiologic signs associated with pain, such as an increase in blood pressure, pulse rate, and respiration. By contrast, *persistent pain* (also referred to as chronic pain) may be intermittent or continuous, lasting more than 6 months. Clinical manifestations of persistent pain are not those of physiologic stress because people adapt to the pain, which may result in symptoms of irritability, depression, and insomnia.[10]

Classification by Pain Pathology

Another way to categorize pain is by the inferred pathology (i.e., nociceptive and neuropathic pain). *Nociceptive pain* results from activation of essentially normal neural systems producing somatic or visceral pain. Somatic pain arises from the stimulation of nerves within structures such as bone, joint, muscle, skin, and connective tissue. Visceral pain, however, arises from the stimulation of nerves within the thoracic, pelvic, or abdominal viscera. When visceral pain is experienced, the person may feel the pain in an area away from the tissue injury or disease. This is called *referred pain* and is experienced because many visceral organs do not have pain receptors. As a result, when sensory nerves carrying pain impulses from visceral organs enter the spinal cord, they stimulate sensory nerves from unaffected organs found in the same spinal cord segment as the nerves where tissue injury or disease is located. For example, gallbladder disease may cause referred pain to the right shoulder, and a myocardial infarction may cause referred pain to the left shoulder, arm, or jaw (especially in men).[9] In contrast, *neuropathic pain* occurs from an abnormal processing of sensory input by the central or peripheral nervous systems. Centrally generated pain may occur after injury to the peripheral nervous system, such as *phantom pain* from an amputated limb or injury to the central nervous system, such as burning pain below a spinal cord lesion. Peripherally generated pain may be felt along the distribution of many peripheral nerves (polyneuropathy), such as with diabetic neuropathy or along the distribution of a single peripheral nerve, such as a nerve root compression.[9]

THE PAIN EXPERIENCE

A person's pain perception and responses are affected by a wide range of factors. Pain occurs when tissues are damaged, but there is no correlation between the amount of tissue damage and the degree or intensity of pain experienced. For example, patients with extensive traumatic injuries may not report the intensity of pain expected, whereas patients with persistent cancer may experience intense pain for which no tissue damage can be found. For this reason, nurses must remember there are variations in how patients interpret and respond to pain even among patients experiencing the same condition. Variations include pain threshold, pain tolerance, cognitive factors, cultural influences, and coping strategies.

Pain Threshold and Pain Tolerance

Both pain threshold and pain tolerance affect a person's pain experience. The *pain threshold* is the point at which a stimulus is perceived as pain. This threshold does not vary significantly over time. By contrast, *pain tolerance* is the duration or intensity of pain that a person endures or tolerates before responding outwardly. A person's culture, experience of pain, expectations, role behaviors, and physical and emotional health influence the tolerance of pain. Pain tolerance decreases with repeated exposure to pain, fatigue, anger, boredom, apprehension, and sleep deprivation. The tolerance increases after alcohol consumption, medication, hypnosis, warmth, and distracting activities, and as a result of strong faith beliefs.[10]

Cognitive Factors and Cultural Influences

A person's pain perception and responses are significantly affected by cognitive factors and cultural influences. This includes the attention individuals give to the pain, the expectation/anticipation of pain, and the judgment/explanation of its occurrence.[11] Patients from different cultures may describe pain using words that are different from those familiar to the nurse. For example, after a painful surgical procedure, a patient denies experiencing "pain" but describes what he feels as an "intolerable ache." Descriptions of pain may be distorted in the translation from a foreign language to English. Some languages have no equivalent for the English word "pain," while others have several equivalents for "pain," each with a different meaning.[12]

People try to explain or make sense of their pain. Those who consider their pain to be an unexplainable mystery and doubt their ability to control or decrease it are less likely to tolerate the pain or use effective coping strategies. Over time, individuals develop cognitive patterns for explaining their pain. These patterns, uniquely defined by one's cultural and environmental background, are constantly changing as new and repeated perceptions of pain are experienced.[11]

Coping Strategies

How a person responds to pain is influenced by coping strategies. Pain coping is a response to reduce the physical, emotional, and psychological burden associated with stressful life events.[13] Two broad categories of pain coping are *problem-focused coping*, which includes efforts to manage or change the stressor and *emotional-focused coping*, which includes managing emotional responses.[13,14]

Problem-Based Coping Strategies

These strategies involve changing activity patterns or intentional self-care activities. Activity patterns include walking, stretching, or yoga. Self-care activities may include taking analgesics, vitamins, or antibiotics. Some people cope by applying the "hot-cold" theory of disease.[13] According to this belief, diseases are caused by a disruption in the balance of hot and cold in the body. Pain is considered a cold disease, which requires treatment with hot foods and medicines.[15] Other self-care activities may include complementary and alternative therapies such as faith healing, herbal remedies, massage therapy, and special diets.[13]

Emotional-Based Coping Strategies

These strategies include religious coping and social support. *Religious coping* includes beliefs (e.g., pain is God's will) and behaviors (e.g., prayer) that provide meaning, promote acceptance of the pain, and can reduce negative emotional responses to pain.[13] Some individuals prefer to talk about their pain with a priest, pastor, or someone else in their place of worship and report praying to God that the pain goes away.[13,15] Others believe destiny, luck, and chance are reasons for which people experience pain or health. Stoicism, defined as bearing pain with dignity and courage and not complaint, is often learned from the family.[13,15] *Social support* from family and friends is sought to reduce the emotional impact of pain.

HEALTH HISTORY

Pain assessment data are gained primarily from an interview. This section presents factors that influence the quality and accuracy of assessment, typical questions included for assessment of pain, and pain assessment tools to enhance the reliability of the assessment.

FACTORS THAT INFLUENCE PAIN ASSESSMENT

Attitudes and beliefs about pain held by nurses can affect how they perceive and respond to the pain of others.[16] Thus nurses need to reflect on and be aware of their own beliefs and attitudes about the pain of others to reduce the introduction of cognitive bias. Inadequate pain management can occur when health care providers inaccurately assess patient pain.[17] Nurses must trust the patient's self-report of pain, even when it appears to be incongruent with the patient's nonverbal behavior or the nurses' individual beliefs. The 2018 ANA position statement, *Ethical Responsibility to Manage Pain and the Suffering it Causes*, confirmed that "nurses have an ethical responsibility to provide clinically excellent care to address a patient's pain."[4,p 6] This position statement further asserts that "nurses have an ethical obligation to assess and address the factors in themselves and their practice environments that constrain their ability and willingness to relieve pain and the suffering it causes."[4,p 7] A survey of 2,949 nurses across the United States found that most nurses understand the principles of pain management. However, the results indicated that assessment of pain is one area in which nurses need additional education. When patients' expressions of pain or reaction to it did not conform to the nurses' beliefs or expectations, the nurses considered the patients' behavior to be inappropriate. The patient's response to pain is not right or wrong; it is merely different from that of the nurse. Although most nurses know that a patient's self-report is the most reliable indicator of pain, many remarks contradicted this. For example, some nurses reported that they try to determine the "real" status of pain in patients who are labeled *drug seeking*, *frequent flyers*, or *clock watchers*. Patients who are thought to be clock watchers are often undertreated and should be labeled *relief seekers* rather than *drug seekers*. Another finding from the survey was the reliance on increases in vital signs as indicators of pain. Although increases in heart and respiratory rates and blood pressures may occur briefly during acute pain, these parameters can increase for many other reasons. Patients with persistent pain do not usually experience any changes in their vital signs because they have adapted to the pain. Increases in vital signs are not always indicators of pain.[18] Box 6.1 contains questions to help nurses assess themselves and determine their cultural beliefs with regard to the assessment of pain.[12]

INTERVIEW QUESTIONS

Nurses interview patients to collect subjective data about their present health and experiences of pain. When obtaining a patient's health history related to pain, the nurse should be sensitive to the influences of culture on communication and responses to pain because pain has psychological, social, spiritual, and physical dimensions.

What are your beliefs about discussing your pain with others? How do you usually communicate your pain to others? To collect data accurately, nurses need to know the patient's preferred way of communicating pain (i.e., verbally or nonverbally), as well as what words or phrases he or she uses to indicate discomfort. Culture influences how people communicate their pain.[16]

Symptom Analysis

Nurses collect data from patients about their pain using a symptom analysis and applying the mnemonic OLD CARTS, which includes the *o*nset, *l*ocation, *d*uration, *c*haracteristics, *a*ggravating factors, *r*elated symptoms, *t*reatment by the patient, and *s*everity (see Box 2.6).

Onset

Pattern

When did the pain begin? What were you doing? Did the pain begin suddenly or gradually? These questions establish onset of pain and are helpful to determine the cause. Acute pain has a sudden onset and is of short duration. Ischemic pain gradually increases in intensity. Persistent pain lasts longer than 6 months.

When you were a child, how did those who cared for you react when you were in pain?
- How did they expect you to behave when you had a minor injury?
- How did they encourage you to cope when you had severe pain?
- How did they encourage you to behave during an injection or procedure?

When those who cared for you as a child were in pain, how did they react?
- Which words did they use to describe the pain?
- How did they cope with their pain?
- Do you tend to follow their example?

Consider a painful experience that you've had as an adult (e.g., childbirth, a fracture, a procedure).
- How did you express (or not express) your pain?
- Did the pain cause you fear? What did you fear?
- How did you cope with the pain?
- How did you want others to react while you were in pain?

Have you ever felt "uncomfortable" with the way a patient was reacting (or not reacting) to pain?
- What did the patient do that concerned you?
- Why did you feel that way?

Do you have "feelings" (make value judgments) about patients in pain who:
- Behave more stoically or expressively than you would in a similar situation?
- Ask for pain medicine frequently or not often enough?
- Choose treatments that you don't believe to be effective or with which you are unfamiliar?
- Belong to a cultural group (ethnic, linguistic, religious, socioeconomic) different from your own?

Do you tend to think that certain reactions to pain are "right" or "wrong"? Why? What about these reactions makes them seem right or wrong?
- Are some expressions or verbalizations of pain "right" or "wrong"?
- Some descriptions of pain?
- Some treatments for pain?

From Narayan M: Culture's effects on pain assessment and management, *AJN* 110:40, 2010.

What do you think is causing your pain? Why do you think the pain started when it did?

Being aware of a patient's insight into the cause of the pain is a patient-centered approach and may assist in pain management.

Location

Where do you feel the pain? Can you point to the location(s)? Does the pain radiate or change its location?

A description of the pain's location may provide information about its cause and type (e.g., somatic versus visceral). The patient may describe the pain location away from the site of the pathology when the pain is referred pain. Chest pain may radiate up the jaw or down the left arm in men, for example.

Duration

Is the pain constant or does it come and go? If it is intermittent, how often does it occur and how long does it last?

Answers to these questions may suggest a cause of the pain. For example, patients with mild peripheral artery disease experience intermittent pain in the legs when walking as a result of ischemia. When they stop walking, their pain is relieved. As the disease progresses, the pain experienced when they are walking becomes constant and is not relieved by rest.

Characteristics

What does the pain feel like (sharp, dull, aching, burning, throbbing, cramping, pressure)?

These descriptors of the pain may provide clues to the underlying cause. For example, somatic pain is usually well localized and described as aching or throbbing. Visceral pain caused by a tumor is described as aching and well localized, but if it is caused by an obstruction, the pain may be poorly localized and described as intermittent cramping.[10]

Aggravating Factors

What makes the pain worse? A change in position or movement? Eating?

The answer may help determine the cause of the pain or understand the impact it may have on the patient. For example, patients with irritable bowel syndrome report that their pain increases after they eat. Patients who have pneumonia may complain of a sharp pain when they take a deep breath (termed *pleuritic chest pain*).

Does the pain seem worse when you feel depressed or anxious?

Some patients experiencing pain also develop feelings of depression and/or anxiety. When these are treated, the patient often requires less pain medication.

Related Symptoms

When you experience the pain, do you notice other symptoms at the same time, such as fluttering or racing of your heart; shortness of breath; sweating; rapid, irregular breathing; nausea; or vomiting?

During low-to-moderate acute pain intensity, the sympathetic nervous system may cause palpitations, dyspnea, diaphoresis, or increasing respiratory rate, whereas during severe or deep pain, the parasympathetic nervous system may cause pallor; rapid, irregular breathing; nausea; and vomiting.

Does the pain interrupt your sleep? Have you noticed any fatigue?

Pain tolerance decreases with sleep deprivation and fatigue. Helping patients with sleeplessness may improve their comfort when awake.

Treatment by the Patient

What have you done to try to alleviate the pain? How do you cope with this pain?

A broad, open-ended question is asked purposefully to encourage patients to report all forms of self-treatments such as medications (i.e., pain relievers), support (i.e., a brace or wrap), lifestyle changes, alternative therapies (i.e., movement therapies, nutritional and herbal remedies, mind-body medicine, energy healing, massage, prayer), or coping strategies.[13,16] All forms of pain relief should be noted, particularly prescriptions and over-the-counter medications taken. Many patients fear adverse effects, as well as potential for addiction to pain medications.[16] Inquiring about the amount of drug taken is important to detect any possible toxic effects, such as drugs that contain acetaminophen, which can be toxic to the liver.

How effective have these methods of pain relief been?

Asking about the effectiveness of pain relief is important because the patient may not volunteer this information and any ineffective medications or other strategies should be reevaluated by the health care provider.

How much pain relief are you expecting?

Patients' cultural beliefs may affect the extent of pain relief expected. When caring for patients who have a low expectation of pain relief, the nurse should ask about their beliefs about pain and whether they are satisfied with the current pain level. A nurse should not assume that patients have the same expectations of pain relief as he or she would have in a similar situation.

Do you have any concerns about taking medication for pain relief?

Patients have reported not taking prescribed pain medication due to fear of addiction, fear of tolerance, concerns about adverse reactions, the need to be a "good patient," and fear of masking symptoms. These concerns can be addressed through patient education.[19]

Severity

How would you describe the intensity, strength, or severity of the pain?

Many individuals will be able to provide these data by using assessment tools such as a numeric rating scale (i.e., a scale of 1 to 10).[19] For patients with persistent pain, functionality may be a better indicator of pain intensity than a numeric scale.[20] Individuals' pain can be documented with their verbal descriptions of pain severity when assessment tools are not useful. Pain assessment tools are described later in the chapter.

How severe do you allow your pain to become before you try some form of pain relief?

This question seeks knowledge about the patient's pain tolerance, which can be influenced by culture and the pain experience, as well as the expectations of pain and its relief. Pain tolerance is increased by medication, warmth, and distracting activities, while it is decreased by fatigue, anger, boredom, apprehension, and sleep deprivation.[10]

Response to Pain

In addition to conducting a symptom analysis, the nurse includes additional questions to gain an understanding regarding the patient's response to pain.

How do you react to your pain? How do you express it (e.g., anger, frustration, crying, or no expression at all)? What do you fear most about your pain? What problems does it cause?

Pain can affect people physically, psychologically, socially, and spiritually. Patients' responses to pain may be influenced by their culture and previous experiences. Pain can evoke a variety of emotional responses, such as anxiety, fear, depression, and anger, and these emotions can exacerbate the experience of pain.[12] The nurse should acknowledge these feelings as the patient's personal response to pain without trying to change them.

Does this pain have any particular meaning for you? If so, what is it?

The meaning of pain is unique for each person. For some people, it is based on a particular action they may have taken that contributed to the pain (e.g., "I should not have tried to steal home base"). To others, the meaning is spiritual or psychological. For example, they may believe that they are being punished or that they have had impure thoughts. In some cultures, people grow up not expecting a great deal of relief from pain because they believe that experiencing pain is part of the healing process. Knowing the meaning of the pain to the patient helps the nurse understand the patient's subjective experience of it. The nurse's role is to encourage the patient to describe the meaning of pain without judging the response.

What has been your past experience with pain and pain relief?

This question addresses the cognitive response to pain. Patients use their past experiences to respond to pain. When nurses know what these experiences are, they can help patients with interventions to meet their goals for pain relief.

How has the pain affected your quality of life? How has it altered your life (e.g., does it interfere with your sleep, appetite, mood, walking ability, work, relationships with others)?

Pain can alter a patient's usual daily activity. Those who have compensated for persistent pain or adjusted to it may perceive a higher quality of life than those who have not adjusted to the pain. However, persistent pain is often associated with a sense of hopelessness and helplessness. Patients with persistent pain may report depression, difficulty in sleeping and eating, fatigue, and a preoccupation with pain.[10]

PAIN ASSESSMENT TOOLS

The patient's self-report is the single most reliable indicator of the existence and severity of pain.[2] Knowing the location and description of pain can provide diagnostic clues for understanding the patient's pathology. Frequently used pain rating scales are the Numeric Rating Scale (NRS) and the Faces Pain Scale Revised (FPS-R),[21] which are validated assessment tools.[22] These rating scales, shown in Fig. 6.2 A and B, give patients the choice of rating their pain on a scale that is a horizontal line with markings from 0 to 10 or on a face that represents their pain, which correlates to a number from 0 to 10.

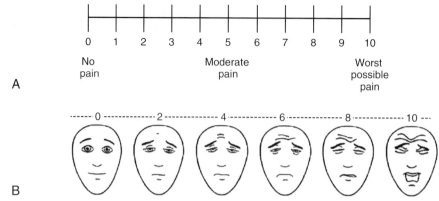

FIG. 6.2 (A) The Numeric Rating Scale (NRS). (B) Faces Pain Scale Revised (FPS-R). (From Pasero C, McCaffery M: *Pain assessment and pharmacologic management*, St Louis, 2011, Elsevier, p 57.)

Cultural groups who read horizontally from left to right are able to use the NRS. However, these numeric scales will produce inaccurate data when used with patients from some cultures like that of China or Japan, where people read vertically. Some Native American patients may select a favorite or sacred number instead of the number that accurately indicates their level of pain.[12]

Assessment tools described above use only the patient's self-reports of pain intensity; however, some health care providers believe that pain intensity alone cannot capture the complexity of the pain experience. A pain assessment tool has been developed called Clinically Aligned Pain Assessment (CAPA). The developers of CAPA believed that pain was more than a number. This tool contains five questions regarding comfort, change in pain, pain control, functioning, and sleep shown on the left side of Table 6.1. On the right of this table are possible answers from a patient. By using this tool, the nurse and patient have a conversation about the pain experience. This pain assessment tool has been approved by TJC for use in hospitals.[23]

TABLE 6.1 FIVE QUESTIONS OF THE CAPA AND SUGGESTED RESPONSES

QUESTION	RESPONSE
Question Comfort	• Intolerable • Tolerable with discomfort • Comfortably manageable • Negligible pain
Change in Pain	• Getting worse • About the same • Getting better
Pain Control	• Inadequate pain control • Partially effective (effective just about right) • Fully effective (would like to reduce medication [why?])
Functioning	• Can't do anything because of pain • Pain keeps me from doing most of what I need to do • Can do most things, but pain gets in the way of some • Can do everything I need to
Sleep	• Awake with pain most of night • Awake with occasional pain • Normal sleep

From Topham D, Ware D: Quality improvement project: Replacing the Numeric Rating Scale with a Clinically Aligned Pain Assessment (CAPA) tool, *Pain Management Nursing* 18(6):363–371, 2017.

EXAMINATION

Most data related to pain assessment are collected during interviews with the patients. However, additional data can be obtained through observations, assessment of vital signs, inspection, and palpation.

Routine Techniques

OBSERVE patient for responses to pain.
LISTEN for sounds the patient makes.
MEASURE blood pressure.
PALPATE pulse.

ASSESS respiratory rate and pattern.
INSPECT site of pain.
PALPATE the site of pain.

Equipment needed

• Stethoscope • Sphygmomanometer • Watch or clock with a second hand

PROCEDURES WITH EXPECTED FINDINGS

ROUTINE TECHNIQUES

PERFORM hand hygiene.

OBSERVE the patient's posture, movement, or any behavior to relieve pain. Notice facial expressions that may suggest pain both when patient is at rest and when the patient's position is changed.

Posture should be relaxed; no movement to relieve pain should be evident. Facial muscles appear relaxed.

LISTEN for sounds the patient makes.

Sounds other than conversation are not expected.

MEASURE the blood pressure.

Blood pressure should be within expected limits for the patient's age.

PALPATE the pulse to assess heart rate.

The heart rate should be within expected limits for the patient's age.

ASSESS the respiratory rate and pattern.

Respirations should be even, quiet, and unlabored. Respiratory rate should be within expected limits for the patient's age.

INSPECT the site of pain for appearance.

Skin should be intact without edema. Skin color should be consistent over the body area inspected.

PALPATE the site of pain for the patient's response.

The patient may report feeling the pressure of the nurse's palpation but should not report tenderness or pain. If the site of pain is an open wound, the nurse should wear gloves during palpation.

ABNORMAL FINDINGS

Guarding of a painful body part, rubbing or pressing the painful area, distorted posture, or fixed or continuous movement may indicate acute pain. Patients may lie very still to avoid movement or they may be restless. Head rocking, pacing, or inability to keep hands still, wrinkled forehead, tightly closed eyes, lackluster eyes, grimacing, clenching of teeth, or lip biting may be other signs of acute pain. Behaviors associated with pain may include agitation, restlessness, irritability, confusion, and combativeness.[5]

Moaning, grunting, screaming, crying, or gasping may indicate acute pain, but some patients make no verbal sounds when they are in pain. Pain may be expressed when moving an affected extremity during an examination.

Systolic blood pressure may be increased by sympathetic stimulation during acute pain.

Heart rate may be elevated during acute pain

Respiratory rate and pattern may vary from slow and deep to rapid and shallow, depending on which provides more comfort to the patient. Some patients may use slow, deep breathing to relax as a pain-relieving strategy.

The area of pain may appear inflamed (red, edematous) and have an incision or visible injury.

Tissue damage or an incision may result in pain on palpation.

AGE-RELATED VARIATIONS

Nurses should adapt their approaches to pain assessment and notice different responses to pain, depending on the age of the patient or situational variation.

INFANTS AND CHILDREN

Neonates respond to pain in a global way, as evidenced by increased heart rate, high blood pressure, decreased oxygenation saturation, pallor, and sweating. Infants and young children are unable to communicate their pain and have difficulty distinguishing between anxiety and pain intensity. School-age children are better able to understand pain and to describe its location. Chapter 19 provides further information about the assessment of pain for this age group.

OLDER ADULTS

Although the transmission and perception of pain may be slowed in older persons, their perception of pain is no different from that of any other adult. Many older adults have a lifetime of experience in coping with pain, but pain is not an expected part of aging. Chapter 21 presents further information about pain assessment in this age group.

SITUATIONAL VARIATIONS

PATIENTS WHO CANNOT COMMUNICATE

Nurses acknowledge that pain cannot be assessed accurately without communicating with the patient. However, patients who are unable to communicate (such as individuals with cognitive impairment, infants and preverbal toddlers, and intubated or unconscious patients) represent a challenge. In such cases, a hierarchy of five pain assessment approaches can be used.

1. Attempt a self-report from the patient or explain why a self-report cannot be used.
2. When patient self-reports are not possible, look for any potential causes of pain, including pathologic conditions and common problems or procedures known to cause pain, such as surgery, rehabilitation, wound care, positioning, blood draws, heel sticks, or any history of persistent pain.
3. List patient behaviors that may indicate pain.
4. Identify behaviors that caregivers and others who are knowledgeable about the patient think may indicate pain, called *proxy reporting.*
5. Attempt an analgesic trial by giving an analgesic ordered by the provider that is appropriate for the estimated intensity of pain based on the patient's pathology and analgesic history, even when the patient cannot communicate pain. Notice any changes in behavior when the analgesic becomes effective.[24]

In addition, a variety of pain scales to assess pain of patients who are unable to communicate have been described. Commonalities among these tools are assessment of facial expressions and movement of arms and legs, including muscle tone and restlessness.[25,26]

CLINICAL APPLICATION AND CLINICAL JUDGMENT

See Appendix B for answers to exercises in this section.

CASE STUDY

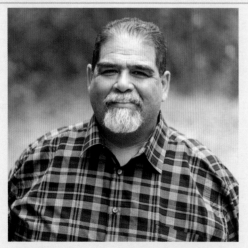

Alberto Cortez comes to the emergency department with a chief complaint of severe abdominal and flank pain on the right side.

Interview Data

He tells the nurse, "The pain came on rather suddenly about an hour ago. I was doing some work at my desk, and it started suddenly." He points to the right flank area as the location of the pain, but it extends into the right lower abdominal area as well. The patient describes the pain as "severe, sharp" pain. On a scale of 0 to 10, he states, "This is off your pain scale—at least a 12." He describes the pain as constant, with intermittent intensity. The other symptom he describes is nausea.

Examination Data

- *General survey:* Blood pressure, 128/96 mm Hg; pulse, 108 beats/min; respirations, 24 breaths/min; temperature, 101.8°F (38.8°C). The patient is curled up on a stretcher in the fetal position, appears uncomfortable, and is groaning.
- *Skin:* Pale, diaphoretic, and warm to touch.
- *Abdomen:* Flat, no scars observed; bowel sounds present; soft, nontender to abdominal palpation. Costovertebral angle (CVA) pain on percussion of the kidneys.

Clinical Judgment

1. What cues do you recognize that suggest a deviation from expected findings, suggesting a need for further investigation?
2. Which additional information should the nurse gather?
3. Which other health care team member could the nurse consult to help relieve this patient's pain?

REVIEW QUESTIONS

1. What is the most reliable way to assess pain in a patient who is awake and alert?
   1. Look at the type and frequency of analgesic medications the patient takes.
   2. Notice the patient's posture and behavior.
   3. Inspect and palpate the site of pain.
   4. Ask the patient to describe the pain.

2. A patient who recently had a knee replacement reports that he has not slept well for several nights. He states that he can't get comfortable and his pain is increasing. What could be a reason for this increase in pain?
   1. Pain after knee surgery varies; it can be mild one day and severe the next.
   2. Pain tolerance decreases with sleep deprivation.
   3. The anesthesia from surgery is wearing off.
   4. The patient is using the pain medication to help him sleep during the day.

3. A patient complains of chest pain. Which question will provide the most useful information at this time?
   1. "What were you doing when the pain first occurred?"
   2. "Do you have shortness of breath with the chest pain?"
   3. "What does the pain feel like?"
   4. "Has anyone in your family ever had similar pain?"

4. A nurse is caring for two women in labor. Janis, who is 18 years old and is having her first baby, has rated her pain as a "7," seems agitated, and has asked for pain medication. Jessica, who is 24 years old, is also having her first baby, also rated her pain as a "7," is calmer, and says she does not need anything for pain at this time. What explains the differences in the outward responses of these women to pain?
   1. Cultural influences and developmental level affect how people react to their pain.
   2. Drug addicts seek medication when there is no indication of actual pain.
   3. Teenagers are immature and have less experience with pain compared to adults.
   4. Preparation for childbirth can prepare women for the pain they will experience.

5. A patient has had persistent back pain for several years. On assessment, the nurse notes that the patient is sitting quietly talking with a companion and does not appear to be in pain. When questioned, the patient rates the pain as a 7 on a scale of 0 to 10. How does the nurse interpret these data?
   1. This patient cannot be believed when he complains of severe pain lasting many months.
   2. This patient is using social support to cope with his current pain.
   3. This patient is drug seeking to maintain an addiction.
   4. This patient is probably not having as much pain as reported initially.

CHAPTER

7

Mental Health Assessment

evolve

http://evolve.elsevier.com/Wilson/assessment

A person's state of mind, reflected by emotional and cognitive responses, is often referred to as the mental status. Assessment of individuals must include their mental health as well as physical health, since the mind and body influence each other. Physical disorders may affect thinking or behavior; likewise, mental health disorders can affect physical health. *Mental health* is defined as a state of well-being in which people realize their own abilities, can cope with normal stresses of life, can work productively, and are able to make contributions to their communities.[1]

CONCEPT OVERVIEW

A number of concepts are represented in this chapter because of the wide range of mental health conditions. These concepts represent potentially serious conditions that can impact one's mental health. *Anxiety* refers to an individual's response to stress—which can range from no anxiety, severe anxiety, and panic. *Stress* represents an individual's perception of and response to a stressor. The response represents the interplay between the way the stressor is perceived and the effectiveness of coping mechanisms. Ineffective coping can lead to anxiety, depression, substance abuse, and addiction. *Mood & Affect* refer to the state of mind, relative to how a person is feeling emotionally and the observable response to those feelings. A person's mood ranges on a spectrum from depression on the low end to mania on the high end. *Addiction* refers to a physiologic and/or psychological dependence on a substance or behavior and can have profound effect on one's mental health. *Cognition*, which is the mental processing of information and decision-making, is affected by severe swings on either end of the mood spectrum and addiction. *Psychosis* refers to a state of impaired cognitive function, impairments in affective response, and the inability to recognize reality and relate to others. *Functional ability* is affected by most of these concepts. When in any mental health crisis, an individual is prone to changes in functional ability. The interrelationships of these seven concepts are depicted in the illustration. Understanding these interrelationships helps the nurse recognize risk factors when conducting a health assessment and is an important step associated with clinical judgment.

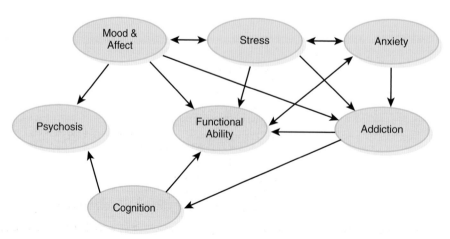

The following case provides a clinical example featuring several of these interrelated concepts and as shown in the illustration.

Ray Harris has an underlying anxiety disorder that has become worse over the past year after quitting his job to open his own business. Initially, he was elated – so happy to be away from a job that made him miserable. Ray knew becoming a small business owner would be a challenge and thought he was well-prepared, but so many issues emerged! The two biggest issues were that he could not keep track of inventory and the projected sales for the first six months were declining. These two factors negatively affected revenue and expenses. His constant worry and stress about not being able to meet his financial obligations and losing the business led to several episodes of panic. After four years of sobriety, he began drinking excessively again to manage his stress. He experienced periods of blackouts after drinking and literally could not remember events from the night before. His girlfriend, frustrated by his behavior, told him he was "impossible to be around" and recently ended their relationship, causing Ray to be severely depressed. Ray feels a complete loss of control over his situation and obsesses over his many failures. He wonders if his life is even worth living.

ANATOMY AND PHYSIOLOGY

Functions of the cerebrum are primarily responsible for a person's mental health. The frontal lobe governs decision-making, problem solving, the ability to concentrate, and short-term memory. Emotions, affect, drive, awareness of self, and autonomic responses related to emotions originate in the frontal lobe. The parietal lobe receives and processes sensory input, while the temporal lobe is responsible for perception and interpretation of sounds and the occipital lobe interprets visual images.[2] The cerebral cortex communicates with the limbic system, also called the *emotional brain*, as shown in Fig. 7.1. This system regulates memory and basic emotions such as fear, anger, and sex drive. Structures of the limbic system include the cingulate gyrus, hippocampus, amygdala, thalamus, and portions of the hypothalamus. These structures enable communication between the limbic system and the cerebral cortex. For example, when a person sees something that jogs a memory about a happy event, communication occurs among the occipital lobe for vision, prefrontal lobe for memory, and limbic system for the happy emotion and the memory.[3]

Neurotransmitters have an essential function in the role of human emotion and behavior. They are chemical vehicles that provide synaptic transmission of messages from neuron to neuron or from neurons to muscle cells. Neurotransmitters affecting mental health include dopamine, norepinephrine, serotonin, histamine, acetylcholine, and gamma-aminobutyric acid (GABA), as described in Table 7.1.

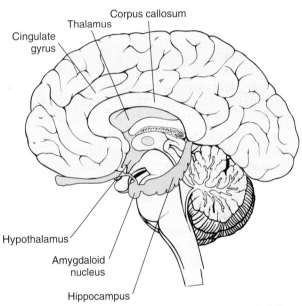

FIG. 7.1 The limbic system. (From McKenry and Salerno, 2003.)

TABLE 7.1 NEUROTRANSMITTERS ASSOCIATED WITH MENTAL ILLNESS

NEUROTRANSMITTER	ASSOCIATION WITH MENTAL ILLNESS
Dopamine (DA)	Decreased in depression Increased in schizophrenia and mania
Norepinephrine (NE)	Decreased in depression Increased in schizophrenia, mania, and anxiety states
Serotonin (5 HT)	Decreased in depression Increased in anxiety states
Histamine	Decreased in depression
Acetylcholine (Ach)	Increased in depression
Gamma aminobutyric acid (GABA)	Decreased in anxiety states mental schizophrenia

From Halter M: *Varcarolis' foundations of psychiatric mental health nursing: a clinical approach*, ed 8, St Louis, 2018, Elsevier.

ETHNIC, CULTURAL, AND SPIRITUAL VARIATIONS

Culturally Relevant Phenomena in Mental Health Nursing

The concept of mental health is formed within a culture, and deviance from cultural expectations can be defined as *illness* by other members of the group. Mental health nursing is based on personality and development theories promoted by Europeans and Americans and grounded in Western cultural ideals and values. Nurses are as influenced by their own professional and ethnic cultures as patients are by theirs and thus must guard against ethnocentric tendencies.

Phenomena include the following:

- *Perception of reality*—Perception may be culturally prescribed, spiritually induced in a traditional healing system, or otherwise sanctioned by the cultural group. For example, a Native American patient may appear to a Caucasian American to have lost touch with reality, but the Native American is practicing his or her spiritual healing ritual, which is important to attain or maintain health.
- *Needs, feelings, thoughts of others and self*—Patients need to attend to their needs, feelings, and thoughts of self and

others. Events considered as stressors vary from one culture to another. For example, Kenyans are taught not to discuss or show their feelings of sadness or pain. If a Kenyan were seen by an American health care provider for a suspected mental health disorder, he or she might not willingly share feelings, which is a large part of the health history for mental health nursing. This patient may be seen as uncooperative, when in fact he or she is complying with the Kenyan culture.

- *Decision-making*—The ability to make decisions may be culturally prescribed so families and cultures designate decision makers, which may include health care decisions. Inability to make decisions is a clinical manifestation of depression and anxiety. For example, in traditional Vietnamese families, the oldest male makes decisions about health care. As a result, a female patient may delay seeking health care until she consults with the oldest male in the family.

From Zoucha R, Wolf K: Cultural implications for psychiatric mental health nursing. In Halter M, editor: *Varcarolis' Foundations of psychiatric mental health nursing: a clinical approach*, ed 8, St Louis, 2018, Elsevier, pp 77–90.

HEALTH HISTORY

Nurses interview patients to collect data about their present health, past health history, family, and psychosocial history, which includes information about their self-concept, interpersonal relationships, stressors, anger, and alcohol and recreational drug use. The history also includes questions about specific mental health problems.

During the interview, notice the patient's appearance (posture, grooming, facial expressions, and body language); behavior (mood, affect, eye contact, and tone of voice); and cognitive functions (orientation, attention span, and recent and remote memory).

GENERAL HEALTH HISTORY

Present Health Status

Do you have any chronic illnesses? If yes, describe.

Patients with chronic disorders (e.g., endocrine disorders such as hypothyroidism or adrenal insufficiency) may experience depression, but may seek health care for their physical symptoms rather than depression.[4]

Are you taking any medications? If yes, describe.

Document medications the patient is taking. Adverse effects of these medications may cause changes in mood and behavior. For example, some oral contraceptives, antihypertensives, or corticosteroids can cause depression.

Do you take any over-the-counter drugs or herbal supplements? If yes, what do you take and how often? What are they for?

Nonprescription drugs and herbal supplements may affect mental health. For example, St. John's wort is an herbal supplement taken to treat mild to moderate depression, although it is not approved by the US Food and Drug Administration (FDA) for that use.

Describe your feelings or mood. Do you consider your present feelings to be a problem in your daily life?

Knowing the patient's feelings or mood may help to identify concerns such as stress, worthlessness, guilt, helplessness, hopelessness, and anger.[5]

Past Health History

Have you ever been treated for mental health problems? If yes, describe.

Patients may have previously been diagnosed and treated for mental health problems that are resolved.

Have you experienced any behaviors that could indicate mental health problems? If yes, describe your experience. How have you coped in the past with these behaviors? How well are these coping strategies working for you?

Identifying the patient's previous problems with mental health provides a baseline. If previous coping strategies are working, they should be continued or resumed. If they have not been successful, other strategies may be suggested or a referral may be needed to a mental health professional.

Family History

Do you have any blood relatives who have behaviors that could indicate a mental health problem, such as mental

illness, alcoholism, or drug abuse? If yes, describe their behaviors.

Some mental illnesses such as anxiety, depression, and schizophrenia have genetic links. Having a family member with a mental illness may be associated with the patient's behavior.

Personal and Psychosocial History

Self-concept

How would you describe yourself to others? What do you like about yourself?

Responses to these questions help to determine how patients perceive themselves. Those with positive self-esteem regard themselves favorably and can name their positive attributes. Those with negative self-esteem tend to list primarily negative attributes and may be at risk for depression.

Interpersonal Relationships

How satisfied are you with your relationships with people? Are there people you can talk with about feelings and problems?

Achieving satisfying interpersonal relationships is needed for mental health. Patients who have few or no interpersonal relationships may be depressed or out of touch with reality. Social support is important for healthy interpersonal relationships.

I am going to ask you four routine questions about abuse that I ask all patients, because abuse and violence are common.

In the last year how often did anyone:
- Hurt you physically?
- Insult or talk down to you?
- Threaten you with physical harm?
- Scream or curse at you?[5]

The first letter from each question forms the acronym, HITS , which is a brief screening for domestic violence.[6] The US Preventive Task Force recommends that all women be screened for intimate partner violence.[7] If the patient gives any answer other than "never," the patient is further screened as described under Problem-Based History later in this chapter. These questions may also apply when the patient is a member of the LGTBQ community or a victim of human trafficking (see Box 2.4).

Stressors

Have there been any recent changes in your life? How have these changes affected your stress level?

Inquire about stressors such as money, intimate relationships, bullying, confinement, loss of freedom, death or illness of a family member or friend, and employment problems.

What are the major stressors in your life now? How do you deal with stress? Are these methods of stress relief currently effective for you?

Coping with the stressors of daily life is essential to maintain mental health. Answers to these questions help identify the patient's stressors and how well they are being managed. Discussing this topic provides an opportunity to teach patients alternative ways to react to their stress. These may include relaxation techniques, meditation, physical exercise, yoga, or journaling. When patients describe difficulty dealing with stress, they can be referred to agencies for care and support. Stressful life events may be a risk factor for depression.[5]

Anger

How do you react when you are angry? Do you react verbally or physically, or do you keep your anger inside? Can you talk about what has caused this anger?

Learning how patients react to anger provides an insight into how healthy their responses are and offers an opportunity to teach them alternative ways to express their feelings (e.g., hit a pillow instead of a person, verbally express anger in an empty room or elevator). Talking about the cause of the anger can be therapeutic and provides an opportunity to make referrals for assistance.

Alcohol Use

How often do you drink alcohol, including beer, wine, or liquor?

Every adult and adolescent should be asked about alcohol consumption to determine if it is a health problem. Additional data are collected when a male patient reports drinking more than two standard drinks daily, a female patient reports more than one standard drink daily, or adults age 65 and older report more than one standard drink daily. Refer to Problem-Based History, Alcohol Use, later in this chapter. Alcohol abuse is a risk factor for depression.

Recreational Drug Use

Some people use recreational drugs. Do you ever use them? If yes, tell me about your drug use.

Every adult and adolescent should be asked about recreational drug use to determine if it is a health problem. Acknowledging that some people use drugs may encourage patients to be honest in reporting their use. When people report recreational drug use, they are asked additional questions as described in Problem-Based History, Drug Use, later in this chapter. Drug abuse is a risk factor for depression.

PROBLEM-BASED HISTORY

Commonly reported symptoms related to mental health include depression, anxiety, altered mental status, alcohol use, drug use, and interpersonal violence. Data from the *General Health History* may indicate the need for additional questions to learn more about these problems that the patient is experiencing.

Depression

Patients who are depressed may neglect their grooming, dressing, and personal hygiene, and have a slumped posture, sad facial expression, or evidence of tearfulness. They may have a sad mood, have a flat affect, avoid eye contact, or speak in a monotone.[5]

RISK FACTORS

Depression

- *Gender:* More women are diagnosed with depression than men, but this may be in part because women are more likely to seek treatment.
- *Age:* Adverse experiences during childhood
- *Substance abuse:* Abuse of alcohol or recreational drugs
- *Genetics:* Blood relatives with a history of depression, bipolar disorder, alcoholism, or suicide may increase risk. Children of parents who have depression are likely to develop the disorder; risk doubles if both parents affected.
- *Psychosocial environment:* People who have a history of trauma, sexual abuse, physical abuse, physical disability, or who have experienced death of a relative, divorce, or financial problems
- *Personal characteristics:* Low self-esteem; being overly dependent or self-critical; being pessimistic; inability to acknowledge personal accomplishment; having a serious illness, few friends or personal relationships; recently given birth (M)
- *Sexuality:* Being lesbian, gay, bisexual, or transgender, or having variations in the development of genital organs that are not clearly male or female, in an unsupportive situation
- *Medical history:* Serious or chronic illness, including cancer, stroke, chronic pain, or heart disease, may put people at risk, as well as a history of other mental health disorders, such as anxiety disorder, eating disorders, or posttraumatic stress disorder.

M = Modifiable risk factor.
From https://www.mayoclinic.org/diseases-conditions/depression/symptoms-causes/syc-20356007. Updated February 8, 2018, Halter M, Kozy M: Depressive disorders. In Halter M, editor: Varcarolis' foundations of psychiatric mental health nursing: a clinical approach, ed 8, St Louis, 2018, Elsevier, pp 242–269.

During the past 2 weeks have you often felt down, depressed, or hopeless? During the past month have you often had little interest or pleasure in doing things?
These two questions are used to screen for major depression. An affirmative answer to either question warrants a follow-up clinical interview.[5]

Are you able to fall asleep and stay asleep without difficulty?
A depressed mood can interrupt sleep habits. Insomnia is reported frequently with variations, including difficulty falling asleep and staying asleep.[5]

Have you noticed any marked changes in your eating habits? Have you recently gained or lost weight without trying?
Appetite changes vary in individuals experiencing depression. Appetite loss is common; however, others eat more and gain weight.[5]

Have you noticed a lack of energy?
Most people with depression experience an abnormal lack of energy; however, some experience agitation manifested by pacing, nail biting, finger tapping, or some other tension-relieving activity.[5]

Have you experienced feelings of elation, increased activity levels, agitation, irritability, or like your thoughts are going very fast?
People with bipolar disorder have mania interspersed with depression. They are more likely to seek help when they are depressed than when experiencing mania or hypomania.[8] For this reason, all patients presenting with depressive symptoms should be assessed for a history of manic or hypomanic symptoms.[9]

Do you have friends who you can trust and who are available when you need them?
Friends can be a source of social support to listen to the patient's feelings and demonstrate their caring for the patient.

Have you had depressive feelings like this before? What did you do about them?
Depression may be a recurring disorder. Treatment that was successful in the past may be useful again.

Have you thought about hurting yourself or taking your own life? Do you have a plan? Do you have the means of carrying out your plan? Is there anything that would prevent you from carrying out your plan?
Always evaluate the person's risk of harm to self or others. Overt hostility is highly correlated with suicide.[5] A patient who has a specific plan for suicide is at higher risk than one who has no plan. Steps must be taken to protect the person who has a plan to hurt himself or herself. In 2016 in the United States, 44,965 people died by suicide, and it remains the 10th leading cause of death for all ages.[10] The age-adjusted suicide rate in the United States was 24% higher in 2014 than in 1999. Increases were reported for both females and males in all ages group under 75 years. For females, the age-adjusted suicide rate increased during this time period for all racial and ethnic groups except Asians and Pacific Islanders. The largest percentage increases were for American Indian or Alaska Native females (89%) and non-Hispanic white females (60%). For males, the age-adjusted suicide rates increased during this time period for American Indians and Alaska Natives (38%) and non-Hispanic white males (28%).[11] Males take their own lives at nearly four times the rate of females.[12] Firearms are the most common method of suicide among males, while poisoning is the most common for females.

What has kept you from hurting yourself in the past?
Reminding the patient of factors that prevented suicide may be useful again. Ambivalence often keeps patients from ending their lives.

Some patients are asked to complete a questionnaire instead of answering questions. One example is the Patient Health Questionnaire-9 (PHQ-9), which contains nine items related to symptoms of depression. Patients are asked to indicate how often they have experienced each symptom during the past 2 weeks. The symptoms include interests, feelings of hopelessness, sleep disturbances, fatigue, changes in appetite,

When patients tell a nurse they want to end their life, the nurse is supposed to ask if they have thoughts about hurting themselves or if they have a plan for hurting themselves. Doesn't that suggest to them that they *should* hurt themselves?

Asking patients about a plan to hurt themselves may seem like a suggestion, but it is not. The purpose of asking the question is to determine if they are depressed or serious enough to make a plan to end their life. If the nurse learns that a patient has a plan, then he or she needs an immediate referral to a mental health professional.

feeling bad about oneself, trouble concentrating, moving or speaking slowly, and thoughts of self-harm. Each response has four possible options ranging from "not at all" to "nearly every day."[5] This questionnaire is available in a PDF format at https://www.uspreventiveservicestaskforce.org/Home/GetFileByID/218.

Anxiety

Do you feel anxious? If yes, how long have you been experiencing this feeling? Have you noticed a change in your feelings? If yes, describe these changes. What do you think initiated them? How did you cope with them?
Feelings of anger, guilt, worthlessness, and anguish often accompany anxiety. The patient may report feeling nervous or anxious or not being able to stop worrying.

Over the last 2 weeks, how often have you had the following experiences?
- Feeling nervous, anxious, or on edge
- Not being able to stop or control worrying
- Worrying too much about different things
- Trouble relaxing
- Having difficulty sitting still
- Being easily annoyed or irritated
- Feeling afraid, as if something awful might happen

These questions comprise items of the Generalized Anxiety Disorder-7 (GAD-7), a valid and efficient tool for screening for anxiety.[13] Patients are asked how often they experience these feelings on a scale from "not at all" to "nearly every day."

Have you had difficulty concentrating or making decisions? Have you been preoccupied or forgetful? Are you able to fall asleep and stay asleep without difficulty?
Anxiety can influence one's ability to concentrate, learn, and solve problems. Sleep deprivation is a risk factor for anxiety.

Have you noticed a change in the amount of energy that you have (fatigue)? Have you been more irritable than usual? Do your muscles seem tense? Do you feel a tightening in your throat?
These are common symptoms of anxiety.[14]

Anxiety

- *Psychosocial environment:* Adults who experience a traumatic event; childhood trauma; illness; or excessive stress (e.g., financial concerns, health, relationships)
- *Genetics:* Anxiety disorders can run in families.
- *Illness:* Having a physical illness can cause significant worry about treatment and prognosis (M)
- *Unrelieved stress:* A significant stressful event or a buildup of smaller stressful life situations may trigger excessive anxiety, such as death in the family, work stress, or worry about finances.
- *Other mental health disorders:* People who have disorders such as depression often have an anxiety disorder.
- *Substance abuse:* Drug and alcohol abuse or withdrawal can cause or worsen anxiety (M).

M = Modifiable risk factor.
From https://www.mayoclinic.org/diseases-conditions/anxiety/symptoms-causzes/syc-20350961. Updated May 4, 2018.

Altered Mental Status

Mental status is defined as the degree of competence that a person shows in intellectual, emotional, psychological, and personality functioning. Alterations may become evident when there are changes in the patient's orientation to person, place, or time; attention span; or memory. Long-term memory can be assessed during the history by asking patients where they were born or about their previous surgeries. Additional data are gathered by determining the patient's orientation, memory, calculation ability, communication skills, judgment, and abstraction.

Orientation

Ask the patient what year it is, where he or she is, and his or her name. Orientation to time is the first orientation to be lost; orientation to place is the second orientation to be lost; and orientation to person is the last orientation to be lost.

Memory

Impaired memory occurs with various neurologic and psychiatric disorders, such as anxiety or depression. Loss of immediate and recent memory with retention of remote memory suggests dementia.[2]

Immediate recall. Ask the patient to repeat the names of three unrelated objects that are spoken slowly, such as "dog," "cloud," and "apple."

Recent memory. Give the patient a short time to view four or five objects and explain that you will ask about these objects in a few minutes. After about 10 minutes, ask the patient to name the objects. All objects should be remembered.

Remote memory. Ask the patient about his or her mother's maiden name, high school attended, or a subject of common knowledge.

Calculation Ability

Calculation ability can be tested by asking the patient about making change. For example, ask a patient, "You buy fruit that costs $2.45 and you give the cashier $3.00. How much change would you expect to receive?"

Calculation should be completed with few errors and within 1 minute when the patient has average intelligence. Impairment of arithmetic skills may be associated with depression or diffuse brain disease.[2]

Communication Skills

Perform this assessment after determining that the patient can see, speak, read, and write. Ask the patient to *name* common objects such as a watch or pencil. *Repetition* is tested by asking the patient to repeat a phrase, such as "No ifs, ands, or buts." *Reading* is tested by asking the patient to read a phrase that is written on a piece of paper and to do what it says, such as, "Lift your right hand." The patient completing this task indicates an ability to read and follow instructions. *Writing* is tested by asking the patient to write a sentence. Do not tell the patient what to write. The sentence must have a subject and a verb to be sensible, but correct punctuation and grammar are not assessed. *Copying* is assessed by asking the patient to copy a drawing of two geometric figures that overlap, such as an intersecting pentagon with about 1 inch on each side. The inability to communicate may indicate poor cognition, dementia, or brain damage.

Judgment and Reasoning

Judgment is considered intact when the patient has a reasonable, appropriate plan for the future and is able to recognize the consequences of actions. Impaired judgment may indicate intellectual disability, emotional disturbance, frontal lobe injury, dementia, or psychosis.[2] Ask the patient about plans for the future.
- Ask the patient for a solution to a hypothetical situation, such as "What would you do if a car was speeding toward you?"

Abstract Reasoning

Ask the meaning of a proverb, such as "A bird in the hand is worth two in the bush." A patient with average intelligence should be able to interpret the proverb. Inability to explain the proverb may indicate poor cognition, dementia, brain damage, or schizophrenia.[2] Another explanation may be that the proverb is not relevant to the patient's culture or generation. When this occurs, the nurse may decide not to use proverbs as an assessment of abstract reasoning or consult with family members or others of the culture to use an appropriate proverb.

Alcohol Use

Patients with an alcohol use disorder often deny or minimize their drinking to avoid being judged by others

Many people drink alcohol. Do you sometimes drink beer, wine, or other alcoholic beverages? If yes, how many times in the past year have you had more than five drinks in a day (for men) or four drinks in a day (for women)?
The National Institute on Alcohol Abuse and Alcoholism (NIAAA) recommends that all health care providers screen every patient for alcohol use disorders (AUD). Not all alcohol

use is dangerous; however, alcohol causes or increases the risk of alcohol-related problems such as cirrhosis and injuries from falls, and complicates the management of other medical problems.

Every adult and adolescent should be asked about alcohol consumption to determine if it is a health problem. According to the Dietary Guidelines for Americans 2015–20, the US Department of Health and Human Services, and US Department of Agriculture, moderate drinking as follows:
- Men: The limit is two alcoholic beverages daily.
- Women: The limit is one alcoholic beverage daily.
- Adults age 65 and older: No more than one standard drink daily.
- Pregnant women: No level of alcohol consumption is safe.[15] The standard drinks are shown in Fig. 7.2.

In the past 2 months, has your drinking repeatedly caused or contributed to
- Risk of bodily harm (e.g., drinking and driving, operating machinery, swimming)?
- Relationship trouble with family or friends?
- Role failure (e.g., interference with home, work, school obligations)?
- Run-ins with the law (e.g., arrests or other legal problems)?
When patients answer "yes" to one or more of these questions, they are abusing alcohol and need to be screened for alcohol dependence.[16] Accurate information about alcohol intake may be difficult to obtain because patients are unwilling to disclose their actual consumption. One tool used to screen for alcoholism is called the Alcohol Use Disorders Identification Test (AUDIT). It has 10 questions that ask about quantity and frequency of drinking, binging, and consequences of drinking (Table 7.2). Another screening tool is the CAGE questions, which is an acronym for Cut down, Annoyed, Guilty, and Eye opener. This tool is available at https://www.uspreventiveservicestaskforce.org/Home/GetFileByID/838.

Have you experienced any symptoms after you stopped drinking, such as headache, hallucinations, or tremors?
These symptoms may indicate one of the stages of alcohol withdrawal syndrome (AWS) that occurs after cessation of drinking. Early detection is important so that prompt treatment can begin. AWS occurs in about 8% of hospitalized patients with AUD, and severe AWS can lengthen the hospital stay.[17] AWS is discussed in "Common Problems and Conditions," later in this chapter.

Drug Use

Patients with drug use disorders are likely to deny or minimize their use to avoid being judged by others. Use a matter-of-fact and nonjudgmental approach when assessing these patients.

Some people use recreational drugs. Have you used drugs in the past? If the patient answers "yes," ask, which of the following substances have you used in your lifetime?
- Cannabis (e.g., marijuana, pot, grass, hash)
- Cocaine (e.g., coke, crack)

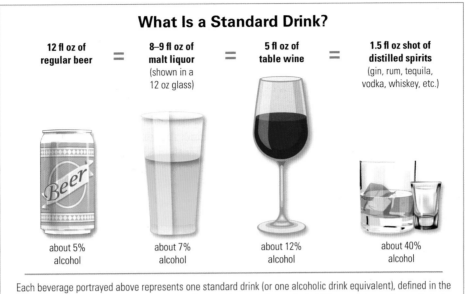

FIG. 7.2 US standard drink equivalents. These are approximate, since different brands and types of beverages vary their actual alcohol content. A standard drink in the United States is any drink that contains about 14 g of pure alcohol (about 0.6 fluid ounces or 1.2 tablespoons). (From National Institute on Alcohol Abuse and Alcoholism [NIAAA]. Available at https://www.niaaa.nih.gov/alcohol-health/overview-alcohol-consumption/what-standard-drink.)

TABLE 7.2 AUDIT STRUCTURED INTERVIEW[a]

QUESTION	SCORE				
	0	1	2	3	4
How often do you have a drink containing alcohol?	Never	Monthly or less	2–4 times/ month	2–3 times/ week	4 or more times/week
How many drinks do you have on a typical day when you are drinking?	None	1 or 2	3 or 4	5 or 6	7–9[b]
How often do you have 6 or more drinks on one occasion?	Never	Less than monthly	Monthly	Weekly	Daily or almost daily
How often during the last year have you found that you were unable to stop drinking once you had started?	Never	Less than monthly	Monthly	Weekly	Daily or almost daily
How often last year have you failed to do what was normally expected from you because of drinking?	Never	Less than monthly	Monthly	Weekly	Daily or almost daily
How often during the last year have you needed a first drink in the morning to get yourself going after a heavy drinking session?	Never	Less than monthly	Monthly	Weekly	Daily or almost daily
How often during the last year have you had a feeling of guilt or remorse after drinking?	Never	Less than monthly	Monthly	Weekly	Daily or almost daily
How often during the last year have you been unable to re-member what happened the night before because you had been drinking?	Never	Less than monthly	Monthly	Weekly	Daily or almost daily
Have you or someone else been injured as a result of your drinking?	Never	Yes, but not in the last year (2 points)		Yes, during the last year (4 points)	
Has a relative, doctor, or other health worker been concerned about your drinking or suggested that you cut down?	Never	Yes, but not in the last year (2 points)		Yes, during the last year (4 points)	

From Report of the US Preventive Services Task Force: *Guide to clinical preventive services*, ed 2, US Department of Health and Human Services, 1996, Washington, DC.

[a]Score of greater than 8 (out of 41) suggests problem drinking and indicates need for more in-depth assessment. Cut-off of 10 points is recommended by some to provide greater specificity.

[b]5 points if response is 10 or more drinks on a typical day.

AUDIT, Alcohol Use Disorders Identification Test.

- Prescription stimulants (e.g., methylphenidate [Ritalin, Concerta], dextroamphetamine [Dexedrine], Adderall, diet pills)
- Amphetamine type stimulants (e.g., speed, diet pills, ecstasy)
- Inhalants (e.g., nitrous, glue, gasoline, paint thinner)
- Sedatives or sleeping pills (e.g., diazepam [Valium], oxazepam [Serax], alprazolam [Xanax])
- Hallucinogens (e.g., D-lysergic acid diethylamide [LSD], acid, mushrooms, phencyclidine [PCP], ketamine [Special K], ecstasy)
- Opioids (e.g., heroin, morphine, codeine, opium)
- Prescription opioids used for nonmedical use (e.g., fentanyl, oxycodone, hydrocodone, methadone, buprenorphine)

Are there any other drugs you have used? If no lifetime drug use is reported, the screening is complete. For each drug use reported, ask the following questions:

- In the past 3 months, how often have you used each of the substances you mentioned?
- How often have you had a strong desire or urge to use?
- How often has your drug use led to health, social, legal, or financial problems?
- How often have you failed to do what was normally expected of you because of your use of this (these) drug(s)?
- Has a friend, relative, or anyone else ever expressed concern about your drug use?
- Have you ever tried and failed to control, cut down, or stop using this (these) drug(s)?
- Have you ever used any drug by injection for nonmedical use?

Screening for drug abuse by asking these questions is an important first step in identifying patients who need to be referred for intervention procedures. Evidenced-based screening and assessment tools for adults and adolescents are available at https://www.drugabuse.gov/nidamed-medical-health-professionals/tool-resources-your-practice/additional-screening-resources.[18]

Interpersonal Violence

Interpersonal violence is not an illness; it is a crime. It is a human rights violation that can have negative impacts on patients' mental and physical health.[19] If a patient answered "yes" to any of the screening questions about interpersonal violence in the history, ask additional questions in private, with only the patient and nurse present. Be calm, matter of fact, and nonjudgmental. Listen carefully and let the patient define the problem. Gather descriptions of the behavior rather than why it happened and what it means. Preface comments by saying: *You are asked about violence because so many people are dealing with this problem in their home. Nobody deserves to be afraid in their home. If abuse is a problem for you, you may talk with me about it safely.*[20]

- Are you in a relationship in which you have been physically hurt or threatened by your partner?
- Are you in a relationship in which you felt you were treated badly? In which ways?
- Has your partner ever destroyed things that you valued?
- Has your partner ever threatened or abused your children?
- Has your partner ever forced you to have sex when you weren't willing? Does he or she force you to engage in sex that makes you feel uncomfortable?
- What happens when you and your partner fight or disagree?
- Do you ever feel afraid of your partner?
- Has your partner ever prevented you from leaving home, seeing friends, getting a job, or continuing your education?
- You mentioned that your partner uses drugs/alcohol. How does he or she act when drinking or using drugs? Is there ever verbal or physical abuse?
- Do you have guns in your home? Has your partner ever threatened to use them?[20]

Assessment tools are available on the Centers for Disease Control, Violence Prevention website (https://www.cdc.gov/violenceprevention/pdf/ipv/ipvandsvscreening.pdf).

HEALTH PROMOTION FOR EVIDENCE-BASED PRACTICE

Substance Abuse, Depression, and Intimate Partner Violence

Recommendations to Reduce Risk (Primary Prevention)
Substance Abuse: National Institute on Drug Abuse
The principles listed as follows are the result of long-term research studies on the origins of drug abuse behaviors and the common elements of effective prevention programs.

1. *Enhance protective factors:* Protective factors include strong, positive bonds within the family; parental monitoring; clear rules of conduct consistently enforced within the family; parent involvement in the lives of children; success in school performance; strong bonds with institutions such as church and school; and adoption of conventional norms regarding drug use.
2. *Reduce risk factors:* Risk factors include a chaotic home environment (especially with parents who have substance abuse problems or mental illness); ineffective parenting; lack of mutual attachments; shy or aggressive behavior in the classroom; failure in school performance; poor social coping skills; association with a deviant peer group; and adoption of attitude that approves of drug use.

Screening Recommendations (Secondary Prevention)
US Preventive Services Task Force
Screening for depression:

- Screening adolescents (12-18 years of age) for major depressive disorder is recommended when systems are in place to ensure accurate diagnosis, psychotherapy (cognitive-behavioral or interpersonal), and follow-up.
- Screening adults for depression is recommended when staff-assisted depression care supports are in place to ensure accurate diagnosis, effective treatment, and follow-up.
- Screening postpartum women for depression providing counseling for pregnant and postpartum women who are at risk for perinatal depression.

Screening for unhealthy substance use:

- Screening and behavioral counseling interventions are recommended to reduce alcohol misuse by adults, including pregnant women, in primary care settings.

Substance Abuse, Depression, and Intimate Partner Violence

- Screen all adults for problematic drinking through a history of alcohol use or use of standardized screening tools such as AUDIT (Alcohol Use Disorders Identification Test).
- Current evidence is insufficient to assess the balance of benefit and harm of screening adolescents, adults, and pregnant women for illicit drug use.

Screening for intimate partner violence:
- Women of reproductive age should be screened for intimate partner violence (IPV).

National Institute on Drug Abuse: DrugFacts: Lessons from Prevention Research, Revised March 2014. Available at https:www.drugabuse.gov/publications/drugfacts/lessons-prevention-research; US Department of Health and Human Services: US Preventive Services Task Force: Recommendations. Available at www.uspreventiveservicestaskforce.org. Webber E, Benedict J: Postpartum depression: a multi-disciplinary approach to screening, management and breastfeed support, *Arch Psychiatr Nurs* 33(6):284, 2019.

EXAMINATION

Most data related to mental health assessment are collected during interviews with patients. However, additional data are obtained through general observations and assessment of vital signs and the eyes.

Routine techniques

- OBSERVE the patient's gait, posture, and movements.
- NOTICE level of consciousness and affect.
- OBSERVE dress and hygiene.
- NOTICE facial expression, voice tone, flow, rate of speech.
- OBSERVE for perspiration and muscle tension.
- MEASURE the blood pressure.
- PALPATE a radial pulse.
- OBSERVE and COUNT respirations.
- MEASURE pupil size.

Equipment needed

- Stethoscope • Sphygmomanometer • Watch or clock with second hand • Penlight with a pupil gauge

PROCEDURES WITH EXPECTED FINDINGS

ROUTINE TECHNIQUES

PERFORM hand hygiene.

OBSERVE the patient's gait, posture, and movements.

Posture should be erect, and the body should be relaxed. Gait and general body movements should be smooth, coordinated, and purposeful.

NOTICE level of consciousness and affect.

The patient should be fully alert, calm, with neutral affect. The patient should be aware of surroundings and respond appropriately to questions and instructions.

ABNORMAL FINDINGS

Shuffling or uncoordinated gait can be associated with impaired cognition. Tense muscles, fidgeting, or pacing may indicate anxiety; a slumped posture and slow movements may indicate depression. Abnormal movements such as tremors may be associated with mental health conditions or adverse effects from drugs.

Indications of reduced consciousness include disorientation to time, place, and person; confusion; sleepiness; lack of response to calling the patient's name, to touch, or to pain.
Extremes in emotional expression, such as mania, crying, or being withdrawn, are considered abnormal findings.

PROCEDURES WITH EXPECTED FINDINGS

ABNORMAL FINDINGS

OBSERVE dress and hygiene.

The clothing worn by the patient should be clean and appropriate for the weather or situation. The patient should show evidence of basic hygiene.

Outlandish dress and makeup may be worn by a patient with cognitive impairment or in a manic phase of a bipolar disorder. Soiled clothing or lack of hygiene may indicate depression or organic brain syndrome.

NOTICE facial expression, voice tone, flow, and rate of speech.

Speech should be smooth, even, and without effort. The conversation should be clear, spontaneous, understandable, and appropriate to the context of the discussion. Facial expression should match verbal expression.

Abnormal findings may include speaking in monotone, slow and unexpressive speech patterns; indistinguishable verbal responses; high-pitched voice and rapid rate of speech; flight of ideas.

OBSERVE for perspiration and muscle tension.

There should be no visible perspiration, and the patient should appear relaxed.

Body tremors, increased muscle tension, perspiration, and sweaty palms are documented.

MEASURE the blood pressure.

Blood pressure varies with gender, body weight, and time of day, but the upper limits for adults are <120 mm Hg systolic and <80 mm Hg diastolic. (See Chapter 4 for measurement of blood pressure.)

Anxiety, especially severe anxiety or panic, may cause elevated blood pressure as a result of sympathetic stimulation.

PALPATE a radial pulse to assess heart rate.

Heart Rate: 60 to 100 beats/min. (See Chapter 12, Box 12.4, for descriptions of pulses.)

Heart rates for patients with anxiety may be elevated as a result of sympathetic stimulation from their anxious thoughts. Substance use may increase pulse rate.

COUNT respirations for rate and OBSERVE breathing pattern.

In adults breathing should occur at a rate of 12 to 20 breaths/min. Evaluate the rhythm or pattern of breathing. It should be smooth and even. The chest wall should symmetrically rise and expand and then relax. It should appear easy, without effort. (See Chapter 4 for measurement of vital signs and Chapter 11 for breathing patterns.)

Respiratory rate may be increased during anxiety as a result of sympathetic stimulation. The patient may appear to be dyspneic. Respiratory rate may be decreased during depression, and the breathing pattern may include frequent, deep sighs.

MEASURE pupil size.

Compare the patient's pupil size with a pupil gauge on the side of a penlight. When you suspect that the patient has drug intoxication, complete the rapid eye test in Box 7.1. (See Chapter 10 for eye examination.)

Use of alcohol and selected illegal substances may cause changes in pupil size as well as redness of sclera, glazing of cornea, edematous eyelids, watering eyes, drooping of the eyelids.

BOX 7.1 RAPID EYE TEST TO DETECT CURRENT DRUG INTOXICATION

General Observation
Look for redness of sclera, ptosis, retracted upper lid (white sclera visible above iris, causing blank stare), glazing, excessive tearing of eyes, and swelling of eyelids.

Pupil Size
Dilated (>6.5 mm) or constricted (<3 mm).

Pupil Reaction to Light
Slow, sluggish, or absent response.

Nystagmus
Hold one finger in the vertical position and have the patient follow it as it moves to the side, in a circle, and up and down.

Positive test is failure to hold gaze or jerkiness of eye movements.

Convergence
Inability to hold the cross-eyed position after an examining finger is moved 1 foot away from the patient's nose and held there for 5 seconds.

Corneal Reflex
Decreased rate of blinking after touching cornea with cotton.

AGE-RELATED VARIATIONS

INFANTS, CHILDREN, AND ADOLESCENTS

Variations for neonates and infants include asking about drug and alcohol use of the mother during the pregnancy. Children are asked about their experiences in school, how they like school, and if they get into trouble at school. They are also asked about the fears of any aspect of their life, including violence in their home. Adolescents are asked about school experience as well. In addition, they are asked about drug and alcohol use, and feelings of depression or anxiety. Assessing the self-esteem of this age group is important. Chapter 19 presents further information regarding the mental health assessment of these age groups.

OLDER ADULTS

The most prevalent mental health disorders of older adults are anxiety, severe cognitive impairment, and mood disorders. Alcohol abuse and dependence are also concerns with this population. Although delirium is common in older adults, it often is unrecognized, which increases the risk of functional decline.[21] Chapter 21 presents further information regarding the mental health assessment of this age group.

COMMON PROBLEMS AND CONDITIONS

MOOD DISORDERS

Major Depression

One of the most common mental health conditions is depression, characterized by a persistently depressed mood lasting a minimum of 2 weeks. The length of a depressive episode may be 5 to 6 months. While people initially experience depression as a single episode, most of have recurrent episodes. Feeling depressed is not the same as the illness of depression. Major depression may interfere with the patient's ability to work, study, sleep, eat, and enjoy pleasurable activities.[5] The prevalence of major depressive episodes in all US adults is estimated at 6.7%, with women having a higher prevalence than men. Those in between the ages of 18 and 25 had the highest prevalence at 10.9%.[22] **Clinical Findings:** A person must have been in a depressed mood or have lost interest or pleasure for at least 2 weeks and have at least five of the following symptoms nearly every day: (1) depressed mood most of the day; (2) markedly diminished interest or pleasure in all, or almost all activities of the day; (3) significant weight loss when not dieting or weight gain or decrease or increase in appetite; (4) psychomotor agitation or retardation; (5) fatigue or loss of energy; (6) feelings of worthlessness, or excessive or inappropriate guilt; (7) diminished ability to think or concentrate or indecisiveness; (8) recurrent thoughts of death, recurrent suicidal ideation without a specific plan; or (9) a suicide attempt or a specific plan for committing suicide.[23]

Postpartum Depression

Postpartum depression (PPD) is a term used to describe depression that occurs during the postpartum period up to 1 year after childbirth and can affect both mother and father. Mothers with PPD may have difficulty initiating breastfeeding and bonding with their infants, which has been found to negatively impact the growth and development of the infants.[24] About 11% of mothers and 4% of fathers experience symptoms of PPD during the first year after birth.[25] **Clinical Findings:** Symptoms of PPD are similar to those of major depression, but may also include crying more often than usual, feeling angry, feeling numb or disconnected from the baby, worrying about the baby, feeling guilty about not being a good mother or doubting the ability to care for the baby, and withdrawing from loved ones.[25]

Bipolar Disorder

This chronic illness is sometimes referred to as manic-depressive disorder. People with bipolar disorder experience recurrent episodes of depression or mania symptoms, which are interspersed by periods of a relatively normal mood. The depressive symptoms are similar to those of major depression. People with bipolar disease are more likely to seek medical help when they are depressed than when experiencing mania. There are two types: bipolar I and bipolar II. Bipolar I disorder is defined by manic episodes lasting at least 7 days or by manic symptoms that are so severe that the person needs immediate hospital care. Usually depressive episodes occur as well, typically lasting at least 2 weeks. By contrast, bipolar II is defined by a pattern of depressive and hypomania episodes, but not the full-blown manic episodes in bipolar I.[26] Hypomania is distinguished from mania by the severity of symptoms. The duration of mood cycles is highly variable over time, but in general, a hypomanic episode may last days to weeks, and a manic episode may last weeks to months.[9] The lifetime prevalence of bipolar disease in the United States is estimated at approximately 4.4%. The mortality rate is high with suicide accounting for 5% of deaths among women and 10% among men compared with 1% and 2% in the general population.[27] **Clinical Findings:** Characteristics of the manic phase are excessive emotional displays, excitement, euphoria, hyperactivity accompanied by elation, boisterousness, impaired ability to concentrate, decreased need for sleep, and limitless energy, often accompanied by delusions of grandeur. By contrast, hypomania is a low-level and less dramatic mania accompanied by excessive activity and energy for at least 4 days. During the depressive phase, people experience marked apathy and feelings of profound sadness, loneliness, guilt, and lowered self-esteem.[28]

PSYCHOTIC DISORDERS

Schizophrenia

This chronic group of mental disorders is characterized by disruptions in thought processes, perception, emotional responsiveness, and social interactions. Precise prevalence estimates are difficult to obtain due to the complexity of diagnosis and overlap with other disorders. The estimated prevalence for schizophrenia and other psychotic disorders in the United States ranges between 0.25% and 0.64%.[29] **Clinical Findings:** Three categories are used to describe clinical findings: positive symptoms, negative symptoms, and cognitive symptoms. Positive symptoms include hallucinations, delusions, thought disorders (dysfunctional thinking), and movement disorders (agitated body movement). Negative symptoms are flat affect, reduced feelings of pleasure, difficulty beginning and sustaining activities, and reduced speaking. Cognitive symptoms include difficulty understanding information and using it to make decisions, difficulty paying attention, and the inability to use information immediately after it is learned.[30]

ANXIETY DISORDERS

The wide variety of anxiety disorders differ by objects or situations that induce them, but share features of excessive anxiety and related behavioral experiences. Anxiety disorders include panic disorder, agoraphobia (fear of being in an open, crowded, or public place), a specific phobia, social anxiety disorder, separation anxiety disorder, generalized anxiety disorder (GAD), obsessive-compulsive disorder (OCD), and posttraumatic stress disorder (PTSD).[14] The latter three are discussed as follows.

Generalized Anxiety Disorder

Anxiety is defined as a feeling of apprehension, uneasiness, uncertainty, or dread resulting from a real or perceived threat. Contrasting it with fear, anxiety is a vague sense of dread related to an unspecified or unknown danger, and fear is a reaction to a specific danger. While the body reacts physiologically in similar ways to both anxiety and fear, the reaction to anxiety invades the core of personality and erodes feelings of self-esteem. Individuals with anxiety disorders experience a degree of anxiety that interferes with personal, occupational, or social functioning. Their response is to use rigid, repetitive, and ineffective behaviors to try to control their anxiety.[14] The prevalence of any anxiety disorder in US adults is 19.1%.[31] **Clinical Findings:** Four levels of anxiety have been described: mild, moderate, severe, and panic. Clinical findings vary based on the level of anxiety the individual is experiencing. Mild anxiety occurs in the normal experience of daily life. A *mildly anxious*

person has a broad perceptual field because the anxiety heightens awareness to sensory stimuli. The person sees more, hears more, and thinks more logically. Learning occurs during mild anxiety. The *moderately anxious* person has a narrower field of perception and uses selective inattention to ignore stimuli in the environment to focus on a specific concern. The *severely anxious* person has reduced perception of stimuli and develops compulsive mechanisms to avoid the anxiety-provoking object or situation. During severe anxiety, the person experiences impaired memory, attention, and concentration; has difficulty solving problems; and is unable to focus on events in the environment. The *panic* level of anxiety is characterized by complete disruption of the perceptual field. The person experiences intense terror and is unable to think logically or make decisions. Physical manifestations of anxiety represent sympathetic nervous system stimulation. The person experiences muscle tension, tachycardia, dyspnea, hypertension, increased respiration, and profuse perspiration.[14]

Obsessive-Compulsive Disorder (OCD)

This disorder is classified as an anxiety disorder because of the anxiety symptoms that develop when the patient tries to resist an obsession or compulsion. *Obsessions* are defined as thoughts, impulses, or images that persist or recur, despite the affected individual's attempts to dismiss them. *Compulsions* are ritualistic behaviors that an individual feels driven to perform in an attempt to reduce anxiety or prevent an imagined calamity. Although obsessions and compulsions can exist separately, they most often occur together.[14] The prevalence of adults with OCD is estimated at 1.2%, with the prevalence in women being three times greater than men.[32] **Clinical Findings:** Common obsessions include fear of germs or contamination, unwanted or forbidden thoughts about sex, religion, and harm; aggressive thoughts toward self or others; or having things symmetric or in perfect order. Common compulsions are excessive cleaning and/or handwashing; arranging things in a particular, precise way; repeatedly checking on things, such as the oven being turned off or the door being locked; and compulsive counting.[33] For example, with an obsession about germs or environmental contaminants, the compulsion might involve excessive handwashing in a certain way or excessive bathing.[14]

Posttraumatic Stress Disorder

A person who is exposed to a potentially traumatic event that is beyond a typical stressor may be at risk for developing a mental disorder called Posttraumatic Stress Disorder (PTSD). Events that may lead to PTSD include violent personal assaults, natural or human-caused disasters, accidents, combat, and other forms of violence. About half of all US adults will experience at least one traumatic event in their lives, but most will not develop PTSD. The lifetime prevalence for PTSD is 3.6% of the US adult population. People with PTSD feel stressed or frightened, even when they are no longer in danger.[34] **Clinical Findings:** Symptoms usually begin within 3 months of the traumatic event. For a diagnosis of PTSD, an adult must have all of the following for at least 1 month:

- At least one re-experiencing symptom: Flashbacks, bad dreams, or frightening thoughts
- At least one avoidance symptom: Staying away from places, events, or objects that are reminders of the experience or avoiding thoughts or feelings related to the traumatic event
- At least two arousal and reactivity symptoms: Being easily startled, feeling tense or "on edge," having difficulty sleeping, and/or having angry outbursts
- At least two cognitive and mood symptoms: Trouble remembering key features of the traumatic event, negative thoughts about oneself or the world, distorted feelings such as guilt or blame; loss of interest in enjoyable activities[35]

SUBSTANCE USE DISORDERS

Repeated use of drugs, including alcohol, that results in functional problems indicates a substance use disorder. There are multiple reasons why people use psychoactive substances. Some people use them because they have pleasurable or desirable effects for the user, while others may use them to block out physical or psychological pain. Stimulants may be used to increase performance, stay awake, or lose weight. The term *substance dependence* is used when a person uses alcohol or other drugs despite extreme negative consequences, such as impairment to their daily lives. Tolerance develops when the person's body becomes less responsive to the drug with repeated use.[36]

The World Health Organization (WHO) developed a screening tool called ASSIST (Alcohol, Smoking and Substance Involvement Screening Test). This screening tool consists of eight questions that provide a risk score for each substance, indicating low, moderate, or high risk. The risk score determines the level of intervention recommended.[36] This tool is available at https://www.who.int/substance_abuse/activities/assist_v3_english.pdf.

Alcohol Abuse

Ethyl alcohol, or ethanol, is a central nervous system depressant found in alcoholic beverages. The blood alcohol level is used to measure the amount of alcohol in blood. The legal intoxication level in most states is 100 mg/dL (0.10%), with some states using 0.08%. In 2018 Utah changed its blood alcohol level to 0.05%.[37] **Clinical Findings:** *Alcohol intoxication* can result in maladaptive behaviors such as impaired judgment, fighting, mood changes, and irritability. Other signs include slurred speech, lack of coordination, unsteady gait, nystagmus, or flushed face. *Alcohol withdrawal syndrome* (AWS) has three phases: minor, moderate, and severe. Symptoms of minor withdrawal include diarrhea, nausea and/or vomiting, hand tremors, insomnia, and headache that begins within 6 hours after cessation of alcohol and lasts up to 4 to 48 hours. Symptoms of moderate withdrawal include hallucinations of visual, tactile, or auditory qualities, illusions while conscious, and seizures that emerge 6 to 48 hours after

the last drink and last up to 6 days. Severe withdrawal is characterized by delirium tremors (DTs) that involve vivid hallucinations, delusions, confusion, and high blood pressure beginning 48 to 72 hours after the last drink and lasting for up to 2 weeks.[17]

Drug Abuse

Stimulants (amphetamines, cocaine); cannabis (marijuana, hashish); hallucinogens and PCP; opioids (heroin, codeine); and sedatives, hypnotics, and anxiolytics (barbiturates, benzodiazepine) are drugs that are commonly abused. **Clinical Findings:** The patient's clinical findings are directly related to the substance used. Physical effects of substance use disorders vary with intoxication, tolerance, and withdrawal.

Intoxication results when a substance is used to excess. *Tolerance* occurs when a person no longer responds to the substance in the way that the person initially responded. Higher doses of the substance are needed to achieve the same level of response initially achieved. *Withdrawal* is a set of symptoms that occur when the person stops using a substance and vary depending on the substance that was used.[38]

NEUROCOGNITIVE DISORDERS

Delirium

This disorder is characterized by a disturbance in attention (i.e., reduced ability to direct, focus, sustain, and shift attention) and awareness (reduced orientation of the environment). Manifestations develop over a short period of time (usually hours to a few days), represent an acute change from baseline attention and awareness, and tend to change in severity during the day. Delirium is a common complication of hospitalized patients, as it is often linked to another medical condition or substance intoxication or withdrawal.[39] It is considered a medical emergency requiring immediate attention to prevent irreversible and serious damage. The reported incidence of delirium in all hospitalized patients is 22% in general medical patients, between 11% and 35% in surgical patients, and up to 80% in patients in intensive care units. In patients over 65 years of age, the incidence is up to 50%. Delirium is often not recognized, which leads to the variability of reported incidences.[40] **Clinical Findings:** Altered level of consciousness; impaired memory, judgment, and calculation; and a fluctuating attention span are indications of delirium. The emotional state can change abruptly and range from fearful to aggressive with hallucinations and delusions. Delirium may worsen at night (sundowning). The sleep cycle may be reversed. Speech may be rapid, inappropriate, and rambling.[40]

Dementia

This chronic, progressive neurocognitive disorder is characterized by failing memory, cognitive impairment, behavioral abnormalities, and personality changes that often begin after the age of 60 years.[2] A disease commonly associated with dementia is Alzheimer disease, which accounts for 60% to 80% of all dementias.[40] (Alzheimer disease is described in

Chapter 21.) Dementia usually is not reversible—a characteristic that distinguishes it from delirium. **Clinical Findings:** Cognitive changes include memory loss, difficulty communicating or findings words, difficulty problem solving, difficulty planning and organizing, and difficulty with coordination and motor functions. Psychological changes include personality changes, depression, anxiety, inappropriate behavior, paranoia, agitation, and hallucinations.[41]

CLINICAL APPLICATION AND CLINICAL JUDGMENT

See Appendix B for answers to exercises in this section.

CASE STUDY

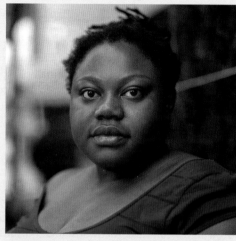

Sarah Ubina comes to the student health clinic with complaints of fatigue. The following data are collected from interview and examination.

Interview Data

Ms. Ubina tells the nurse that she has constantly felt tired, and all she wants to do is sleep. She says that she doesn't have time to be tired because final examinations are approaching, and she is very concerned about her grades. She begins to cry. "I'm so afraid that I won't pass my classes. If I don't pass, my parents won't help me with school anymore." When asked to describe herself, Sarah replies, "Friendly, but not very smart."

Ms. Ubina tells the nurse that she has a boyfriend but only sees him occasionally because he lives in another state. When asked about other friends, Ms. Ubina replies, "I know all of the people in my class."

Examination Data

- *General survey:* Well-nourished, overweight young woman appearing unkempt, with slightly swollen red eyes from crying. Makes infrequent eye contact.
- *Vital signs:* Blood pressure, 128/84 mm Hg; pulse, 96 beats/min; respirations, 22 breaths/min; temperature, 98.6°F (36.7°C); height: 5 ft 3 in (160 cm); weight: 148 lbs (67 kg).
- Pupils are equal and 4 mm in size.
- *Mental status:* Oriented to person, place, and time. Slow speech pattern with flat affect.
- All body system findings are within expected limits.

Clinical Judgment

1. What cues do you recognize that suggest deviations from normal findings, suggesting to the nurse that Ms. Ubina may have a mental health issue?
2. What additional information should the nurse ask about or assess for?
3. Based on the data, which risk factors for depression does this patient have?
4. With which other health care team members could you collaborate to help this patient?

REVIEW QUESTIONS

1. Which question is appropriate for a nurse to ask at the beginning of a mental health history?
   1. "Have you been feeling anxious or sad?"
   2. "How have you been feeling about yourself?"
   3. "Are you alone a lot, or do you socialize with friends?"
   4. "How are you dealing with the stressors in your life?"

2. During a history, the patient says that she is so uncomfortable with her life that she wishes that it was over. Which is an appropriate follow-up question from the nurse?
   1. "Have you thought of hurting yourself?"
   2. "Oh, I've felt that way many times."
   3. "That feeling will go away; just give it some time."
   4. "In which ways has your life been uncomfortable?"

3. During a health history, a patient says, "Stressors? Oh, yeah, I have stressors. I got a promotion at work, and with the extra income, I'm going to move into a new house. But that has been delayed because my mother is in the hospital and my son is going off to college. To get through this time, I just keep using my support systems, exercising, and meditating." How does a nurse interpret these comments by this patient?
   1. Flight of ideas
   2. Moderate anxiety
   3. Positive coping strategies
   4. Rationalization and denial

4. Which technique does a nurse use to assess the mental status of patients?
   1. Ask them about any of their relatives who have mental health disorders.
   2. Have them calculate the change to expect after making a purchase.
   3. Ask them to recall how they cope with stress on a daily basis.
   4. Have them describe the moods and emotions they experience on a usual day.

5. During a sports physical of an 18-year-old girl, the nurse asks which questions to collect data about drug use?
   1. "Many teenagers have tried street drugs. Have you tried any?"
   2. "Tell me which street drugs your friends have offered you."
   3. "Do your friends tell you about the street drugs they use?
   4. "Your high school has a reputation for students using street drugs. Do you use these drugs?"

6. A patient reports nausea and vomiting, and the nurse observes hand tremors, agitation, and sweating. In view of these findings, which additional cues would the nurse need to collect?
   1. Which fears or stressors the patient has been experiencing
   2. When the patient last took illegal drugs and which drug(s) was (were) taken
   3. Which kinds of obsessions or compulsions the patient has been experiencing
   4. When the patient last drank alcohol and how much was consumed

CHAPTER

8

Nutritional Assessment

evolve

http://evolve.elsevier.com/Wilson/assessment

CONCEPT OVERVIEW

The concept for this chapter is *Nutrition*, which represents the optimal intake and metabolism of nutrients. Individuals can be well nourished or develop malnourishment from either inadequate or excessive nutrient intake or altered metabolism of nutrients. Malnourishment is associated with poor health outcomes. Many important concepts associated with nutrition are represented in the illustration. Understanding the interrelationships among these concepts helps the nurse recognize risk factors and thus increases awareness when conducting a health assessment. Nutrition has a close relationship with elimination, hormonal regulation, immunity, tissue integrity, and sensory perception. Problems with sensory perception can impact the ability to prepare foods, impaired elimination can interfere with appetite, and impaired hormonal regulation can lead to problems with the metabolism of nutrients. Poor nutritional status may lead to impaired immunity and problems with tissue integrity. The following case provides a clinical example featuring several of these interrelated concepts.

William Washington is a 72-year-old man who has been obese for most of his life. He has a 20-year history of type 2 *diabetes, a condition characterized by impaired glucose regulation. Over the past 2 months, he has had an infected diabetic foot ulcer that won't heal. His blood glucose levels and A_{1C} have remained high, and he has "given up" trying to manage his disease through dietary measures. He has been eating what he wants and gaining weight. Without appropriate intervention, Mr. Washington is at risk for serious and exacerbated health complications.*

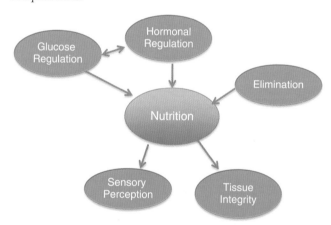

ANATOMY AND PHYSIOLOGY

Nutrients are necessary to provide the body calories for energy, build and maintain body tissues, and regulate body processes. The term kilocalorie (kcal) is the scientific term used to measure a unit of food energy and represents 1000 "small calories" of energy. However, the common term *calorie* is often used interchangeably. The base energy requirement is called the *basal metabolic rate* (BMR), which is influenced by several factors. Activity levels, illness, injury, infection, ingestion of food, and starvation can all affect the BMR. When caloric intake meets energy needs, no weight change occurs.

When energy needs exceed caloric intake, weight loss occurs. When caloric intake exceeds energy needs, weight gain occurs. Nutrients are classified into one of three groups: macronutrients, micronutrients, and water.

MACRONUTRIENTS

Nutrients that are required in large amounts are referred to as *macronutrients*. The three categories of macronutrients are carbohydrates, proteins, and fats.

Carbohydrate

The main source of energy and fiber in the diet comes from *carbohydrates*. Fiber passes through the digestive tract partially undigested, providing bulk that stimulates peristalsis. The two main sources of carbohydrates are plant foods (fruits, vegetables, and grains) and lactose (from milk). Although small amounts of carbohydrates are stored in the liver and muscle in the form of glycogen (to serve as energy reserves between meals), moderate amounts of carbohydrates must be ingested at regular intervals to meet the energy demands. If more carbohydrates are ingested than required, the excess is stored as fat. Each gram of carbohydrate provides 4 calories of energy. The recommended daily allowance (RDA) for carbohydrate intake is 130 g/day for children and adults, but increases to 175 g/day during pregnancy and 210 g/day for lactating women.[1] Carbohydrates should account for 55% to 60% of total calories. Many carbohydrate sources are classified as high energy, non-nutrient dense. Examples include sugar-sweetened beverages, desserts, and candy. Sedentary people should decrease consumption of energy-dense carbohydrates to maintain an ideal body weight.[1]

Protein

While also a source of energy, protein plays an essential role in facilitating the growth and repair of body tissues. The simplest form of protein is an amino acid. There are 20 different amino acids that combine in different ways to form proteins. Ten of the amino acids are considered essential in the diet because the body does not synthesize them. A complete-protein food contains all of the essential amino acids and is also referred to as a high–biologic value protein. Foods containing complete proteins are the highest-quality proteins and come from animal sources (meat, fish, poultry, milk, and eggs). Foods that contain incomplete proteins include cereals, legumes, and some vegetables. Combinations of incomplete-protein foods can provide all the essential amino acids. If more protein is ingested than needed, the extra is used to supply energy or is stored as fat. Each gram of protein provides 4 calories of energy. The RDA for protein intake in the adult diet is 0.8 g/kg of body weight, or an average of 56 g/day for adult males, 46 g/day for adult females, and 71 g/day for pregnant or lactating females.[1] Ideally, protein should account for 12% to 20% of total calories. These requirements are based on ideal body weight.

Fat

Fat is the main source of fatty acids, which are essential for normal growth and development. Other functions of fat include synthesis and regulation of certain hormones, tissue structure, nerve impulse transmission, energy, insulation, and protection of vital organs. There are two essential fatty acids for metabolic processes: linoleic (or omega 6) and alpha-linolenic (or omega 3) acids. Fat is the major form of stored energy in the body. One gram of fat yields 9 calories of energy. If energy needs exceed carbohydrate intake, fat can be converted to glucose by a process known as gluconeogenesis. If more fat is ingested than needed, it is stored in adipose tissue. Ideally, fats should account for 20-30% of total calories.[1]

MICRONUTRIENTS

Micronutrients are nutrients required in small quantities. The two groups of micronutrients, vitamins and minerals, are essential for growth, development, and metabolic processes that occur continuously throughout the body.

Vitamins are classified as water soluble or fat soluble (Table 8.1). Water-soluble vitamins cannot be stored in the body; thus they must be ingested in the diet daily. Fat-soluble vitamins can be stored in the body, and vitamin toxicity can result if they are taken in large quantities. Deficiencies or toxicities in micronutrients result in nutritionally-based diseases; these deficiencies are usually a late sign of depletion.

Minerals are grouped into two categories: major minerals and trace minerals (Table 8.2). Major minerals are present in the body in large amounts with a required intake of more than 100 mg/day. Trace minerals are present in smaller amounts with a required intake of under 100 mg/day.

WATER

Water comprises of 60% to 79% of total body weight, making it a critical component of the body. The body requires fluid for metabolic and cellular processes; cells depend on a well-hydrated environment for optimal functioning. Water intake typically occurs through the ingestion of fluids and foods. Water is lost from the body in a number of ways, including

TABLE 8.1 VITAMINS

FAT-SOLUBLE VITAMINS	WATER-SOLUBLE VITAMINS
Vitamin A	Vitamin C
Vitamin D	B vitamins
Vitamin E	Thiamin
Vitamin K	Riboflavin
	Niacin
	Pyridoxine (B_6)
	Pantothenic acid
	Biotin
	Folate
	Cobalamin (B_{12})

TABLE 8.2 MINERALS

MAJOR MINERALS	TRACE MINERALS
Calcium	Iron
Phosphorus	Iodine
Magnesium	Zinc
Sodium	Copper
Potassium	Manganese
Chloride	Chromium
Sulfur	Cobalt
	Selenium
	Molybdenum
	Fluoride

through urine and through insensible fluid losses (from the lungs, skin, and feces). Fluid loss occurs continually; thus fluid replacement is required on an ongoing basis—in fact, humans can survive only a few days in the complete absence of water intake. The average adult should consume 2.5 to 3 L of water every day in the form of both foods and fluids, although fluid needs are increased in certain situations, such as exposure to a hot climate or illness, especially fever, infection, gastrointestinal (GI) losses, respiratory illness, and draining wounds.

HEALTH HISTORY

A nutritional assessment is an integral part of a total health assessment because foods and fluids are basic biologic needs. Collecting data specifically related to nutritional status and identifying risk factors for nutritional problems are included in the health history. The nurse asks questions to elicit information about current health status, past health history, family history, personal and psychosocial history, and risk factors. Specific questions are asked to assess the patient's actual or potential nutritional needs and to assess for nutrition-related problems. Data gained from the history are used to evaluate the adequacy of the diet and identify areas needed for patient education to make necessary dietary modifications.

GENERAL HEALTH HISTORY

Present Health Status

Do you have any chronic illnesses? If so, what are your conditions? Are you on a special diet or have dietary restrictions as part of the management of the health condition?
Many chronic illnesses are associated with nutritional problems. For example, individuals with GI disease are at greater risk for malnutrition.[2] Individuals may also be following a prescribed dietary plan to manage a particular health condition such as diabetes mellitus, cystic fibrosis, phenylketonuria, celiac disease, heart failure, renal failure, or cancer.

Do you take any medications (prescription or over-the-counter) or herbal supplements? If so, what do you take, what dose, how often, and for what reason?
Many medications can affect nutritional status. Some medications affect appetite; others may cause GI discomfort such as nausea, a feeling of fullness, constipation, or diarrhea. Some medications are affected by foods ingested; thus food restrictions may be necessary. For example, warfarin, an anticoagulant, has a moderate interaction with alcohol and foods that have a high amount of vitamin K per portion (such as kale, spinach, collards, and other vegetables).

Do you take vitamins or dietary supplements? If so, what do you take, how often, and for what reason?
Many individuals use vitamins and/or nutritional supplements as health-promotion measures or to manage nutritional deficiencies. Iron deficiency occurs among many adolescents and women of childbearing years. Many older women take calcium and vitamin D supplementation to treat or prevent osteoporosis. Overuse of fat-soluble vitamins (A, E, D, and K) can lead to toxicities. Dietary supplements and vitamins are not intended to serve as a substitute food intake, but are useful sources of nutrients.[3]

Do you have any food allergies or intolerances? If so, describe.
Food allergies are very common, estimated to affect 4% of adults, and 4% to 6% of children.[4] A food allergy occurs when ingested food triggers an immune system reaction that can range from mild (hives) to life-threatening anaphylaxis. Lifetime prevalence of food intolerance is estimated to be 5% to 10%.[5] A food intolerance occurs when ingested food causes unpleasant side effects usually affecting the GI system (such as nausea, bloating, cramping, and diarrhea) but can also cause other symptoms such as headaches, cough, and runny nose. Table 8.3 presents foods that commonly cause allergies and intolerances.

Have you noticed any unexplained changes in your weight (weight gain or weight loss) in the last 6 months? If so, describe.
Weight should remain fairly stable over time. Significant or rapid changes in weight require further evaluation, especially if the patient has experienced unexplained weight loss of more than 10 pounds in 6 months.

TABLE 8.3 COMMON FOODS ASSOCIATED WITH ALLERGIES AND INTOLERANCE	
FOODS ASSOCIATED WITH ALLERGIES	**FOODS ASSOCIATED WITH INTOLERANCE**
Milk	Lactose
Eggs	Wheat
Shellfish	Gluten
Fish	Caffeine
Peanut	Histamines
Tree Nut (i.e., walnut, pecan, almond)	Food additives (multiple—such as sweeteners,
Wheat	nitrates, sulfites,
Soy	preservatives, colorings)

Information from: American College of Asthma, Allergy, and Immunology. https://acaai.org/allergies/types/food-allergy; Nordqvist C: What is a food intolerance? *Medical News Today.* MediLexicon, Intl., December 20, 2017. Retrieved from: https://www.medicalnewstoday.com/articles/263965.php

Past Health History

Have you ever had problems or concerns in the past related to your weight or problems eating? If so, what have you tried to resolve the problems (e.g., diet modification, exercise, medications, surgery)? How effective were these measures?

A personal history of excessive weight gain (such as during pregnancy) or weight loss during an illness is important to note. Many individuals who have experienced weight gain try to lose weight. Determine which measures they have used or attempted in the past and if they were effective.

Have you ever had surgery that has affected your nutritional intake or nutritional status? What has the impact been on your overall health?

Surgical procedures, particularly abdominal surgery, can affect nutritional intake and metabolism of nutrients. Individuals who have had bariatric surgery as a treatment for morbid obesity have the most weight loss during the first year after surgery. By 2 years after surgery, about half of patients have regained some weight back.[6] Several nutritional issues can result from bariatric surgery, especially B_{12} deficiency.

Have you ever had nutrition-related problems such as obesity or diabetes mellitus?

Obesity is the prime risk factor for type 2 diabetes mellitus.

Have you suffered from an eating disorder such as compulsive eating disorders, bulimia, or anorexia nervosa?

Eating disorders commonly occur during adolescence and may cause lingering macro and micronutrient deficiency or psychological problems in adulthood.

Family History

Has anyone in your family ever had nutrition-related problems such as obesity or diabetes mellitus?

Obesity in one or both parents makes an individual at higher risk for excessive weight, which is partly genetic and partly from learned patterns of behavior in relation to eating. Individuals with a family history of diabetes are at risk of developing the disease.

Has anyone in your family suffered from an eating disorder?

Eating disorders tend to run in families and are thought to have a genetic basis.[7]

Personal and Psychosocial History

Describe your activity level and exercise pattern.

Physically active people have a reduced risk of becoming overweight or obese. Specifically, sedentary lifestyle is a known risk factor for weight gain and obesity. Children and adults should avoid inactivity and are encouraged to meet the 2018 Physical Activity Guidelines for Americans.[8]

Do you follow a specific diet based on personal preferences and/or as part of your cultural or spiritual practices?

Many individuals independently adopt specific diets (e.g., vegetarian, vegan, low carbohydrate, ketogenic, or mediterranean) as a personal choice. Dietary practices may also be

ETHNIC, CULTURAL, AND SPIRITUAL VARIATIONS

Dietary Practices

Dietary practices are often influenced by religious beliefs and practice. The following are some examples of traditional dietary practices by religious groups.

- **Buddhism:** Tend to follow vegetarian diet; avoidance of alcohol.
- **Catholic:** Avoid meat on certain holy days such as Ash Wednesday, Good Friday, and during Lent.
- **Hinduism:** Preference for vegetarian diet; tend to avoid animal meat/flesh, especially beef and pork; fasting on certain holy days.
- **Islam:** Avoid foods that are non-halal. Examples include pork, pork products, alcoholic beverages/products. Other meat consumption allowed if it has been prepared according to Islamic law.
- **Judaism:** Avoid pork and shellfish; other meats should be certified kosher. Meat and dairy cannot be combined.
- **Mormonism:** Encouraged to avoid overindulging on food; avoidance of consumption of tea, coffee, alcohol. Monthly fast first Sunday of each month.
- **Seventh Day Adventist:** Promote vegetarian diet; animal products (eggs, dairy) should be consumed in moderation. If meats are consumed, they must be "clean meats"—similar to kosher.

influenced by cultural or religious beliefs, as shown in the *Ethnic, Cultural, and Spiritual Variations* Box.

Do you have any problems obtaining, preparing, or eating foods? If so, describe.

Food insecurity refers to a lack of consistent access to enough food for an active healthy life. An estimated 11.8% of households in the United States experienced food insecurity at some point in 2017, most commonly affecting low-income groups, the elderly, or those with disabilities.[9] Many individuals with physical disabilities or illness may have difficulty in procuring and preparing food. If this is an issue, assess their support systems (someone willing to purchase and prepare food) or assess for community resources (e.g., Meals on Wheels).

Do you use street drugs or drink alcohol? If so, describe.

The use of drugs or alcohol can contribute to nutritional deficiencies. Alcohol is a source of "empty" calories (i.e., calories that supply no nutrients), which in turn suppresses the appetite. Alcohol also impairs the absorption of nutrients. Furthermore, money spent on drugs or alcohol may replace money available for the purchase of food. Patients with a history of substance abuse often underreport alcohol consumption and drug use. Refer to Chapter 7 for alcohol and drug-abuse assessment.

PROBLEM-BASED HISTORY

Commonly reported symptoms related to nutrition include weight loss, weight gain, difficulty in chewing and swallowing, and nausea or loss of appetite. As in all areas of health assessment, the nurse completes a symptom analysis using the mnemonic OLD CARTS from Box 2.6, which includes *O*nset, *L*ocation, *D*uration, *C*haracteristics, *A*ggravating Factors, *R*elated Symptoms, *T*reatment, and *S*everity.

Weight Loss

When did the weight loss start? What is your normal weight? What is your weight now? How many pounds have you lost in the last 6 months?
Establish the total weight loss and the time frame over which it occurred.

To what do you attribute the weight loss? Was it intentional or unintentional? If intentional, what have you done to lose the weight? If unintentional, what do you think is causing the weight loss?
Intentional weight loss may be the result of a change in eating habits or an increase in exercise (or both). Strict calorie intake, fasting, bulimia, laxative abuse, and excessive exercise are indications of an unhealthy preoccupation with body weight or a possible eating disorder. Unintentional weight loss may be caused by loss of appetite, vomiting, illness, stress, or medications. Individuals may be able to explain factors contributing to weight loss. Advanced age is a known risk factor for undernutrition.

Have you had any symptoms associated with the loss of weight such as fatigue, headaches, bruising, constipation, hair loss, or cracks in the corners of the mouth?
Excessive weight loss may cause a number of symptoms because of inadequate energy and protein, and deficiency in vitamins and minerals.

Weight Gain

When did you start gaining weight? What do you consider your normal weight? What is your weight now? How many pounds have you gained in the last 6 months?
Establish the total weight gained and the time frame over which it occurred, whether sudden or gradual.

To what do you attribute your weight gain? Has it been intentional? Unintentional?
Intentional weight gain usually occurs from an increase in caloric intake or use of dietary supplements (or both). Intentional weight gain may result from a decrease in activity levels, change in eating habits, increased appetite, or smoking cessation. It may also be associated with fluid retention as a result of certain medical conditions (e.g., heart failure) or as a side effect of certain medications (e.g., corticosteroids).

Difficulty in Chewing or Swallowing

What kind of problem are you experiencing with chewing or swallowing? When did the problem begin? What other symptoms are you experiencing?
Determine the time frame over which the chewing or swallowing difficulties have occurred. Choking and coughing are common symptoms associated with impaired swallowing.

Do you find certain foods more difficult to eat than others? If so, describe.
Thin liquids and foods requiring forceful chewing (such as meat) may not be tolerated well.

Which types of foods are you able to consume without difficulty?
Foods that are soft and highly viscous are chewed and swallowed most easily.

Has your weight changed since this problem developed?
Weight loss, particularly if unintentional, may be an indication that food intake is hampered by chewing or swallowing difficulties.

Loss of Appetite or Nausea

Tell me about the problems you are experiencing with appetite or nausea (or both). When did you first notice the problem? Is the problem constant, or does it come and go?
Establish the nature and onset of the problem—this may provide clues to the cause and potential nutritional deficiencies.

RISK FACTORS

Nutrition

OBESITY	PROTEIN-CALORIE MALNUTRITION	EATING DISORDERS
• Sedentary lifestyle (M)	• Age	• Preoccupation with weight (M)
• High-fat diet (M)	• Acute or chronic illness	• Perfectionist (M)
• Genetics	• Side effects from medications or treatments	• Poor self-esteem (M)
• Ethnicity/race	• Hospitalization for acute illness	• Self-image disturbances (M)
• Female	• Resident of long-term care facility (M)	• Peer pressure (M)
• Low socioeconomic status (M)	• Low socioeconomic status (M)	• Athlete—drive to excel (M)
		• Compulsive or binge eating (M)
		• First-generation relative with eating disorder or alcoholism

M, Modifiable risk factor.
From Grodner, M. *Nutritional foundations and clinical applications*, ed 5, St. Louis, 2012, Elsevier; Center for Disease Control, Fact Sheet: Health Disparities in Obesity, 2015, available from: http://www.cdc.gov/minorityhealth/reports/CHDIR11/FactSheets/Obesity.pdf

Appetite may fluctuate from time to time. A reduction in appetite over an extended period of time may result in nutritional deficiencies.

To what do you attribute your loss of appetite or nausea (e.g., medications, illness, pregnancy, depression)?
The patient may have an idea of what is causing a change in appetite or nausea. Medications, pregnancy, certain chronic illnesses, and depression can all contribute to changes in appetite or nausea.

Which types of foods are the most offensive or intolerable? Which types of foods are you able to consume without difficulty?
In some cases, an individual may avoid an entire food group and eat from another. Determining which nutrients the patient is consuming and identifying any possible deficiencies in the diet are important.

Has your weight changed since these problems developed?
A significant change in weight indicates a problem and may suggest nutritional deficiencies as well.

ASSESSMENT OF DIETARY INTAKE

To complete an individual nutritional assessment, nurses collect information about the patient's dietary intake. Obtaining accurate information about total dietary intake is a challenge because of the high incidence of underreporting, the wide variation in day-to-day intake, and variations in serving portions. Thus a "snapshot" of nutrient intake over 1 day, or even over a course of several days, may not be an accurate reflection of intake over a long period of time.

Dietary intake is usually assessed using retrospective or prospective approaches with both methods associated with benefits and challenges.[10] Retrospective approaches involve recalling intake or completing food frequency questionnaires. A common retrospective approach is the 24-hour recall where the patient describes what was eaten in the last 24 hours. Although this is an easy approach from a patient's perspective, it may not reflect the typical daily intake, with underreporting a common issue. Prospective approaches involve recording food as it is eaten during a specified time. In a food diary, the patient records every food or drink consumed in a designated period of time. Many electronic devices, software, and web-based tools, such as the Supertracker or Fitbit website, make the process easier, but it may not always be convenient. Data are more accurately recorded in two nonconsecutive 1-day recordings as opposed to a 2-day or a 3-day consecutive record.[11]

Short dietary assessment instruments, often called screeners, may be useful when the frequency of eating various categories of foods is desired rather than an assessment of the total diet. Dietary intake estimates from short dietary assessment instruments tend to be less accurate as compared with a food diary.[12]

In addition to determining nutrient intakes, ask patients about their appetite, food preferences, food dislikes, and food intolerances. Specifically, ask patients about special diets they may be following and the use of dietary supplements or herbs. Diets may be followed for weight loss, weight gain, or disease control (e.g., low-salt diet) or as part of cultural/religious practice.

Once the patient's dietary intake is obtained, the nurse can use several methods to determine if it is adequate. Comparing dietary intake with the US Department of Agriculture *MyPlate* guide is the simplest approach to dietary assessment.[13] Determine the portion of food on a typical plate for a rough comparison with the recommended intake (Fig. 8.1). An internet-based interactive program and additional information for consumers and health care professionals are easily located at: http://www.choosemyplate.gov/.

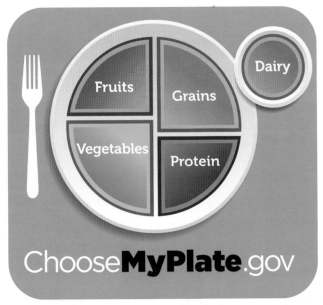

FIG. 8.1 MyPlate. (From the US Department of Agriculture, www.choosemyplate.gov/.)

EXAMINATION

The nutritional examination includes anthropometric measurements, biochemical tests, and nutrition-focused assessment. Although data collection varies with age groups and various stages in the life cycle (such as pregnancy), the nurse's general approach should be consistent for patients of all ages. Many nutritional deficiencies may become apparent through routine examination. However, sometimes, assessment findings associated with nutritional deficiencies may be caused by non–nutritionally related problems. For example, multiple bruises could be associated with nutritional deficiency, be related to tissue trauma, or be caused by low platelet count. For this reason, findings must be considered in association with a detailed history. Table 8.4 summarizes common findings associated with nutritional deficiencies.

Routine techniques

- MEASURE height and weight to calculate body mass index.
- ASSESS general appearance and orientation.
- INSPECT skin.
- PALPATE skin.
- INSPECT hair and nails.
- PALPATE hair and nails.
- INSPECT eyes.
- INSPECT oral cavity.
- INSPECT extremities.
- PALPATE extremities.

Special circumstances

- CALCULATE desirable body weight.
- CALCULATE percentage change in weight.
- CALCULATE waist-to-hip ratio.
- ESTIMATE body fat by measuring triceps skinfold.
- ASSESS nutritional status by reviewing laboratory tests (if available).

Equipment needed

- Weight and height scale • Calculator • Tape measure • Tongue blade • Penlight • Examination gloves • Skinfold calipers

TABLE 8.4 CLINICAL MANIFESTATIONS OF VARIOUS NUTRIENT DEFICIENCIES

AREA OF EXAMINATION	CLINICAL MANIFESTATION	POTENTIAL NUTRIENT DEFICIENCY
Hair	Alopecia	Zinc, essential fatty acids
	Easy pluckability	Protein, essential fatty acids
	Lackluster	Protein, zinc
	"Corkscrew" hair	Vitamin C, vitamin A
	Decreased pigmentation	Protein, copper
Eyes	Xerosis of conjunctiva	Vitamin A
	Corneal vascularization	Riboflavin
	Keratomalacia	Vitamin A
	Bitot spots	Vitamin A
Gastrointestinal tract	Nausea, vomiting	Pyridoxine
	Diarrhea	Zinc, niacin
	Stomatitis	Pyridoxine, riboflavin, iron
	Cheilosis	Pyridoxine, iron
	Glossitis	Pyridoxine, zinc, niacin, folate, vitamin B_{12}
	Magenta tongue	Riboflavin
	Swollen, bleeding gums	Vitamin C
	Fissured tongue	Niacin
	Hepatomegaly	Protein
Skin	Dry and scaling	Vitamin A, essential fatty acids, zinc
	Petechiae/ecchymoses	Vitamin C, vitamin K
	Follicular hyperkeratosis	Vitamin A, essential fatty acids
	Nasolabial seborrhea	Niacin, pyridoxine, riboflavin
	Bilateral dermatitis	Niacin, zinc
Extremities	Subcutaneous fat loss	Kilocalories
	Muscle wastage	Kilocalories, protein
	Edema	Protein
	Osteomalacia, bone pain, rickets	Vitamin D
	Arthralgia	Vitamin C
Neurologic	Disorientation	Niacin, thiamin
	Confabulation	Thiamin
	Neuropathy	Thiamin, pyridoxine, chromium
	Paresthesia	Thiamin, pyridoxine, vitamin B_{12}
Cardiovascular	Congestive heart failure, cardiomegaly, tachycardia	Thiamin
	Cardiomyopathy	Selenium

From Ross Products Division, Abbott Laboratories. In Seidel HM et al: *Mosby's guide to physical examination*, ed 7, St Louis, 2011, Mosby.

PROCEDURES WITH EXPECTED FINDINGS

ROUTINE TECHNIQUES

PERFORM hand hygiene.

MEASURE height and weight for body mass index (BMI).

BMI is a weight-to-height ratio that is significantly correlated with total body fat. It is an alternative to the traditional height-weight tables for assessing nutritional status. BMI can be estimated using a BMI table (Table 8.5) or using BMI calculators readily available online. BMI can also be calculated using the formula in Box 8.1.

The normal range for BMI is 18.5 to 24.9.

ASSESS general appearance and orientation.

A well-nourished individual is alert and has a well-proportioned body that is within an acceptable weight range.

ABNORMAL FINDINGS

Patients increase their risk of developing nutrition-related problems the farther their weight varies from the normal range.
- BMI <18.5: underweight
- BMI 25–29.9: overweight
- BMI 30–34.9: obesity class I
- BMI 35–39.9: obesity class II
- BMI >40: obesity class III (extreme obesity)

Excessive obesity or generalized edema is an obvious indicator of poor nutritional status. Prominent cheek and clavicle bones or wasted-appearing limbs (cachexia) suggest malnutrition. A patient with insufficient caloric intake may be irritable or have a flat affect. Disorientation can be caused by niacin deficiency.

TABLE 8.5 BODY MASS INDEX CHART

BMI	19	20	21	22	23	24	25	26	27	28	29	30	31	32	33	34	35
HEIGHT (INCHES)								BODY WEIGHT (POUNDS)									
58	91	96	100	105	110	115	119	124	129	134	138	143	148	153	158	162	167
59	94	99	104	109	114	119	124	128	133	138	143	148	153	158	163	168	173
60	97	102	107	112	118	123	128	133	138	143	148	153	158	163	168	174	179
61	100	106	111	116	122	127	132	137	143	148	153	158	164	169	174	180	185
62	104	109	115	120	126	131	136	142	147	153	158	164	169	175	180	186	191
63	107	113	118	124	130	135	141	146	152	158	163	169	175	180	186	191	197
64	110	116	122	128	134	140	145	151	157	163	169	174	180	186	192	197	204
65	114	120	126	132	138	144	150	156	162	168	174	180	186	192	198	204	210
66	118	124	130	136	142	148	155	161	167	173	179	186	192	198	204	210	216
67	121	127	134	140	146	153	159	166	172	178	185	191	198	204	211	217	223
68	125	131	138	144	151	158	164	171	177	184	190	197	203	210	216	223	230
69	128	135	142	149	155	162	169	176	182	189	196	203	209	216	223	230	236
70	132	139	146	153	160	167	174	181	188	195	202	209	216	222	229	236	243
71	136	143	150	157	165	172	179	186	193	200	208	215	222	229	236	243	250
72	140	147	154	162	169	177	184	191	199	206	213	221	228	235	242	250	258
73	144	151	159	166	174	182	189	197	204	212	219	227	235	242	250	257	265
74	148	155	163	171	179	186	194	202	210	218	225	233	241	249	256	264	272
75	152	160	168	176	184	192	200	208	216	224	232	240	248	256	264	272	279
76	156	164	172	180	189	197	205	213	221	230	238	246	254	263	271	279	287

To use the table, find the appropriate height in the left-hand column. Move across to a given weight. The number at the top of the column is the BMI at that height and weight. Pounds have been rounded off.

From National Institutes of Health/National Heart, Lung, and Blood Institute: *Clinical guidelines on the identification, evaluation, and treatment of overweight and obesity in adults: the evidence report,* June 1998. NIH Publication 98-4093. Available at www.nhlbi.nih.gov/guidelines/obesity/ob_gdlns.pdf.

BOX 8.1 CALCULATION OF BODY MASS INDEX (BMI)

Calculation Using Kilograms and Meters

$$BMI = \frac{Weight\ (kg)}{Height\ (M^2)}$$

Calculation Using Pounds and Inches

$$BMI = \frac{Weight\ (lb) \times 705}{Height\ (in^2)}$$

Example: A woman is 65 inches tall and weighs 156 pounds.

$$156 \times \frac{705}{65^2} = \frac{109980}{4225}\ BMI\ 26.03$$

FREQUENTLY ASKED QUESTIONS

Why is body mass index (BMI) used instead of the height and weight tables?

BMI takes into account height and weight, but the difference is that a mathematic formula is applied to these data so the same range is used for all individuals. A person with a BMI between 18.5 and 25 is within the normal range, regardless of whether he or she is 5 feet 2 inches or 6 feet 7 inches tall.

PROCEDURES WITH EXPECTED FINDINGS

INSPECT the skin for surface characteristics and lesions.

The skin should be without lesions, cracks, or bruising. (See further information regarding skin assessment in Chapter 9.)

PALPATE the skin for surface characteristics and skin turgor

The skin should be smooth and elastic. (Fig. 8.2). (See further information regarding skin assessment in Chapter 9.)

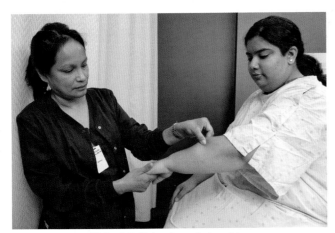

FIG. 8.2 Palpation of the skin.

INSPECT the hair and nails for appearance.

In well-nourished individuals, hair appears shiny. Nails should be pink, intact, and without deformity.

PALPATE the hair and nails for texture.

In well-nourished individuals, hair and nails should feel smooth and firm (Fig. 8.4).

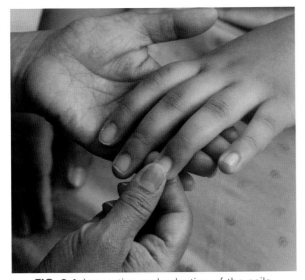

FIG. 8.4 Inspection and palpation of the nails.

ABNORMAL FINDINGS

Multiple bruises are associated with vitamin C and K deficiencies; essential fatty acid deficiencies lead to dry flaking skin and eczema.

The presence of edema indicates fluid retention (which may reflect protein depletion), whereas dry skin and decreased skin turgor may reflect dehydration. (Refer to Chapter 12 for assessment of edema.). Follicular hyperkeratosis is associated with vitamin A deficiency and creates rough patches and small bumps on the skin (Fig. 8.3).

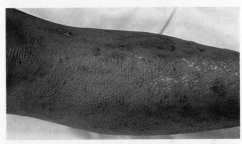

FIG. 8.3 Follicular hyperkeratosis associated with vitamin a deficiency. Note multiple clusters of follicular papules. (From Noguera-Morel et al., 2018.)

Hair that is dull and falls out easily or observable hair loss indicate protein and fatty acid deficiencies.

Spoon-shaped nails may be associated with iron deficiency (Fig. 8.5).

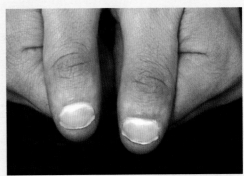

FIG. 8.5 Spoon-shaped nails. (From Thornton et al., 2010.)

PROCEDURES WITH EXPECTED FINDINGS

INSPECT the eyes for surface characteristics.

Mucous membranes (conjunctivae) around the eyes should be pink, moist, and free of lesions or drainage. The corneas should be clear and shiny (Fig. 8.6).

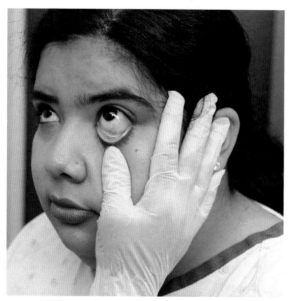

FIG. 8.6 Inspection of the conjunctiva.

INSPECT the oral cavity for dentition and intact mucous membranes.

Don examination gloves. A penlight and tongue blade are used to improve visualization of the oral cavity. The teeth should be present, clean, and intact; dentures, if present, should be assessed for fit. The mucous membranes and gums should be moist, pink, and free of lesions. The tongue and lips should be pinkish-red, smooth, and without lesions (Fig. 8.8).

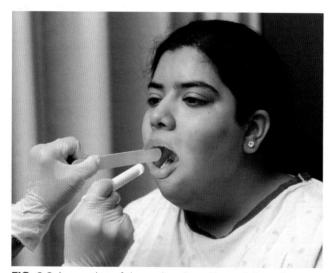

FIG. 8.8 Inspection of the oral cavity with penlight and tongue depressor.

ABNORMAL FINDINGS

Pale conjunctivae may be a sign of anemia. Excessively red conjunctivae may indicate riboflavin deficiency. Foamy-looking areas on the eyes (known as Bitot spots) or excessively dry eyes are caused by vitamin A deficiency; with further deficiency, the cornea becomes dry and hard—a condition known as xerophthalmia (Fig. 8.7).

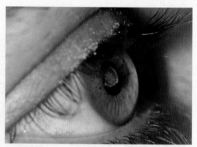

FIG. 8.7 Xerophthalmia. (Courtesy Lemmi and Lemmi, 2013.)

Poor dentition and painful oral lesions can negatively affect food intake. Dry mucous membranes may indicate dehydration. Bleeding gums may be a sign of vitamin C or vitamin K deficiency; vitamin B complex deficiency can cause cracks in the corners of the mouth or on the lips or an excessively red tongue. A reddish-purple tongue can be caused by riboflavin deficiency.

PROCEDURES WITH EXPECTED FINDINGS

INSPECT the upper and lower extremities for shape, size, and coordinated movement.

Well-developed muscles should be observed, and these should be bilaterally equal. The patient should have coordinated muscle movement.

PALPATE the upper and lower extremities for muscle strength and sensation.

The patient should have full muscle strength and full sensation to the extremities (Fig. 8.9).

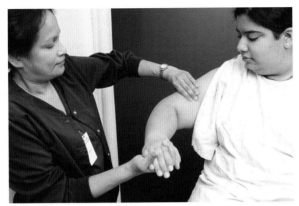

FIG. 8.9 Palpation of the extremities for muscle mass as an indication of nutritional status.

SPECIAL CIRCUMSTANCES

CALCULATE desirable body weight (DBW).

Calculate the patient's DBW and compare this to the actual body weight. These calculations allow you to express the current weight as a percentage of the DBW.

DBW is calculated using the formula in Box 8.2. The calculated weight can be increased or decreased by 10% to account for bone structure and amount of muscle or fat tissue. Ideally, the patient falls between 90% and 110% of DBW.

BOX 8.2 CALCULATION OF DESIRABLE BODY WEIGHT (DBW)

Females: 100 lb (45.5 kg) for the first 5 feet (60 inches); 5 lb (2.27 kg) for each inch greater than 5 feet; ±10%
Males: 106 lb (48 kg) for the first 5 feet (60 inches); 6 lb (2.7 kg) for each inch greater than 5 feet; = ±10%
  Express current weight as a percentage of DBW by dividing the current weight by DBW and multiplying by 100. % of DBW = Current Weight / DBW × 100

Example: A woman is 5'3" tall and weighs 130 pounds. Her desirable body weight is 115 lbs, and she is currently 113% of her DBW.

ABNORMAL FINDINGS

Muscle wasting may be a sign of inadequate protein intake or excessive protein wasting. Uncoordinated muscle movements may interfere with the ability to feed oneself. Vitamin D deficiency can cause skeletal malformation.

Muscle weakness may be a sign of inadequate protein intake or excessive protein wasting. Thiamin deficiency can cause peripheral neuropathy and paresthesia.

Patients increase their risk of developing nutrition-related problems the further their weight varies from desired body weight.
- Severely underweight: 70% or less of DBW
- Moderately underweight: 70%–80% or less of DBW
- Mild obesity: 20%–40% above DBW
- Moderate obesity: 40%–100% above DBW
- Morbid obesity: over 100% above DBW or more than 45 kg higher than DBW

PROCEDURES WITH EXPECTED FINDINGS

CALCULATE percentage change in weight.

Document the amount of weight loss over a period of time to determine the severity of weight loss.

To determine the rate of weight loss, calculate the percentage change of weight by dividing current body weight by the usual body weight (UBW) and multiplying by 100.

$$\frac{\text{Total Weight Lost}}{\text{UBW}} \times 100 = \% \text{ Weight Loss}$$

CALCULATE waist-to-hip ratio.

Waist-to-hip ratio is an indication of the risk of unhealthy fat distribution and is indicated for individuals with excessive fat on their hips or abdomen.
To obtain the waist-to-hip ratio, measure the waist at the narrowest point and the hips at the widest point. Calculate the waist-to-hip ratio using the following formula:

$$\frac{\text{Waist (inches [cm])}}{\text{Hips (inches [cm])}}$$

For example, if a man has a 44-inch (112 cm) waist and 40-inch (101 cm) hips, the calculation would be as follows:

$$\frac{112\text{cm}}{101\text{cm}} = 1.1 \text{ Waist-to-hip ratio}$$

The desired waist-to-hip ratio for women is 0.8 or less and for men is 1 or less.

ESTIMATE body fat by measuring triceps skinfold.

Skinfold measurements provide an estimate of total body fat and are typically indicated when body weight falls outside normal ranges.

Triceps skinfold measurements are made with skinfold calipers (Fig. 8.11). The nurse uses the thumb and index finger to grasp and lift a fold of skin and fat about ½ inch (1.27 cm) on the posterior aspect of the patient's arm halfway between the olecranon process (tip of the elbow) and acromial process on the lateral aspect of the scapula. The opened caliper jaws are placed horizontal to the raised skinfold; the nurse releases the lever of the calipers to make the measurement to the nearest millimeter.

Two or three measurements at the same site should be taken, and the numbers averaged. Normal ranges for triceps skinfold fat measurements for men and women are included in Table 8.6. The desired skinfold measurement falls at or near the 50th percentile. The accuracy of this measurement is related to the nurse's skill in using the calipers. Furthermore, these measurements are not useful in patients who are acutely ill because of shifts in fluid.

ABNORMAL FINDINGS

- Moderate weight loss: 1%–2% weight change over 1 week
- Severe weight loss: >2% weight change over 1 week
- Moderate weight loss: 5% weight loss over 1 month
- Severe weight loss: >5% weight loss over 1 month, >7.5% weight loss over 3 months, or >10% weight loss over 6 months[14]

A ratio that exceeds the desired ratio indicates obesity. This increases the risk of developing health problems related to obesity (e.g., diabetes, hypertension, coronary artery disease, gallbladder disease, osteoarthritis, and sleep apnea). Women typically accumulate fat on their hips, giving their bodies a pear (gynecoid) shape. However, men build up fat around their waists, giving them an apple (android) shape (Fig. 8.10).

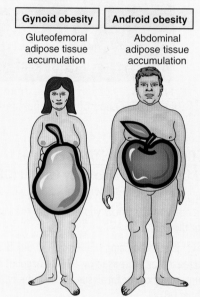

Gynoid obesity	Android obesity
Gluteofemoral adipose tissue accumulation	Abdominal adipose tissue accumulation

FIG. 8.10 Distribution of body fat. *Left,* Pear shape. *Right,* Apple shape. (From Lewis et al., 2011.)

Values significantly higher than normal can indicate increased fat mass. Values significantly lower than normal can indicate decreased fat mass secondary to an increase in lean mass or depleted fat stores.

PROCEDURES WITH EXPECTED FINDINGS

ABNORMAL FINDINGS

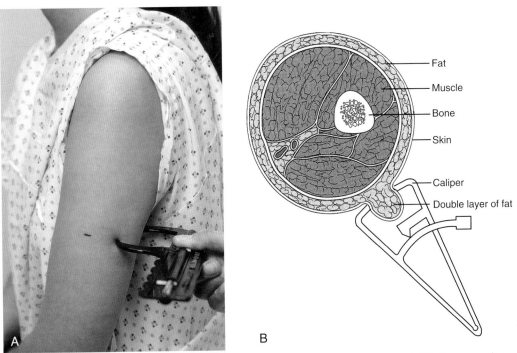

FIG. 8.11 (A) Placement of calipers for triceps skinfold thickness measurement. (B) Cross-section of arm with triceps skinfold measurement. (B, From Barkauskus et al., 2002.)

TABLE 8.6 PERCENTILES FOR TRICEPS SKINFOLD MEASUREMENTS (ADULTS)

GENDER	TRICEPS SKINFOLD		
	5TH	50TH	95TH
Males			
18–19	4	9	24
19–25	4	10	22
25–34	5	12	24
35–45	5	12	23
45–54	6	12	25
55–64	5	11	22
65–74	4	11	22
Females			
18–19	10	18	30
19–25	10	18	34
25–34	10	21	37
35–45	12	23	38
45–54	12	25	40
55–64	12	25	38
65–74	12	24	36

From Frisancho AR: New norms of upper limb fat and muscle areas for assessment of nutritional status, *Am J Clin Nutr* 34:2540–2545, 1981.

ASSESS nutritional status by reviewing laboratory tests (if available).

Laboratory tests provide additional information regarding nutritional status that may not be apparent during physical examination.
Many laboratory tests are helpful in the assessment of nutritional status. Not all of these tests are indicated for all situations. Nutritional tests include serum albumin, prealbumin, hemoglobin and hematocrit, blood glucose, lipid profile, blood urea nitrogen/creatinine ratio, and urine specific gravity.

Table 8.7 summarizes the normal ranges of laboratory tests, their purposes, and significance of abnormal findings in adults.

TABLE 8.7 LABORATORY TESTS USED FOR NUTRITIONAL ASSESSMENT

TEST AND NORMAL VALUEª	PURPOSE	SIGNIFICANCE OF ABNORMAL FINDINGS
Serum Albumin 3.5–5 g/dL or 35–50 g/L (SI units)	Serum albumin measures circulating protein; levels can be affected by fluid status, blood loss, liver function, trauma, and surgery. Fluctuations in albumin levels occur over a 3- to 4-week period.	Low albumin levels suggest protein-calorie malnutrition. Levels between 2.8 and 3.5 g/dL are consistent with moderate protein deficiency; levels below 2.5 g/dL represent severe protein depletion. Rapid changes in albumin are most likely caused by factors other than nutrition.
Prealbumin 15–36 mg/dL or 150–360 mg/L (SI units)	Prealbumin is a reflection of protein and calorie intake for the previous 2–3 days.	A deficiency of either calories or protein can cause prealbumin to decline. A malnourished individual undergoing refeeding therapy can produce rises in prealbumin levels.
Hemoglobin (Hgb) and Hematocrit (Hct) Male: Hgb 14–18 g/dL or 8.7–11.2 mmol/L (SI units); Hct 42%–52% or 0.42–0.52 volume fraction (SI units) Female: Hgb 12–16 g/dL or 7.4–9.9 mmol/L (SI units); Hct 37%–47% or 0.37–0.47 volume fraction (SI units) Pregnancy: Hgb >11 g/dL; Hct >33%	Hgb and Hct provide information regarding erythrocytes. These are clinically useful to screen for anemia caused by dietary deficiency such as iron, folate, and vitamin B_{12}. Hematocrit is also useful in evaluation of hydration.	Low Hgb and Hct levels suggest anemia. Causes of anemia are numerous, but dietary deficiencies of iron, vitamin B_{12}, or folate are a few possible causes. Elevated Hgb and Hct levels may occur in dehydration, chronic anoxia, and polycythemia.
Blood Glucose 70–105 mg/dL or 3.9–5.8 mmol/L (SI units)	Blood glucose reflects carbohydrate metabolism. A fasting glucose level is used to screen for the presence of diabetes mellitus or glucose intolerance.	Hypoglycemia (blood glucose level less than 70 mg/dL) may indicate inadequate caloric intake. Hyperglycemia (blood glucose level over 126 mg/dL) may be an indication of diabetes mellitus.
Lipid Profile *Serum Cholesterol* <200 mg/dL or 5.2 mmol/L (SI units) *Serum Triglyceride* Male: 40–160 mg/dL or 0.45–1.81 mmol/L Female: 35–135 mg/dL or 0.40–1.52 mmol/L *High-Density Lipoproteins (HDLs)* Male: >45 mg/dL or >0.75 mmol/L Female: >55 mg/dL or >0.91 mmol/L *Low-Density Lipoproteins (LDLs)* Male and female: <130 mg/dL or <3.37 mmol/L *Cholesterol to HDLs* Male: 5.0 Female: 4.4	Lipid profile includes several tests that are indicators of lipid metabolism and important determinants of risk factors for cardiovascular disease. A lipid profile includes total cholesterol and triglyceride levels, HDL level, LDL level, and cholesterol/HDL ratio. The cholesterol-to-HDL ratio is calculated by dividing the total cholesterol value by the HDL value.	Values ≥200 mg/dL for total cholesterol and triglyceride levels indicate that the patient is at increased risk for vascular disease. Elevations of LDL are associated with increased risk of developing coronary heart disease; elevated HDL levels reduce the risk.
BUN/Creatinine Ratio Up to 20:1	Blood test is used as an indication of hydration.	Levels 21:1-24:1 are associated with impending dehydration; levels >25:1 indicate dehydration.
Urine Specific Gravity	Urine test is used as an indication of hydration.	Levels >1.029 are associated with dehydration.

Data from Pagana KD, Pagana TJ, Pagana TN: *Mosby's diagnostic and laboratory test reference*, ed 13, St Louis, 2017, Mosby; and National Cancer Institute Short Dietary Assessment Instruments. 2014. http://appliedresearch.cancer.gov/diet/screeners/

ªValues for adults only; refer to a laboratory reference for other age groups.

BUN, Blood urea nitrogen; *g/dL*, gram per deciliter; *g/L*, gram per liter; *Hct*, hematocrit; *HDL*, high-density lipoprotein; *Hbg*, hemoglobin; *LDL*, low-density lipoprotein; *mg/dL*, milligram per deciliter; *mmol/L*, millimole per liter; *SI units*, International System of Units.

AGE-RELATED VARIATIONS

INFANTS AND CHILDREN

The pediatric nutritional assessment includes many of the components described for the adult, although some specific differences exist, including assessing feeding patterns; body weight; plotting weight, length, and head circumference on a growth chart; observing for the presence of rooting reflex, effective suck effort, and swallowing in infants; and observing for the presence of tooth decay in children. Childhood obesity is one of the most significant of all nutritional concerns. Chapter 19 presents further information regarding the nutritional assessment in this age group.

OLDER ADULTS

The nutritional assessment for an older adult is essentially the same as that previously described for adults with a few exceptions, including the ability to acquire and prepare food, social interactions, and general functional assessment. Chapter 21 presents further information regarding the nutritional assessment of older adults.

COMMON PROBLEMS AND CONDITIONS

OBESITY

Obesity occurs when there is greater energy intake than energy expenditure. This condition is caused by genetics, overeating, and inactivity. The number of overweight or obese children, adolescents, and adults has become an epidemic and contributes to significant morbidity and mortality. In the United States, more than two-thirds of adults are classified as overweight or obese; 7.6% of the adult population is extremely obese.[15] Obesity may increase the risk for health problems such as type 2 diabetes mellitus, hypertension, heart disease, cerebrovascular accidents, arthritis, and sleep apnea.[16] **Clinical Findings:** Obesity is characterized by excessive adipose tissue on the face and neck, trunk, and extremities (Fig. 8.12). Overweight, obesity, and extreme obesity are clinically defined as BMI greater than 25, 30, and 40, respectively.

HYPERLIPIDEMIA

This condition is associated with elevated serum lipids that can include cholesterol, triglycerides, and phospholipids. Causes include excessive dietary fat and genetics. An estimated 95 million American adults have total blood cholesterol values of 200 mg/dL and higher, and an estimated 29 million adult Americans have total cholesterol levels higher than 240 mg/dL.[17] **Clinical Findings:** Hyperlipidemia is not associated with any clinical symptoms until a significant cardiovascular event occurs. Biochemical indications include elevations in serum lipids. In adults, total cholesterol levels from 200 to 239 mg/dL are considered borderline high; levels of 240 mg/dL or higher are considered high.[18]

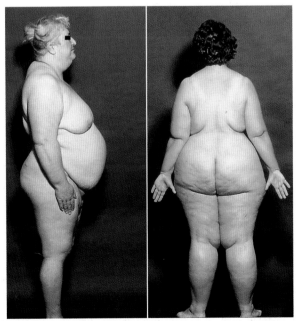

FIG. 8.12 Obesity. (From Forbes and Jackson, 2003.)

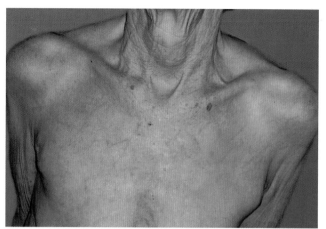

FIG. 8.13 Loss of subcutaneous fat and muscle wasting. (Courtesy Lemmi and Lemmi, 2013.)

PROTEIN-CALORIE MALNUTRITION

Protein-calorie malnutrition (PCM) refers to the state of inadequate protein and calorie intake. PCM is the most common form of undernutrition and can result from poor or limited food intake, a wasting disease (such as cancer), malabsorption syndromes, endocrine imbalances, or poor living conditions. Among the hospitalized elderly, up to 65% are undernourished; up to 60% of elderly who live in an institutional setting are undernourished.[19]

Clinical Findings: The malnourished individual often appears thin with muscle wasting and a loss of subcutaneous fat (Fig. 8.13) and other protein deficiency findings presented in Table 8.4. One is considered underweight when one's body mass index is less than 18.5 or if more than 10% below desired body weight. Biochemical indications such as low serum levels of albumin or protein may exist.

EATING DISORDERS

Eating disorders refer to a group of psychiatric conditions resulting in altered food consumption. Three prevalent

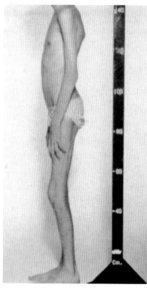

FIG. 8.14 Extreme weight loss associated with anorexia nervosa. (From Taylor, 1995.)

eating disorders are anorexia nervosa, bulimia nervosa, and binge-eating disorder. An estimated 9% of women and 3% of men experience anorexia nervosa during their lifetime; the lifetime bulimia nervosa prevalence is 5% of women and 1% of men. Binge eating disorders affect an estimated 2% of men and women.[20]

Clinical Findings: The clinical manifestations vary based on the type of eating disorder. *Anorexia nervosa:* refusing to eat, extreme thinness, along with other symptoms of PCM (Fig. 8.14). *Bulimia nervosa:* recurrent binge-and-purge eating cycles, electrolyte imbalances, chronic irritation or erosion of the pharynx, esophagus, and teeth (from exposure to hydrochloric acid). *Binge-eating disorder:* consumption of large quantities of food until uncomfortably full. Frequently the individual experiences feelings of being out of control during the binge episodes.

CLINICAL APPLICATION AND CLINICAL JUDGMENT

See Appendix B for answers to exercises in this section.

CASE STUDY

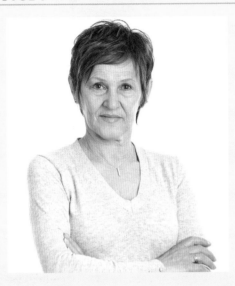

Marian Parker is a 45-year-old woman who is brought to the hospital after an episode of fainting.

Interview Data

Ms. Parker states that she has been very tired lately and gets short of breath and tires very easily. She also complains of cracks in the corners of her mouth that won't heal. When asked about her diet, she tells the nurse that she is a "new vegetarian." She states that she started a vegetarian diet about 4 months ago "to prevent diseases and because animals are unclean." She acknowledges weight loss since starting the diet but states, "I am healthy because of what I eat and because I am thin." She refuses foods that contain meat or animal products. Her diet is described as "healthy"; she typically eats beans, rice, breads, and salad. She is not specific about portions, stating, "I eat until I'm full." Her fluid intake consists of coffee, tea, and water. She does not use drugs or alcohol. She also tells the nurse that her financial resources are very limited.

Examination Data

- *Vital signs and other measurements:* blood pressure, 118/76 mm Hg; pulse, 92 beats/min; respirations, 20 breaths/min; temperature, 98.2°F (36.8°C); height, 5 feet 4 inches (162 cm); weight, 110 lb (50 kg)
- *General observation:* Very thin, protruding bony prominence to cheeks and clavicles
- *Skin:* Warm, very dry with scaling—especially on arms and legs
- *Hair:* Brown, thin, dull, easily plucked
- *Oral cavity:* Pink, moist mucous membranes without lesions; teeth present, in good repair; cracks noted in corners of mouth
- *Eyes:* Pale conjunctivae; no drainage or lesions
- *Extremities:* Bilaterally equal; extremities thin; small amount of muscle mass noted; muscle strength 4/5

Clinical Judgment

1. What cues do you recognize that suggest a deviation from normal findings, prompting a need for further investigation?
2. For which additional information should you ask or assess?
3. Which risk factors for nutritional problems can be identified?
4. Which additional health care professionals should you consider collaborating with to meet her health care needs?

REVIEW QUESTIONS

1. The nurse calculates the body mass index of a patient at 31.8. What is the most appropriate action of the nurse?
   1. Refer the patient for behavioral interventions for weight loss.
   2. Estimate body fat using tricep skinfold measurement.
   3. Calculate the percent of change in weight since the last visit.
   4. Calculate grams of fat that patient consumed daily.

2. A man weighs 265 pounds and is 6 feet 4 inches tall. Based on these data, how does the nurse classify his weight?
   1. Overweight
   2. Class I obesity
   3. Class II obesity
   4. Class III obesity

3. An older woman is 5 feet 2 inches tall and weighs 100 pounds. To best understand her dietary intake, which question is most appropriate?
   1. "Who prepares your meals on a daily basis?"
   2. "What are your favorite foods?"
   3. "How do you get to the grocery store each week?"
   4. "What you eat on a typical day?"

4. Why does the nurse ask about medications taken as part of a nutritional assessment?
   1. Medications must be taken with food to avoid irritation to the gastrointestinal system.
   2. Actions of many drugs require adjustments to the diet.
   3. The absorption and bioavailability of some medications are affected by food.
   4. Some medications taste bad and may interfere with the appetite.

5. A patient reports "a lot" of unintentional weight loss over the past 4 months. The nurse measures his height and weight (5 feet 11 inches, 170 pounds) and determines that his body mass index is 22.7. Which action is most appropriate to better evaluate his recent weight loss?
   1. Calculate his desirable body weight.
   2. Ask, "What is your usual body weight?"
   3. Record what he ate in the last 24 hours.
   4. Determine his hip-to-waist ratio.

Skin, Hair, and Nails

evolve

http://evolve.elsevier.com/Wilson/assessment

CONCEPT OVERVIEW

The feature concept for this chapter is *Tissue Integrity*. This concept represents the structural intactness and physiologic function of tissues and conditions that affect integrity. In this chapter the tissues referred to are skin, hair, and nails. Several concepts are interrelated to tissue integrity and include perfusion, gas exchange, nutrition, motion, tactile sensory perception, elimination, and pain. These are shown in the illustration.

The maintenance of tissue integrity requires adequate perfusion to carry oxygenated blood and nutrients to tissues; interference with perfusion results in tissue injury or necrosis. Adequate nutrition is also required to maintain tissues. Sustained pressure over tissue may occur if an individual has limited motion and/or limited tactile sensory perception. Urinary or bowel incontinence can also contribute to impairment of tissue integrity. Finally, a loss of tissue integrity often results in pain. Understanding the interrelationships among these concepts helps the nurse recognize risk factors and thus increases awareness when conducting a health assessment.

The following case provides a clinical example featuring several of these interrelated concepts.

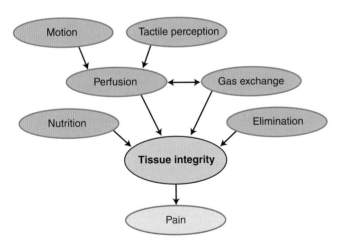

Roberta is a 24-year-old female who has been confined to a wheelchair for the last 2 years as a result of a spinal cord disease that has left her partially paralyzed. She has been very depressed, resulting in poor appetite and weight loss over the last 18 months. She has developed skin breakdown over her sacrum as a result of sustained pressure that impaired perfusion (caused by reduced motion and tactile sensation); the condition is exacerbated by her poor nutritional status.

ANATOMY AND PHYSIOLOGY

The skin and the accessory structures (i.e., hair, nails, sweat glands, and sebaceous glands) form what is referred to as the *integumentary system.* The skin is an elastic, self-regenerating cover for the entire body. Because they are composed of several tissues that perform specialized tasks, the skin and related structures are considered a body organ. The skin has several important functions. The primary functions are to protect the body from microbial and foreign-substance invasion and to protect internal body structures from minor physical trauma.

The skin also helps retain body fluids and electrolytes; without skin, an individual would suffer tremendous water loss. The skin provides the body with its primary contact with the outside world, providing sensory input about the environment. Its sensitive surface detects and reports comfort factors such as temperature and surface textures, enabling the body to adapt through either temperature regulation or position changes. This regulation of body temperature is accomplished continuously through radiation, conduction, convection, and

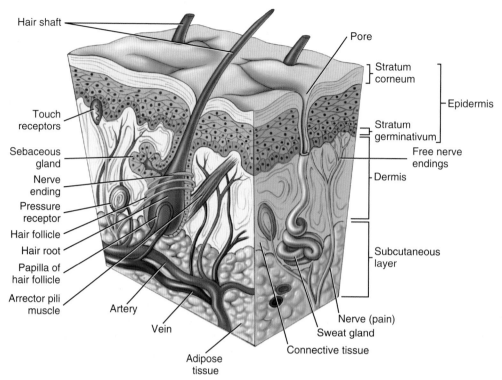

FIG. 9.1 Anatomic structures of the skin and hair. (From Herlihy, 2011.)

evaporation. Other functions of the skin include production of vitamin D; excretion of sweat, urea, and lactic acid; expression of emotion (e.g., blushing); and even repair of its own surface wounds through the normal process of cell replacement. The skin and appendages often mirror systemic disease and thus may provide valuable clues to an internal disorder such as jaundice resulting from liver disease.

SKIN

The skin is composed of three layers that are functionally related: the epidermis; the dermis; and the subcutaneous layer, also known as the *hypodermis*. The main components of each of these layers and their functional and spatial relationships are shown in Fig. 9.1.

Epidermis

The epidermis is the thin, outermost layer of the skin and is composed of stratified squamous epithelium. This layer of skin is *avascular*, meaning that it has no direct blood supply. The deepest aspect of the epidermis is the stratum germinativum. This layer lies adjacent to the dermis, which provides a rich supply of blood. Within this deepest layer of epidermis, active cell generation takes place. As cells are produced, they push up the older cells toward the skin surface. As the cells move toward the surface, they undergo a process known as *keratinization*, in which keratin (a protein) is deposited, causing the cells to become flat, hard, and waterproof. The outermost aspect of the epidermis, the stratum corneum, is composed of 30 layers of

these flattened, keratinized cells. This exposed layer serves as the protective barrier and regulates water loss. The cells are continuously sloughed off and replaced by new cells moving up from the underlying epidermal layers. The entire process takes approximately 30 days.

Melanocytes, located in the basal cell layer of the epidermis, secrete melanin, which provides pigment for the skin and hair and serves as a shield against ultraviolet radiation.

Dermis

The dermis comprises of highly vascular connective tissue. The blood vessels dilate and constrict in response to external heat and cold and internal stimuli such as anxiety or hemorrhage, resulting in the regulation of body temperature and blood pressure. The dermal blood nourishes the epidermis, and the dermal connective tissue provides support for the outer layer. The dermis also contains sensory nerve fibers that react to touch, pain, and temperature. The arrangement of connective tissue enables the dermis to stretch and contract with body movement. Dermal thickness varies from 1 to 4 mm in different parts of the body.

Subcutaneous Layer

The subcutaneous tissue (hypodermis) is not actually skin tissue but a support structure for the dermis and epidermis—literally acting as an anchor for these upper layers. This layer is composed primarily of loose connective tissue interspersed with subcutaneous fat. These fatty cells help to retain heat, provide a protective cushion, and provide calories.

APPENDAGES

Hair, nails, and glands (the eccrine sweat glands, the apocrine sweat glands, and the sebaceous glands) are considered appendages. These structures are formed at the junction of the epidermis and the dermis.

Hair

Epidermal cells in the dermis form hair. Each hair consists of a root, a shaft, and a follicle (the root and its covering). At the base of the follicle is the papilla, a capillary loop that supplies nourishment for growth. Melanocytes within the hair shaft provide color. Variations in hair color, density, and pattern of distribution vary considerably as a result of age, gender, race, and hereditary factors. Structures of the hair follicle are shown in Fig. 9.1.

Nails

Nails are really epidermal cells converted to hard plates of keratin. The nails assist in grasping small objects and protect the fingertips from trauma. The nail is composed of a free edge, the nail plate, and the nail root (i.e., the site of nail growth). The white, crescent-shaped area at the base, the lunula, represents new nail growth (Fig. 9.2). Skin tissue adjacent to the nail is referred to as *paronychium;* the cuticle is epidermal tissue (stratum corneum) that grows on the nail plate at the nail base. Tissue directly under the nail plate is highly vascular, providing clues to oxygenation status and perfusion.

Eccrine Sweat Glands

Eccrine sweat glands regulate body temperature by water secretion through the surface of the skin. They are the most numerous and widespread sweat glands on the body. They

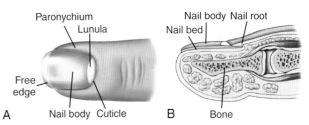

FIG. 9.2 Structures of the nail. (A) External structures. (B) Internal structures. (From Herlihy, 2011.)

are distributed almost everywhere throughout the surface of the skin, found in greatest numbers on the palms of the hands, the soles of the feet, and the forehead. Sweat glands are controlled primarily by the nervous system.

Apocrine Sweat Glands

These structures are much larger and deeper than the eccrine glands and are found only in the axillae, nipples, areolae, anogenital area, eyelids, and external ears. They begin secretion at puberty and are strongly influenced by hormones. In response to emotional stimuli, the glands secrete an odorless fluid containing protein, carbohydrates, and other substances. Decomposition of apocrine sweat produces what we associate with body odor.

Sebaceous Glands

These glands secrete a lipid-rich substance called *sebum,* which keeps the skin and hair lubricated. The greatest distribution of sebaceous glands is found on the face and scalp, although they are found in all areas of the body with the exception of the palms and soles. Sebum secretion, stimulated by sex hormone activity, accelerates during puberty and varies throughout the life span.

HEALTH HISTORY

Nurses interview patients to collect subjective data about their present health and any past experiences. In addition to present health status, past health history, family history, and personal and psychosocial history, nurses ask patients about their home environment, occupational environment, and travel, which may affect the health condition of their skin, hair, and nails.

GENERAL HEALTH HISTORY

Present Health Status

Do you have any chronic illnesses? If so, describe.
Some chronic illnesses (e.g., liver failure, renal failure, venous insufficiency, autoimmune disease) cause changes to the skin such as pruritus, excessive dryness, discoloration, and skin lesions.

Do you take any medications (prescription or over-the-counter) or herbal supplements? If so, what do you take and how often? What are the medications for?

Medications can cause a number of adverse effects that are manifested in the skin, including allergic reactions, lesions associated with photosensitivity, or other systemic effects such as acne, thinning of the skin, and stretch marks. The nurse should document medications that are used to treat skin problems.

Do you have any allergies to medications, foods, or things in the environment?
Allergic reactions can be triggered by a number of substances that often manifest as hives or rashes on the skin.

Have you noticed any changes in the way your skin, hair, or nails look or feel? Any changes in the sensation of your skin? If so, where? Describe.
Ask patients if they have noticed changes as opposed to asking them if they have any problems, because they may not perceive skin or hair changes as a "problem." The development of lesions or other changes such as how the skin feels may indicate a skin condition or an underlying systemic disease.

Past Health History

Have you ever had problems with your skin such as skin disease, infections involving the skin or nails, or trauma involving the skin? If so, describe.

Past skin injuries and conditions may provide clues to current skin lesions or findings.

Family History

Has anyone in your family ever had skin-related problems such as skin cancer or autoimmune-related disorders such as systemic lupus erythematosus?

A family history helps determine predisposition to certain skin disorders. Some skin disorders (such as skin cancer) have familial or genetic links.[1] Autoimmune disorders tend to be familial and may manifest in a number of ways, including rash and alopecia.

Personal and Psychosocial History

What do you do to keep your skin healthy (e.g., hygiene measures, use of lotions, protection from sun exposure, use of sunscreen)?

Health care practices may provide clues for underlying skin problems and areas for education. Specifically determine products and the frequency they are used. Excessive exposure to sun and ultraviolet light is a known risk factor for skin cancer.[1]

What type of work do you do? To your knowledge are you exposed to chemicals at home or in the workplace? If so, describe.

Dangerous chemicals are found in the home and in the workplace. According to the Centers for Disease Control and Prevention, an estimated 13 million workers in the United States are potentially exposed to chemicals that can be absorbed through the skin and can lead to adverse health.[2] Occupations with highest incidence of chemical exposures to the skin include food service, cosmetology, health care, agriculture, cleaning, painting, mechanics, printing/lithography, and construction.[3,4]

RISK FACTORS

Skin Cancer

- Personal history of skin cancer
- Family history of skin cancer
- Older age
- Exposure to ultraviolet (UV) radiation
  - Lifetime sun exposure (M)
  - Severe, blistering sunburns, especially at early age (M)
  - Indoor tanning (M)
- Fair skin; blond or red hair
- Blue or green eyes
- Moles (large numbers of common moles or a dysplastic nevus)

M, Modifiable risk factor.
Center for Disease Control: What are the Risk Factors for Skin Cancer? 2020. Available at www.cdc.gov/cancer/skin/basic_info/risk_factors.htm

---

PROBLEM-BASED HISTORY

Commonly reported symptoms of skin disease include pruritus, rashes, pain, lesions, changes in skin color and texture, and wounds. Data about changes or symptoms related to hair and nails are also reported. As with symptoms in all areas of health assessment, the nurse completes a symptom analysis using the mnemonic OLD CARTS, which stands for the *O*nset, *L*ocation, *D*uration, *C*haracteristics, *A*ggravating factors, *R*elated symptoms, *T*reatment, and *S*everity (Box 2.6).

Skin

Pruritus (Itching)

When did the itching first start? Did it start suddenly or gradually? Where did it start? Has it spread?

Understanding the onset and location of the pruritus may provide clues to the cause.

Does anything make the itching worse? Is there anything that relieves it? What have you done to treat yourself?

Document characteristics and aggravating and alleviating factors of the pruritus; these data may provide clues to the cause. For example, if taking an antihistamine relieves the itch, the cause may be an allergy.

What were the circumstances when you first noticed the itching? Taking medications? Contact with possible allergens such as animals, foods, drugs, plants? Do you have dry or sensitive skin?

Common factors causing pruritus include excessively dry or sensitive skin; an allergic response (hives); exposure to chemicals; or infestation of scabies, lice, or insect bites. Systemic diseases such as biliary cirrhosis and some types of cancer such as lymphoma may also cause pruritus.[5]

Rash

When did the rash start? Where did you first notice the rash? Describe the appearance of the rash initially: Flat? Raised? Has the rash been there constantly or does it come and go?

Determining onset, location, and duration of the rash may provide clues to the cause.

Does the rash itch or burn? What makes it better? Worse? What have you done to treat it? Have you noticed any other symptoms associated with this rash such as joint pains, fatigue, or fever?

Document related symptoms, aggravating factors, and self-treatment measures to better understand the cause.

Do you have any known allergies to plants, skin/hair products, laundry detergent, chemicals, or animals? Does anyone else in your family have a similar rash? Have you been exposed to others with a similar rash?

A rash is not generally a disease in itself but rather a symptom of an allergic response, skin disorder, or systemic illness. Some of these questions help differentiate the cause of the rash.

Pain

When did the pain start? Describe its location. Does the pain spread anywhere? Does the pain stay on the skin surface, or does it go deep inside?
There are multiple causes of skin pain; onset and location are important factors in determining the cause.

Describe the pain (e.g., sharp, dull, achy, burning, itching). How bad is your pain on a scale of 0 to 10? Is it constant, or does it come and go? If constant, does the pain vary? If pain comes and goes, how long does it last?
Document characteristics of the pain to better understand the cause.

What triggers the pain? Are there things that make it worse? Better?
Document aggravating factors and measures of self-treatment for the pain.

Lesion or Changes in Mole

Describe the lesion with which you are concerned. Where is the lesion? When did you first notice it? Do you have any symptoms associated with the lesion such as pain, pruritus, or drainage? If so, describe.
Lesions may result from acne, trauma, infections, exposure to chemicals or other irritants, tumors, or other systemic disease.

Describe the changes you have noticed in the mole (i.e., color, shape, texture, tenderness, bleeding, or itching).
A changing or irregular mole may be a sign of a malignant lesion.[6]

Change in Skin Color

Have there been any generalized changes in your skin color such as a yellowish tone or paleness?
Changes in overall skin color or tone may be reported such as pale tone, yellowish tone, reddish color, and brown. Skin color changes can be caused by medications, anemia, poor circulation, and systemic disease.

Have there been any localized changes in your skin color such as redness, discoloration of one or both feet, or areas of bruises or patches? What do you think caused the change in skin color?
Localized changes may be associated with changes in tissue perfusion, causing a discoloration to the affected area, cyanosis, bruising (may be a sign of a hematologic condition, abuse, frequent falls), or vitiligo (i.e., a loss of pigmentation in the skin).

Skin Texture

In what way has the texture of your skin changed (e.g., skin thinning, fragile, excessive dryness)?
Changes in the skin texture may be expected (e.g., associated with aging) or may indicate a metabolic or nutritional problem.

Do you have excessively dry (xerosis) or oily (seborrhea) skin? If so, is it seasonal, intermittent, or continuous? What do you do to treat it?
A history of dry skin may provide information about an existing systemic disease (e.g., thyroid disease), or it may be related to an environmental condition such as low humidity. Dry skin may also be associated with poor skin lubrication.

Wounds

Where is your wound located? What caused it? How long have you had it? Do you have any associated symptoms such as pain or drainage? If so, describe.
The location of a wound and how long it has been there may provide clues to its cause. For example, chronic wounds on the lower legs suggest problems with peripheral perfusion. Leg ulcers associated with venous insufficiency tend to recur after healing.[7] If the explanation for the cause of the wound does not seem to fit, suspect interpersonal violence.

What have you done to treat the wound?
Self-treatment of a wound may provide insight to the appearance, particularly if the patient reports problems associated with wound healing.

Do you typically have problems with wound healing?
A history of problems associated with wound healing can point to nutritional or metabolic problems, infection, or poor circulation.

Hair

What changes or problems with your hair are you experiencing? When did you notice the changes? Did they occur suddenly or gradually?
Establish the type of problem, the onset, and the nature of the changes with the hair. Common problems associated with hair include excessive dryness, brittleness, hair loss, and pain/dryness to the scalp.

Can you think of any factors contributing to the problems or changes? Have you recently experienced stress? Fever? Other illness? Itching? What kind of hair products have been used recently?
Reports of changes in the hair such as excessive dryness or brittle hair may indicate stress or systemic disease. Exposure to hair care products may account for changes in texture or condition of hair.

Has there been a change in your diet in the last few months?
Nutritional deficiencies may be observed by changes in hair appearance or texture. For example, dullness and hair that is easily plucked could be caused by a protein deficiency.

Have you noticed any changes in the distribution of hair growth on your arms or legs?
A decrease in hair growth on an extremity, particularly the lower extremity, may be associated with aging or may

indicate underlying medical conditions such as hypothyroidism, immune system conditions, and reduced peripheral circulation.[8] Increased hair growth may be caused by an ovarian or adrenal tumor.

Nails

What type of problems or changes are you experiencing with your nails? When did you first notice them?
The appearance and consistency of the fingernails and toenails may be important signs about the patient's general health. Hyperthyroidism may cause the nail to separate from the nail bed and make the nail appear "dirty."

Are your nails brittle? Have you noticed a pitting type of pattern to your nails?
Pitting, brittle nails, crumbling, and changes in color can be caused by nutritional deficiencies, systemic diseases, or localized fungal infections.

Do you chew your nails? Do you now have, or have you ever had, an infection of the nail or around the nail bed? If so, describe.
Patients who have a habit of nail biting may use the biting as an unconscious way to handle stress. The nails may show signs of local infection such as fungal infection.

HEALTH PROMOTION FOR EVIDENCE-BASED PRACTICE

Skin Cancer

Skin cancer is the most common cancer, accounting for almost half of all cancers. The number of nonmelanoma (basal and squamous cell) skin cancers is difficult to estimate because reporting these types of cancers is not required. However, estimates are that more than 3 million cases are diagnosed per year. An estimated 100,350 new cases of melanoma were diagnosed in the United States in 2020. The estimated number of skin cancer–related deaths in 2020 was 11,480, of which 6800 were related to melanoma. In the elderly, melanoma tends to be diagnosed at a later stage and is more likely to be lethal.

Recommendations to Reduce Risk (Primary Prevention)
American Cancer Society
- Skin should be protected from sun exposure by
  - Wearing clothing made of tightly woven material and wearing a wide-brimmed hat.
- Applying sunscreen that has sun protection factor (SPF) of 15 or higher to exposed skin (even on cloudy or hazy days).
- Wearing sunglasses to protect the skin around the eyes.
- Seeking shade (especially at midday) whenever possible.
- Avoiding sunbathing and indoor tanning.

United States Preventative Services Task Force
- Recommends counseling parents of children and young adults about minimizing exposure to ultraviolet radiation between ages 6 months to 24 years to reduce cancer risk.

Screening Recommendations (Secondary Prevention)
American Cancer Society
- Adults should examine their skin periodically; new or unusual lesions should be evaluated promptly by a health care provider.
- Use the ABCDE mnemonic for evaluating lesions (see Box 9.1).

From American Cancer Society: *Cancer facts & figures 2020*, Atlanta, 2020, American Cancer Society; United States Preventive Services Task Force: Skin Cancer Prevention: Behavioral Counseling, 2018. Retrieved from https://www.uspreventiveservicestaskforce.org/Page/Document/UpdateSummaryFinal/skin-cancer-counseling2?ds=1&s=skin%20cancer.

EXAMINATION

Routine Techniques
- INSPECT the skin.
- PALPATE the skin.
- INSPECT and PALPATE the scalp and hair.
- INSPECT facial and body hair.
- INSPECT and PALPATE the nails.

Techniques for Special Circumstances
- INSPECT and PALPATE skin lesions.

Equipment needed
- Light source (e.g., overhead light, penlight) • Centimeter ruler • Magnifying lens if required • Gloves (if open lesions present)
- Wood's lamp

PROCEDURES WITH EXPECTED FINDINGS	ABNORMAL FINDINGS

ROUTINE TECHNIQUES

Start with a general survey, noticing the color of the skin, general pigmentation, vascularity or bruising, and lesions or discoloration. Note any unusual odors. Next inspect and palpate the skin more closely, moving systematically from the head and neck to the trunk, arms, legs, and back. In a head-to-toe assessment you can examine the skin in conjunction with other body systems. Before you begin, be sure to have adequate lighting so that subtle changes are not missed. Be alert for cuts, bruises, scratches, and welts that may indicate interpersonal violence, especially when the explanation for their cause does not seem to fit the lesions observed.

PERFORM hand hygiene.
INSPECT the skin for general color.

Inspect the skin for general color and uniformity of color. The skin color should be consistent over the body surface, with the exception of vascular areas such as the cheeks, upper chest, and genitalia, which may appear pink or have a reddish-purple tone. The normal range of skin color varies from whitish pink to olive tones to deep brown. Table 9.1 compares clinical findings of patients with light and dark skin. Sun-exposed areas may show evidence of slightly darker pigmentation.

Abnormal skin color may be evidence of local or systemic disease. Common abnormal findings of particular importance include *cyanosis, pallor,* and *jaundice* (see Table 9.1). Less common findings include:
- *Hypopigmentation,* also known as *albinism* (a complete absence of pigmentation; pale white skin tone is noted over the entire body surface).
- *Hyperpigmentation* (increased melanin deposition) may be an indication of an endocrine disorder (e.g., Addison's disease) or liver disease.

TABLE 9.1 COMPARISON OF SKIN-RELATED FINDINGS IN LIGHT- AND DARK-SKINNED PATIENTS

CLINICAL SIGN	LIGHT SKIN	DARK SKIN
Cyanosis	Grayish-blue tone, especially in nail beds, earlobes, lips, mucous membranes, palms, and soles of feet	Ashen-gray color most easily seen in the conjunctiva of the eye, oral mucous membranes, and nail beds
Ecchymosis (bruise)	Dark red, purple, yellow, or green color, depending on age of bruise	Deeper bluish or black tone; difficult to see unless it occurs in an area of light pigmentation
Erythema	Reddish tone with evidence of increased skin temperature secondary to inflammation	Deeper brown or purple skin tone with evidence of increased skin temperature secondary to inflammation
Jaundice	Yellowish color of skin, sclera of eyes, fingernails, palms of hands, and oral mucosa	Yellowish-green color most obviously seen in sclera of eye (do not confuse with yellow eye pigmentation, which may be evident in dark-skinned patients), palms of hands, and soles of feet
Pallor	Pale skin color that may appear white	Skin tone appears lighter than normal; light-skinned African Americans may have yellowish-brown skin; dark-skinned African Americans may appear ashen; specifically evident is a loss of the underlying healthy red tones of the skin
Petechiae	Lesions appear as small, reddish-purple pinpoints	Difficult to see; may be evident in the buccal mucosa of the mouth or sclera of the eye
Rash	May be visualized and felt with light palpation	Not easily visualized but may be felt with light palpation
Scar	Narrow scar line	Frequently has keloid development, resulting in a thickened, raised scar

PROCEDURES WITH EXPECTED FINDINGS

INSPECT the skin for localized variations in skin color.

Almost all healthy individuals have natural variations in skin pigmentation. A common intentional localized variation in skin color is a tattoo. If a tattoo is present, its location and the characteristics of the surrounding areas should be examined and documented. Normal localized variations of the skin pigmentation include the following:

- *Pigmented nevi (moles):* Moles are considered an expected finding; most adults have between 10 and 40 moles scattered over the body. They are commonly located above the waist on sun-exposed body surfaces (chest, back, arms, legs, and face). They tend to be uniformly tan to dark brown, are typically less than 5 mm in size, and may be raised or flat. The expected shape of a mole is round or oval with a clearly defined border (see Table 9.2 later in this chapter).
- *Freckles:* Freckles are small, flat, hyperpigmented macules that may appear anywhere on the body, particularly on sun-exposed areas of the skin. Common locations are on the face, arms, and back.
- *Patch:* A patch is an area of darker skin pigmentation that is usually brown or tan and typically is present at birth (birthmarks). Some of these patches fade, but many do not change over time (see Table 9.2 later in the chapter).
- *Striae:* Striae are silver or pink "stretch marks" secondary to weight gain or pregnancy.

BOX 9.1 EARLY SIGNS OF MELANOMA

To help you remember the early signs of melanoma, use the mnemonic ABCDE

A—Asymmetry (not round or oval)
B—Border (poorly defined or irregular border)
C—Color (uneven, variegated)
D—Diameter (usually greater than 6 mm)
E—Evolving (a skin lesion that looks different from others or is changing in size, shape, or color)

ABNORMAL FINDINGS

Melanoma: The nurse should be familiar with abnormal characteristics of pigmented moles that might point to melanoma (Box 9.1). Moles located below the waist or on the scalp or breast are rarely "normal" moles.

Vitiligo is an acquired condition associated with the development of unpigmented patch or patches; it is more common in dark-skinned races and is thought to be an autoimmune disorder (see Table 9.2 later in this chapter).

Localized areas of hyperpigmentation may be associated with endocrine disorders (pituitary, adrenal) and autoimmune disorders (systemic lupus erythematosus).

Look for areas of maceration, discoloration, or rashes under skinfolds (Fig. 9.3).

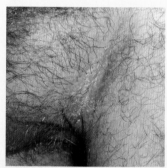

FIG. 9.3 Maceration in a skinfold. (From Habif, 2010.)

⊕ ETHNIC, CULTURAL, AND SPIRITUAL VARIATIONS

Coining and Cupping

- Coining is a treatment practiced by various cultures particularly in southeastern Asian. The body is rubbed vigorously with a coin or scraped with a spoon while exerting pressure until red marks appear over the bony prominence of the rib cage on the back and chest. Marks created by this treatment have been mistaken as signs of abuse or mistreatment.
- Cupping is an alternative medicine therapy for arthritis, stomach aches, bruises, and paralysis. Glass cups with negative pressure are applied to the skin; the negative pressure may be achieved by heating the air in the cups before application. As a result of the heat, the cup adheres to the skin and may leave a reddened area or mark. An alternative mechanism is the use of a rubber pump that creates a vacuum. This is practiced by Latin American and Russian cultures.

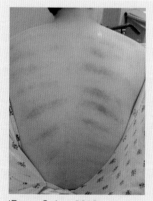

(From Saks, 2016.)

From Vitale SA, Prashad T: Cultural awareness: coining and cupping, *International archives of Nursing and Health Care* 3(3), 2017. DOI 10.23937/2469-5823/1510080

PROCEDURES WITH EXPECTED FINDINGS	ABNORMAL FINDINGS

PALPATE the skin for texture, temperature, moisture, mobility, turgor, and thickness.

Texture

The skin should be smooth, soft, and intact, with an even surface. Expected variations include calluses over the hands, feet, elbows, and knees.

Excessive dryness, flaking, cracking, or scaling of the skin may occur secondary to environmental conditions or may be signs of systemic disease or nutritional deficiency.

Temperature

The skin temperature is best evaluated using the dorsal aspect of your hands. The skin should be warm. The skin temperature should be consistent for the entire body with the exception of the hands and feet, which may be cooler, particularly in a cool environment.

Cool skin: Generalized cool or cold skin is an abnormal finding and may be associated with shock or hypothermia. Localization of cold skin, particularly in the extremities, may be an indication of poor peripheral perfusion.

Hot skin: Generalized hot skin may reflect hyperthermia, associated with a fever, increased metabolic rate (e.g., hyperthyroidism), or exercise. Localized areas of skin that are hot may reflect an inflammation, infection, traumatic injury, or thermal injury such as sunburn.

Moisture

The skin is normally dry. There should be minimal perspiration or oiliness, although increased perspiration may be an expected finding associated with increased environmental temperatures, strenuous activity, or anxiety.

Diaphoresis (excessive sweating) is an abnormal finding in the absence of strenuous activity. This may indicate hyperthermia, extreme anxiety, pain, or shock. Excessively moist skin may often be seen with metabolic conditions such as hyperthyroidism.[9]

Mobility and Turgor

Skin mobility and turgor are assessed by picking up and slightly pinching the skin on the forearm or under the clavicle. The skin should be elastic (i.e., move easily when lifted) and return to place immediately when released. The technique and expected findings for skin turgor are shown in Fig. 9.4.

Edema, excessive scarring to the skin, or some connective tissue disorders (such as scleroderma) reduce skin mobility. Poor skin turgor is noted if "tenting" is observed or the skin slowly recedes back into place. Decreased turgor may result from dehydration or may be a finding in an individual who has experienced significant weight loss (Fig. 9.5).

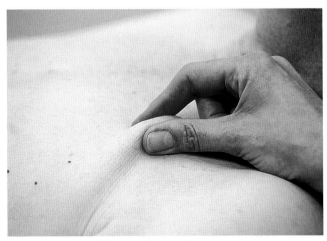

FIG. 9.4 Elastic skin turgor.

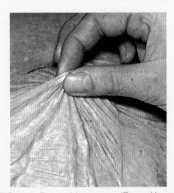

FIG. 9.5 Poor skin turgor. (From Kamal and Brocklehurst, 1991.)

PROCEDURES WITH EXPECTED FINDINGS

Thickness

Skin thickness varies based on age and area of the body. Skin thickens until adulthood and decreases in thickness after age 20. The skin is thickest over the palms of hands and soles of feet and thinnest over the eyelids. A callus is an area of excessive thickening of skin that is an expected variation associated with friction or pressure over a particular surface area. A callus is commonly found on the hands or feet.

INSPECT the scalp and hair for surface characteristics, hair distribution, quantity, and color and PALPATE the scalp and hair for texture.

The scalp should be smooth to palpation and show no evidence of flaking, scaling, redness, or open lesions. The hair should be shiny and soft. The texture of the hair may be fine or coarse. Note the quantity and distribution of the hair for balding patterns and isolated areas of hair loss. If there are areas of isolated hair loss, note whether the hair shaft is broken off or absent completely. Men may show a gradual, symmetric hair loss on the scalp caused by genetic disposition and elevated androgen levels.

INSPECT facial and body hair for distribution, quantity, and texture.

Examine the quantity and distribution of facial and body hair. Men generally have noticeable hair present on the lower face, neck, nares, ears, chest, axilla, back, shoulders, arms, legs, and pubic region. The noticeable hair distribution in women is usually limited to the arms, legs, axillae, pubic region, and around the nipples. Women may also have fine or light-colored hair on the back, face, and shoulders. The women in some cultural groups may also have facial or chin hair. Fine vellus hair covers the body; whereas coarser hair is found on the eyebrows and lashes, pubic region, axillary area, male beards, and to some extent the arms and legs. The male pubic hair configuration is an upright triangle, with the hair commonly extending midline to the umbilicus. The female pubic hair configuration forms an inverse triangle; the hair may also extend midline to the umbilicus. Transgender women may use techniques to remove hair from face, chest, back, and abdomen.

INSPECT the nails for shape, contour, and color; PALPATE the nails for thickness and firmness.

Inspect and palpate the nail edges. Note the length of the nails. The edge of the nail should be smooth and rounded.
The nail surface should be smooth and flat in the center and slightly curved downward at the edges.

ABNORMAL FINDINGS

An increase in skin thickness is seen in patients with diabetes mellitus and is thought to be caused by abnormal collagen resulting from hyperglycemia.[10] Excessively thin skin may take on a shiny or transparent appearance and is seen in hyperthyroidism, arterial insufficiency, and aging.

Dull, coarse, and brittle hair is seen with nutritional deficiencies, hypothyroidism, and exposure to chemicals in some hair products and bleach. Hyperthyroidism makes the hair texture fine.[9] *Parasitic infection* with lice is characterized by the presence of nits (eggs) found on the scalp at the base of the hair shaft. *Alopecia* (hair loss) often occurs as a manifestation of many systemic diseases, including autoimmune disorders, anemic conditions, and nutritional deficiencies, or treatment with radiation or antineoplastic agents.

Hair loss on the legs may indicate poor peripheral perfusion. Thinning of the eyebrows is a prominent finding in hypothyroidism.[11] *Hirsutism* (hair growth in women with an increase of hair on the face, body, and pubic area) may be a sign of an underlying endocrine disorder. Pubic hair distribution that deviates from typical gender patterns may indicate a hormonal imbalance.

Note excessive length or damage to edges.

Note grooves, depressions, pitting, and ridges. Pitting of the nail is commonly associated with psoriasis (Fig. 9.6). Minor pitting may also be seen in persons with no health care problems.

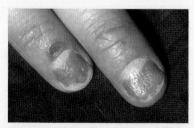

FIG. 9.6 Nail pitting. (From White and Cox, 2000.)

PROCEDURES WITH EXPECTED FINDINGS

In light-skinned individuals nail beds are pink. Individuals with darker-pigmented skin typically have nails that are yellow or brown, and vertical banded lines may appear (Fig. 9.8). The use of artificial nails and nail polish is common and may limit direct evaluation of nail surface.

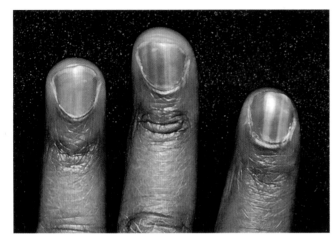

FIG. 9.8 Nail bed color of a dark-skinned person. Pigmented bands occur as a normal finding in more than 90% of African Americans. (From Herlihy, 2011.)

The skin adjacent to the nail should be intact, the same color as adjacent skin and without edema.

Inspect the nail base angle (i.e., the angle of the proximal nail fold and the nail plate). The expected angle of the nail base is 160 degrees.

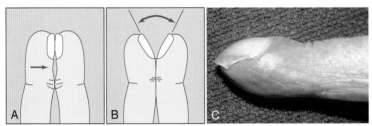

FIG. 9.10 Assessment of finger clubbing. (A) Normally when opposing fingers are placed together, a small space is visible between the place where the fingers and the nail beds meet. (B) With finger clubbing, no space is observed between the fingers and the nail beds angle away from one another. (C) With finger clubbing, the base of the nail is enlarged and curved. (A and B, From Seidel et al., 2011; C, From White and Cox, 2000.)

Examine the thickness of the nail itself. The nail should have a uniform thickness. Finally, palpate the nail to ensure that the nail base feels firm and adheres to the nail bed.

ABNORMAL FINDINGS

Beau's lines manifest as a groove or transverse depression running across the nail. They result from a stressor such as trauma that temporarily impairs nail formation. The groove first appears at the base of the nail by the cuticle and moves forward as the nail grows out.

Koilonychia (spoon nail) presents as a thin, depressed nail with the lateral edges turned upward (Fig. 9.7). This is associated with anemia or may be congenital.[12]

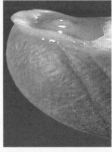

FIG. 9.7 Severe spooning with thinning of the nail. (From Beaven and Brooks, 1994.)

Leukonychia appears as white spots on the nail plate (Fig. 9.9). This is usually caused by minor trauma or manipulation of the cuticle.

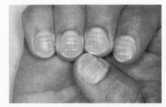

FIG. 9.9 Leukonychia punctata. Transverse white bands result from repeated minor trauma to the nail matrix. (From Baran, Dawber, and Levene, 1991.)

Inflammation characterized by edema and erythema of the folds of the finger tissue may indicate infection.

Clubbing is present when the angle of the nail base exceeds 180 degrees (Fig. 9.10). It is caused by proliferation of the connective tissue, resulting in an enlargement of the distal fingers. Clubbing is commonly associated with chronic respiratory or cardiovascular disease.

Thinning or brittleness of the nail may be secondary to poor peripheral circulation or inadequate nutrition.

PROCEDURES WITH EXPECTED FINDINGS	ABNORMAL FINDINGS

SPECIAL CIRCUMSTANCES

INSPECT and PALPATE skin lesions.

An in-depth examination of lesions is not performed routinely during every health assessment; however, when the patient has a new lesion or when a lesion has changed (i.e., changed in appearance or become painful), it should be examined.[13]

A strong light source to determine the exact color, elevation, and borders and a centimeter ruler to measure the size of lesions are helpful. The lesion is documented based on its characteristics, including location, distribution, color, pattern, shape, edges, depth, size, and other characteristics such as presence of exudate (Fig. 9.11 and Box 9.2). Lesions are classified as primary, secondary, or vascular.

Primary Lesions

Many primary lesions are considered expected variations of the skin and include moles, freckles, patches, and comedones (acne) among adolescents and young adults. These have been discussed in previous sections (see Table 9.2).

Use a Wood's lamp to identify fluorescing lesions, indicating fungal infection. Darken the room and shine the light on the area to be examined. If there is no fungal infection, the light tone on the skin appears soft violet.

Some primary lesions are considered abnormal findings and are associated with a specific disease process or injury (see Table 9.2).

A yellow-green or blue-green fluorescence indicates the presence of fungal infection.

Secondary Lesions

Some secondary lesions are considered expected variations (Table 9.3). For example, a scar is a common variation caused by injury to the skin. A multitude of skin injuries can cause a scar; thus in many cases scars lack significance.

Abnormal secondary lesions result from changes in a primary lesion or trauma to a primary lesion (Table 9.3). Although scars can be an expected finding, they also may be an indication of past physical abuse. Examples may include excessive scars or those that appear on skin surfaces typically protected. Scarring caused by needle-track marks generally indicates intravenous drug use.

Vascular Lesions

Many vascular lesions are considered common variations (Table 9.4). Ecchymosis (bruising) on a bony prominence is generally considered a common finding secondary to the activities of daily living. Other vascular lesions include the following
- *Telangiectasia:* A fine, irregular, red line caused by permanent dilation of a group of superficial blood vessels.
- *Cherry angioma:* A small, slightly raised, bright red area that typically appears on the face, neck, and trunk of the body. These increase in size and number with advanced age (see Table 9.4).

Abnormal vascular lesions are presented in Table 9.4. A *hematoma* forms when there is a leakage of blood in a confined space caused by a break in a blood vessel. Bruising over soft tissue areas of the body in the absence of injury or the presence of multiple bruises on the body in various stages of healing is considered an abnormal finding warranting further investigation. Possible causes include physical abuse or a bleeding disorder.

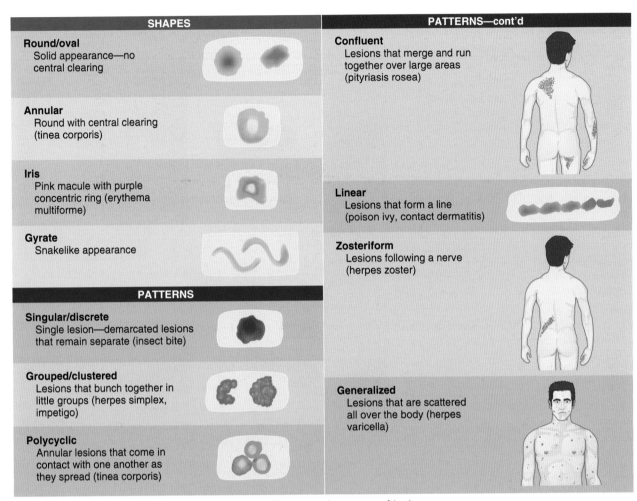

SHAPES	PATTERNS—cont'd
Round/oval Solid appearance—no central clearing	**Confluent** Lesions that merge and run together over large areas (pityriasis rosea)
Annular Round with central clearing (tinea corporis)	
Iris Pink macule with purple concentric ring (erythema multiforme)	**Linear** Lesions that form a line (poison ivy, contact dermatitis)
Gyrate Snakelike appearance	**Zosteriform** Lesions following a nerve (herpes zoster)
PATTERNS	
Singular/discrete Single lesion—demarcated lesions that remain separate (insect bite)	
Grouped/clustered Lesions that bunch together in little groups (herpes simplex, impetigo)	**Generalized** Lesions that are scattered all over the body (herpes varicella)
Polycyclic Annular lesions that come in contact with one another as they spread (tinea corporis)	

FIG. 9.11 Shapes and patterns of lesions.

BOX 9.2 LESION CHARACTERISTICS TO BE NOTED DURING EXAMINATION

- Note the **location** and **distribution** of the lesion. Is the lesion generalized over the entire body or section of the body, or is it localized to a specific area such as around the waist, under a piece of jewelry, or in the hair?
- Describe the **color** of the lesion and how this lesion may be different in color from other lesions noted on the body (e.g., a mole or freckle). Has the patient noticed a change in the color of the lesion?
- What is the **pattern** of the lesion(s)? Are the lesions clustered? Are they in a line? How does the patient describe the development of the pattern of the lesions? (See Fig. 9.11.)
- What is the **shape** of the lesion? Is the lesion round, oval, or annular? Does it have concentric rings? Is it shaped like a wavy line?

- What does the **edge** of the lesion look like? Is the edge regular or irregular? Has the patient noticed a change in the shape of the lesion?
- What is the **depth** of the lesion? Is the lesion flat, raised, or sunken?
- What is the current **size** of the lesion? Measure using a centimeter ruler. Has the patient noticed a change in the size?
- What are the **characteristics** of the lesion? Is it hard, soft, or fluid-filled? If there is an exudate, what is the color of the drainage fluid? Does the exudate have an odor? Has the patient noticed a change in either the characteristics or drainage of the lesion? If so, how and when?

TABLE 9.2 PRIMARY SKIN LESIONS

SKIN LESIONS	EXAMPLES		
Macule Flat, circumscribed area that is a change in the color of the skin; less than 1 cm in diameter	Freckles, flat moles (nevi), petechiae, measles, scarlet fever	**Macule** 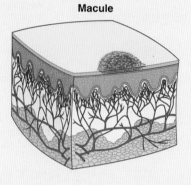	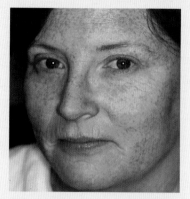 Freckles. (Courtesy Lemmi and Lemmi, 2013.)
Papule Elevated, firm, circum-scribed area less than 1 cm in diameter	Wart (verruca), ele-vated moles, lichen planus, cherry angi-oma, neurofibroma, skin tag	**Papule** 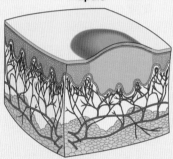	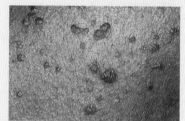 Moles. (Courtesy Lemmi and Lemmi, 2013.)
Patch A flat, nonpalpable, irregular-shaped macule more than 1 cm in diameter	Vitiligo, port wine stains, Mongolian spots, café-au-lait spots	**Patch** 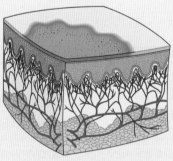	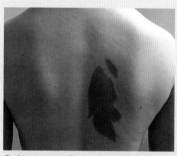 Café-au-lait. (Courtesy Lemmi and Lemmi, 2013.)
Plaque Elevated, firm, and rough lesion with flat top surface greater than 1 cm in diameter	Psoriasis, seborrheic and actinic kerato-ses, eczema	**Plaque** 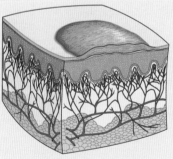	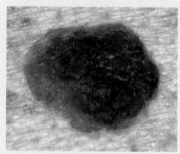 Seborrheic keratoses. (Courtesy Lemmi and Lemmi, 2013.)

TABLE 9.2 **PRIMARY SKIN LESIONS—cont'd**

SKIN LESIONS	EXAMPLES

Wheal

Elevated irregular-shaped area of cutaneous edema; solid, transient; variable diameter

Insect bites, urticaria, allergic reaction, lupus erythematosus

Wheal

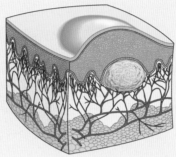

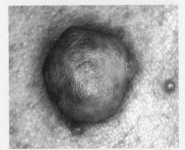

Allergic reaction to the skin. (Courtesy Lemmi and Lemmi, 2013.)

Nodule

Elevated, firm, circumscribed lesion; deeper in dermis than a papule; 1 to 2 cm in diameter

Dermatofibroma erythema nodosum, lipomas, melanoma, hemangioma, neurofibroma

Nodule

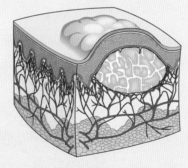

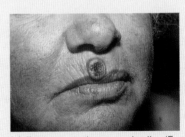

Dermatofibroma. (Courtesy Lemmi and Lemmi, 2013.)

Tumor

Elevated and solid lesion; may or may not be clearly demarcated; deeper in dermis; greater than 2 cm in diameter

Neoplasms, lipoma, hemangioma

Tumor

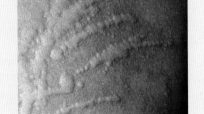

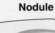

Malignant neoplasm on the lip. (From Goldstein and Goldstein, 1997.)

Vesicle

Elevated, circumscribed, superficial, not into dermis; filled with serous fluid; less than 1 cm in diameter

Varicella (chickenpox), herpes zoster (shingles), impetigo, acute eczema

Vesicle

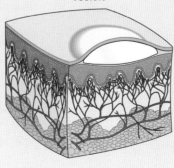

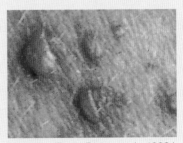

Varicella. (From Farrar et al., 1992.)

Continued

TABLE 9.2 **PRIMARY SKIN LESIONS—cont'd**

SKIN LESIONS   **EXAMPLES**

Bulla

Vesicle greater than 1
  cm in diameter

Blister, pemphigus
  vulgaris, lupus ery-
  thematosus, impe-
  tigo, drug reaction

Bulla

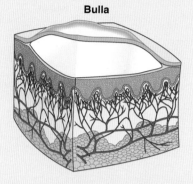
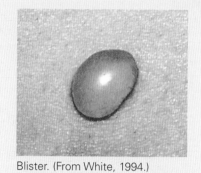

Blister. (From White, 1994.)

Pustule

Elevated, superficial
  lesion; similar to a
  vesicle but filled
  with purulent fluid

Impetigo, acne,
  folliculitis, herpes
  simplex

Pustule

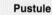
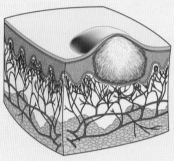
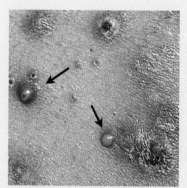

Acne. (From Weston, Lane, and
  Morelli, 2002.)

Cyst

Elevated, circumscribed,
  encapsulated lesion;
  in dermis or subcuta-
  neous layer; filled with
  liquid or semisolid
  material

Sebaceous cyst,
  cystic acne

Cyst

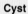
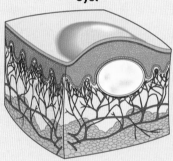
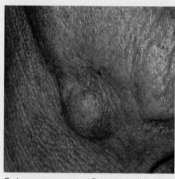

Sebaceous cyst. (Courtesy Lemmi
  and Lemmi, 2013.)

TABLE 9.3 SECONDARY SKIN LESIONS

SKIN LESIONS	EXAMPLES		

Scale

Heaped-up keratinized cells; flaky skin; irregular; thick or thin; dry or oily; variation in size

Flaking of skin with seborrheic dermatitis following scarlet fever or flaking of skin following a drug reaction; dry skin, pityriasis rosea, eczema, xerosis

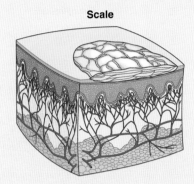

Scale

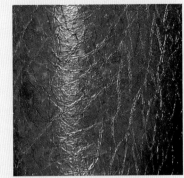

Scaling. (From White, 2004).

Lichenification

Rough, thickened epidermis secondary to persistent rubbing, pruritus or skin irritation; often involves flexor surface of extremity

Chronic dermatitis, psoriasis

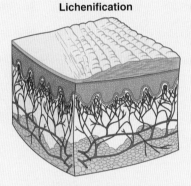

Lichenification

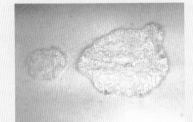

Psoriasis. (Courtesy Lemmi and Lemmi, 2013.)

Keloid

Irregular-shaped, elevated, progressively enlarging scar; grows beyond the boundaries of the wound

Keloid formation following surgery

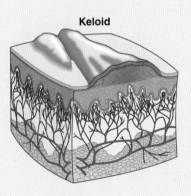

Keloid

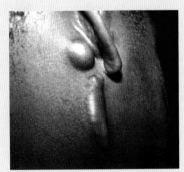

Keloid. (From Weston, Lane, and Morelli, 2002.)

Scar

Thin-to-thick fibrous tissue that replaces normal skin following injury or laceration to the dermis

Healed wound or surgical incision

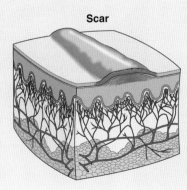

Scar

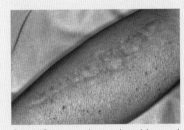

Scar. (Courtesy Lemmi and Lemmi, 2013.)

Continued

TABLE 9.3 **SECONDARY SKIN LESIONS—cont'd**

SKIN LESIONS	EXAMPLES		

Excoriation

Loss of the epidermis; linear hollowed-out crusted area

Abrasion or scratch, scabies

Excoriation

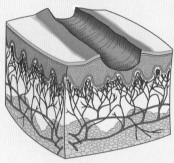

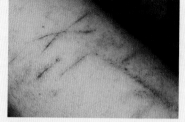

Scratches on skin surface. (Courtesy Lemmi and Lemmi, 2000.)

Fissure

Linear crack or break from the epidermis to the dermis; may be moist or dry

Athlete's foot, cracked skin, chapped hands, eczema, intertrigo labialis

Fissure

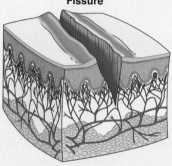

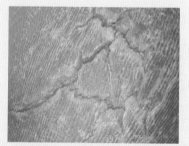

Cracked skin on foot. (Courtesy Lemmi and Lemmi, 2000.)

Crust

Dried drainage or blood; slightly elevated; variable size; colors variable—red, black, tan, or mixed

Scab on abrasion, eczema

Crust

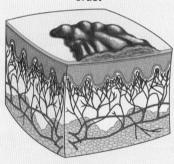

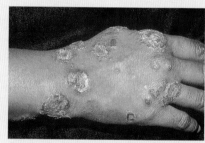

Eczema. (From White and Cox, 2006.)

Erosion

Loss of part of the epidermis; depressed, moist, glistening; follows rupture of a vesicle or bulla

Varicella, variola after rupture, candidiasis, herpes simplex

Erosion

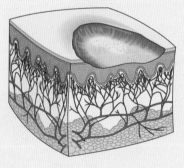

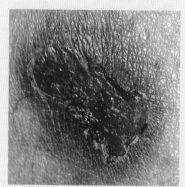

Ruptured vesicle. (Courtesy Lemmi and Lemmi, 2013.)

TABLE 9.3 SECONDARY SKIN LESIONS—cont'd

SKIN LESIONS	EXAMPLES		
Ulcer Loss of epidermis and dermis; concave; varies in size	Pressure ulcer, stasis ulcers, syphilis chancre	**Ulcer** 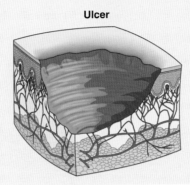	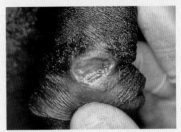Syphilis chancre. (From Goldstein and Goldstein, 1997.)

FREQUENTLY ASKED QUESTIONS

What is the best way to memorize all the different types of skin lesions?

Learning to accurately describe a lesion is more important than memorizing the types of lesions themselves. As you become more proficient with descriptions, you will also begin to remember the names. When you describe a lesion, be sure to include the following information:

- Location, size, and color of the lesion
- Shape (oval, round, irregular) and borders (regular or irregular)
- Elevation (flat, raised, sunken)
- Characteristics (e.g., hard, soft, fluid-filled)
- Pattern (e.g., discrete, clustered, linear, generalized)

TABLE 9.4 VASCULAR SKIN LESIONS

SKIN LESIONS	CAUSE/EXAMPLES		
Petechiae Tiny, flat, reddish-purple, nonblanchable spots in the skin less than 0.5 cm in diameter; appear as tiny red spots pinpoint to pinhead in size	Causes: tiny hemorrhages within the dermal or submucosa—caused by intravascular defects and infection	**Petechiae** 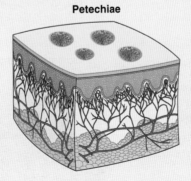	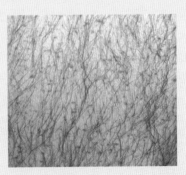Dermal petechiae. (Courtesy Lemmi and Lemmi, 2013.)

Continued

TABLE 9.4 **VASCULAR SKIN LESIONS—cont'd**

SKIN LESIONS	CAUSE/EXAMPLES		

Purpura

Flat, reddish-purple, nonblanchable discoloration in the skin greater than 0.5 cm in diameter

Causes: infection or bleeding disorders resulting in hemorrhage of blood into the skin

Examples: senile, actinic purpura, progressive pigmented purpura, vasculitis purpura, thrombocytopenic purpura

Purpura

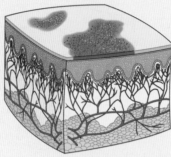

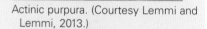

Actinic purpura. (Courtesy Lemmi and Lemmi, 2013.)

Ecchymosis (Bruise)

Reddish-purple, nonblanchable spot of variable size

Cause: trauma to the blood vessel resulting in bleeding under the tissue

Bruise

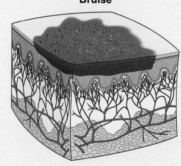

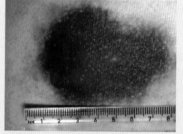

Bruise. (Courtesy Lemmi and Lemmi, 2000.)

Angioma

Benign tumor consisting of a mass of small blood vessels; can vary in size from very small to large

Examples: cherry angioma, hemangioma, cavernous hemangioma, strawberry hemangioma

Angioma

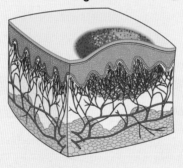

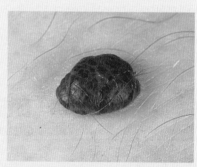

Angioma. (From Dinulos, 2018.)

Capillary Hemangioma (Nevus Flammeus)

Type of angioma that involves the capillaries within the skin producing an irregular patch that can vary from light red to dark red to purple in color

Cause: congenital vascular malformation of capillaries

Example: port wine stain, stork bite

Capillary Hemangioma

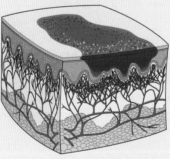

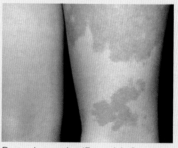

Port wine stain. (From McCance and Huether, 2002.)

TABLE 9.4 VASCULAR SKIN LESIONS—cont'd

SKIN LESIONS	CAUSE/EXAMPLES		

Telangiectasia

Permanent dilation of preexisting small blood vessels (capillaries, arterioles, or venules) resulting in superficial, fine, irregular red lines within the skin

Causes: rosacea, collagen vascular disease; actinic damage, increased estrogen levels
Examples: essential telangiectasia, hereditary hemorrhagic telangiectasia

Telangiectasia

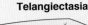

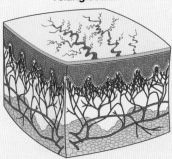

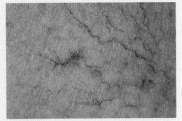

Essential Telangiectasia. (Courtesy Lemmi and Lemmi, 2000.)

Vascular Spider (Spider Angioma)

Type of telangiectasia characterized by a small central red area with radiating spider-like legs; this lesion blanches with pressure

Causes: may occur in absence of disease, with pregnancy, in liver disease, or with vitamin B deficiency

Vascular Spider

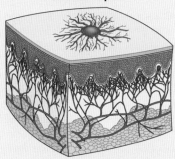

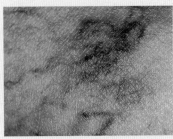

Spider Angioma. (Courtesy Lemmi and Lemmi, 2013.)

Venous Star

Type of telangiectasia characterized by a nonpalpable bluish, star-shaped lesion that may be linear or irregularly shaped

Cause: increased pressure in the superficial veins

Venous Star

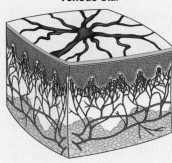

Venous Star. (Courtesy Lemmi and Lemmi, 2000.)

DOCUMENTING EXPECTED FINDINGS

The skin is the expected color for race: it is smooth, soft, warm, dry, and intact with an even surface and elastic turgor. Freckles are noted on the face, back, arms, and legs. Hair on the scalp is red, shiny, soft, and fine. Facial and body hair are consistent with female distribution. Nails are clean, pink, smooth, and unpolished.

CLINICAL JUDGMENT

Skin

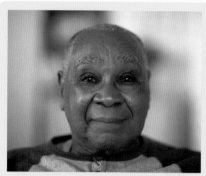

Case Presentation
Blake Ferguson, a 76-year-old man with a 27-year history of type 2 diabetes mellitus (DM), hypertension, and peripheral artery disease (PAD), presents at a community clinic with a redness and pain to his left lower leg just above the ankle. His vital signs are within normal limits.

Reflecting
The nurse reflects on Mr. Ferguson's clinical presentation and this clinical encounter. He was seen by a family practice physician and diagnosed with cellulitis of the left lower leg. He was prescribed an antibiotic and instructed to take acetaminophen for pain, with instructions to follow up with his primary care provider. This experience contributes to the nurse's expertise when encountering a similar situation.

Noticing / Recognizing Cues
Based on the presenting information, the experienced nurse recognizes that Mr. Ferguson's age and medical conditions increase his risk for inflammation due to impaired peripheral perfusion and impaired immunity. Mr. Ferguson tells the nurse that the pain started several days ago and has become progressively worse. Upon assessment, the nurse observes a large area of redness and edema over the medial aspect of the left lower leg, just above the ankle. Mr. Ferguson confirms the leg is very tender when the nurse lightly palpates the affected area; the nurse also notices that the area is warmer than other parts of his skin.

Responding / Taking Action
The nurse initiates appropriate initial interventions to reduce the inflammation and coordinates care to ensure that Mr. Ferguson receives immediate and follow up care, including instructions about how to treat and prevent infections.

Interpreting / Analyzing Cues & Prioritizing Hypotheses
Following the cognitive cues, the nurse considers two possible causes of the inflammation to the leg: potential deep vein thrombosis or infection. To determine whether either has any probability of being correct, the nurse gathers additional data.
- Has there been a recent injury to the area, creating a mechanism for bacterial entrance into the skin?

When asked about recent injury to his leg, Mr. Ferguson recalls scratching his leg on a stick the previous week while cutting weeds. "It wasn't any big deal – it was just a scratch," he tells the nurse.

The experienced nurse not only recognizes inflammation and infection by the presenting signs (erythema, heat, edema) and symptom (pain) but also interprets this information in the context of a skin injury to an extremity in an individual with type 2 DM and PAD.

AGE-RELATED VARIATIONS

The discussion thus far has featured the assessment of skin, hair, and nails for the adult patient. This assessment is performed for individuals across the life span. In general, the approach is the same, but there are variations in findings.

INFANTS AND CHILDREN

The assessment of skin among infants and children follows the same general principles as previously described for the adult. Skin lesions common to infants and children include milia, erythema toxicum, diaper rash, and rashes associated with allergens. Chapter 19 presents further information regarding the assessment of skin, hair, and nails for these age groups.

ADOLESCENTS

The most common skin lesions of concern among adolescents are acne because of the increase in sebaceous gland activity. Not only are these lesions painful, but they are also of concern to the patient because of personal appearance. Chapter 19 presents further information.

OLDER ADULTS

The skin and hair undergo significant changes with aging. Many lesions found on older adults are considered expected variations associated with the aging process. Inspection of sun-exposed areas is important because the incidence of skin cancer increases with age. Further information related to changes of the skin and lesions commonly found among older adults is presented in Chapter 21.

SITUATIONAL VARIATIONS

PATIENTS WITH LIMITED MOBILITY

Risk for skin breakdown secondary to pressure and body fluid pooling increases for patients with limited mobility, because of an inability to feel pressure or a decreased ability to independently change position to relieve pressure. A pressure ulcer is a localized injury to the skin and/or underlying tissue usually over a bony prominence as a result of pressure or pressure in combination with shear and/or friction.[14] The nurse should examine the patient's skin, especially over bony prominences. The nurse may need assistance to turn the patient so that a complete skin assessment may be performed. In addition, patients who operate their own manual wheelchairs are at high risk for developing hand calluses. Therefore special care should be taken to examine the patient's hands.

Assessing for pressure ulcers gained additional importance in 2006 when the Centers for Medicaid and Medicare Services (CMS) eliminated payment to hospitals for conditions deemed "reasonably preventable," also referred to as *never events*. Because hospital-acquired pressure ulcers are included as never events, the skin of all patients admitted is carefully assessed for pressure ulcers.[15] When found, these patients' ulcers are photographed to document their presence at the time of admission as opposed to being hospital acquired. In addition, to prevent pressure ulcers from developing, nurses assess patients at risk for them (e.g., those who are immobile, are incontinent of urine or stool, or have nutritional deficiencies). Nurses then implement preventive interventions such as keeping the skin clean, dry, and free of prolonged pressure. Furthermore, nurses collaborate with dietitians to plan a diet to maintain skin integrity (e.g., a diet including protein, vitamin C, and zinc). If nurses assess a pressure ulcer after admission to the hospital, they collaborate with a wound care nurse for prompt, early interventions to prevent further skin damage and regain skin integrity.

Expected and Abnormal Findings

Inspect and palpate all pressure points for patients who have limited mobility (Fig. 9.12). When a red area of skin is noted, blanch the skin by applying gentle pressure over the red areas. If the skin becomes white (blanches) when pressure is applied and reddens again after pressure is relieved, the circulation to that area is sufficient, and the redness will disappear.

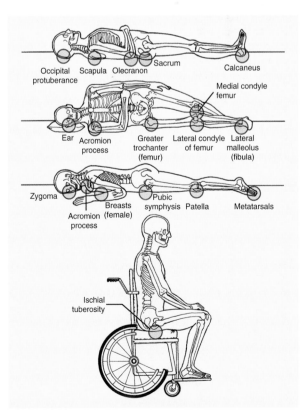

FIG. 9.12 Bony prominences vulnerable to pressure.

Pressure ulcers are staged in four categories, I through IV (Table 9.5). Stage I is recognized by prolonged redness with unbroken skin; if the skin does not blanch when pressure is applied, a stage I pressure ulcer has developed. Stage II is characterized by partial-thickness skin loss that appears as a shallow, open ulcer with pink wound bed. Stage III involves full-thickness skin loss with damage to the subcutaneous tissue with no bone, tendon, or muscle exposed. Stage IV is full-thickness tissue loss with exposed bone, muscle, or tendon.

Eschar or slough may be present in some parts of the wound bed. If the entire wound bed is covered by slough or eschar, the wound is considered unstageable.[14] Underlying soft tissue damage resulting from pressure or shear force injury can occur without disruption to the skin surface. This may appear as an area of discolored (purple or maroon) intact skin or blood-filled blister; the wound may also become covered with eschar. This type of tissue wound may be difficult to detect among individuals with dark skin tone.

TABLE 9.5 STAGING OF PRESSURE ULCERS

DESCRIPTION	CLINICAL PRESENTATION
Stage I Intact skin with nonblanchable redness, usually over a bony prominence. The area may be painful, firm, soft, warmer, or cooler compared to adjacent tissue. May be difficult to detect in individuals with dark skin tones.	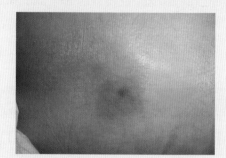
Stage II Partial-thickness loss of dermis. Presents as a shiny or dry shallow open ulcer with pink wound bed without slough or bruising. May also present as an intact or open/ruptured serum-filled blister.	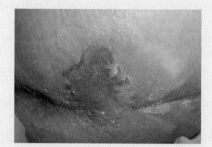
Stage III Full-thickness skin loss involving damage to or necrosis of subcutaneous tissue. Subcutaneous fat may be visible, but bone, tendon, or muscles are not exposed. Slough may be present; wound may include undermining and tunneling. Depth of a stage III ulcer varies by anatomic location because of variation in presence and depth of subcutaneous tissue.	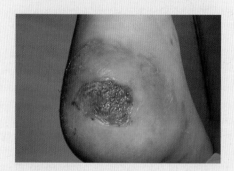
Stage IV Full-thickness tissue loss with exposed bone, tendon, or muscle. Slough or eschar may be present within the wound bed. Undermining and tunneling often present. Depth of a stage IV ulcer varies by anatomic location because of variation in presence and depth of subcutaneous tissue.	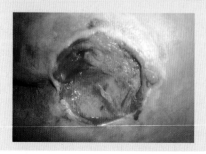

TABLE 9.5 STAGING OF PRESSURE ULCERS—cont'd

DESCRIPTION   **CLINICAL PRESENTATION**

Unstageable Ulcer

Full-thickness tissue loss in which base of ulcer is covered by slough (yellow, tan, gray-green, or brown) and/or eschar (tan, brown, or black). True depth of the wound cannot be determined until the slough and/or eschar is/are removed to expose the base of the wound.

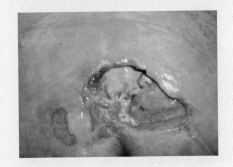

Suspected Deep Tissue Injury

Localized area of discolored (purple or maroon) intact skin or blood-filled blister caused by underlying soft tissue damage resulting from pressure or shear. May be difficult to detect among individuals with dark skin tone. May include a blister over a dark wound bed; wound may become covered with eschar.

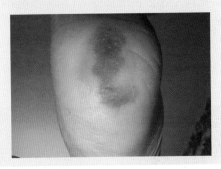

Used with permission from the National Pressure Injury Advisory Panel (NPIAP). Copyright 2020 NPIAP.

COMMON PROBLEMS AND CONDITIONS

SKIN

Clavus (Corn)

A corn is a lesion that develops secondary to chronic pressure from a shoe over a bony prominence. **Clinical Findings:** This lesion is a flat or slightly raised, painful, and generally has a smooth, hard surface (Fig. 9.13). A "soft" corn is a whitish thickening commonly found between the fourth and fifth toes. A "hard" corn is clearly demarcated and has a conical appearance.

Atopic Dermatitis

The term *dermatitis* is used to describe a variety of superficial inflammatory conditions of the skin that can be acute or chronic. Atopic dermatitis is a chronic superficial inflammation of the skin with an unknown cause; however, it is commonly associated with hay fever and asthma and is thought to be familial. While seen in all age groups, it is more common in infancy and childhood. **Clinical Findings:** During infancy and early childhood, red, weeping, crusted lesions appear on the face, scalp, extremities, and diaper area (Fig. 9.14). In older children and adults, lesion characteristics include erythema, scaling, and lichenification. The lesions are associated with intense pruritus and are usually localized to the arms and hands (particularly at the antecubital fossa) and the legs and feet (in the popliteal space).

Contact Dermatitis

Contact dermatitis is an inflammatory reaction of the skin that develops in response to irritants or allergens such as metals, plants, chemicals, or detergent. This condition affects people of all ages and ethnic groups. **Clinical Findings:** Contact dermatitis develops in an area exposed to the causative irritant or allergen and appears as localized erythema that

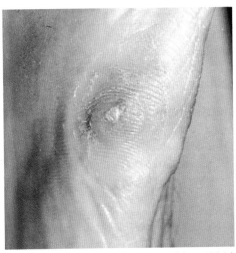

FIG. 9.13 Corn (Clavus). (From White, 1994.)

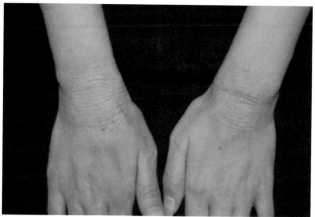

FIG. 9.14 Atopic dermatitis on back of hands, wrists. Note erythema and lichenification. (From Kabashima-Kubo, et al., 2012.)

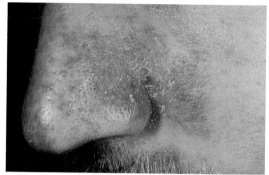

FIG. 9.16 Seborrheic dermatitis. (From James, et al., 2017.)

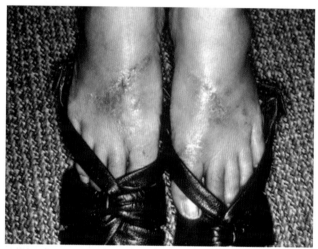

FIG. 9.15 Contact dermatitis caused by an allergic reaction to shoes. (From James, et al., 2017.)

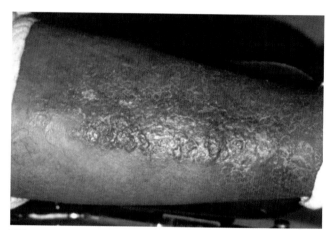

FIG. 9.17 Stasis dermatitis on lower leg. (From Brinster et al., 2011.)

may also include edema, wheals, scales, or vesicles that may weep, ooze, and become crusted (Fig. 9.15). Pruritus is a common symptom. The inflammatory response is highly individualized; it can vary from no-to-extreme reaction.

Seborrheic Dermatitis

This chronic inflammation of the skin has no known cause and affects individuals throughout their lives, often with periods of remission and exacerbation. (In infants this condition is known as cradle cap.) **Clinical Findings:** The lesions appear as scaly, white, or yellowish plaques involving skin on the scalp, eyebrows, eyelids, nasolabial folds, ears, axillae, chest, and back. Lesions typically cause mild pruritus; lesions on the scalp cause dandruff (Fig. 9.16).

Stasis Dermatitis

Commonly seen in older adults, stasis dermatitis is an inflammation of the skin usually affecting the lower legs. **Clinical Findings:** Initially this condition is characterized by an area or areas of erythema and pruritus followed by scaling, petechiae, and brown pigmentation (Fig. 9.17). Stasis dermatitis progresses to ulcerated lesions (known as stasis ulcers) if untreated.

Psoriasis

This is a common chronic skin disorder that can occur at any age but usually develops by age 20. An inflammatory process causes lesions of psoriasis, and the disease can range from mild to severe. **Clinical Findings:** The lesions appear as well-circumscribed, slightly raised, erythematous plaques with silvery scales on the surface. They appear frequently on the elbows, knees, buttocks, lower back, and scalp. A specific characteristic of this condition is the observance of small bleeding points if the lesion is scratched. Other symptoms include pruritus, burning, and bleeding of the lesions and pitting of the fingernails (Fig. 9.18).

Pityriasis Rosea

Pityriasis rosea is a common, acute, self-limiting inflammatory disease that usually occurs in young adults during the winter months. **Clinical Findings:** The initial manifestation is a lesion referred to as a *herald patch* (i.e., a single lesion, usually located on the trunk, resembling tinea corporis) (Fig. 9.19A). At 1 to 3 weeks following the initial lesion, a generalized eruption of pale, erythematous, and macular lesions occurs on the trunk and extremities (Fig. 9.19B); occasionally they appear as vesicular lesions. The patient generally feels well but may complain of mild pruritus.

Warts (Verruca)

A wart is a small benign lesion caused by human papillomavirus (HPV) and transmitted by contact. Because there are more than 60 different types of HPV, many different types of warts occur in many locations and in many sizes. They may appear at any age. **Clinical Findings:** Common warts (ver-

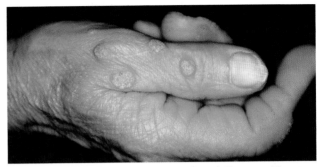

FIG. 9.20 Common warts on hand and fingers. (Courtesy Alexandra Geusau.)

rucae vulgaris) are round or irregular-shaped papular lesions that are light gray, yellow, or brownish black. They commonly appear on fingers, hands, elbows, and knees (Fig. 9.20). Plantar warts are found on the sole of the foot and are typically tender to pressure.

Herpes Simplex

The term *herpes simplex* represents a group of eight deoxyribonucleic acid (DNA) viruses. Herpes simplex virus (HSV) is a chronic, noncurable condition transmitted by contact during an outbreak when the infected person is shedding the virus; between outbreaks the virus is dormant. Outbreaks are triggered by a number of factors, including sun exposure, stress, and fever. **Clinical Findings:** Before the onset of lesions, many patients report a sensation of slight stinging and increased sensitivity. The classic manifestation of HSV is the development of grouped vesicles on an erythematous base. The lesions are very painful and highly contagious after direct contact with skin. Lesions caused by herpes simplex virus type 1 (HSV-1) often appear on the upper lip (often referred to as a *cold sore*), nose, around the mouth, or on the tongue (Fig. 9.21). HSV type 2 (HSV-2) lesions usually appear on the genitalia. As the lesions erupt, they move through maturational stages of vesicles, pustules, and finally crusting. They typically last for approximately 2 weeks. (See Chapter 17 for further discussion of HSV-2.)

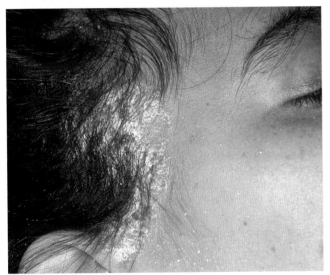

FIG. 9.18 Psoriasis on the scalp. (From Lemmi and Lemmi, 2013.)

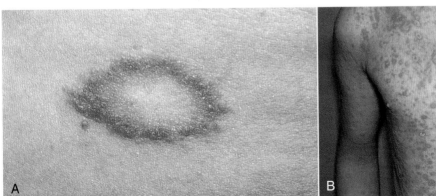
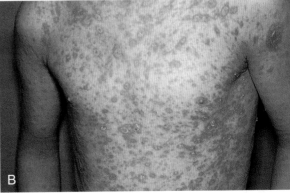

FIG. 9.19 Pityriasis rosea. (A) Large herald patch on the chest. (B) Many oval lesions on the chest. (A, From Cohen, 1993. B, Courtesy Lemmi & Lemmi, 2013.)

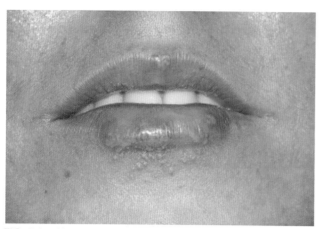

FIG. 9.21 Herpes simplex. Typical manifestation with vesicles appearing on the lips and extending onto the skin. (From Regezi et al., 2017.)

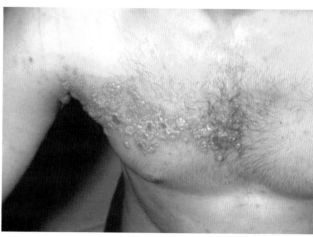

FIG. 9.23 Herpes zoster (Shingles). (From Nawas et al., 2018.)

Herpes Varicella (Chickenpox)

This is a highly communicable viral infection that spreads by droplets. It commonly occurs in children but can also infect adults who did not have the infection as children. **Clinical Findings:** The lesions first appear on the trunk and then spread to the extremities and the face. Initially, the lesions are macules; they progress to papules and then vesicles, and finally the old vesicles become crusts. The lesions erupt in clusters over a period of several days. For this reason, lesions in various stages are seen concurrently. The period of infectivity is from a few days before lesions appear until the final lesions have crusted, usually about 6 days after the first lesions erupt (Fig. 9.22A and B).

Herpes Zoster (Shingles)

A dormant herpes varicella virus causes herpes zoster, which is an acute inflammation by reactivation of the virus. Herpes zoster follows years after the initial varicella infection in some individuals. **Clinical Findings:** Linearly grouped vesicles appear along a cutaneous sensory nerve line (dermatome) (Fig. 9.23). As the disease progresses, the vesicles turn into pustules followed by crusts. This painful condition is generally unilateral and commonly appears on the trunk and face. Pain may precede lesion eruption by several days.

Tinea Infections

These infections are caused by a number of dermatophyte fungal infections involving the skin, hair, and nails that affect children and adults. **Clinical Findings:** *Tinea corporis* (ringworm) involves generalized skin areas (excluding scalp, face, hands, feet, and groin) and appears as circular, well-demarcated lesions that tend to have a clear center (Fig. 9.24A). They are hyperpigmented in light-colored skin and hypopigmented in dark-skinned persons. *Tinea cruris* ("jock itch") affects the

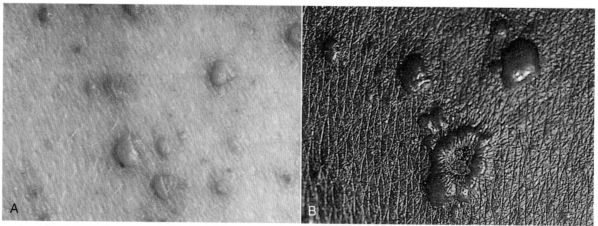

FIG. 9.22 Herpes varicella (Chickenpox). Lesions in various stages of development, including red papules, vesicles, umbilicated vesicles, and crusts. (A) Light-skinned person. (B) Dark-skinned person. (From Farrar et al., 1992.)

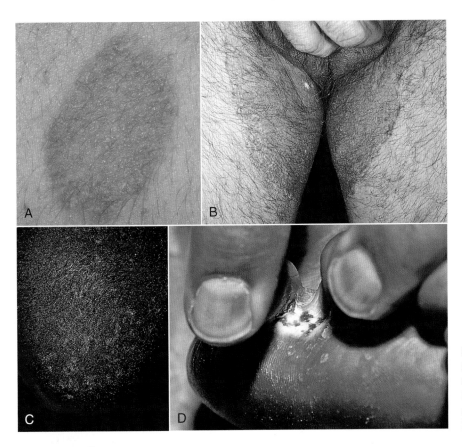

FIG. 9.24 Fungal infections. (A) Tinea corporis on chest—pink, oval-shaped with scaling. (B) Tinea cruris. (C) Tinea capitis. (D) Tinea pedis. (A and B, courtesy Lemmi and Lemmi, 2013; C and D, from White, 2004.)

groin area and is characterized by small erythematous and scaling vesicular patches with a well-defined border spreading over the inner and upper surfaces of the thighs (Fig. 9.24B). *Tinea capitis* involves the scalp, causing scaling and pruritus with balding areas resulting from hair that breaks easily (Fig. 9.24C). *Tinea pedis* is a chronic infection involving the foot ("athlete's foot"). It initially appears as small weeping vesicles and painful macerated areas between the toes and sometimes on the sole of the foot. As the lesions develop, they may become scaly and hard and cause discomfort and pruritus (Fig. 9.24D).

Candidiasis

This fungal infection is caused by *Candida albicans* and is normally found on the skin, mucous membranes, gastrointestinal tract, and vagina. It can develop under certain conditions such as a favorable environment (warm, moist, or tissue maceration); disease states (diabetes mellitus, Cushing syndrome, debilitated states, immunosuppression); and systemic antibiotic administration. **Clinical Findings:** A *Candida* infection affects the superficial layers of skin and mucous membranes. It appears as a scaling red rash with sharply demarcated borders. The area is generally a large patch but may have some loose scales. Common areas for candidiasis involving the skin include the genitalia, the inguinal areas, and along gluteal folds (Fig. 9.25).

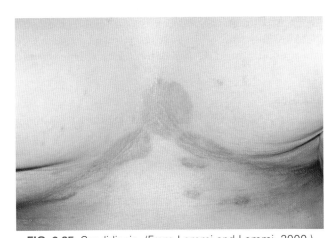

FIG. 9.25 Candidiasis. (From Lemmi and Lemmi, 2000.)

Cellulitis

The term cellulitis refers to an acute infection of the skin and subcutaneous tissue usually caused by streptococcal or staphylococcal pathogens. Cellulitis can occur at any age and can involve any skin area on the body. **Clinical Findings:** The skin is red, warm to the touch and tender, and appears to be indurated. There may be regional lymphangitic streaks and lymphadenopathy (Fig. 9.26).

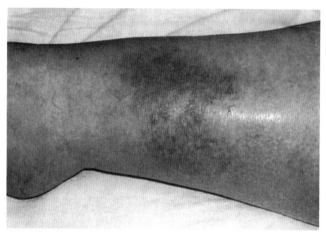

FIG. 9.26 Cellulitis to the lower leg.

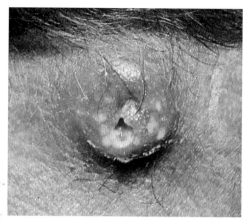

FIG. 9.27 Furuncle. (From Thompson et al., 2002. Courtesy JA Tschen, MD, Baylor College of Medicine, Department of Dermatology, Houston, Tex.)

Folliculitis

This is an inflammation of hair follicles. **Clinical Findings:** An acute lesion appears as an area of erythema with a pustule surrounding the hair follicle, commonly on the scalp and extremities. A chronic condition occurs when deep hair follicles are infected (usually seen in bearded areas).

Furuncle

Also known as an *abscess* or *boil*, a furuncle is a localized bacterial lesion caused by a staphylococcal pathogen. Furuncles often develop from folliculitis. **Clinical Findings:** Initially a furuncle is a nodule surrounded by erythema and edema. As it progresses, it becomes a pustule and the center (or core) fills with a sanguineous purulent exudate. The skin around a furuncle is red, hot, and extremely tender (Fig. 9.27).

Scabies

Scabies is a highly contagious infestation associated with the mite *Sarcoptes scabiei*. The female mite burrows into the superficial layer of skin and lays eggs. Transmission usually occurs with direct skin-to-skin contact. **Clinical Findings:** Severe pruritus is the hallmark of scabies caused by a hypersensitivity to the mite and its feces. The lesions are small papules, vesicles, and burrows that result from the mite entering the skin to lay eggs. The burrows appear as short, irregular marks that look as if they were made by the end of a pencil. Areas commonly affected include the hands, wrists, axillae, genitalia, and inner aspects of the thigh.

Lyme Disease

Lyme disease occurs after a bite from a tick infected with a spirochete, *Borrelia burgdorferi*, and is the most commonly reported vectorborne illness in the United States, with an estimated 30,000 new cases each year. The large majority of Lyme disease cases in the United States occur in the northeast states.[16] **Clinical Findings:** The classic manifestation of Lyme disease is the development of an expanding raised erythemic rash with central clearing at the site of the tick bite (Fig. 9.28).

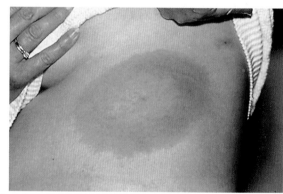

FIG. 9.28 Lyme disease. Note expanding erythematous lesion with central clearing on trunk. (From Goldstein and Goldstein, 1997. Courtesy John Cook, MD.)

This rash has been called a bullseye rash and typically exceeds 5 cm and persists for several weeks. Most individuals also have flulike symptoms (e.g., fever, headache, muscle aches).

Spider Bites

The bites of the black widow and the brown recluse spiders are of concern to humans. Black widow spiders are found throughout the United States; brown recluse spiders are found predominantly in the central and south-central United States. **Clinical Findings:** Minimal symptoms occur at the time of the bite of either the black widow or brown recluse spiders. The initial lesion of a black widow spider bite appears as an area of erythema with two red puncta at the bite site. Within a few hours, symptoms of severe abdominal pain and fever typically develop. The bite of a brown recluse spider initially appears as a lesion with erythema and edema that evolves into a necrotic ulcer with erythema and purpura. Other symptoms include fever, nausea, and vomiting.

Basal Cell Carcinoma

The most common form of skin cancer is basal cell carcinoma. It predominantly afflicts light-skinned individuals

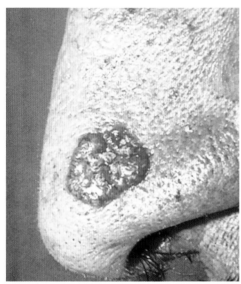

FIG. 9.29 Basal cell carcinoma. (From Thompson et al., 1993. Courtesy Gary Monheit, MD, University of Alabama at Birmingham School of Medicine.)

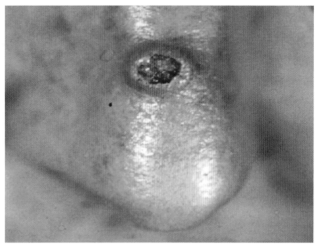

FIG. 9.30 Squamous cell carcinoma. (From Kwiek, et al., 2016.)

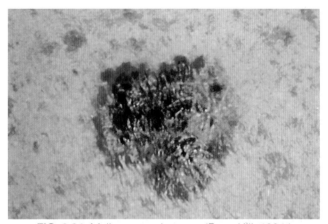

FIG. 9.31 Malignant melanoma. (From Hill, 1994.)

between ages 40 and 80. This malignancy is locally invasive and rarely metastasizes. The incidence increases with age and is more common in males than females.[17] **Clinical Findings:** The lesion has different forms but usually appears as a nodular pigmented lesion with depressed centers and rolled borders. In some cases, the center is ulcerated. This malignancy is usually found in areas that have had repeated exposure to the sun or ultraviolet light such as the face (Fig. 9.29).

Squamous Cell Carcinoma

The second-most frequent form of skin cancer is squamous cell carcinoma. It is an invasive skin cancer that typically appears on the head and neck and occurs as a result of excessive sun or ultraviolet light exposure. Those commonly affected are individuals over the age of 50 who have blue eyes and childhood freckling (light pigmentation). Men are more commonly affected than women.[17] **Clinical Findings:** Initially this cancer appears as a red, scaly patch that has a sharply demarcated border. As the lesion develops further, it becomes soft, mobile, and slightly elevated. As the tumor matures, a central ulcer may form with surrounding redness (Fig. 9.30).

Melanoma

Melanoma is the most serious form of skin cancer, responsible for a large majority of skin cancer-related deaths.[17] It is a malignant proliferation of pigmented cells (melanocytes). These lesions typically arise from already present nevi. **Clinical Findings:** The mnemonic ABCDE (see Box 9.1) is used to remember the classic manifestations of melanoma: *A*symmetry, *B*order irregularity, *C*olor variation, *D*iameter greater than 6 mm, *E*volving (recent changing in size, shape, or color). The lesion may have a flaking or scaly texture; its color may vary from brown to pink to purple, or it may have mixed pigmentation (Fig. 9.31).

Skin Lesions Caused by Abuse

Injuries to the skin are among the most easily recognized signs of physical abuse. When abuse is suspected, compare the type of injury or injuries to the history and the developmental level (if it involves an infant or child). Injuries to the skin are generally recognized in three forms: bruises, bites, and burns.

Bruise (Ecchymosis)

A bruise is a discoloration of the skin or mucous membrane caused by blood seeping into the tissues as a result of a trauma to the area. It can indicate superficial or deep injury such as injury to muscle or abdominal organs. Consider the location, appearance, and pattern of bruises and the type of mark made. **Clinical Findings:** A recent bruise (1 to 3 days old) is purple to deep black in appearance. A bruise that is 3 to 6 days old is green to brown in color, whereas an older bruise (6 to 15 days old) changes from green to tan to yellow and then fades (Fig. 9.32). Look for a pattern in the bruise markings. Bruises associated with abuse may be caused by

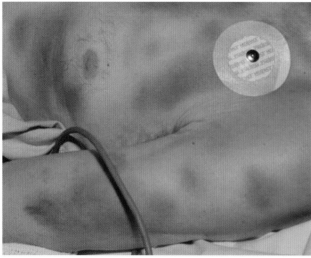

FIG. 9.32 Extensive bruising on the chest is caused by abuse. (From Gibbs, 2014.)

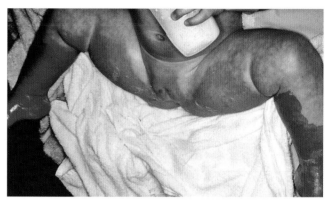

FIG. 9.34 Stocking burn patterns to perineum, thighs, legs, and feet. (From Zitelli, McIntire, and Nowalk, 2012. Courtesy Thomas Layton, MD.)

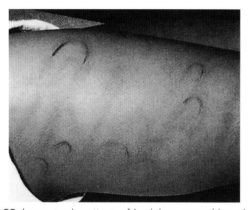

FIG. 9.33 Loop mark pattern of bruising caused by whipping with an electrical cord. (From Monteleone, 1996.)

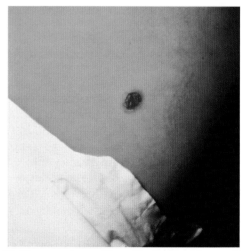

FIG. 9.35 Cigarette burn. (From Zitelli, McIntire, and Nowalk, 2012.)

objects that leave distinctive patterns, such as a loop pattern from being hit with a cord (Fig. 9.33).[18]

Bites

Bites are always intentional and are a common injury associated with abuse. Bite marks are ovoid with tooth imprints that may or may not break the skin. They may have a suck mark (bruising) in the middle. The size of the bite mark is important to note to determine the age of the person who may have left the mark (i.e., child versus adult). Bite marks on infants and children are frequently located on the genitals or buttocks.[18]

Burns

Burns are frequently associated with abuse. The most common type is an immersion burn. This is easily recognizable by a "glove" or "stocking" burn pattern (a line of demarcation) in which the child is immersed into scalding hot water. Look for this pattern on hands and arms, feet and legs, and buttocks (Fig. 9.34). Another common type of burn associated with abuse is a *contact burn* (i.e., a burn caused by intentionally placing a hot object such as a cigarette, light bulb, lighter, or hot iron on the skin) (Fig. 9.35). Intentional contact burns are easily recognizable because they literally leave a "branded pattern" on the skin. An accidental burn with an object typically leaves a glancing burn pattern with a nonuniform pattern.[19]

HAIR

Pediculosis (Lice)

Lice are parasites that invade the scalp, body, or pubic hair regions. Lice on the body are called *pediculosis corporis*, and pubic lice are called *pediculosis pubis*. Infestations are spread commonly by close person-to-person contact.[20] **Clinical Findings:** The eggs (nits) are visible as small, white particles at the base of the hair shaft. The skin underlying the infested area may appear red and excoriated.

Alopecia Areata

This is a chronic inflammatory disease of the hair follicles resulting in hair loss on the scalp. The cause is unknown, but it is associated with autoimmune disorders, metabolic disease, and stressful events. **Clinical Findings:** Hair loss is observed in multiple round patch areas of the scalp. The affected areas are either completely smooth or have short shafts of hair. The poorly developed and fragile hair shafts break and generally grow back within 3 to 4 months, although some individuals suffer total scalp hair loss.

Hirsutism

This condition is associated with an increase in the growth of facial, body, or pubic hair in women. Hirsutism has familial tendency and can be associated with endocrine disorders; polycystic ovarian disease; menopause; and side effects of medications, especially corticosteroid or androgenic steroid therapy.[21] **Clinical Findings:** An increase of body or facial hair is seen; the amount of hair varies. Hirsutism is more pronounced among individuals with darkly pigmented hair. Increased hair growth may or may not be associated with other signs of virilization when secondary male sexual characteristics are acquired by females.

NAILS

Onychomycosis

This is a fungal infection of the nail plate caused by tinea unguium. Although the prevalence varies, it occurs in up to 14% of the population in North America.[22] **Clinical Findings:** The nail plate turns yellow or white as hyperkeratotic debris accumulates. As the problem progresses, the nail separates from the nail bed, and the nail plate crumbles (Fig. 9.36).

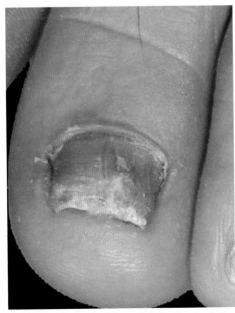

FIG. 9.36 Onychomycosis (Fungal Infection) of the toenail. (From Welsh et al., 2010.)

Paronychia

Paronychia involves an acute or chronic infection of the cuticle. The infection is usually caused by staphylococci and streptococci, although *Candida* may also be the causative organism. **Clinical Findings:** Acute infection involves the rapid onset of very painful inflammation at the base of the nail, often after minor trauma to the area. In some cases an abscess may form. With chronic paronychia the inflammation develops slowly, usually starting at the base of the nail within the cuticle and progressing along the sides of the nails (lateral nail folds). Frequent exposure of the hands to moisture is a risk factor for chronic paronychia (Fig. 9.37).

Ingrown Toenail

A relatively common problem, an ingrown toenail occurs when the nail grows through the lateral nail fold and into the skin. This condition usually involves the great toe and is usually caused by cutting the nail too far down the sides, wearing shoes that fit too tightly, or injury.[23] **Clinical Findings:** The individual experiences pain, redness, and edema. An acute infection may occur, resulting in purulent drainage (Fig. 9.38).

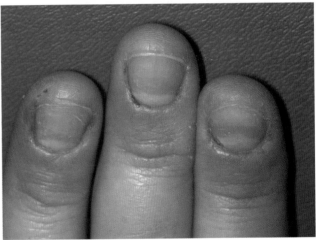

FIG. 9.37 Chronic paronychia with swollen posterior nail folds and nail dystrophy. (Courtesy Lemmi and Lemmi, 2013.)

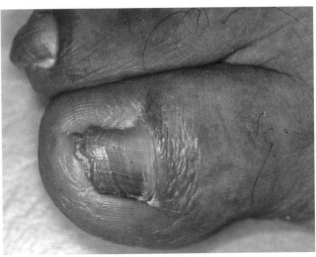

FIG. 9.38 Ingrown toenail. (Courtesy Lemmi and Lemmi, 2013.)

CLINICAL APPLICATION AND CLINICAL JUDGMENT

See Appendix B for answers to exercises in this section.

CASE STUDY

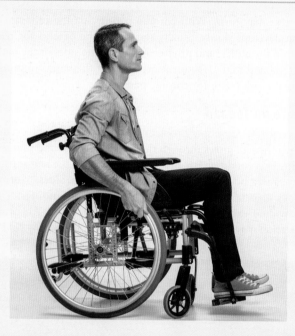

Don Hillerman is a 38-year-old male paraplegic admitted to the hospital for unexplained weakness and depression. The following data are collected by the nurse during an interview and assessment.

Interview Data

Don states that he became a paraplegic 2 years ago after a motorcycle accident. He claims that he is fully independent and needs no assistance. However, for about the past month he has felt weak and has had a loss of appetite. Normally he is able to transfer himself in and out of a wheelchair but admits that he has engaged in very little activity during the last few weeks. His mother and father keep telling him that he is depressed, and this makes him feel very angry. He has no other medical problems and no allergies to medications.

Examination Data

- *General survey:* Alert, very thin male with flat affect lying in a supine position. Height, 6 ft 2 in (188 cm); weight, 153 lb (69.5 kg). Slight foul-smelling odor noted.
- *Skin:* Skin color is pale. No evidence of bruising, no skin discoloration. Presence of stage 2 skin breakdown involving the epidermis over the left greater trochanter and sacrum.
- *Hair:* Full hair distribution on head with soft texture.
- *Abdomen:* Active bowel sounds. Abdomen soft, nondistended, nontender.
- *Musculoskeletal:* Paralysis, atrophy to both lower extremities; upper extremities have full range of motion and adequate muscle strength and tone.

Clinical Judgment

1. What cues do you recognize that suggest a deviation from normal findings, suggesting a need for further investigation?
2. For which additional information should the nurse ask or assess?
3. Which risk factors for pressure ulcers does this patient have?
4. With which interdisciplinary team members can the nurse collaborate to help meet this patient's needs?

REVIEW QUESTIONS

1. A patient has edema and redness of the skin surrounding the nail on his right index finger. Which data elicited from his history best explains this condition?
   1. He has a family history of fungal infections of the nails.
   2. There has been a scabies outbreak among his family members.
   3. He has a new full-time job as a dishwasher at a restaurant.
   4. He recently had several warts removed from each of his hands.

2. When examining a 16-year-old male patient, the nurse notes multiple pustules and comedones on the face. The nurse recognizes that increased activity of which cells or glands produce these manifestations?
   1. Epidermal cells
   2. Eccrine glands
   3. Apocrine glands
   4. Sebaceous glands

3. A patient with darkly pigmented skin has been admitted to the hospital with hepatitis. How does the nurse assess for jaundice in this patient?
   1. Inspect the color of the sclera.
   2. Inspect genitalia for color.
   3. Blanch the fingernails.
   4. Jaundice cannot be assessed in patients with darkly pigmented skin.

4. A patient has multiple solid, red, raised lesions on her legs and groin that she describes as "itchy insect bites." How does the nurse document these lesions?
   1. Wheals
   2. Bulla
   3. Tumors
   4. Plaques

5. The nurse observes multiple red circular lesions with central clearing that are scattered all over the abdomen and thorax. How does the nurse document the shape and pattern of these lesions?
   1. Gyrate and linear
   2. Annular and generalized
   3. Iris and discrete
   4. Oval and clustered

6. Which disorder is an example of a vascular lesion?
   1. Dermatofibroma
   2. Vitiligo
   3. Sebaceous cyst
   4. Port wine stain

7. A 60-year-old male patient states that he has a sore above his lip that has not healed and is getting bigger. The nurse observes a red scaly patch with an ulcerated center and sharp margins. These findings are commonly associated with which malignancy?
   1. Kaposi's sarcoma
   2. Malignant melanoma
   3. Basal cell carcinoma
   4. Squamous cell carcinoma

8. A 48-year-old woman asks the nurse how to best protect herself from excessive sun exposure while at the beach. Which response would be most appropriate?
   1. "Limit your time in the sun to 5 minutes every hour."
   2. "Wear a wet suit that covers your arms and legs."
   3. "Apply a waterproof sunscreen (SPF 15 or higher) to exposed skin surfaces; reapply at least every 2 hours."
   4. "Apply sunscreen with a minimum SPF 50 to all skin surfaces before leaving for the beach; this will provide all-day coverage."

CHAPTER

10

Head, Eyes, Ears, Nose, and Throat

evolve

http://evolve.elsevier.com/Wilson/assessment

CONCEPT OVERVIEW

The feature concept for this chapter is *Sensory Perception.* This concept refers to the ability to understand and interact with the environment through senses (sight, hearing, smell, taste, and touch) and conditions that negatively affect these perceptions. Sensory perception occurs through a variety of body systems, and complex interactions between sensory structures and neurologic function. The illustration shows the interrelationships among the concepts that are impacted by sensory perception and the relationship that sensory perception has to neurologic function. The importance of intracranial regulation on sensory perception is shown as a bidirectional arrow. The other concepts are affected by disruptions in sensory perception, shown as a single directional arrow. For example, a child with chronic ear infections may be impacted by pain, interrupted sleep, and developmental delay. An individual with a visual disturbance may experience changes in mobility. Having an understanding of the interrelationships of these concepts helps the nurse recognize potential risk factors and thus increases awareness when conducting a health assessment. This understanding is an important step associated with clinical judgment. The following case provides a clinical example featuring several of these interrelated concepts.

Mr. Rodriquez is a 79-year-old man who lives alone. He has a long history of diabetes mellitus and hypertension. Over the past 8 years, he has experienced a progressive loss of vision as a result of retinopathy (a complication from diabetes). His reduced vision has resulted in frequent falls, and because he no longer cooks for himself, he has lost weight. He also has hearing loss and tinnitus (ringing in the ears), which interferes with his sleep. Mr. Rodriquez has become progressively withdrawn to the point where his grown children are exploring alternative living arrangements for him.

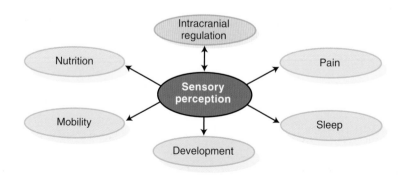

ANATOMY AND PHYSIOLOGY

The head and neck regions contain multiple structures that make the examination of these areas complex. The skull encloses the brain; facial structures include the eyes, ears, nose, and mouth. Structures of the neck include the upper portion of the spine, the esophagus, the trachea, the thyroid gland, arteries, veins, and lymph nodes. Because of the regional relationship, all of these structures are presented in this chapter.

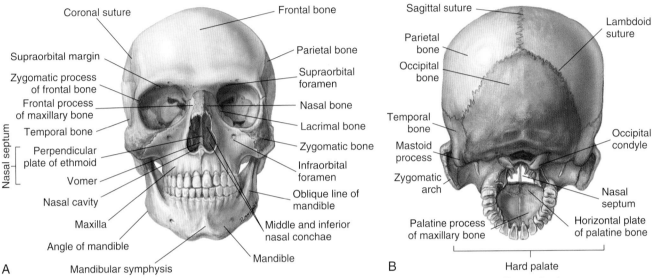

FIG. 10.1 Bones of the skull and face. (A) Anterior view. (B) Posterior view. (From Seeley, Stephens, and Tate, 1995. The McGraw Hill Companies.)

THE HEAD

The skull is a bony structure that protects the brain and upper spinal cord (Fig. 10.1). The special senses of vision, hearing, smell, and taste are also contained within the brain. Six bones form the skull (one frontal bone, two parietal bones, two temporal bones, and one occipital bone) and are fused together at sutures. The skull is covered by scalp tissue, which is typically covered with hair.

The face consists of 14 bones that protect facial structures, including the eyes, ears, nose, and mouth; these structures are generally symmetric. Like the skull, these bones are immobile and are fused at sutures, with the exception of the mandible. The mandible articulates with the temporal bone of the skull at the temporomandibular joint, allowing for movement of the jaw up, down, in, out, and from side to side. The facial muscles are innervated by cranial nerves V (trigeminal) and VII (facial).

THE EYES

External Ocular Structures

The external eye is composed of the eyebrows, upper and lower eyelids, eyelashes, conjunctivae, and lacrimal glands (Fig. 10.2). The opening between the eyelids is termed the *palpebral fissure*. The eyelashes curve outward from the lid margins, filtering out dirt. Two thin, transparent mucous

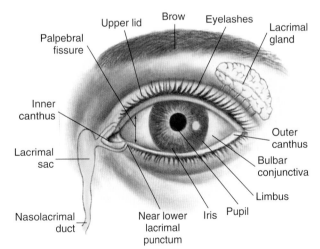

FIG. 10.2 External ocular structures. (From Thompson et al., 2002.)

membranes termed *conjunctivae* lie between the eyelids and the eyeball. The bulbar conjunctiva covers the scleral surface of the eyeballs. The palpebral conjunctiva lines the eyelids and contains blood vessels, nerves, hair follicles, and sebaceous glands. One of the sebaceous glands, the meibomian gland, secretes an oily substance that lubricates the lids, prevents excessive evaporation of tears, and provides an airtight seal when the lids are closed. Tears, formed by the lacrimal

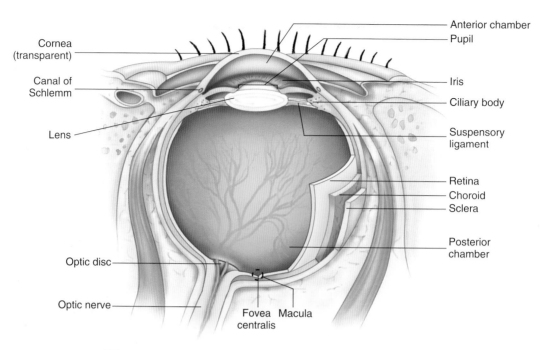

FIG. 10.3 Anatomy of the human eye. (From Lewis et al., 2014.)

glands, combine with sebaceous secretions to maintain a constant film over the cornea. In the inner (or medial) canthus small openings termed the *lacrimal puncta* drain tears from the eyeball surface through the lacrimal sac into the nasolacrimal ducts.

Ocular Structures

The globe of the eye, also known as the "eyeball," is surrounded by three separate layers: the sclera, uvea, and retina (Fig. 10.3). The *sclera* is a tough, fibrous outer layer commonly referred to as the "white of the eye." The sclera merges with the cornea in front of the globe at a junction termed the *limbus*. The cornea covers the iris and the pupil. It is transparent, avascular, and richly innervated with sensory nerves via the ophthalmic branch of the trigeminal nerve (cranial nerve V). The constant wash of tears provides the cornea with oxygen and protects its surface from drying. An important corneal function is to allow light transmission through the lens to the retina. The area between the cornea and the iris is called the anterior chamber.

The middle layer, termed the *uvea*, consists of the choroid posteriorly and the ciliary body and iris anteriorly. The choroid layer is highly vascular and supplies the retina with blood. The iris is a circular, muscular membrane that regulates pupil dilation and constriction via the oculomotor nerve (cranial nerve III). The central opening of the iris, the pupil, allows light transmission to the retina through the transparent lens. The ciliary body is a thickened region of the choroid that has two functions: it adjusts the shape of the lens to accommodate vision at varying distances, and it produces transparent aqueous humor—a fluid that helps maintain the intraocular pressure and metabolism of the lens and posterior cornea. Aqueous humor fills the anterior chamber

between the cornea and lens and flows between the lens and the iris.

The inner layer of the eye, the *retina*, is an extension of the central nervous system. This transparent layer has photoreceptor cells, termed *rods* and *cones,* scattered throughout its surface. As the term *photoreceptor* suggests, these cells perceive images and colors in response to varying light stimuli. Rods respond to low levels of light, and cones to higher levels of light. Although these rods and cones are scattered throughout the retina, they are not evenly distributed. The macula lutea, a pigmented area about 4.5 mm in diameter, is densely packed peripherally with rods. The fovea centralis, a small depression in the center of the macula lutea on the posterior wall of the retina, is concentrated with cones but contains no rods (see Fig. 10.29).

Perforating the retina is the optic disc, which is the head of the optic nerve (cranial nerve II). It contains no rods or cones, causing a small blind spot located about 15 degrees laterally from the center of vision. The central retinal artery and central vein bifurcate at the optic disc and feed into smaller branches throughout the retinal surface as shown in Fig. 10.3 (see Fig. 10.29).

Ocular Function

Vision, the primary function of the eyes, occurs when rods and cones in the retina perceive images and colors in response to varying light stimuli. The lenses are constantly adjusting to stimuli at different distances through accommodation. When the lenses bring an image into focus, nerve impulses transmit the information from the retina along the optic nerve and optic tract, reaching the visual cortex (located in the occipital lobe of each cerebral hemisphere) for cognitive interpretation.

Six extraocular muscles and three cranial nerves allow for eye movement in six directions. The medial, inferior, and superior rectus muscles and the inferior oblique muscles, guided by the oculomotor nerve (cranial nerve III), control upward outer, lower outer, upward inner, and medial eye movements. The superior oblique muscle controls lower medial movement, innervated by the trochlear nerve (cranial nerve IV). The lateral rectus muscle controls lateral eye movement, innervated by the abducens nerve (cranial nerve VI).

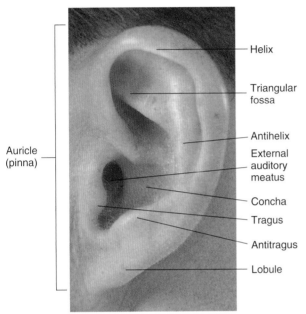

FIG. 10.4 Anatomic structure of the auricle (Pinna).

THE EARS

External Ear

The external ear is composed of the auricle (pinna) and the external auditory ear canal. The auricle is composed of cartilage and skin. The helix is the prominent outer rim; the concha is the deep cavity in front of the external auditory meatus (Fig. 10.4). The bottom portion of the ear is referred to as the *lobule*. The auricle is attached to the head by skin, extension cartilage to the external auditory canal cartilage, ligaments, and muscles (the anterior, superior, and posterior auricular muscles). The auricle serves three main functions: collection and focus of sound waves, location of sound (by turning the head until the sound is loudest), and protection of the external ear canal from water and particles.

The external ear canal of the adult is an S-shaped pathway leading from the outer ear to the tympanic membrane (TM), commonly known as the *eardrum* (Fig. 10.5). The lateral one third of the ear canal has a cartilaginous framework; the medial two thirds of the canal is surrounded by bone. The skin covering the cartilaginous portion of the auditory canal has hair follicles surrounded by sebaceous glands that secrete cerumen (earwax). The hair follicles and cerumen protect the middle and inner ear from particles and infection.

Middle Ear

The middle ear is an air-filled cavity separated from the external ear canal by the TM. The TM, composed of layers of skin, fibrous tissue, and mucous membrane, is shiny and pearl gray. It is translucent, permitting limited visualization of the middle ear cavity. The middle ear contains three tiny

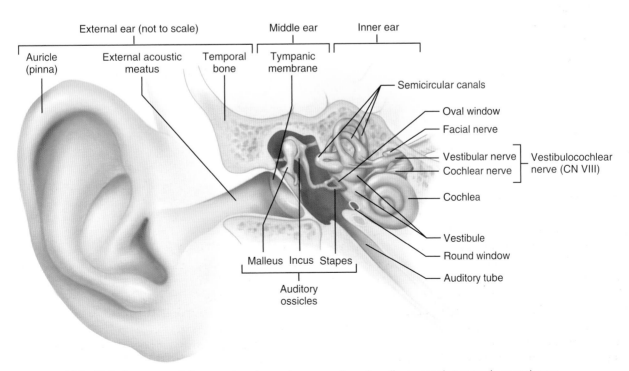

FIG. 10.5 Anatomy of the ear showing outer ear, external auditory canal, tympanic membrane, and structures of the middle and inner ear. (From Lewis et al., 2014.)

bones—the malleus, incus, and stapes—that are collectively known as ossicles (see Fig. 10.5). Lying between the nasopharynx and the middle ear is the eustachian tube. It opens briefly during yawning, swallowing, or sneezing to equalize the pressure of the middle ear to the atmosphere.

The function of the middle ear is the amplification of sound. Sound waves cause the TM to vibrate; this vibration is transmitted through the ossicles to the inner ear. The amplification results from the ossicles vibration and from the size (area) difference between the TM and the oval window (an oval-shaped aperture in the wall of the middle ear leading to the inner ear).

Inner Ear

The inner ear is encased in a bony labyrinth that contains three primary structures: the vestibule, the semicircular canals, and the cochlea (see Fig. 10.5). The vestibule and the semicircular canals contain receptors responsible for balance and equilibrium. The coiled snail-shaped cochlea contains the organ of Corti, the structure that is responsible for hearing. Specialized hair cells on the organ of Corti act as sound receptors. Sound waves that reach the cochlea cause movement of the hair cells, which in turn transmit the impulses along the cochlear nerve branch of the acoustic nerve (cranial nerve VIII) to the temporal lobe of the brain, where the interpretation of sound occurs.

THE NOSE

The nose serves as a passageway for inspired and expired air. It humidifies, filters, and warms air before it enters the lungs and conserves heat and moisture during exhalation. Other functions of the nose include identifying odors and giving resonance to laryngeal sounds.

The upper third of the nose is encased in bone, and the lower two thirds are composed of cartilage. The floor of the nasal cavity is the hard palate. The septal cartilage maintains the shape of the nose and separates the nares (nostrils), which maintain an open passage for air. The nasal cavity is lined with highly vascular mucous membranes containing cilia (nasal hairs) that trap airborne particles and prevent them from reaching the lungs. The inferior, middle, and superior turbinates (also referred to as *concha*) line the lateral walls of the nasal cavity, providing a large surface area of nasal mucosa for heat and water exchange as air passes through the nose. The space between the inferior and middle turbinates is the middle meatus, which is an outlet for drainage from the frontal, maxillary, and anterior ethmoid sinuses. The nasolacrimal ducts drain into the inferior meatus, and the posterior ethmoid sinus drains into the middle and superior meatus (Fig. 10.6).

Paranasal sinuses extend out of the nasal cavities through narrow openings to the skull bones to form four paired, air-filled cavities (i.e., sphenoid, frontal, ethmoid, and maxillary) that make the skull lighter (Fig. 10.7A and B).

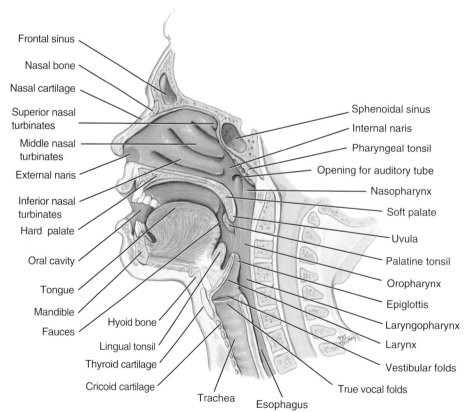

FIG. 10.6 Cross-sectional view of structures of the nose and nasopharynx. (From Applegate, 2011.)

They are lined with mucous membranes and cilia that move secretions along excretory pathways.

THE MOUTH AND OROPHARYNX

Within the mouth are several structures, including the lips, tongue, teeth, gums, and salivary glands (Fig. 10.8A and B). The roof of the mouth consists of the hard palate, near the front portion of the oral cavity, and the soft palate, toward the back of the pharynx. The tongue has hundreds of taste buds (papillae) on its dorsal surface. The taste buds distinguish sweet, sour, bitter, and salty tastes. The ventral (bottom) surface of the tongue is smooth and highly vascular.

Humans have two sets of teeth: deciduous teeth (baby teeth) and permanent teeth. There are 32 permanent teeth: 12 incisors, 8 premolars, and 12 molars. Teeth are tightly encased in fibrous gum tissue covered by mucous membranes and rooted in the alveolar ridges of the maxilla and mandible.

Three pairs of salivary glands—the parotid, submandibular, and sublingual—release saliva through small openings (ducts) in response to the presence of food (see Fig. 10.8). The parotid glands lie anterior to the ears, immediately above the mandibular angle, and drain into the oral cavity through *Stensen*'s ducts (parotid gland openings). These are visible adjacent to the upper second molars. The submandibular glands are tucked under the mandible and lie approximately

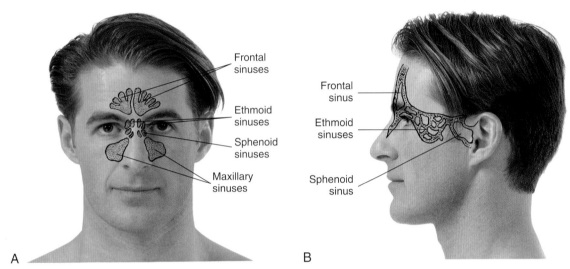

FIG. 10.7 Paranasal sinuses. (A) Front view. (B) Side view.

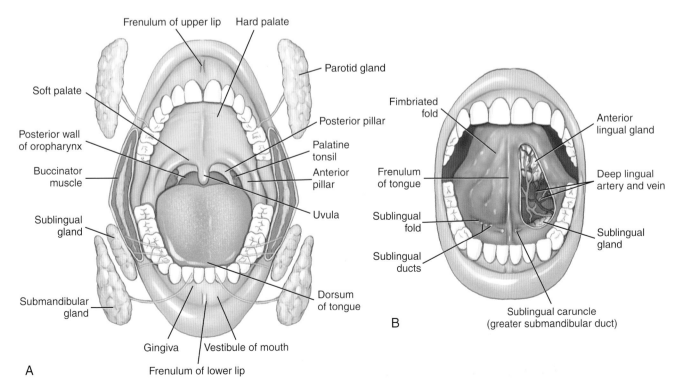

FIG. 10.8 Structures of the mouth. (A) View of dorsal tongue surface. (B) View of ventral tongue surface.

midway between the chin and the posterior mandibular angle. *Wharton*'s ducts, the openings for the submandibular glands, are visible on either side of the lingual frenulum under the tongue. The sublingual glands, the smallest salivary glands, lie on the floor of the mouth and drain through 10 to 12 tiny ducts that cannot be seen with the naked eye.

Located at the back of the mouth, the oropharynx includes several structures that are visible on examination: the uvula, the anterior and posterior pillars, the tonsils, and the posterior pharyngeal wall (see Fig. 10.8A). The uvula is suspended midline from the soft palate, which extends out to either side to form the anterior pillar. The tonsils are masses of lymphoid tissue that are tucked between the anterior and posterior pillars. These may be atrophied in adults to the point of being barely visible. The posterior pharyngeal wall is visible when the tongue is extended and depressed. This wall is highly vascular and may show color variations of red and pink because of the presence of small vessels and lymphoid tissue. The epiglottis, a cartilaginous structure that protects the laryngeal opening, sometimes projects into the pharyngeal area and is visible as the tongue is depressed.

THE NECK

Structures within the neck include the cervical spine, sternocleidomastoid and trapezius muscles, hyoid bone, larynx, trachea, esophagus, thyroid gland, lymph nodes, carotid arteries, and jugular veins (Fig. 10.9). The neck is formed by the bones within the upper spine (cervical vertebrae), which are supported by ligaments and the sternocleidomastoid and trapezius muscles. These structures allow for the extensive movement within the neck. The relationship of neck muscles to one another and to adjacent bones creates anatomic landmarks called *triangles* (Fig. 10.10). The medial borders of

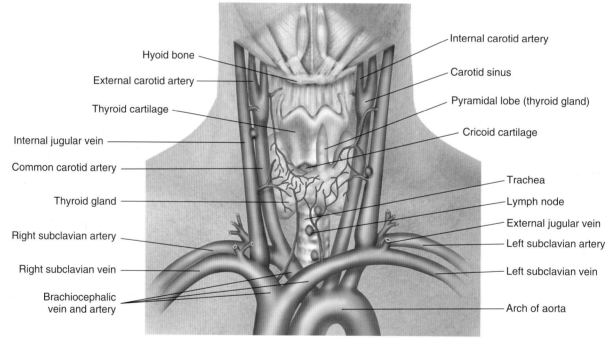

FIG. 10.9 Underlying structures of the neck.

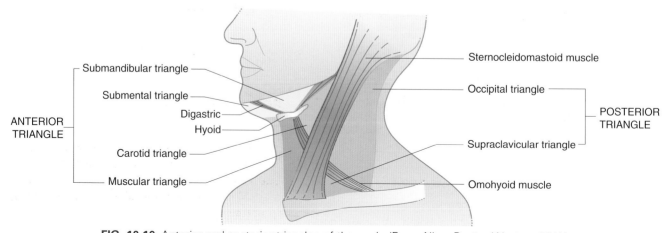

FIG. 10.10 Anterior and posterior triangles of the neck. (From Allan, Baxter, Weston, 2011.)

sternocleidomastoid muscles and the mandible form the anterior triangle. Inside this triangle lie the submandibular triangle, the carotid triangle, and the muscular triangle. Structures within the anterior triangle include the thyroid and cricoid cartilage, larynx, trachea, esophagus, and anterior cervical lymph nodes. The hyoid bone is a U-shaped bone at the base of the mandible that anchors the tongue. It is the only bone in the body that does not articulate with another bone.

The posterior triangle is formed by the trapezius and sternocleidomastoid muscles and the clavicle. Inside the posterior triangle are the occipital triangle and the supraclavicular triangle. The primary structures of the posterior triangle are the posterior cervical lymph nodes.

Larynx

The larynx (also known as the *voice box*) lies just below the pharynx and just above the trachea. It acts as a passageway for air (into the trachea) and allows for vocalization with the vocal cords. The largest component of the larynx is the thyroid cartilage (also known as the *Adam's apple*), located in the anterior portion of the neck (see Fig. 10.9). The thyroid cartilage is a tough, shield-shaped structure with a notch in the center of its upper border that protrudes in the front of the neck, protecting the other structures within the larynx (epiglottis, vocal cords, and upper aspect of the trachea).

Thyroid Gland

The largest endocrine gland in the body, the thyroid produces two hormones, thyroxine (T_4) and triiodothyronine (T_3), both of which regulate cellular metabolism. Mental and physical growth and development depend on thyroid hormones. The thyroid gland is positioned in the anterior portion of the neck, just below the larynx, situated on the front and sides of the trachea (see Fig. 10.9). The right and left lobes of the thyroid gland are butterfly-shaped, joined in the middle by the isthmus. The isthmus lies across the trachea under the cricoid cartilage (the uppermost ring of the tracheal cartilages) and tucks behind the sternocleidomastoid muscle.

Cardiovascular Structures

The carotid arteries and internal jugular veins lie deep and parallel to the anterior aspect of the sternocleidomastoid

muscle (see Fig. 10.9). The carotid pulses are palpated along the medial edge of the sternocleidomastoid muscle in the lower third of the neck. See Chapter 12 for further information about these vessels.

Lymph Nodes

The tiny oval clumps of lymphatic tissue, usually located in groups along blood vessels, are referred to as lymph nodes. Nodes located in subcutaneous connective tissue are called *superficial nodes*; those beneath the fascia of muscles or within various body cavities are called *deep nodes*. Superficial nodes are accessible and can become enlarged and tender, providing early signs of inflammation. Deep nodes, however, are not accessible to inspection or palpation.

In the head, lymph nodes are categorized as preauricular, postauricular, occipital, parotid, retropharyngeal (tonsillar), submandibular, submental, and sublingual. In the neck, lymph nodes are found in chains and are named according to their relation to the sternocleidomastoid muscle and the anterior and posterior triangles of the neck. Lymph nodes in the neck include the anterior and posterior cervical chains, sternomastoid nodes, and the supraclavicular nodes (Fig. 10.11).

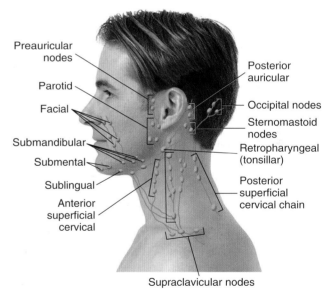

FIG. 10.11 Lymph nodes of the head and neck.

HEALTH HISTORY

Nurses interview patients to collect subjective data about their present health status, past health history, family history, and personal and psychosocial history, which may affect the health condition of their head, eyes, ears, mouth, and neck.

GENERAL HEALTH HISTORY

Present Health Status

Have you noticed any changes in your overall health or changes to your head, eyes, ears, nose, or mouth?
The patient may have noticed a change but may not consider it a "problem." This question allows you to potentially identify problems.

Do you have any chronic conditions that specifically affect your head, eyes, ears, nose, mouth, head, or neck regions (e.g., cataracts, glaucoma, headaches, hearing loss, hypothyroidism)?

There are many chronic conditions specific to the eyes, ears, nose, mouth, and head/neck regions that may be noted during a history and examination. For example, a person with cataracts may experience reduced visual acuity, and a cataract may be observed during the examination.

Do you have other chronic conditions that indirectly affect your head, eyes, ears, nose, mouth, or neck (e.g., hypertension, diabetes mellitus, autoimmune disorders)?

Chronic diseases can lead to many clinical findings in the head and neck regions. For example, diabetes mellitus can lead to poor vision due to retinopathy; hypertension is a risk factor for macular degeneration, and autoimmune disorders are linked to hearing loss.[1]

Do you take any medications (prescription or over-the-counter) or herbal supplements? If so, what do you take and how often? What are the medications for?

Adverse effects of medications can cause symptoms associated with the head and neck regions. Taking ototoxic medications such as aminoglycosides (an antibiotic) increases one's risk for hearing loss.[2] Long-term corticosteroid use is a known risk factor for glaucoma and cataracts. Headaches, dizziness, changes in vision, ringing in the ears, and dry mouth are all examples of medication adverse effects.

Do you use corrective devices for vision (e.g., contact lenses, glasses), hearing (e.g., hearing aids), or use dentures? If so, are any of the devices effective?

The use of corrective devices such as glasses and hearing aids is very common. This question helps establish baseline conditions but also the effectiveness of the treatment.

Past Health History

Have you ever had an injury to your head, eyes, ears, mouth, or neck? If so, describe when and what happened. Do you continue to have any problems related to the injury?

Injuries, either recent or past, may provide information relevant to a patient's clinical findings. Although not common, some individuals have lost an eye as a result of disease or injury and have an eye prosthesis.

Have you had surgery involving your eyes, nose, ears, mouth, or neck? If so, what was the purpose of the surgery and when did this occur?

Knowledge of past surgeries may provide information that may be applied to clinical findings. Teeth extraction and removal of tonsils are common surgical procedures that affect findings within the mouth. Common surgical procedures on the eyes include cataract surgery and surgery for corrective vision. Myringotomy is a common surgical procedure of the ears among children.

Family History

Is there a history of cancer involving the mouth, throat, lymph nodes, or thyroid in your family? If so, which family member(s)? Which kind of cancer was diagnosed?

The patient could have a genetic predisposition to cancer.

Does anyone in your family have conditions impacting hearing, vision, or thyroid?

Cataracts, glaucoma, presbycusis, Meniere disease, and hyperthyroidism are examples of conditions that have familial tendencies and may increase a patient's risk. Hearing loss has also been tied to genetic mutations of the GJB2 gene.[3]

Personal and Psychosocial History

When were your last routine examinations (dental, vision, hearing)?

This question helps describe a patient's health promotion practices. Routine dental examinations and examination of the eyes and ears are recommended. The frequency of examinations depends on the patient's age, underlying medical conditions, and the use of corrective devices.

Describe some of your daily practices to maintain the health of your eyes, ears, and mouth (e.g., brushing and flossing teeth, cleaning contact lenses, wearing sunglasses).

These questions help describe a patient's health promotion practices and potential risks.

Do you know of any occupational or recreational risks for injury to your eyes, ears, or mouth?

Assessment of environmental risk factors that can contribute to vision or hearing loss is an important component of a health history. Patients should be encouraged to take protective action to minimize injury, such as avoiding loud sounds, wearing earplugs, wearing goggles, and wearing eye and/or mouth protection when engaging in contact sports. Regulatory agencies such as the Occupational Safety and Health Administration have guidelines and regulations to reduce injuries in the work environment.[4]

Do you use nicotine products or drink alcohol? If so, how much and how often?

These questions help describe a patient's potential risks for problems involving the head, eyes, and mouth. Chronic alcohol intake and smoking are risk factors for many problems, including cataracts, glaucoma, and cancers of the oropharynx.

PROBLEM-BASED HISTORY

Commonly reported symptoms related to the head and related structures (eyes, ears, nose, throat, and neck) include headache, dizziness, difficulty with vision, hearing loss, ringing in the ears, earache, nasal discharge, sore throat, mouth lesions, and toothaches. As with symptoms in all areas of health assessment, a symptom analysis is completed using the mnemonic OLD CARTS, which includes the *Onset, Location, Duration, Characteristics, Aggravating factors, Related* symptoms, *Treatment,* and *Severity* (see Box 2.6).

Headaches

How long have you been having headaches? How often do you have a headache? How long does it last? Does it follow a pattern?

Many times a headache may be a sign of stress. At other times, it may be a sign of chemical imbalance in the body or even of a more serious pathologic condition. Identification of headache patterns may help determine aggravating factors and causes. Cluster headaches occur more than once a day and last for less than an hour to about 2 hours. They may follow this pattern for a couple of months and then disappear for months or years. Migraine headaches may occur at periodic intervals and may last from a few hours to 1 to 3 days.

What is the location of the headaches? Is the pain in one area, or is it generalized? What does it feel like? How severe is it on a scale of 0 to 10?

Sinus headaches may cause tenderness over frontal or maxillary sinuses. Tension headaches tend to be located in the front or back of the head, and migraine and cluster headaches are usually unilateral. Cluster headaches produce pain over the eye, temple, forehead, and cheek. Tension headaches are described as viselike, migraine headaches produce throbbing pain, and cluster headaches cause a burning or stabbing feeling behind one eye.

Can you think of any factors that trigger headaches? If so, describe. What other symptoms do you experience with the headaches?

Possible triggers include stress, fatigue, exercise, food, and alcohol. Box 10.1 lists common foods that trigger headaches for some individuals. Conditions that can precipitate headaches include hypertension, hypothyroidism, and vasculitis.

Migraines may be accompanied by visual disturbances, nausea, and vomiting. Cluster headaches may occur with nasal stuffiness or discharge, red teary eyes, or drooping eyelids.

How do you treat the headache or what relieves the headaches? If you use medication, what kind is used? How often do you take the medication? How effective is this treatment?

Patients may report using medications, massage, lying in a dark room, or applying a warm or cold cloth to relieve their headache. Knowing what brings relief may help in determining the cause of the headache. Rest can help relieve migraine headaches, whereas movement helps relieve cluster headaches.

Dizziness

Describe the sensation of dizziness that you are experiencing. When did it first begin? How often does it occur? How long does it last?

Ask the patient to define what he or she means when reporting a history of dizziness because *dizziness* is a term used by patients to describe a number of things. Box 10.2 provides a useful distinction of differentiating terms. Nearly all patients who self-report a sensation of motion have vertigo.[5]

Does dizziness interfere with your normal daily activities? Do you experience these symptoms when driving a car or operating machinery? Have you ever fallen as a result of dizziness?

Knowing the effect on activities of daily living (ADLs) helps determine the extent to which dizziness is interfering with the patient's life and the frequency of the problem. Vertigo and dizziness are particularly disabling among older adults.[6] Assessing the patient's risk of falling during periods of dizziness is important. If the patient describes symptoms consistent with vertigo, he or she should be advised about the potential hazard of driving or operating machinery.

BOX 10.1 HEADACHE-TRIGGERING FOODS

- Alcohol
- Beans (broad beans, lima beans, fava beans, snow peas)
- Caffeine (coffee, tea, chocolate)
- Cultured dairy products (yogurt, sour cream buttermilk)
- Fruits
  - Fresh fruits (citrus fruits, ripe bananas, raspberries, kiwi, pineapple, red plums, avocado)
  - Dried fruits (figs, raisins, dates)
- Monosodium glutamate (soy sauce, meat tenderizers, seasoned salt)
- Nitrates and nitrites—commonly found in processed meats (ham, hot dogs, pepperoni, bacon, sausage)
- Nuts (especially peanuts, almonds)
- Onions
- Pizza
- Sunflower seeds
- Tyramine-rich foods (strong or aged cheese, cured or smoked meats, beers on tap)

From National Headache Foundation: Diet and Headache—Foods, 2019. Retrieved from: https://headaches.org/2007/10/25/diet-and-headache-foods/

BOX 10.2 DIFFERENTIATING DIZZINESS

Dizziness is a symptom used by many patients to describe a wide range of sensations, including faintness, light-headedness, feeling as if their head is spinning, or the inability to maintain normal balance in a standing or seated position. The following terms differentiate reports of dizziness.

Presyncope: Feeling of faintness and impending loss of consciousness—sometimes referred to as "near faint." This is often a cardiovascular symptom.

Disequilibrium: Feeling of falling—often a vestibular function disorder.

Vertigo: Sensation of movement, usually rotational motion such as whirling or spinning. Subjective vertigo is the sensation that one's body is rotating in space; objective vertigo is the sensation that objects are spinning around the body. Vertigo is the cardinal symptom of vestibular dysfunction.

Light-headedness: Vague description of dizziness that does not fit any of the other classifications.

Difficulty With Vision

What type of difficulty are you having with vision? Does the problem affect one eye or both? When did it begin? Did it begin suddenly or gradually? Is it constant, or does it come and go?

The patient's description is essential in determining the cause of visual difficulty. The sudden onset of visual symptoms may indicate a detached retina and requires an emergency referral. The involvement of both eyes tends to indicate a systemic problem, whereas the involvement of one eye is a localized problem.

What other symptoms are you experiencing? What makes your vision worse? What treatment have you tried for the vision difficulty? How effective was the treatment?

Headaches, dizziness, and nausea are symptoms commonly associated with visual difficulty. Knowing what makes the vision problem worse may help identify its cause. Determining which therapies have been used successfully or unsuccessfully helps discern the problem and guides treatment strategies.

Has your vision problem interfered with your daily life? If so, describe how.

Determine the impact that this visual difficulty has had on the patient's quality of life and evaluate the adjustments the patient has made to lifestyle and routines.

RISK FACTORS

Glaucoma

- Age: Prevalence increases sharply each year over age 60.
- Gender: Women have a higher prevalence than men.
- Ethnicity: African Americans have the highest prevalence.
- Family history: Those with a history of glaucoma in a first-degree relative have three times the risk.
- Medication: Long-term corticosteroid use (M).
- Chronic disease: Diabetes mellitus and hypertension.

M, Modifiable risk factor.
From National Eye Institute, National Institutes of Health: https://nei.nih.gov/

Hearing Loss

How long have you had trouble hearing? Does the problem affect one ear or both? What tones or sounds are difficult for you to hear? Did the hearing loss occur suddenly or gradually? Have you noticed other symptoms associated with the hearing loss?

Establish the onset of the problem. A sudden hearing loss in one or both ears that is not associated with an ear infection or upper respiratory infection requires further evaluation. Hearing loss associated with aging (presbycusis) occurs gradually and increases with advancing age, particularly with high frequencies.

RISK FACTORS

Hearing Loss

- Age: Incidence increases across life span especially after age 50
- Gender: Men have a greater risk
- Environmental noise (repeated exposure to loud noise >80 dB) (M)
- Ototoxic medications (aminoglycosides, salicylates, furosemide) (M)
- Family history (sensorineural hearing loss)
- Autoimmune disorders (sensorineural hearing loss)
- History of congenital hearing loss

M, Modifiable risk factor.
From Blazer D, Domnitz S, Liverman C: *Hearing health care for adults: priorities for improving access and affordability,* 2016, National Academy of Sciences.

To what degree does your hearing loss bother you? Does it interfere with your daily routine or create problems on the job or in social interactions?

Hearing loss may cause individuals to withdraw or become isolated because they cannot hear or they are embarrassed. This may lead to reduced interpersonal communication, depression, and exacerbation of coexisting psychiatric conditions.

Ringing in the Ears (Tinnitus)

Describe the noise that you are hearing. Is it ringing, hissing, crackling, or buzzing? When did it first begin? Does the sound occur all of the time, or does it come and go? If it comes and goes, does it occur with certain activities or at the same time of day?

Ringing of the ears (tinnitus) is a sensation or sound heard only by the affected individual. It can manifest differently with a variety of sounds or sensations.[7] Establish the pattern of the symptom; this may provide clues to determine the cause of the problem.

Earache

How long have you had an earache? Does the problem affect one ear or both? Is the pain deep inside the ear or on the surface of the ear? What does the pain feel like (dull, sharp)? On a scale of 0 to 10, how would you rate the severity of your ear pain? Is it constant, or does it come and go? If it comes and goes, how often does it occur and how long does it last?

Determine the onset, location, and duration of pain. Ear pain can be unilateral or bilateral; it can be internal or external. If the pain is intermittent, explore possible triggering mechanisms. Ear pain can be related to an infection in the mouth, sinuses, or throat. Pain caused by an ear infection involving the external ear or ear canal increases with movement of the ear; pain caused by otitis media does not change with manipulation of the ear.

Is there any discharge from the ear? If so, what does it look like? Does it have an odor?

A description of ear discharge might help determine the cause of the symptoms. Ear discharge may be a sign of bacterial otitis media.

Nasal Discharge/Nose Bleed

When did the nasal discharge/nose bleed begin? How would you describe the discharge (color, consistency, odor)? Is it coming from one side of your nose or both?

A thick or purulent green-yellow, malodorous discharge usually results from a bacterial infection. A foul-smelling discharge, especially unilateral discharge, is associated with a foreign body or chronic sinusitis. Profuse watery discharge is typically seen with allergies. A bloody discharge may result from a neoplasm, trauma, or an opportunistic infection such as a fungal disease. A nose bleed (epistaxis) may occur secondary to trauma, chronic sinusitis, malignancy, or a bleeding disorder; it may also result from cocaine use.

What other symptoms do you have?

Related symptoms consistent with allergic rhinitis include itching, swelling, discharge from the eyes, postnasal drip, and cough.[8] Fatigue, fever, and pain may be symptoms associated with infection.

What have you done to treat the discharge/bleeding? How effective is the treatment?

Determining what has been used successfully in the past may guide current treatment strategies and provide an opportunity for teaching. If the patient uses nasal spray other than normal saline, alert him or her that it should be used for only 3 to 5 days to avoid causing rebound congestion.

Sore Throat

How long have you had a sore throat? Describe what it feels like (e.g., a lump, burning, scratchy). Does it hurt to swallow? Are others in your home ill or have they just recovered from a sore throat or cold?

The onset and description of the symptoms the patient is experiencing may help determine the underlying cause. Often edema and pain associated with throat infections make swallowing difficult. Sore throats are usually caused by viral infections and resolve within a few days. Less common causes are environmental factors such as inhalation of dust, fumes, or excessively dry air.

Do you have any other symptoms such as a fever, cough, fatigue, painful lymph nodes?

A sore throat may have many causes, from nasal congestion or sinus drainage to an infection or allergy. Commonly related symptoms include fever and fatigue. Nasal congestion that requires mouth breathing during the night may cause a sore throat in the morning.

Mouth Sores or Lesions

Where is the mouth sore? How long has it been present? Is it painful? Is there just one sore or are there others?

Mouth lesions can be located anywhere in the mouth (lips, tongue, gums, buccal mucosa, palate) and caused by many things, including trauma, infection, nutritional deficits, immunologic problem, or cancer. Some mouth lesions are very painful, while some are painless.

Does the sore bother you when eating or talking? Have you had any other symptoms? Are there sores anywhere else on your body such as in the vagina? In the urethra? On the penis? In the anus?

Bleeding, lumps, and thickened areas in the mouth are possible symptoms of oral cancer. Enlarged lymph nodes might be associated with cancer or an infection. Painful ulcerations may impair adequate nutritional intake. Sexually transmitted diseases (including chlamydia, gonorrhea, syphilis, herpes, and human papillomavirus) can be transmitted through oral sex.[9]

RISK FACTORS

Oropharyngeal Cancer

- Tobacco use (M)
- Alcohol use (M)
- Age: Incidence is increased after age 55, with peak incidence between ages 64 and 74.
- Gender: There is a 2:1 male-to-female incidence.
- Human papillomavirus (HPV) infection of the mouth
- Exposure to ultraviolet (UV): increased risk for lip cancers among those with prolonged exposure to the sun. (M)
- Immunosuppression increases risk.

*Note: Tobacco and alcohol use are two greatest risk factors. Individuals who smoke and use alcohol are estimated to have 100 times the risk compared with those who do not smoke or drink. *M*, Modifiable risk factor.
From American Cancer Society, www.cancer.org, 2018.

Toothache

Which tooth or teeth are hurting? How long have you had the pain? What does the pain feel like? (Dull, sharp, throbbing?) Is the pain constant or does it come and go?

Toothaches can be attributed to several factors, including tooth decay, gum disease, tooth fracture, damaged filling, or an abscess. Establishing the onset and character of the pain may provide clues to help determine the underlying cause.

Do you recall a specific incident that may have caused the pain? What other symptoms have you noticed (bleeding gums, fever, heat or cold sensitivity)? Does the pain interfere with eating?

Determining the precipitating and aggravating factors may provide clues to the underlying cause. A fever could be associated with an abscess; trauma to the mouth could suggest a tooth fracture. Tooth decay can cause pain over a long period of time and worsen as the decay progresses.

HEALTH PROMOTION FOR EVIDENCE-BASED PRACTICE

Hearing

An estimated 28 million people in the United States have a hearing impairment. These impairments are caused by a number of factors, including genetics (congenital), exposure to excessive noise (noise-induced hearing loss), trauma, infections (especially otitis media), and certain drugs. Hearing is a necessary component for child development; therefore identification of hearing impairment at an early age is critical. Newborn hearing screening is required by law in many states.

Recommendations to Reduce Risk (Primary Prevention)
- Wear hearing protection when exposed to loud or potentially damaging noise at work, in the community, or at home.
- Limit periods of exposure to noise.

- Reduce volume when using stereo headsets or listening to amplified music in a confined place such as a car.
- Be aware of and minimize noise in the personal environment. Consider noise rating when purchasing recreational equipment, children's toys, household appliances, and power tools; look for those items with lower noise ratings.

Screening Recommendations (Secondary Prevention)
The Centers for Disease Control and Prevention recommend screening for hearing loss in all newborn infants, not later than 1 month of age. If loss is identified, perform audiologic evaluation by age 3 months and enroll in appropriate intervention services by age 6 months as needed.

From Centers for Disease Control and Prevention: *Screening and diagnosis of hearing Loss*, 2018. Available at https://www.cdc.gov/ncbddd/hearingloss/screening.html

EXAMINATION

Routine Techniques

Head
- INSPECT the head.
- INSPECT the facial structures.

Eyes
- TEST visual acuity.
- ASSESS visual fields for peripheral vision.
- INSPECT the external ocular structures.
- INSPECT the corneal light reflex.
- INSPECT each sclera.
- INSPECT the cornea transparency and surface characteristics of each eye.
- INSPECT each iris.
- INSPECT the pupils.

Ears
- ASSESS hearing.
- INSPECT the external ears.
- INSPECT each external auditory meatus.

Nose
- INSPECT the external nose.

Mouth
- INSPECT the lips.
- INSPECT the teeth and gums.
- INSPECT the tongue.
- INSPECT the buccal mucosa and anterior and posterior pillars.
- INSPECT the palate, uvula, posterior pharynx, and tonsils.

Techniques for Special Circumstances

Head
- PALPATE the structures of the skull.
- PALPATE the bony structures of the face and jaw.
- PALPATE the temporal arteries.
- AUSCULTATE the temporal arteries.

Eyes
- ASSESS eye movements: Six cardinal fields of gaze and cover-uncover test.
- PALPATE the eyes, eyelids, and lacrimal puncta.
- EVERT the eyelids.
- TEST the corneal reflexes.
- INSPECT the anterior chambers.
- INSPECT intraocular structures.

Ears
- PALPATE the external ears and mastoid areas.
- INSPECT the internal ear structures.
- TEST auditory function.

Nose
- PALPATE the nose.
- INSPECT the internal nasal cavity.
- PALPATE the paranasal sinuses.
- TRANSILLUMINATE the sinuses.

Mouth
- PALPATE the teeth, inner lips, and gums.
- PALPATE the tongue.

Routine Techniques	Techniques for Special Circumstances
Neck • INSPECT the neck. • ASSESS the range of motion. • ASSESS neck muscle strength.	**Neck** • PALPATE the trachea. • PALPATE the thyroid gland. • PALPATE the lymph nodes.

Equipment needed

• Ophthalmoscope • Otoscope with pneumatic bulb • Stethoscope • Penlight • Snellen chart or Snellen "E" chart • Handheld vision screener (Rosenbaum or Jaeger) • Cover card (opaque) • Tuning fork • Audioscope • Watch with second hand • Nasal speculum • Examination gloves • Tongue blade • 4 × 4 gauze • Transilluminator

PROCEDURES WITH EXPECTED FINDINGS

ROUTINE TECHNIQUES: HEAD

PERFORM hand hygiene.

INSPECT the head for size, shape, and position. INSPECT skin and scalp for surface characteristics.

Look at the head in relation to the neck and shoulders for size and shape. *Normocephalic* is the term designating that the skull is symmetric and appropriately proportioned for the size of the body. The head should be held upright in a straight position. To inspect the scalp, part the hair in various locations. The scalp should be intact, without lesions, redness, or flakes.

INSPECT the facial structures for size, symmetry, movement, skin characteristics, facial expression, and skin tone.

The facial bones and features (eyes and eyebrows, palpebral fissures, nasolabial folds, and sides of the mouth) should appear appropriately proportioned and symmetric. Facial movement should be smooth, symmetric with a calm facial expression (Fig. 10.12). The overlying skin should be smooth and without lesions or edema; even skin tone, and appropriate presence of facial hair for age and gender.

ABNORMAL FINDINGS

Microcephaly is an abnormally small head. *Macrocephaly* is an abnormally large head.

Note asymmetric facial bones or facial features (Fig. 10.13). Note facial expression associated with stress or anxiety or abnormal facial movements (tics). Note abnormal skin color, uneven skin pigmentation or skin tone, skin lesions, coarse facial hair (in women), and edema.

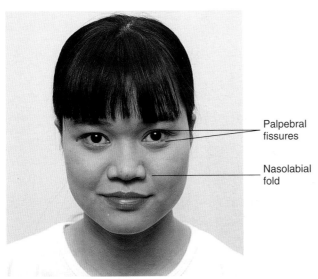

Palpebral fissures

Nasolabial fold

FIG. 10.12 Symmetry of facial features.

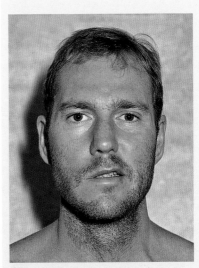

FIG. 10.13 Right facial palsy causing asymmetry of facial features. (From Swartz, 2010.)

PROCEDURES WITH EXPECTED FINDINGS	ABNORMAL FINDINGS

SPECIAL CIRCUMSTANCES: HEAD

PALPATE the structures of the skull for symmetry, tenderness, and intactness.

Palpation of the skull is done when there is a suspected injury, observed irregularity or abnormality, or reported pain.

Procedure: Palpate the skull from front to back using a gentle rotary motion using your finger pads. Examination gloves should be worn if the patient has scalp lesions, injury, or poor hygiene.

Findings: The skull should be symmetric, intact, and feel firm without tenderness.

Lumps, marked protrusions, or tenderness should be differentiated to determine if they are on the scalp or actually part of the skull. Depressions or unevenness of the skull may occur secondary to skull injury.

PALPATE the bony structures of the face and jaw, noting jaw movement and tenderness.

Palpation of the face and jaw is done when there is suspected injury, observed irregularity, or a reported problem such as pain or jaw clicking.

Procedure: To palpate movement of the temporomandibular joint (TMJ), place two fingers in front of each ear and ask the patient to slowly open and close the mouth and move the lower jaw from side to side (Fig. 10.14).

Findings: The jaw should move smoothly and without pain.

Limited movement, pain with movement, and a jaw that clicks or catches with movement may indicate TMJ disease.[10] Pain associated with palpation of facial structures should be explored further.

PALPATE the temporal arteries for pulsation, texture, and tenderness and AUSCULTATE the temporal arteries for sounds.

Temporal arteries are examined if the patient reports headache/pain in the temporal area.

Procedure: Using your finger pads, palpate over the temporal bone on each side of the head lateral to each eyebrow for the temporal artery. Use the bell of the stethoscope to auscultate the temporal arteries, if indicated.

Findings: The artery should be smooth and nontender, with pulsation noted. No sound is expected with auscultation.

Tender, edematous, or hardened temporal arteries with redness over the temporal region suggest temporal arteritis. A bruit (a low-pitched blowing sound) heard during auscultation indicates a vascular abnormality.

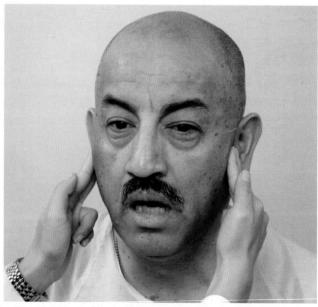

FIG. 10.14 Position fingers in front of each ear to palpate the temporomandibular joint.

PROCEDURES WITH EXPECTED FINDINGS

ROUTINE TECHNIQUES: EYES

TEST visual acuity (distance vision).

Procedure Using Snellen Eye Chart: Place the Snellen chart on the wall in a well-lighted room. The patient may sit or stand at the appropriate distance (based on chart instructions). If the patient wears contact lenses or glasses, he or she should leave them in place. Notice the ease with which the patient reads the letters.

- Have the patient cover one eye with an opaque card and read the line of smallest letters that is possible to read. Test the other eye and then test both eyes using the same procedure.
- Document the line read completely by the patient, using the fraction printed at the end of the line; also indicate if the patient was wearing glasses or contacts.
- Next, to assess perception ask the patient to use both eyes to distinguish which of the two horizontal lines is longer. Finally, ask the patient to name the colors of the two horizontal lines to document red and green color perception.
- Note: A Tumbling E chart is used for patients who cannot read letters. The patient is asked to indicate the direction in which the "E" points (see Fig. 3.15C).

Findings: The reading pattern should be smooth. The expected finding is 20/20.

TEST visual acuity (near vision).

Assess near vision for people over 40 years of age or for those who think that they have difficulty reading. Ask the patient to cover one eye, hold a Jaeger or Rosenbaum card about 14 inches from the eyes, and read the smallest line possible (see Fig. 3.16). Repeat the assessment, covering the other eye. Document the line read completely using the fraction at the end of the line. The findings are the same as those for the Snellen chart.

ASSESS the visual fields for peripheral vision (confrontation test).

Procedure: Face the patient, standing or sitting at a distance of 2–3 feet (60–90 cm). Ask the patient to cover one eye with an opaque card and look directly at you; cover your own eye directly opposite the patient's covered eye.

- Hold a pencil or use your finger and extend it to the farthest periphery and gradually bring the object close to the midline (equal distance between you and the patient). Ask the patient to report when he or she first sees the object; you should see the object at the same time.
- Slowly move the object inward from the periphery in four directions. Move your fingers superiorly (from above the head down into field of vision), inferiorly (from upper chest up toward field of vision), temporally (move in laterally from behind the patient's ear into field of vision), and nasally (move medially into field of vision; Fig. 10.15).

Note: This test assumes that the nurse has normal peripheral visual fields.

Findings: Normal values are 50 degrees superiorly, 70 degrees inferiorly, 90 degrees temporally, and 60 degrees nasally. The temporal value is greater than the nasal value because of the position of the opaque card covering one of the eyes.

ABNORMAL FINDINGS

Note any hesitancy, squinting, leaning forward, blinking, or facial expressions indicating that the patient is struggling to see. The larger the denominator, the poorer the vision. As an example, a finding of 20/40 means that the patient can read at 20 feet what a person with normal vision can read at 40 feet. If the patient can read all but one letter in the 20/40 line, document the finding as 20/40−1.

If vision is poorer than 20/30 or if the patient is unable to distinguish colors or line length, refer him or her to an ophthalmologist or optometrist. A person is considered legally blind when the best corrected visual acuity is 20/200.

With age there is a loss of elasticity of the lens of the eye; this finding is termed *presbyopia*. As a result, the patient needs to move the Jaeger or Rosenbaum card farther away to see it clearly.

If the patient cannot see the pencil or finger at the same time that you see it, peripheral field loss is suspected. Refer the patient to an ophthalmologist or optometrist for more precise testing.

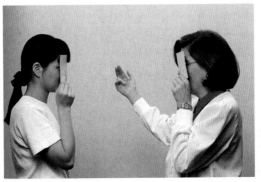

FIG. 10.15 Testing peripheral vision.

PROCEDURES WITH EXPECTED FINDINGS

INSPECT the eyebrows, eyelashes, and eyelids for symmetry, skin characteristics, and discharge.

Skin should be intact and eyebrows symmetric. Note whether the eyebrow extends over the eye. Eyelashes should be distributed equally and curled slightly outward. Palpebral fissures (the opening between eyelids) should be equal bilaterally. The color of the eyelids should correspond to skin color. The eyelid margins should be pale pink and fit flush against the eyeball surfaces; the upper lid should cover part of the iris but not the pupil; the lower lid generally covers to just below the limbus (Fig. 10.16). Lid closure should be complete, with a smooth, easy motion. Blinking is typically frequent and bilateral with involuntary movements, averaging 15–20 blinks per minute.

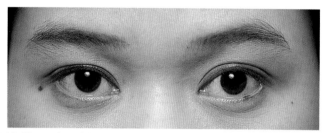

FIG. 10.16 Normal position of eyes and eyelids with symmetric light reflection in both corneas.

🌐 ETHNIC, CULTURAL, AND SPIRITUAL VARIATIONS

Eyes

- The palpebral fissures are horizontal in non-Asians, whereas Asians normally have an upward slant to the palpebral fissures (see Fig. 10.12).
- In Caucasian patients, the eyeball does not protrude beyond the supraorbital ridge of the frontal bone. In African American patients it may protrude slightly beyond the supraorbital ridge.
- The sclera appears white except in darker-skinned patients, in whom it is normally a darker shade. Tiny black dots of pigmentation may be present near the limbus in dark-skinned individuals. In light-skinned individuals, there may be a slight yellow cast.

ABNORMAL FINDINGS

Flakiness, loss of eyebrows or lashes, scaling, and unequal alignment of movement are abnormal as are asymmetric palpebral fissures. The lid of either eye covering part of the pupil is known as *ptosis* (Fig. 10.17). Sclera is visible between the upper lid and iris in hyperthyroid exophthalmos (Fig. 10.18). Closure of the lid that is incomplete or accomplished only with pain or difficulty may occur with infections. Edema of the lid (periorbital edema) may occur with trauma or infection. The presence of lesions, nodules, erythema, flaking, crusting, excessive tearing, or discharge should be documented. Note inward deformity of the lid and lashes. This is a finding seen in enophthalmos (Fig. 10.19).

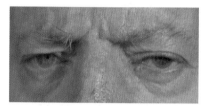

FIG. 10.17 Ptosis. Patient with ptosis to left eye. Note that lid is covering a portion of the pupil. (Courtesy Lemmi and Lemmi, 2013.)

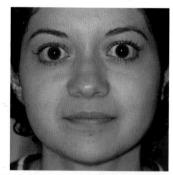

FIG. 10.18 Exophthalmos. (Courtesy Lemmi and Lemmi, 2013.)

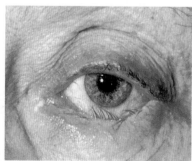

FIG. 10.19 Enophthalmos. The eyelid and lashes are rolled in. (From Bedford, 1986.)

PROCEDURES WITH EXPECTED FINDINGS

INSPECT each conjunctiva for color, drainage, and lesions.

Procedure: Don examination gloves. Ask the patient to look up. Gently separate the lids widely with the thumb and index finger, exerting pressure over the bony orbit surrounding the eye. Have the patient look up, down, and to each side. Next, evert the lower lid; ask the patient to look up (Fig. 10.20).

Findings: The bulbar conjunctiva should be pink and clear; tiny red vessels are often noted.

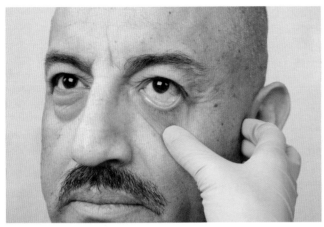

FIG. 10.20 Inspection of the conjunctiva of the lower eyelids.

INSPECT the corneal light reflex for symmetry (Hirschberg test).

Ask the patient to stare straight ahead with both eyes open. Shine a penlight toward the bridge of the nose at a distance of 12–15 inches (30–38 cm). Light reflections should appear symmetrically in both corneas (see Fig. 10.16). *Note:* When an imbalance is found in the corneal light reflex, perform the cover-uncover test (discussed in the following sections).

INSPECT each sclera for color and surface characteristics.

Sclera should be white and clear, although slight yellowing may be seen in darkly pigmented individuals.

ABNORMAL FINDINGS

Red conjunctiva, particularly with purulent drainage, may indicate conjunctivitis (see Fig. 10.61 later in this chapter). A sharply defined area of blood adjacent to normal-appearing conjunctiva may indicate subconjunctival hemorrhage. Lesions, nodules, and foreign bodies are abnormal findings.

If light reflections appear at different spots in each eye (asymmetrically), it may indicate weak extraocular muscles.

Yellow sclera may indicate jaundice caused by liver disease or obstruction of the common bile duct. Redness within the sclera suggests inflammation or hemorrhage (Fig. 10.21). A blue tone to the sclera may be caused by osteogenesis imperfecta. The appearance of a pink growth of conjunctiva over the sclera is a pterygium (Fig. 10.22).

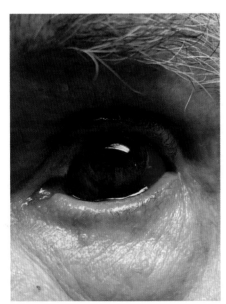

FIG. 10.21 Subconjunctival hemorrhage.

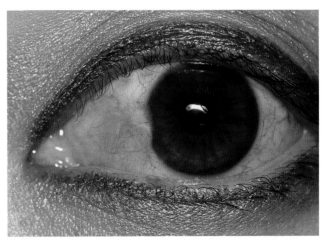

FIG. 10.22 Pterygium. (Courtesy Lemmi and Lemmi, 2013.)

PROCEDURES WITH EXPECTED FINDINGS

INSPECT each cornea for transparency and surface characteristics.

Use oblique lighting and slowly move the light reflection over the corneal surface. Observe for transparent quality and a smooth surface that is clear and shiny.

INSPECT each iris for shape and color.

The iris should be round with consistent coloration. Some people may have a normal variation in color in which each iris is a different color. This is caused by genetic factors.

INSPECT the pupils for size, shape, reaction to light, consensual reaction, and accommodation.

Procedure: To determine the *pupil size*, use a pupil gauge like the one found at the bottom of a Rosenbaum pocket vision screener (see Fig. 3.16).

To assess *reaction to light and consensual reaction*, dim the room lights if possible. Ask the patient to hold the eyes open and fix his or her gaze on an object across the room. Approach with a penlight beam from the side and shine it directly on the pupil. Observe the pupil receiving the light for the direct reaction and the other pupil for the consensual reaction. Repeat with the other eye.

To test *accommodation*, ask the patient to fix his or her gaze on a distant object across the room. Then ask the patient to shift his or her gaze to your finger, placed about 6 inches from the patient's nose.

Findings: The pupil diameter is normally between 2 and 6 mm. Pupils should be round and equal in size. The illuminated pupil should constrict (direct response); the other pupil should constrict simultaneously (consensual response). The pupils should dilate when visualizing a distant object and constrict when focusing on a near object. Box 10.3 provides tips used to document the expected findings of pupils.

ABNORMAL FINDINGS

Note opacities, irregularities in light reflections, lesions, abrasions, or foreign bodies. Especially note a white, opaque ring encircling the limbus, termed *corneal arcus*, seen in many patients over 60 years old and individuals with hyperlipidemia.

Patients who have had an iridectomy or iridotomy to correct glaucoma have a section of the iris missing. Coloboma is a congenital defect of the iris. Blunt trauma to the eye can cause an iridodialysis (tearing of the iris from the sclera).

A pupil diameter less than 2 mm or greater than 6 mm is an abnormal finding Table 10.1. Failure of either one or both eyes to constrict to light in speed or magnitude indicates dysfunction of the oculomotor nerve (cranial nerve III). If the pupillary response is unequal to light, note whether larger or smaller pupil reacts more slowly, or not at all.

BOX 10.3 DOCUMENTATION TIPS FOR PUPILS

PERRLA
Pupils are **E**qual and **R**ound and **R**eact to **L**ight and **A**ccommodation.

Remembering Cs and Ds for Expected Findings for Accommodation
Pupils **C**onstrict when focusing on a **C**lose object
Pupils **D**ilate when focusing on a **D**istant object

TABLE 10.1 PUPIL ABNORMALITIES

ABNORMALITY	CONTRIBUTING FACTORS	APPEARANCE
Miosis (pupils <2 mm)	Miotic eyedrops such as pilocarpine given for glaucoma	
Mydriasis (pupils >6 mm)	Mydriatic or cycloplegic drops such as atropine; midbrain (reflex arc) lesions or hypoxia; oculomotor (cranial nerve III) damage; acute-angle glaucoma (slight dilation)	
Anisocoria (unequal size of pupils)	Congenital (20% of population have minor differences in pupil size, but reflexes are normal); eye medications (constrictors or dilators); eye disease such as amblyopia, or unilateral sympathetic or parasympathetic pupillary pathway destruction.	

From Ball et al., 2015. Figures from Thompson, 2002.

PROCEDURES WITH EXPECTED FINDINGS

SPECIAL CIRCUMSTANCES: EYES

ASSESS eye movements for the six cardinal fields of gaze (tests cranial nerves III, IV, and VI).

This procedure is done as part of a neurologic exam or when the corneal light reflex is not symmetric.

Procedure: While the patient is looking at you, position your finger 10–12 inches (25–30 cm) from the patient's nose. Ask the patient to keep the head still and use the eyes only to follow your finger or an object in your hand (Fig. 10.23).

- Move the object slowly from its center position to upper outer extreme, hold there, move back to center, to lower inner extreme, and hold there.
- Move the object slowly to temporal-nasal extremes, holding there momentarily. Move the object slowly to opposite upper outer extreme and back to the opposite lower inner extreme.
- An alternative method is to move your finger slowly in a circle to each of the six directions. Stop in each position so the patient can hold the gaze briefly before moving to the next position.

Findings: There will be parallel tracking of the object with both eyes, documented as extraocular movements (EOM) intact. Mild nystagmus at extreme lateral gaze may be noticed.

ABNORMAL FINDINGS

Unequal movement or failure of eyes to move in parallel indicates weakness of the extraocular muscles or an abnormality associated with the cranial nerve. *Nystagmus is* the involuntary movement of the eyeball in a horizontal, vertical, rotary, or mixed direction. It may be congenital or acquired from multiple causes.

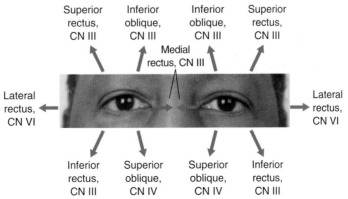

FIG. 10.23 Six cardinal fields of gaze. *CN*, cranial nerve. (From Sanders, 2007.)

PROCEDURES WITH EXPECTED FINDINGS

PERFORM the cover-uncover eye test.

Perform this test if the corneal light reflex is asymmetric.

Procedure and Findings: Ask the patient to stare straight ahead. Cover one of the patient's eyes with the opaque card. Observe the uncovered eye. No deviation or movement from a steady, fixed gaze is observed (Fig. 10.24A). Remove the card from the covered eye; observe if this eye moves to try to focus. The eye should not move (Fig. 10.24B). Repeat steps with the other eye.

ABNORMAL FINDINGS

An eye that moves to focus after being uncovered indicates strabismus (Fig. 10.25), which is caused by extra-ocular muscle weakness or paralysis, difficulty focusing, refractive errors.

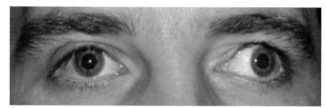

FIG. 10.25 Strabismus with left eye drift. (Courtesy of Kammi Gunton, MD.)

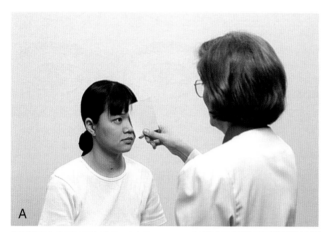

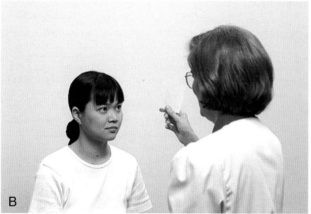

FIG. 10.24 The cover-uncover test is used to evaluate function of eye muscles. (A) Left eye covered; observe right eye. (B) Left eye uncovered; observe it for movement.

PALPATE the eyes, eyelids, and lacrimal puncta for firmness, tenderness, and discharge.

This procedure is done when inflammation is observed or pain is reported.

Procedure and Findings: Ask the patient to look down with lids closed. Gently palpate the upper lid over the eyeball; it should indent with slight pressure. Avoid direct pressure for any length of time. Palpate the lower orbital rim near the inner canthus. This pressure slightly everts the lower lid. Puncta are seen as small elevations on the nasal side of the upper and lower lid margins.

Eyes should be moist, without excessive tearing. Gently palpate the upper and lower lids for tenderness or nodules; there should be no pain or nodules.

An eyeball that is very firm and resists palpation may occur in glaucoma. Lacrimal puncta that are clogged with mucus or particles cause inflammation (dacryocystitis). Fluid or purulent material may be discharged from the puncta in response to pressure. Excessive tearing (epiphora) may be caused by blockage of the nasolacrimal duct. Tenderness, nodules, or irregularities to the lids indicate a problem.

PROCEDURES WITH EXPECTED FINDINGS	ABNORMAL FINDINGS

EVERT each upper eyelid to inspect the conjunctiva of the upper eyelid.

Occasionally eversion of the upper eyelid is necessary when inspection of the conjunctiva of the upper lid is required (such as when patients complain of eye pain or a foreign body is suspected).

Procedure: Wearing gloves, gently grasp the upper eyelashes and pull downward gently while the patient is looking down with the eyes slightly open. Place a cotton-tipped applicator stick about 1 cm above the upper lid margin and push gently down with the applicator while still holding the lashes to evert the lid (Fig. 10.26A). Hold the lashes of the everted lid against the upper ridge of the bony orbit, just below the eyebrow, and examine the lid (Fig. 10.26B). Return the lid to its normal position by moving the lashes slightly forward and asking the patient to look up and then blink.

Finding: The conjunctiva should be pink and clear.

Lesions or foreign bodies may be present and are considered abnormal findings.

TEST each corneal reflex.

Test the corneal reflex *only* in selected cases such as unconscious patients.

Procedure: Lightly touch the cornea with cotton. This reflex tests the sensory reception of the ophthalmic branch of the trigeminal nerve (cranial nerve V) and the motor branch of the facial nerve (cranial nerve VII), which create a blink.

Findings: The lids of both eyes blink when either cornea is touched.

Edema of the brainstem might impair the function of cranial nerves V and VII and may occur after head injury, cerebral hemorrhage, or tumor.

INSPECT the anterior chamber for transparency, iris surface, and chamber depth of each eye.

Perform this procedure when the cornea is not clear and to inspect the depth of the anterior chamber when closed-angle glaucoma is suspected.

Procedure: Using a penlight or an ophthalmoscope, shine light from the side across the iris (Fig. 10.27).

Findings: Anterior chambers should be transparent, irises flat, and a rough estimation of the depths of the chamber is made.

Cloudiness, visible material, or blood may be noted. The iris should not bulge toward the cornea. A narrow anterior chamber may indicate closed-angle glaucoma (Fig. 10.27B). Also note iris or pupil shapes other than round, inconsistent iris coloration, and unequal pupil sizes.

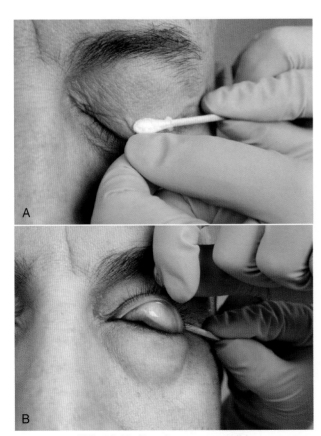

FIG. 10.26 Everting upper eyelid.

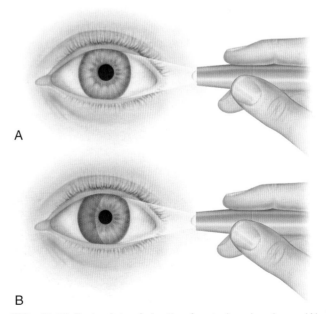

FIG. 10.27 Evaluation of depth of anterior chambers. (A) Normal anterior chamber. (B) Shallow anterior chamber.

PROCEDURES WITH EXPECTED FINDINGS

INSPECT intraocular structures of each eye (ophthalmoscopic examination).

This examination, usually performed by nurses working in a specialty practice, is indicated to assess for the presence of many eye conditions such as cataracts, macular degeneration, and retinopathy.

Procedure: Darken the room to help dilate the patient's pupils. Have the patient remove glasses; contact lenses may be left in. Turn on the ophthalmoscope light and set the diopter wheel to 0.

To examine the patient's right eye, hold the ophthalmoscope in your right hand and use your right eye. To examine the patient's left eye, hold the ophthalmoscope in your left hand and use your left eye. Place your index finger on the diopter wheel so you can change the focus as needed to visualize the internal structures. Red numbers (minus or negative) compensate for the patient's myopia (nearsighted), and black numbers (plus or positive) compensate for hyperopia (farsighted). With the ophthalmoscope against your eye, your field of vision is reduced. To help orient yourself, place your free hand on the patient's shoulder or forehead.

Direct the patient to continuously gaze at a point across the room and slightly above your shoulder. Begin about 10 inches (25 mm) from the patient's eye at a 15-degree angle lateral to his or her line of vision. Shine the light of the ophthalmoscope on the pupil while looking through the viewing lens.

INSPECT for a red reflex.

Procedure and Findings: The red reflex is a red or orange glow over the patient's pupil created by light illuminating the retina. Keep the red reflex in sight and move closer to the eye, adjusting the lens with the diopter wheel as needed to focus; there should be no interruption in the red reflex. Absence of the red reflex may be caused by movement of the light away from the pupil; correct by repositioning the light.

INSPECT the optic disc for discrete margin, shape, color, and physiologic cup.

Procedure: After seeing the red reflex, continue to move closer until you nearly touch foreheads with the patient (Fig. 10.28). Focus varies, depending on the refractive state of both the nurse and the patient; adjust your focus with the diopter wheel. When a blood vessel is located, follow it inward toward the nose until the optic disc is seen.

ABNORMAL FINDINGS

Decreased or irregular red reflex, dark spots, and opacities should be noted. Dark shadows or black dots may indicate opacities that occur with cataracts or may be caused by hemorrhage in the vitreous humor.

Cataracts prevent inspection of the optic disc because the light cannot penetrate the opacity of the lens.

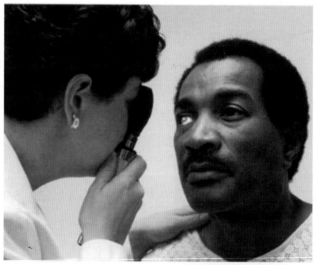

FIG. 10.28 Ophthalmoscopic examination using an ophthalmoscope. (From Linton, 2007).

PROCEDURES WITH EXPECTED FINDINGS

Findings: The margin of the disc should have a distinct, sharp outline. Scattered or dense pigment deposits may be seen at the border. A gray crescent may appear at the temporal border.

The optic disc should be round or slightly oval vertically. Marked myopic refractive errors may make the disc appear larger, and hyperopic errors may make it appear smaller. The color of the optic disc should be creamy yellow to pink, lighter than the retina, possibly with tiny blood vessels visible on the surface (Fig. 10.29).

The physiologic cup is a small depression just temporal to the disc center that does not extend to the border. It usually appears lighter than the rest of the disc. The horizontal diameter of the physiologic cup occupies less than one half of the horizonal diameter of the disc (referred to as the cup-to-disc ratio). Vessels entering the disc may drop abruptly into the cup or appear to fade gradually.

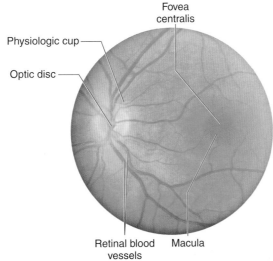

FIG. 10.29 Retinal structures of the left eye. (From Newell, 1992.)

INSPECT the retinal vessels for color, arteriolar light reflex, artery-to-vein ratio, and arteriovenous crossing changes.

Procedure and Findings: From the optic disc follow each of the four sets of retinal vessels from the disc to the periphery. Arteries are, on average, one-fourth narrower than veins; artery-to-vein width should be 2:3–4:5. Arteries are light red and may have a narrow band of light in the center. By contrast, veins are larger than arteries and have no light reflex. They are darker, and venous pulsations may be visible (see Fig. 10.29). Overall the caliber of both arteries and veins should be regular and uniformly decreasing in size as they branch and move toward the periphery. Artery and vein crossing should give no evidence of constricting either vessel.

INSPECT the retinal background for color, presence of microaneurysms, hemorrhages, and exudates.

Procedure and Findings: Look at the overall appearance of the retinal background. The color is uniform throughout and may be pink, red, or orange; it varies with skin color. The retinal surface should be finely granular, with tiny vessels possibly visible. Movable light reflections may appear on the surface, usually in young people.

ABNORMAL FINDINGS

Blurred margin may indicate papilledema, which is caused by increased intracranial pressure relayed along the optic nerve.

Irregular disc or discs that differ in size or shape between the two eyes should be noted. Impaired blood flow may cause the disc to appear whiter than expected. Hyperemic discs with engorged or tortuous vessels on the surface are abnormal.

The depression of the physiologic cup should not extend to the border of the disc and should not occupy more than one half of the diameter of the disc. A large cup suggests open-angle glaucoma. The appearance (size or placement) of the physiologic cup should not differ between eyes.

Extremely narrow arteries are abnormal. The width of the light reflex should not cover more than one third of the artery. Arteries should not be pale or opaque.

Irregularities of caliber, either dilation or constriction, should be noted. Indentations or pinched appearances where veins and arteries cross occur with hypertension and are termed *arteriovenous nicking*.

Pale fundus in either general or localized areas, or hemorrhages (linear, flame-shaped, round, dark red, large, or small) is abnormal. Note microaneurysms, which appear as fine red dots, and any exudates (i.e., soft, hard, fuzzy, or well defined).

PROCEDURES WITH EXPECTED FINDINGS

INSPECT the macula lutea for color and surface characteristics.

Procedure and Findings: Ask the patient to look directly into the ophthalmoscope light. The macula is about one disc diameter (DD) in size and lies about two DDs temporal to the optic disc. The macula and its center should be slightly darker than the rest of the retina. Tiny vessels may appear on the surface. Fine pigmentation and granular appearance may be visible. *Note:* The macula may be difficult to see if the patient's pupil has not been dilated chemically.

ROUTINE TECHNIQUES: EARS

ASSESS hearing based on responses from conversation.

During the history, note the patient's ability to hear by noticing patterns of communication. A patient's ability to engage in conversation is considered an expected finding. Relying on the patient's self-report of hearing ability could result in failure to detect hearing loss.[11] *Note:* Perform further tests for hearing if findings suggest a hearing deficit (described in the following Special Circumstances section).

INSPECT the external ears for alignment, position, size, symmetry, skin color, skin intactness, and presence of lesions or deformities.

The top of the pinna of the ear should align directly with the outer canthus of the eye and be angled no more than 10 degrees from a vertical position (Fig. 10.30).

The ears should be between 4 and 10 cm in length and appear the same bilaterally. If the ears are pierced, note the skin around the piercing for skin intactness, edema, or discharge. The skin should be an even skin tone, with color about the same as that noted on the face. It should be intact and without lesions. A small, painless nodule, called *Darwin tubercle*, is a normal deviation and may be noted at the helix of the ear (Fig. 10.31).

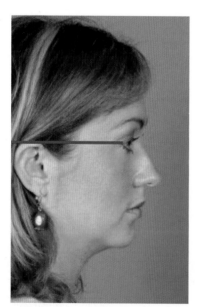

FIG. 10.30 Normal ear position and alignment. (From Totonchi et al, 2018.)

ABNORMAL FINDINGS

Drusen bodies are deposits that form within the layer under the retina and appear as small, discrete spots in the retina. They become yellow as the spots enlarge. When drusen bodies increase in size or number, they may contribute to macular degeneration.

Subtle indications of hearing loss include the patient who asks you to repeat questions, repeatedly misunderstands questions asked, has garbled speech sounds with word distortion, leans forward or tilts his or her head, watches your lips as you speak, or speaks in a loud monotone voice.

Low-set ears (the pinnae are located below the external corner of the eye) or ears that are misaligned (the ear is angled more than 10 degrees from a vertical position) should be considered abnormal. Low-set ears are seen in persons with congenital diseases such as Down syndrome.

If the ears are smaller than 4 cm in length, they are referred to as *microtia* ears. If the ears are larger than 10 cm in length, they are referred to as *macrotia* ears.
Other abnormal findings include lesions or deformities such as nodules, cancerous lesions, sebaceous cysts, cauliflower ear, hematoma, or edema (Table 10.2).

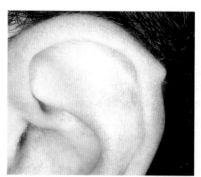

FIG. 10.31 Darwin tubercle. (From Bingham, Hawke, and Kwok, 1992.)

TABLE 10.2 ABNORMAL FINDINGS OF THE EXTERNAL EAR

CAULIFLOWER EAR

Appears as a thickened, disfigured auricle resulting from repeated episodes of minor or major blunt trauma.

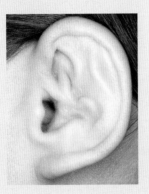

CARCINOMA

Appears in the form of progressive ulcer (as shown) or a patch of crusty skin (squamous cell) or a waxy bump or flat lesion (basal cell).

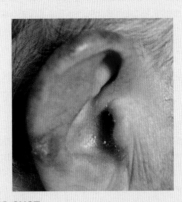

HEMATOMA

Is commonly caused by direct trauma, usually from a contact sport (e.g., football, rugby, wrestling) or a blow to the side of the head (e.g., trauma from a motor vehicle accident, assault).

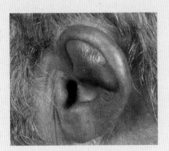

SEBACEOUS CYST

Manifests as a nodule usually found behind the earlobe in the postauricular fold. It is very painful if it becomes infected.

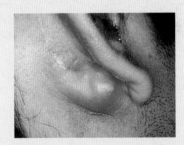

PROCEDURES WITH EXPECTED FINDINGS

INSPECT each external auditory meatus for discharge or lesions.

There should be no lesions or discharge.

SPECIAL CIRCUMSTANCES: EARS

PALPATE the external ears and mastoid areas for characteristics, tenderness, and edema.

Palpation of the ear is usually done in the presence of deformity, injury, inflammation, and/or reported pain.

Findings: The upper part of the ear should be firm and flexible; the earlobe should be soft. All areas should be without tenderness or edema. Gently pull on the helix of the ear to determine if there is any discomfort or pain. There should be none.

ABNORMAL FINDINGS

Discharge from the ear is always an abnormal finding. A bloody or clear discharge from the ear accompanied by a history of head injury may indicate a skull fracture. A purulent or crusty discharge usually indicates infection or the presence of a foreign body.

Tenderness of the mastoid area may indicate mastoiditis. Pain when the helix of the ear is pulled may indicate an inflammation within the auditory canal.

PROCEDURES WITH EXPECTED FINDINGS

INSPECT the ear structures of each ear.

Inspection of the ear canal and internal structures is indicated when inflammation, foreign body, or obstruction of the ear canal is suspected.

Procedure: Use an otoscope to inspect the outer and middle ear. If a variety of speculum sizes are available, choose the largest speculum that comfortably fits into the external auditory meatus. Proper technique using the otoscope is necessary to optimize visualization and prevent discomfort or injury. Turn the light source on before beginning.

- When examining the patient's right ear, grasp the top of the ear with the left hand and gently pull upward and slightly toward the back of the head, and hold the scope in the right hand (Fig. 10.32A). This straightens the S-shaped curve of the auditory canal.
- Holding the otoscope with the handle upside down in the right hand, insert the speculum of the otoscope 1–1.5 cm into the patient's external auditory canal. Rest the back of the right hand against the patient's cheek to steady the positioning of the otoscope (Fig. 10.32B). Alternatively, many nurses hold the otoscope in a handle-down position. Either way, be careful not to insert the otoscope speculum into the canal too far because the bony section of the ear canal is very sensitive.
- When examining the patient's left ear, grasp the top of the ear with the right hand and gently pull upward and slightly toward the back of the head, and hold the scope in the left hand. Rest the back of the left hand against the patient's head to steady the positioning of the otoscope. Use the same procedure described previously.

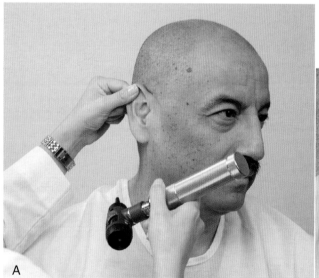
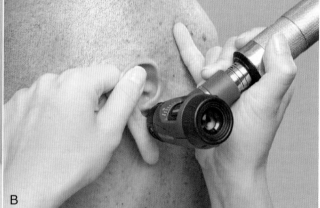

FIG. 10.32 Use of an otoscope. (A) Pull the top of the ear upward and slightly toward the back of the head. (B) Hold the otoscope either vertically or upside down (as shown). Stabilize the otoscope by resting the back of your hand against the patient's temple area.

PROCEDURES WITH EXPECTED FINDINGS

INSPECT each ear canal for cerumen, odor, edema, erythema, discharge, and foreign bodies.

Once the otoscope is properly positioned, look through the lens to visualize the walls of the canal.

Findings: Cerumen is almost always in the canal (Fig. 10.33). Note the characteristics of the cerumen. The color may be black, brown, dark red, creamy, or brown-gray. The texture ranges from moist to dry and flaky to hard. White and dark—skinned races have cerumen that is moist, sticky, and dark. Asians, Native Americans, and Alaskan Natives have cerumen that is lighter in color and generally sparse, dry, and flaky. There should be no odor, edema, erythema, discharge, or foreign bodies in the ear canal.

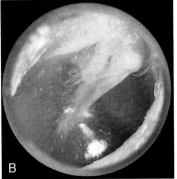

FIG. 10.33 Cerumen (Earwax) in the external ear canal. (From Bingham, Hawke, and Kwok, 1992.)

INSPECT each tympanic membrane for landmarks, color, contour, translucence, and fluctuation.

Continue looking through the lens to visualize the TM.

Findings: Most of the TM is taut and is known as the *pars tensa;* a smaller, less taut (flaccid) part is the *pars flaccida,* and the dense fibrous ring around the membrane is the *annulus.* The cone of light may be seen downward and anteriorly. Using an example of a clock face, the cone of light is seen at the 5 o'clock location in the right ear and the 7 o'clock location in the left ear. Part of the malleus and incus may be visualized through the TM (Fig. 10.34). Note the color and contour. It should be a translucent, pearly gray color.

ABNORMAL FINDINGS

Erythema and edema of the auditory canal may be an indication of otitis externa. The infection may cause the canal to become occluded.

Purulent discharge may occur secondary to otitis externa or with rupture of the tympanic membrane (TM) associated with acute otitis media (AOM). Clear fluid or frank bloody drainage following a head injury may indicate a basilar skull fracture. Other abnormal findings in the auditory canal include the presence of foreign bodies, excessive cerumen, an odor, or a polyp. If an excessive amount of cerumen is present in the ear, it may occlude the entire ear canal.

Absence or distortion of the landmarks on the TM should be considered abnormal. A hole in the TM is referred to as a perforation (Fig. 10.35), which occurs with untreated AOM, a blow to the head, or penetration by a foreign body. Variations in the color and characteristics of the TM indicating an abnormality are presented in Box 10.4.

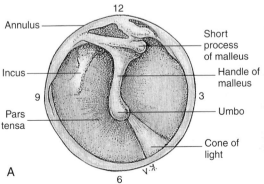

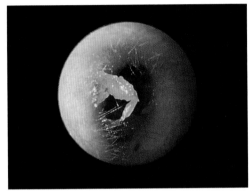

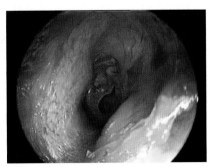

FIG. 10.34 Tympanic membrane. (A) Landmarks of tympanic membrane with "clock" superimposed (right ear). (B) Photograph of a normal-appearing tympanic membrane. (A, From Potter and Perry, 1991. B, Courtesy Dr. Richard A. Buckingham, Clinical Professor, Otolaryngology, Abraham Lincoln School of Medicine, University of Illinois, Chicago. From Barkauskas et al., 2002.)

FIG. 10.35 Perforated tympanic membrane. (From Nassif, 2015.)

BOX 10.4 ABNORMAL APPEARANCE OF THE TYMPANIC MEMBRANE AND POSSIBLE CAUSES

- **Yellow/amber:** Serous fluid in the middle ear, which may indicate otitis media with effusion
- **Redness:** Infection in the middle ear such as acute purulent otitis media
- **Chalky white:** Infection in the middle ear such as otitis media
- **Blue or deep red:** Blood behind the tympanic membrane (TM), which may have occurred secondary to injury
- **Red streaks:** Injected/increased vascularization may be caused by allergy
- **Dullness:** Fibrosis or scarring of the TM secondary to repeated infections
- **White flecks/plaques:** Healed inflammation of the TM

PROCEDURES WITH EXPECTED FINDINGS

Mobility of the TM is evaluated by attaching a pneumatic bulb to the otoscope. To perform this procedure, make sure that the speculum is fully inserted into the canal and the speculum is large enough to completely occlude the canal. Gently squeeze the bulb so puffs of air are transmitted to the TM.

Findings: The expected response is that the TM slightly fluctuates with the puffs of air. This procedure can be performed with any age group but is commonly done when examining infants and young children because they are unable to provide a history regarding the pain they are experiencing.

TEST the acoustic cranial nerves (VIII) to evaluate auditory function.

The following tests are indicated when hearing loss is suspected.

Whispered Voice Test

Procedure: Stand behind the patient to prevent lip reading. Instruct the patient to occlude one ear with his or her hand so one ear may be tested at a time. Softly whisper several monosyllabic (e.g., ball, chair, cat) and disyllabic (e.g., streetcar, baseball, highchair) words and ask the patient to repeat what is heard. Repeat the procedure with the other ear. Although this test is simple, standardization of the results is difficult because of variance of the loudness of whispers among nurses.

Findings: The patient should be able to hear and repeat at least 50% of all words whispered.

Finger-Rubbing Test

Stand directly in front of the patient with outstretched arms so that hands are positioned 3–4 inches from the patient's ears. The patient has eyes closed and is instructed to listen to indicate on which side the rubbing is heard. Using your right or left hand, briskly rub your index finger against your thumb. The patient should be able to hear the noise generated by rubbing the fingers together. Repeat the technique with the other ear using the other hand.

Weber Test

Procedure: This test uses a tuning fork to assess hearing. Activate the tuning fork by holding it by the base stem and striking the prongs against the base of the palm of the hand. Immediately place the base of the fork on the midline of the patient's skull. Ask the patient to indicate in which ear the sound is heard louder.

Findings: Because sound is transmitted along the skull to the inner ear, the patient should hear the tone equally in both ears (Fig. 10.36). However, studies show that up to 40% of normal-hearing persons have sound lateralize to one side.[12]

ABNORMAL FINDINGS

Bulging of the TM with no mobility indicates pus or fluid behind the TM. Retraction of the TM with no mobility indicates obstruction of the eustachian tube.

Increased mobility of only one part of the TM (as determined with the pneumatic bulb) indicates an area of healed TM perforation.

When the patient cannot repeat at least 50% of the spoken words, the findings are considered abnormal. Consider each ear separately.

Patients with a high-frequency hearing loss may not be able to hear the noise generated from finger rubbing.

If the sound lateralizes to one side (i.e., the patient hears the tone better in one ear than the other), the test should be considered abnormal. Lateralization of sound to the affected ear suggests conductive hearing loss (Fig. 10.37A). Lateralization of sound to the unaffected ear suggests sensorineural hearing loss (Fig. 10.37B).

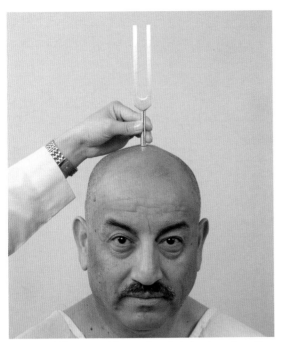

FIG. 10.36 Weber test. The tuning fork is placed on the midline of the skull.

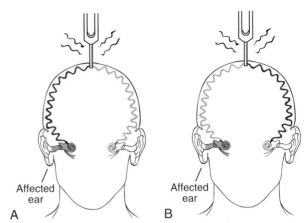

FIG. 10.37 Weber test abnormal findings. (A) Patient with conduction loss; sound lateralizes to the defective ear because the sound transmits through the bone rather than air. (B) Patient with sensorineural loss; sound lateralizes to the unaffected ear.

PROCEDURES WITH EXPECTED FINDINGS

Rinne Test

The Rinne (pronounced "RIN-neh") test also uses a tuning fork to assess hearing by comparing air conduction (AC) of sound to bone conduction (BC) of sound. The AC route through the ear canal is a more sensitive route.

Procedure: Explain the procedure and ask the patient to indicate when the sound is no longer heard when the activated tuning fork is placed on the bone and when it is placed in the front of the ear.

- Activate the tuning fork by holding it by the base stem and striking the prongs against the base of the palm of the hand. Immediately place the base of the tuning fork directly on the patient's mastoid process (Fig. 10.38A).
- Use a watch with a second hand to time the seconds. The patient should be able to hear the tone. Instruct the patient to indicate when the tone can no longer be heard.
- When the patient indicates the tone can no longer be heard, note the number of seconds counted; quickly remove the fork from the mastoid process and hold the vibrating prongs about 2.5 cm (1 inch) in front of the patient's ear Fig. 10.38B).
- Begin timing again. The patient should be able to hear the tone again. Instruct the patient to indicate when the tone is no longer heard.
- When the patient no longer hears the tone, note the number of seconds counted.

Findings: The tone heard in front of the ear should last twice as long as the tone heard when the fork was on the mastoid process (AC > BC by 2:1). This is the expected (positive) response. Repeat the test with the other ear.

ABNORMAL FINDINGS

Consider the test abnormal when the sound is heard longer by bone conduction than air conduction (BC > AC). Patients with conductive hearing loss have bone conduction longer than air conduction in the affected ear (Fig. 10.39A). Patients with sensorineural hearing loss have air conduction longer than bone conduction (AC > BC) in the affected ear, but it will be less than a 2:1 ratio (Fig. 10.39B).

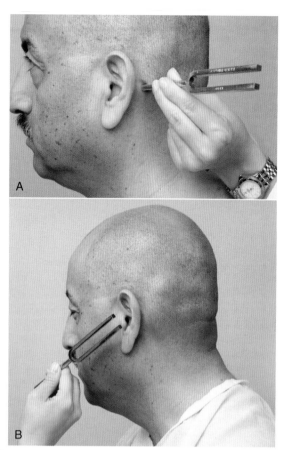

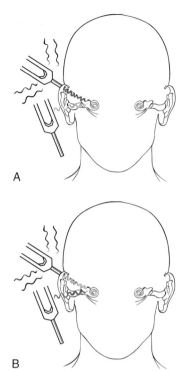

FIG. 10.38 Rinne test. (A) The tuning fork is placed on the mastoid bone for bone conduction. (B) The tuning fork is placed in front of the ear for air conduction.

FIG. 10.39 Rinne test abnormal findings. (A) Patient with conduction loss hears bone conduction longer than air conduction (BC > AC). (B) Patient with sensorineural loss hears air conduction longer than bone conduction (AC > BC).

PROCEDURES WITH EXPECTED FINDINGS

Audioscope

Use an audioscope to measure the degree of hearing loss (see Fig. 3.19).

Procedure: Select a speculum that best fits the ear canal (a snug fit is desired to screen out surrounding noise). Attach the speculum to the probe and insert it in the ear, sealing the external auditory canal. As tones are delivered at each frequency, the patient indicates if the tone can be heard, thus providing an objective measurement of hearing. Because of the high degree of accuracy and ease of use, the audioscope is often used for hearing screening in the primary care setting.

Findings: The patient who hears well is able to hear all tones at all frequencies delivered by the audioscope.

ROUTINE TECHNIQUES: NOSE

INSPECT the external nose for appearance, symmetry, and discharge.

The skin should be smooth and intact, and the skin color should match the rest of the face. The nose should be symmetric and midline. The nostrils should be symmetric, not flaring or narrowed. There should be no nasal discharge present.

ABNORMAL FINDINGS

A 20-dB loss in high frequencies results in difficulty hearing high-pitched consonants. A 40-dB loss in all frequencies causes moderate difficulty in hearing normal speech.

Lesions, erythema, and discoloration may be signs of a systemic illness. Marked asymmetry of the nose and septal deviation causing asymmetry of the nostrils (Fig. 10.40) may be the result of current or past injury. Edema, nasal discharge, and crusting are possible signs of infection, allergy, or injury. Watery, unilateral nasal discharge following a history of head injury may indicate a skull fracture. Unilateral, purulent, thick nasal drainage may indicate a foreign body.

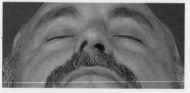

FIG. 10.40 Deviated septum. (From Monahan & Neighbors, 1998.)

PROCEDURES WITH EXPECTED FINDINGS

SPECIAL CIRCUMSTANCES: NOSE

PALPATE the nose for tenderness and to assess patency.

This procedure is indicated in the presence of injury or reported pain or obstruction.

Procedure: Palpate the bridge and soft tissue of the nose. Apply pressure to occlude one nostril; ask the patient to close his or her mouth and sniff through the opposite nostril; repeat on the other side.

Findings: The nose should not be tender with palpation. There should be noiseless, free exchange of air on each side.

INSPECT the nasal cavity for color, surface characteristics, lesions, erythema, discharge, and foreign bodies.

This procedure is indicated in the presence of injury or reported pain or obstruction.

Procedure: The internal nasal cavity is inspected using an otoscope with a short, wide tip or a nasal speculum and a light source. Hold the otoscope in the palm of the hand and use the index finger to stabilize it against the side of the nose. Turn on the light and insert the tip slowly and carefully (Fig 10.41). When using a nasal speculum, hold it in the palm of one hand and use the index finger to stabilize it against the side of the nose. Open the speculum slowly on a slightly oblique axis (not horizontally) because direct pressure on the septum is painful. Use the other hand to hold the light source (Fig. 10.42A).

Findings: With the patient's head erect, note the floor of the nose, inferior turbinate, nasal hairs, and mucosa, which should be slightly darker red than the oral mucosa. The patient's nasal septum should be intact and midline. With the patient's head back, inspect the middle meatus and middle turbinate (Fig. 10.42B). Turbinates and meatus should be a deep pink color, similar to the color of the surrounding tissue.

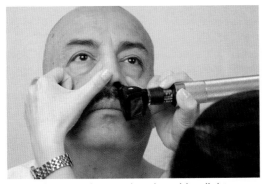

FIG. 10.41 Inspect the nasal cavity with a light source.

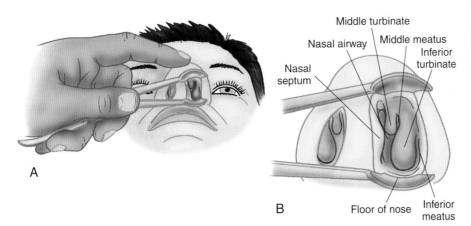

FIG. 10.42 (A) Inspecting the nasal cavity with a nasal speculum. (B) View of the Nasal Mucosa. (From Seidel et al., 2006.)

ABNORMAL FINDINGS

Narrowing of the nostrils when the patient inhales may be associated with chronic obstruction that may necessitate mouth breathing. Noisy or obstructed breathing may occur secondary to nasal congestion, trauma to the nasal passage, polyps, or allergies. Instability or tenderness from trauma or inflammation may be noted on palpation.

Foreign bodies, discharge, perforations, bleeding, or crusting are abnormal findings. A perforation of the nasal septum (Fig. 10.43) appears as a hole within the septum wall. Erythema and edema may occur as a result of infection or inflammation.

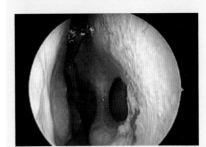

FIG. 10.43 Perforated nasal septum. (From Jennings, et al., 2019.)

PROCEDURES WITH EXPECTED FINDINGS

PALPATE the frontal and maxillary paranasal sinus areas for tenderness.

This procedure is indicated in the presence of injury or reported pain over the sinuses. (Refer to Fig. 10.8 for the location of sinuses.)

Procedure: To palpate the frontal sinuses, press upward on the frontal sinuses with the thumbs on the supraorbital ridge just below the eyebrows. Be careful not to press directly over the eyeballs (Fig. 10.44A). To palpate the maxillary sinuses, press over the sinus area above the cheekbones (Fig. 10.44B).

Findings: There should be no tenderness or pain with palpation over the sinuses.

Tenderness on palpation may indicate sinus congestion or infection. If the patient complains of sinus pain or shows signs of sinus congestion, transilluminate the sinuses (described in the next section).

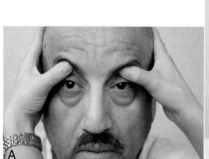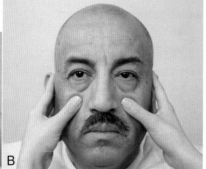

FIG. 10.44 Palpation of sinuses. (A) Frontal. (B) Maxillary.

TRANSILLUMINATE the sinus areas for a dim red glow.

If the patient complains of sinus pain or shows signs of sinus congestion, transilluminate the frontal and maxillary sinuses using a transilluminator or bright penlight.

Procedure and Findings: To transilluminate the maxillary sinuses, darken the room and place the source of light lateral to the nose, just beneath the medial aspect of the eye. Look through the patient's open mouth for illumination of the hard palate. Transilluminate the frontal sinuses by placing the light source against the medial aspect of each supraorbital rim. A dim red glow is transmitted above the eyebrows.

An absence of a glow during transillumination of the sinuses may indicate that one or more sinuses congested and filled with secretions or that it never developed.

ROUTINE TECHNIQUES: MOUTH

INSPECT the lips for color, symmetry, moisture, and texture.

Lips should appear pink and symmetric both vertically and laterally. They should be smooth and moist and have slight vertical linear markings. There should be a distinct border between the lips and the facial skin (vermillion border).

Pale lips may indicate anemia or shock. Cyanotic (bluish) lips and circumoral cyanosis (bluish tint surrounding the mouth) may indicate hypoxemia or hypothermia. Dry, flaking, or cracked lips may be caused by dehydration or exposure to dry air or wind. Cracks and erythema in the corners of the mouth may be caused by vitamin B deficiencies.[13] Lesions, plaques, vesicles, nodules, or ulcerations may be signs of infection, irritation (such as lip biting), or skin cancer. Lips may be edematous because of an allergic reaction.

PROCEDURES WITH EXPECTED FINDINGS

INSPECT the teeth and gums for color, surface characteristics, condition, and alignment.

Procedure and Findings: The teeth should be white, yellow, or gray, with smooth edges. Inspect the condition of the teeth, making note of caries and broken, loose, and missing teeth.

Observe alignment by asking the patient to clench the teeth and smile. The upper back teeth should rest directly on the lower back teeth, with the upper incisors slightly overriding the lower ones. The teeth should be evenly spaced.

The gingiva around the base of the teeth should have a pink, moist appearance with a clearly defined margin at each tooth. For patients who wear dentures, observe the gum line beneath the dentures.

🌐 ETHNIC, CULTURAL, AND SPIRITUAL VARIATIONS

Mouth

- About 30% of Asian Americans, 15% of Native Americans, and 10% of Caucasians have a congenital absence of the third molar and thus have only 28 teeth as adults. This pattern is rare in African Americans. Caucasians have the smallest teeth; African Americans tend to have larger teeth than Caucasians; Asians and Native Americans have the largest teeth.
- Darker-skinned persons often have darker oral pigmentation and may have a patchy brown pigmentation of the gums. There may also be a dark brown to black pigmented line along the gingival margin.
- A split uvula occurs in up to 10% of Asians and 18% of some Native American groups.

ABNORMAL FINDINGS

Missing teeth may occur secondary to tooth extraction or trauma. Darkened or stained teeth may occur secondary to coffee, medications, poor dental care, or frequent vomiting. Brown spots in the crevices or between the teeth may indicate caries. Excessively exposed tooth neck (the narrowed part of the tooth between the crown and the root) with receding gums may occur secondary to aging or gingival disease. Malocclusion refers to a misalignment of teeth. Common variations of malocclusion include protrusion of the upper incisors (also known as overbite; Fig. 10.45), protrusion of the lower jaw (known as prognathism; Fig. 10.46), or misalignment of teeth (Fig. 10.47).

The presence of debris usually occurs because of poor dental hygiene. Redness, edema, and bleeding of the gums may occur secondary to gingivitis, systemic disease, hormonal changes, and drug therapy (see Fig. 10.68).

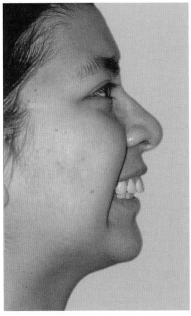

FIG. 10.45 Malocclusion of teeth: overbite. (Courtesy Lemmi and Lemmi, 2013.)

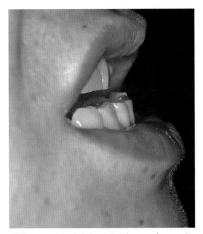

FIG. 10.46 Malocclusion of teeth: prognathism. (Courtesy Lemmi and Lemmi, 2013.)

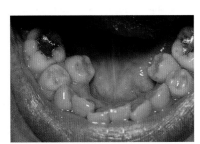

FIG. 10.47 Misalignment of teeth in lower jaw. (Courtesy Lemmi and Lemmi, 2013.)

PROCEDURES WITH EXPECTED FINDINGS

INSPECT the tongue for movement, symmetry, color, and surface characteristics.

Procedure: Ask the patient to stick out his or her tongue. (This maneuver also tests cranial nerve XII—the hypoglossal nerve.)

Findings: The forward thrust should be smooth and symmetric, and the tongue itself should appear symmetric. The tongue should be pink and moist with a glistening surface dorsally and laterally. The surface may appear slightly rough because of the papillae on the dorsal surface of the tongue.

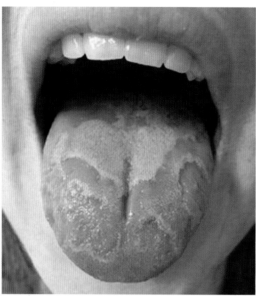

FIG. 10.48 Geographic tongue. (From Ogueta et al., 2019.)

INSPECT the buccal mucosa and anterior and posterior pillars for color, surface characteristics, and odor.

Procedure and Techniques: Ask the patient to open the mouth widely to allow for inspection of the buccal mucosa with gloved hands using a penlight and tongue blade. Inspect the anterior and posterior pillars. Note the color of the mucosa and the symmetry of the pillars.

Findings: The color of the tissue should be pale coral or pink with slight vascularity. Using a tongue blade, gently pull the buccal mucosa away from the molars. It should be smooth, with a transverse occlusion line appearing adjacent to where teeth meet. Clear saliva should cover the surface. The parotid gland duct opening (also known as Stensen duct) is on the buccal mucosa adjacent to the upper second molar. It appears as a slightly elevated pinpoint red mark. Also note the odor of the breath. The mouth should have a slightly sweet odor or none at all.

ABNORMAL FINDINGS

Note edema or variation in size, color, coating, or ulceration. Atrophy of the tongue on one side or deviation of the tongue may be a sign of a neurologic disorder. A smooth or beefy-red-colored, edematous tongue with a slick appearance may indicate B vitamin deficiency.[13] A tongue with irregular patches with a map-like appearance is referred to as a geographic tongue (Fig. 10.48). A hairy tongue with yellow-brown-to-black, elongated papillae may occur secondary to antibiotic therapy, superinfection, or pipe smoking. An enlarged tongue may be seen in patients with Down syndrome or hypothyroidism. Lesions and sores are always considered abnormal.

Aphthous ulcers on the buccal mucosa appear as white, round, or oval ulcerative lesions with a red halo (see Fig. 10.71). Leukoplakia is a white patch or plaque found on the oral mucosa that cannot be scraped off. Erythroplakia is a red patch found on the oral mucosa. An excessively dry mouth or excessive salivation may indicate salivary gland blockage or may occur secondary to medications, dehydration, or stress.

An acetone odor on the breath may indicate diabetic ketoacidosis. A fetid odor may occur secondary to gum disease, caries, poor dental care, or sinusitis.

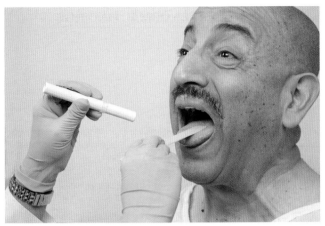

FIG. 10.49 Displace the tongue with a tongue depressor for inspection of the pharynx.

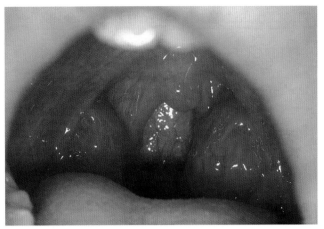

FIG. 10.50 Tonsil enlargement in healthy adolescent. (Courtesy Lemmi and Lemmi, 2013.)

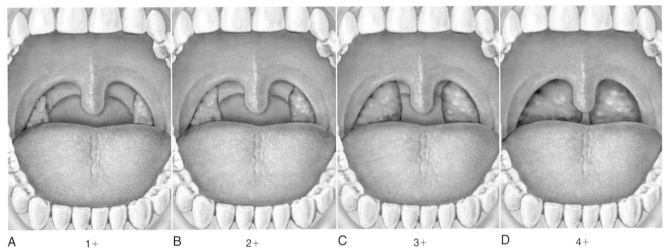

A 1+   B 2+   C 3+   D 4+

FIG. 10.51 Grading tonsil enlargement. (A) 1+, visible; (B) 2+, halfway between tonsillar pillars and uvula; (C) 3+, nearly touching the uvula; (D) 4+, touching one another.

PROCEDURES WITH EXPECTED FINDINGS

INSPECT the palate, uvula, posterior pharynx, and tonsils for texture, color, surface characteristics, and movement.

Procedure and Techniques: Continue use of a penlight and tongue blade. With gloved hands, instruct the patient to tilt his or her head back so the palate and uvula can be inspected. The hard palate should be smooth, pale, and immovable with irregular transverse rugae. The soft palate and uvula should be smooth and pink, with the uvula in a midline position. Instruct the patient to say "ah." If necessary, depress the tongue with a tongue depressor. (This tests cranial nerve X, the vagus nerve.) Observe if the soft palate rises symmetrically with the uvula remaining in the midline position. (This tests cranial nerve IX, glossopharyngeal nerve.) Using a tongue depressor to hold the tongue down, examine the posterior wall of the pharynx (Fig. 10.49). The tissue should be smooth and have a glistening pink coloration. The tonsils extend beyond the posterior pillars. They should appear slightly pink with an irregular surface. Enlarged, noninflamed tonsils are a normal variation among adolescents as shown in Fig. 10.50. *Note:* Touching the posterior pharynx with the tongue depressor may initiate a gag reflex but is not part of a routine exam.

ABNORMAL FINDINGS

Nodules observed on the palate may indicate a tumor. Lesions may be present on both the hard and soft palates. Opportunistic infections may occur when an individual has been on antibiotics or is immunosuppressed. Failure of the soft palate to rise bilaterally and uvula deviation during vocalization may indicate a neurologic problem.

Exudate or mucoid film on the posterior pharynx may be present secondary to postnasal drip or infection. A grayish tinge to the membrane may occur with allergies or diphtheria. Edematous, erythematous tonsils with or without exudate may indicate infection. Tonsil enlargement is graded from 1+ to 4+ (Fig. 10.51).

PROCEDURES WITH EXPECTED FINDINGS	ABNORMAL FINDINGS

SPECIAL CIRCUMSTANCES: MOUTH

PALPATE the teeth, inner lips, and gums for condition, stability, and tenderness.

This technique is indicated in the presence of injury, lesions, or reported pain.

Procedure and Findings: Wearing examination gloves, palpate the teeth and inner aspects of the lips and upper and lower gingivobuccal fornices and gingivae (gums). The teeth should be anchored firmly.

Marked movement of the teeth may be secondary to either periodontal disease or trauma. Gum tenderness or thickening may indicate that the dentures do not fit well or the presence of lesions.

PALPATE the tongue for texture.

This technique is indicated in the presence of injury, lesions, or reported pain.

Procedure and Findings: Wearing examination gloves, grasp the tongue with a 4 × 4-inch gauze pad, and palpate all sides (Fig. 10.52). During palpation note any lumps, nodules, or areas of thickening. The tongue should feel relatively smooth and even. Papillae create slight roughness on the dorsum of the tongue.

Lumps, nodules, or masses may indicate local or systemic disease or oral cancer.

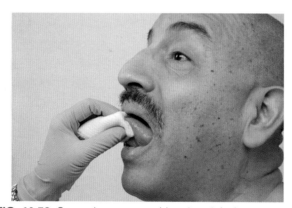

FIG. 10.52 Grasp the tongue with a 4 × 4–inch gauze pad.

ROUTINE TECHNIQUES: NECK

INSPECT the neck position in relation to the head and trachea.

The neck should be centered, and the trapezius and sternocleidomastoid muscles should be bilaterally symmetric (Fig. 10.53). The trachea should be midline.

Note rhythmic movements or tremor of the neck and head. Observe also for tics or spasms. Tracheal deviation suggests displacement by a mass in the chest.

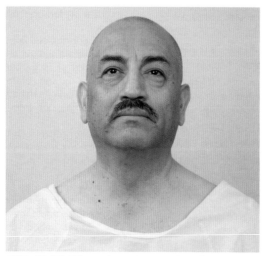

FIG. 10.53 Bilateral symmetry of neck muscles.

PROCEDURES WITH EXPECTED FINDINGS

INSPECT the neck for skin characteristics, presence of lumps, masses.

The skin color should match other skin areas. In some individuals (particularly thin men) the thyroid cartilage may protrude enough to be visible. The thyroid gland is usually not visualized clearly.

ESTIMATE the range of motion (ROM).

Procedure and Findings: Ask the patient to move the neck forward (chin to chest, 45 degrees), backward (toward the ceiling, 55 degrees), and side to side (ear to shoulder, 40 degrees). The shoulders should remain stationary during the assessment. Next, ask the patient to rotate the head laterally to the right and left (70 degrees in both directions). All movements should be controlled, smooth, and painless.

ASSESS neck muscle strength.

Technique and Findings: Assess sternocleidomastoid muscle strength by asking the patient to turn his or her head from side to side against the resistance of your hand placed against the patient's cheek and jaw (see Fig. 14.15). Assess trapezius muscle strength by asking the patient to shrug the shoulders against the resistance of your hands pressing down on his or her shoulders (see Fig. 14.20). This technique also assesses the spinal accessory nerve (cranial nerve XI). Palpation of the neck muscles helps assess for areas of muscle tenderness. The muscles should be firm and nontender with palpation.

ABNORMAL FINDINGS

Lesions or masses on the neck are abnormal. A goiter (enlarged thyroid) may be seen as fullness in the neck (Fig. 10.54).

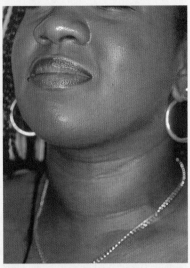

FIG. 10.54 Goiter. Note visible enlargement over the anterior neck. (Courtesy Lemmi and Lemmi, 2013.)

Limited range of motion or pain during movement may indicate either a systemic infection with meningeal irritation, a musculoskeletal problem such as muscle spasm, or degenerative vertebral disks. Note weakness of muscles or tremors. Note if the patient complains of pain throughout the movement or at particular points.

Unilateral or bilateral muscle weakness is an abnormal finding.
Tenderness, muscle spasms, and edema are abnormal findings and may suggest injury.

PROCEDURES WITH EXPECTED FINDINGS

ABNORMAL FINDINGS

SPECIAL CIRCUMSTANCES: NECK

The following procedures are indicated if abnormalities are observed or if the patient reports pain, masses, or reduced range of motion.

Procedure and Findings: Ask the patient to move the neck forward (chin to chest, 45 degrees), backward (toward the ceiling, 55 degrees), and side to side (ear to shoulder, 40 degrees). The shoulders should remain stationary during the assessment. Next, ask the patient to rotate the head laterally to the right and left (70 degrees in both directions). All movements should be controlled, smooth, and painless.

Limited range of motion or pain during movement may indicate either a systemic infection with meningeal irritation, a musculoskeletal problem such as muscle spasm, or degenerative vertebral disks. Note weakness of muscles or tremors. Note if the patient complains of pain throughout the movement or at particular points.

PALPATE the neck for anatomic structures and trachea.

Procedure and Findings: Palpate the neck and trachea just above the suprasternal notch. Palpate for the tracheal rings, cricoid cartilage, and thyroid cartilage. All structures should be midline and nontender.

Abnormalities include tenderness or masses on palpation or location of the structures away from the midline position.

PALPATE the thyroid gland for size, consistency, tenderness, and presence of nodules.

This procedure is indicated when patients report an enlarged mass in their neck or when they display symptoms of hyperthyroidism or hypothyroidism.

Procedure: The thyroid may be palpated using either an anterior or a posterior approach. The technique used is the choice of the nurse. Use a gentle touch to palpate the thyroid. Fingernails should be well trimmed at or below the fingertips. Nodules and asymmetric position are more difficult to detect if the pressure is too hard. In either technique, the patient should flex the neck slightly forward and toward the side being examined to relax the sternocleidomastoid muscle.

Posterior approach (Fig. 10.55A): Stand behind the patient. Have him or her sit straight with the head slightly flexed. Reach from behind, around the patient's neck, and place your fingers on either side of the trachea below the cricoid cartilage. Use two fingers of the left hand to push the trachea to the right. Instruct the patient to swallow while you use the finger pads of the right hand to feel for the right lobe of the thyroid gland, between the right sternocleidomastoid muscle and the trachea. Repeat the technique using the right hand to push the trachea to the left. Instruct the patient to swallow while your left hand feels for the left lobe of the thyroid.

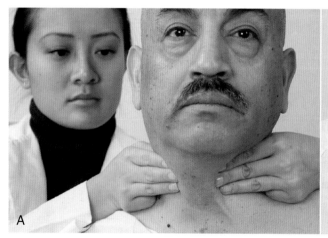
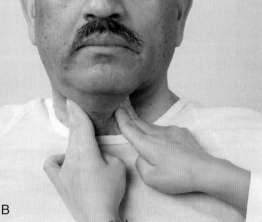

FIG. 10.55 Palpation of thyroid gland. (A) Posterior approach. (B) Anterior approach.

PROCEDURES WITH EXPECTED FINDINGS

Anterior approach (Fig. 10.55B): Stand in front of the patient. Ask him or her to sit up straight and bend the head slightly forward and to the right. Push the patient's trachea to the right with the left thumb. Palpate the thyroid gland below the cricoid process. Instruct the patient to swallow; the patient's displaced right thyroid lobe may be palpated between the sternocleidomastoid muscle and the trachea by the finger pads of your left index and middle fingers. Use the same examination techniques with reversed hand position to examine the left thyroid lobe.

Findings: The thyroid gland is a little larger than the size of the thumb pad. It often is not detected, and this is considered a normal finding. If the thyroid is felt, it should feel small, smooth, and soft; and the gland should move freely during swallowing. The thyroid should be nontender.

PALPATE the lymph nodes for size, consistency, mobility, and tenderness.

Lymph nodes are palpated when an inflammatory process or malignancy is suspected, or if the patient reports pain. Regional lymph nodes include occipital, preauricular, postauricular, anterior and posterior cervical chain, parotid, retropharyngeal (tonsillar), submental, submandibular, and supraclavicular nodes.

Procedure: Palpate the nodes using the pads of the second, third, and fourth fingers. Use both hands, one on each side of the head and neck, to compare the findings. However, the submental nodes are easier to palpate with one hand.

Begin by palpating the preauricular nodes (Fig. 10.56), followed by the parotid, postauricular, occipital, retropharyngeal, submandibular, and submental nodes. Next, examine the anterior and posterior cervical chain by tipping the patient's head toward the side being examined (Fig. 10.57); palpate the anterior chain on either side of the sternocleidomastoid muscle and the deep posterior cervical nodes at the anterior border of the trapezius muscle. Palpate the supraclavicular nodes by having the patient hunch the shoulders forward and flex the chin toward the side being examined. Place the fingers into the medial supraclavicular fossa. Ask the patient to take a deep breath while you press deeply behind the clavicles to detect nodes.

Findings: Lymph nodes may or may not be palpable. If they are palpable, they should be soft, mobile, nontender, and bilaterally equal.

ABNORMAL FINDINGS

A thyroid that is easily palpable before swallowing is enlarged—a common finding in hyperthyroidism. If the thyroid gland is enlarged, use the bell of the stethoscope to auscultate it for vascular sounds. A bruit indicates an abnormally large volume of blood flow and suggests a goiter. Lumps, nodules, or tenderness are abnormal findings.

Lymph nodes that are enlarged, tender, and firm but freely movable may suggest an infection of the head or throat. Malignancy may be suspected when nodes are hard, asymmetric, fixed, and nontender.

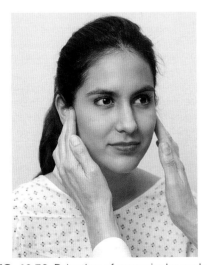

FIG. 10.56 Palpation of preauricular nodes.

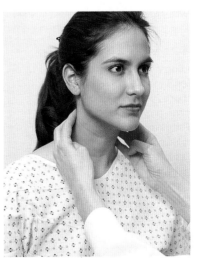

FIG. 10.57 Palpation of posterior superficial cervical chain nodes.

DOCUMENTING EXPECTED FINDINGS

Head: Head symmetric and proportioned for body size. Scalp clean, intact with male-pattern balding. Face and jaw symmetric and proportional. The temporomandibular joint moves smoothly. Temporal arteries palpable bilaterally with a regular rate and rhythm, 2+.

Eyes: Distance and near vision 20/20 both eyes with contact lens. Horizontal and color perceptions intact. Eyebrows symmetric, with eyelashes evenly distributed and curled upward. Palpebral fissures equal bilaterally, and eyelid color appropriate for race. Eyelid margins pale pink, covering the top of the brown iris. Lid closure complete with frequent, bilateral, and involuntary blinking. Bulbar conjunctiva pink and clear. Corneal light reflex symmetric. Sclera white, clear, and moist; corneas transparent. PERRLA, consensual reaction present. Peripheral vision present. Extraocular movements intact. Eyeballs indent with slight pressure, no tenderness of eyelids. Irises clear, with no shadow noted. *Ophthalmic examination:* Red reflex present; disc margins distinct; round, yellow, physiologic cup temporal to disc center; artery-to-vein ratio 2:3, retina red uniformly; macula and fovea slightly darker.

Ears: Hearing present with conversation. Pinna aligned with outer canthus of eyes. Upper part of ear firm, flexible, and soft without discomfort; ears symmetric. Cerumen in auditory canal; TM pearly gray, cone of light reflex present. Whispered words repeated correctly, tone heard bilaterally in Weber test, AC:BC = 2:1.

Nose: Skin smooth, intact, and oily. Nasal passages patent, turbinates pink without exudate, septum midline, sinuses nontender.

Mouth, Throat, and Neck: Breath without odor. Lips symmetric, moist, smooth; 32 white, smooth, aligned teeth. Tongue symmetric, pink, moist, and movable. Gingiva pink and moist, symmetric pillars, clear saliva. Hard palate smooth, pale; soft palate smooth, pink, and rises as expected; uvula midline; posterior pharynx pink, smooth tonsils pink with irregular surface. Trachea midline; thyroid smooth, soft, moves freely with swallow. Neck centered with full range of motion, no palpable lymph nodes.

CLINICAL JUDGMENT

Head and Neck

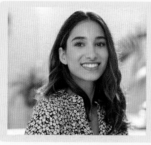

Case Presentation
Sarina Cortez, 21-year-old female college student presents to the student health clinic reporting that she is not feeling well. She states she has a headache and has pain "under her cheeks and forehead" for the last several days along with nasal drainage and reduced appetite.

Reflecting
The nurse reflects on Sarina's care. She was seen by a nurse practitioner; her diagnosis was sinus infection and was prescribed an antibiotic and an anti-inflammatory agent. This experience contributes to the nurse's expertise when encountering a similar situation.

Noticing / Recognizing Cues
The nurse observes a healthy-appearing woman who is calm, with adequate air exchange, and appears well-hydrated. The nurse is aware that Sarina has presented with common findings associated with inflammation of the sinuses.

Responding / Taking Action
The nurse initiates appropriate initial interventions, determines the type of health care provider for Sarina, and ensures she has appropriate follow-up care including fever management, drinking plenty of fluids, and medication management.

Interpreting / Analyzing Cues & Forming Hypotheses
Following the cognitive cues, the experienced nurse recalls that the two most common causes of sinus pain are allergies and sinus infection. To determine if either has any probability of being correct, the nurse gathers additional data:

- *Does the patient have a history of allergies, and is it allergy season?*
Sarina confirms she has a history of seasonal allergies. Currently the airborne pollen count is low.
- *What color is the nasal drainage?*
Sarina reports thick yellow nasal discharge.
- *Does she have a fever?*
The nurse takes a set of vital signs and confirms that Sarina's temperature is 100.7°F (38.0°C).

The experienced nurse not only recognizes sinus inflammation (based on the presenting symptoms) but also interprets this information in the context of additional presenting data (fever and thick yellow nasal discharge) as a probable sinus infection. The nurse eliminates the likelihood that seasonal allergies are causing her symptoms based on the time of year, the description of nasal discharge, and the presence of fever.

AGE-RELATED VARIATIONS

This chapter discusses assessment techniques with adult patients. These data are important to assess for individuals of all ages, but the approach and techniques used to collect the information may vary depending on the patient's age.

INFANTS AND CHILDREN

The nurse should be aware of several important differences when conducting an assessment of the head, eyes, ears, nose, and throat of infants and young children. These differences include interview questions to ask, anatomic differences,

examination procedures, and findings. Refer to Chapter 19 for a detailed discussion related to assessment for this age group.

OLDER ADULTS

Multiple changes occur as a consequence of advancing age; many of these age-related changes impact assessment findings presented within this chapter. See Chapter 21 for further information about the differences of assessment for this age group.

COMMON PROBLEMS AND CONDITIONS

HEAD

Headaches

Headaches are one of the most common medical complaints of humans. Most recurrent headaches are symptoms of a chronic primary headache disorder; but they can also be associated with other problems such as ophthalmologic problems, dental problems, sinusitis, infections, adverse effects from medications, cerebral hemorrhage, or tumors. The pain associated with headaches can be mild or severe. Typically headaches can be classified based on the symptoms and history.

Tension Headache

A tension headache is the most common type of headache experienced by adults between 20 and 40 years of age. **Clinical Findings:** It is usually bilateral and may be diffuse or confined to the frontal, temporal, parietal, or occipital area. The onset may be very gradual and may last for several days. The headache may be accompanied by contraction of the skeletal muscles of the face, jaw, and neck. Patients frequently describe this headache as feeling a tight band around their head.[14]

Migraine Headache

The second most common headache syndrome in the United States is the migraine headache. These headaches can occur in childhood, adolescence, or early adult life; young women are more susceptible. **Clinical Findings:** The headache generally starts with an aura caused by a vasospasm of intracranial arteries and is described as a throbbing unilateral distribution of the headache pain.[15] Accompanying signs and symptoms may include feelings of depression, restlessness or irritability, photophobia, and nausea or vomiting. The headache may last up to 72 hours.

Cluster Headache

A cluster headache is considered to be the most painful of primary headaches. Cluster headaches are most common from adolescence to middle age. **Clinical Findings:** This type of headache is characterized by intense episodes of excruciating unilateral pain. A cluster headache may last from 30 minutes to 1 hour but may repeat daily for weeks at a time (hence the term *cluster*) followed by periods of remission, during which the person is completely free from the attacks. On average, a cluster period lasts from 6 to 12 weeks; and remissions last for an average of 12 months, although they may last for years.[16] The pain is described as "burning," "boring," or "stabbing" pain behind one eye and may be accompanied by unilateral ptosis, ipsilateral lacrimation, and nasal stuffiness and drainage. In general, the headaches occur without warning, although some report a vague premonitory warning such as slight nausea.

Posttraumatic Headache

This headache occurs secondary to a head injury or concussion. **Clinical Findings:** A posttraumatic headache is characterized by a dull, generalized head pain. Accompanying symptoms may be a lack of ability to concentrate, giddiness, or dizziness.

Hydrocephalus

Hydrocephalus is the abnormal accumulation of cerebrospinal fluid (CSF) that may develop from infancy to adulthood. In infants, hydrocephalus is usually a result of an obstruction of the CSF drainage in the head. In adults, it may be caused by obstruction of CSF circulation or resorption. **Clinical Findings:** In infants a gradual increase in intracranial pressure occurs, leading to an actual enlargement of the head (Fig. 10.58). As the head enlarges, the facial features appear

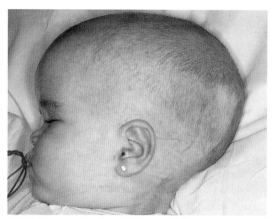

FIG. 10.58 Three-month-old infant with hydrocephalus. (From Bowden, 1998.)

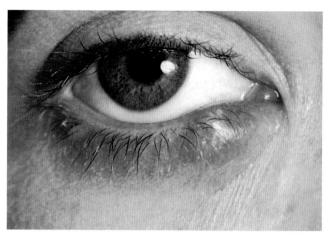

FIG. 10.60 Hordeolum (Stye). (From Bedford, 1986.)

small in proportion to the cranium; fontanels may bulge, and the scalp veins dilate. In adults, the signs of increased intracranial pressure (decreased mental status, headache) are noted because the skull is unable to expand.

EYES

External Eye

Chalazion

A chalazion is a nodule of the meibomian gland in the eyelid. It may be tender if infected and often follows hordeolum or chronic inflammation such as conjunctivitis, blepharitis, or meibomian cyst (Fig. 10.59). **Clinical Findings:** A firm, nontender nodule is observed in the eyelid.

Hordeolum (Stye)

An acute infection originating in the sebaceous gland of the eyelid is termed a *hordeolum*. It is usually caused by *Staphylococcus aureus* (Fig. 10.60). **Clinical Findings:** The affected area is usually painful, red, and edematous.

Conjunctivitis

An inflammation of the palpebral or bulbar conjunctiva is termed *conjunctivitis*. It is caused by local infection of bacteria or virus and by an allergic reaction, systemic infection, or chemical irritation (Fig. 10.61). **Clinical Findings:** The eye appears red. Bacterial conjunctivitis produces a purulent exudate causing a stickiness of eyelids in the morning, viral conjunctivitis produces a watery exudate, and allergic conjunctivitis produces a stringy mucoid discharge and itchiness of the eyes.[12]

Corneal Abrasion or Ulcer

Disruptions of the corneal epithelium and stroma create a corneal abrasion or ulcer. It is caused by fungal, viral, or bacterial infections or desiccation (dryness) because of incomplete lid closure or poor lacrimal gland function. It can also be caused by scratches, foreign bodies, or contact lenses that are poorly fitted or overworn. **Clinical Findings:** The patient feels intense eye pain, has a foreign body sensation, and reports photophobia. Tearing and redness are observed.

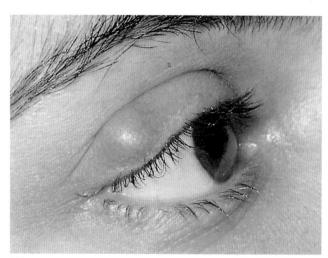

FIG. 10.59 Chalazion (Right upper eyelid). (From Newell, 1992.)

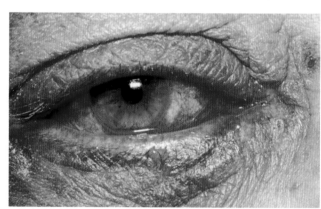

FIG. 10.61 Acute conjunctivitis. (From Krachmer and Palay, 2014.)

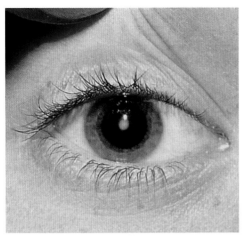

FIG. 10.62 Cataract. Note cloudy white spot over pupil. (From Zitelli, McIntire, and Nowalk, 2012.)

Internal Eye

Cataract

An opacity of the crystalline lens is referred to as a cataract. It commonly occurs from denaturation of lens protein caused by aging, but it can also be congenital or caused by trauma (Fig. 10.62). An estimated 50% of Americans will have a cataract by age 75.[17] **Clinical Findings:** Patients report cloudy or blurred vision; glare from headlights, lamps, or sunlight; and diplopia. They also report poor night vision and frequent changes in their glasses prescriptions. A cloudy lens can be observed on inspection. The red reflex is absent because the light cannot penetrate the opacity of the lens.

Glaucoma

Glaucoma is a group of diseases characterized by an increase in intraocular pressure. Untreated it causes damage to the optic nerve and leads to blindness. Types of glaucoma include open-angle (most common), closed-angle, congenital, and glaucoma caused by drugs or other medical conditions (leads to open- or closed-angle glaucoma). **Clinical Findings:** No specific symptoms accompany open-angle glaucoma. Patients may report gradual and painless loss of peripheral vision, and the eye may be very firm to palpation. The most reliable indicator is an intraocular pressure measurement. Patients with closed-angle glaucoma complain of sharp eye pain and seeing a halo around lights. Clinical findings associated with congenital glaucoma usually begin during infancy within the first few months of life and include cloudiness over the pupil, red-appearing eye, eye enlargement (compared with the other eye), and light sensitivity.

EARS

Foreign Body

A foreign body within the ear is frequently seen in children, although it may occur in all age groups. A foreign body can be any small object such as a small stone, a small part of a toy, or even an insect. **Clinical Findings:** The patient feels a sense of fullness in the ear and experiences decreased hearing. If the foreign body is a live insect, the patient may report hearing the insect move and often experiences severe pain. In this case, symptoms may also include fever. An inspection of the auditory canal reveals the foreign body (Fig. 10.63).

Infection

Acute Otitis Media

AOM is an infection of the middle ear. It can occur at any age but is one of the most common childhood infections for which antibiotics are prescribed.[18] **Clinical Findings:** The major symptom associated with AOM is ear pain (otalgia). Infants unable to verbally communicate pain may demonstrate irritability, fussiness, crying, lethargy, and pulling at the affected ear. Associated manifestations include fever, vomiting (infants), and decreased hearing (older children and adults). On inspection in the early stages, the TM appears inflamed; it is red and may be bulging and immobile (Fig. 10.64). Later stages may reveal discoloration (white or yellow drainage) and opacification to the TM. Purulent drainage from the ear canal with a sudden relief of pain suggests perforation of the TM.

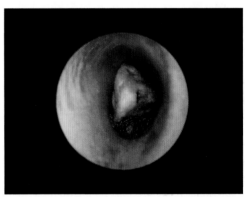

FIG. 10.63 Foreign body in ear canal. Patient inserted a small stone into the deep part of the external ear canal. It is lying against the tympanic membrane. (From Bingham, Hawke, and Kwok, 1992.)

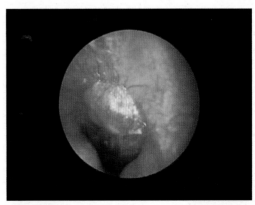

FIG. 10.64 Acute otitis media. Acute otitis media with redness and edematous swelling of the pars flaccida, shown in the central part of the illustration (left ear). (From Bingham, Hawke, and Kwok, 1992.)

Otitis Media With Effusion

Otitis media with effusion (OME) is an inflammation of the middle ear space resulting in the accumulation of serous fluid in the middle ear. **Clinical Findings:** Common symptoms include a clogged sensation in the ears and problems with hearing and balance. Some report clicking or popping sounds within the ear. Because OME is not associated with acute inflammation (as with AOM), fever and ear pain are absent. Upon examination, the TM is often retracted and is yellow or gray with limited mobility (Fig. 10.65).

Hearing Loss

Conductive Hearing Loss

Interference of air conduction to the middle ear results in a conductive hearing loss. It can result from blockage of the external auditory canal (such as a cerumen impaction), problems with the TM (perforations, retraction pockets, or tympanosclerosis), or problems within the middle ear (OME, otosclerosis, trauma, or cholesteatoma).[19] **Clinical Findings:** Typically the chief complaint is a decreased ability to hear and the report of muffled tones. Other findings depend on the cause; obstructions within the auditory canal or problems with the TM may be visible with otoscopic examination, whereas problems within the middle ear may not be visible. During a Weber test, the patient reports sound heard only in the affected ear. During a Rinne test, the patient hears bone conduction longer than air conduction (BC>AC).

Sensorineural Hearing Loss

Sensorineural hearing loss (SNHL) is caused by structural changes, disorders of the inner ear, or problems with the auditory nerve. SNHL accounts for over 90% of hearing loss cases.[19] Presbycusis, the most common cause of SNHL, is caused by atrophy and deterioration of the cells in the cochlea or atrophy, degeneration, and stiffening of cochlear

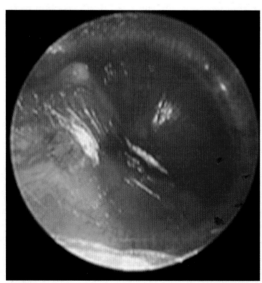

FIG. **10.65** Otitis media with effusion. (From Robb and Williamson, 2016.)

motion. **Clinical Findings:** Presbycusis usually manifests as a gradual and progressive bilateral deafness with a loss of high-pitched tones. Patients with presbycusis have difficulty filtering background noise, making listening difficult. During a Weber test, the patient reports sound only in the unaffected ear. During a Rinne test, the patient hears air conduction longer than bone conduction (AC>BC), but it will be less than a 2:1 ratio.

NOSE

Epistaxis

The term *epistaxis* means bleeding from the nose. Epistaxis occurs in all age groups but commonly affects the elderly[20] and is one of the most common conditions of the nose. Frequent causes of nosebleeds include forceful sneezing or coughing, trauma, picking the nose, or heavy exertion. Some nosebleeds occur spontaneously without an obvious causative event. **Clinical Findings:** The primary sign is bleeding from the nose. Bleeding can be mild or heavy. Most nosebleeds are located in the highly vascular Kiesselbach area located in the anterior aspect of the septum; however, bleeds from the posterior septum may also occur and tend to be more severe.

Inflammation/Infection

Allergic Rhinitis

The term *rhinitis* refers to inflammation of the nasal mucosa. Chronic rhinitis affects millions of individuals and is usually caused by an inhalant allergy, which may be a seasonal allergy or a year-round sensitivity to dust and molds. A strong family history is associated with allergic rhinitis. **Clinical Findings:** After exposure to the allergen the individual experiences sneezing, nasal congestion, and nasal drainage. Other symptoms can include itchy eyes, cough, and fatigue.[8] Turbinates are often enlarged and may appear pale or darker red.

Acute Sinusitis

This is an infection of the sinuses that typically occurs as a result of pooling of secretions within the sinuses, which often occurs after an upper respiratory infection. These pooled secretions provide a medium for bacterial growth. **Clinical Findings:** The most common findings are throbbing pain within the affected sinus and tenderness of the sinus during palpation. The patient may also have fever; thick purulent nasal discharge; and edematous, erythematous nasal mucosa.[20] If transillumination is performed, the absence of a red glow is noted in the affected sinus.

MOUTH

Inflammation/Infection

Herpes Simplex

A cold sore is a highly contagious, common viral infection caused by the herpes simplex virus type 1 (HSV-1). The closely related herpes simplex virus type 2 (HSV-2) is associated with genital herpes but can also cause herpes sores on the face or mouth.[22] It is spread by direct contact. Recurrent infections occur following a stimulus of sun exposure, cold temperature, fever, or allergy. Herpes simplex lesions also can occur in the mouth. **Clinical Findings:** The patient typically has a prodromal burning, tingling, or pain sensation before the outbreak of the lesions. Lesions usually appear on the lip-skin junction as groups of vesicular lesions with an erythematous base. Like other herpes infections, the lesions progress from vesicles, to pustules, and finally to crusts (Fig. 10.66). Herpes simplex lesions in the mouth appear as white ulcerations (Fig. 10.67).

Gingivitis

A common condition among adults, gingivitis is an inflammation of the gingivae (gums). It can be acute, chronic, or recurrent. The most common cause is poor dental hygiene,

leading to the formation of bacterial plaque on the tooth surface at the gum line, resulting in inflammation. **Clinical Findings:** Hyperplasia of the gums, erythema, and bleeding with manipulation are the most common signs (Fig. 10.68).[22] Edema of the gum tissue deepens the crevice between the gingivae and teeth, allowing for the formation of gingival pockets where food particles collect, causing further inflammation. Periodontitis occurs when the inflammatory process causes erosion of the gum tissue and loosening of the teeth.

Tonsillitis

Tonsillitis is an infection of the tonsils. Common bacterial pathogens include β-hemolytic and other streptococci. **Clinical Findings:** The classic presentation of tonsillitis includes sore throat, pain with swallowing (odynophagia), fever, chills, and tender cervical lymph nodes. Some patients may also complain of ear pain.[24] Upon inspection, the tonsils appear enlarged and red and may be covered with white or yellow exudates (Fig. 10.69).

Candidiasis (Thrush)

Candidiasis is an opportunistic infection typically caused by *Candida albicans.* Thrush is commonly seen among individuals who are chronically debilitated, in patients who are immunosuppressed, or as a result of antibiotic therapy. **Clinical Findings:** Oral candidiasis appears as soft, white plaques on

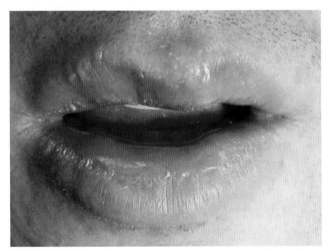

FIG. 10.66 Herpes simplex lesion on upper lip. (From Jong, 2012.)

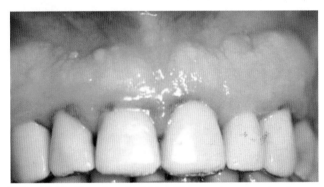

FIG. 10.68 Chronic gingivitis. Note enlargement of gum tissue and inflammation at teeth margins. (From Fiorellini, et al., 2019.)

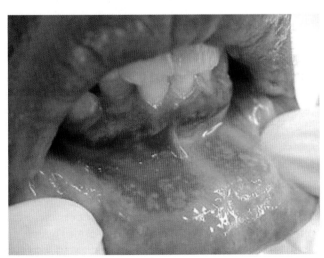

FIG. 10.67 Herpes simplex lesions on the mucous membranes in mouth. (From Fatahzadeh and Schwartz, 2007.)

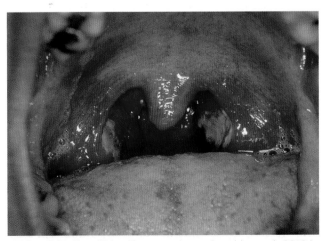

FIG. 10.69 Tonsillitis. (Courtesy Lemmi and Lemmi, 2013.)

the tongue, buccal mucosa, or posterior pharynx (Fig. 10.70). If the lesion is peeled off, a raw, bleeding, erythematous, eroded, or ulcerated surface results.

Lesions

Aphthous Ulcer (Canker Sore)

A canker sore is a common oral lesion with an unknown etiology that affects up to 66% of the population.[25] **Clinical Findings:** These lesions are very painful and appear on the buccal mucosa, the lips, the tongue, or the palate as round or oval ulcerative lesions with a yellow-white center and an erythematous halo (Fig. 10.71). The ulcers may last up to 2 weeks.

Oral Cancer

Oral cancers can occur on the lip or within the oral cavity and oropharynx. An estimated 53,260 new cases will be diagnosed in 2020.[26] **Clinical Findings:** Oral cancer lesions are often subtle and asymptomatic in early stages; premalignant changes of the oral mucosa such as white or red patches (leukoplakia and erythroplakia) may be seen. These lesions progress to painless, nonhealing ulcers (Fig. 10.72). Later-stage signs and symptoms include enlarged, hard, nontender cervical chain or submental lymph nodes; noticeable mass;

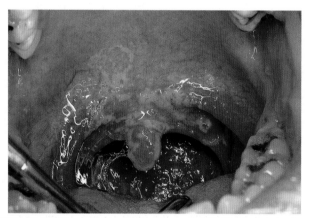

FIG. 10.70 Candidiasis. (From Regezi, Sciubba, and Jordan, 2012.)

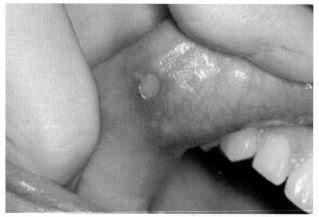

FIG. **10.71** Aphthous ulcer inside upper lip. (From Ali et al., 2016.)

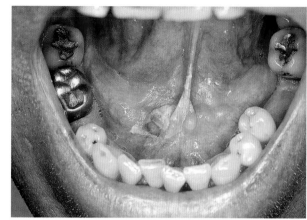

FIG. 10.72 Early squamous cell carcinoma on the floor of the mouth. (From Regezi, Sciubba, and Jordan, 2003.)

bleeding; loosening of teeth; difficulty wearing dentures; and difficulty swallowing.

NECK

Thyroid Disorders

Hyperthyroidism

Hyperthyroidism is a condition associated with excessive production and secretion of thyroid hormone. Of the several diseases that can cause hyperthyroidism, Graves disease, a familial autoimmune disorder, is the most common cause.[27] **Clinical Findings:** Because thyroid hormone affects all body tissue, most body systems are affected. The signs and symptoms reflect increased metabolism and may include enlargement of the thyroid gland and exophthalmos (see Fig. 10.18). Auscultation of the goiter may reveal a bruit.

Hypothyroidism

The most common problem associated with thyroid function is hypothyroidism, characterized by a decreased production of thyroid hormone. Several etiologies have been linked to hypothyroidism, including autoimmune thyroiditis, decreased secretion of thyroid-releasing hormone from the hypothalamus, congenital defects, a result of treatment for hyperthyroidism (i.e., antithyroid drugs or surgical resection of thyroid tissue), atrophy of the thyroid gland, and iodine deficiency.[28] **Clinical Findings:** A decreased metabolism is noted; patients seem to be in "slow motion," with a depressed affect. Goiter may be seen with hypothyroidism because of increases in thyroid-stimulating hormone (see Fig. 10.54).

Thyroid Cancer

As the most common endocrine-related cancer, thyroid cancer was diagnosed in an estimated 52,890 people in 2020.[26] **Clinical Findings:** Thyroid cancer frequently does not cause symptoms. Typically it is first discovered as a small nodule on the thyroid gland. As the tumor grows, changes in the voice and problems with swallowing or breathing may be experienced because of invasion of the tumor into the larynx, esophagus, and trachea, respectively.

CLINICAL APPLICATION AND CLINICAL JUDGMENT

See Appendix B for answers to exercises in this section.

CASE STUDY

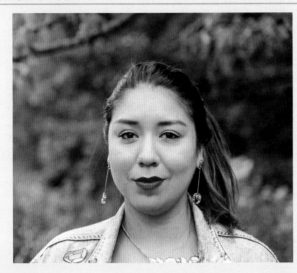

Trudy Neinto is a 25-year-old female who was brought to the clinic by her sister. The following data are collected by the nurse during an interview and examination.

Interview Data

The patient tells the nurse, "My left ear is hurting very badly, and last night I had drainage from my ear on my pillow. I might have a fever too." She adds, "My earache started yesterday, and it is getting worse. I wanted to get it checked yesterday, but I couldn't get a ride to the clinic." Trudy also tells the nurse, "I have been treated many times for this problem."

Examination Data

- *General survey:* Healthy-appearing adult female. Temperature: 101.8°F (38.8°C).
- *External ear examination:* Symmetric position of ears bilaterally. Left ear pinna red. Dried purulent drainage noted on the left external ear and in the left external canal. Grimaces when the left ear is touched. Right ear unremarkable.
- *Internal canal and tympanic membrane:* Dried drainage noted in the left ear canal. TM perforated. Right ear unremarkable.
- *Hearing examination:* Whisper test in right ear 80%; whisper test in left ear 0%.

Clinical Judgment

1. What cues do you recognize that suggest a deviation from normal findings, suggesting a need for further investigation?
2. For which additional information should the nurse ask or assess?
3. Based on the data, which risk factors for hearing loss does Trudy have?
4. With which additional health care professionals should you consider collaborating to meet her health care needs?

REVIEW QUESTIONS

1. A patient describes a recent onset of frequent and severe unilateral headaches that last about 1 hour. Based on these symptoms, the nurse suspects which type of headache?
   1. Cluster headache
   2. Migraine headache
   3. Tension headache
   4. Sinus headache

2. During a physical examination, the nurse is unable to feel the patient's thyroid gland with palpation from an anterior approach. What is the appropriate action of the nurse at this time?
   1. Recognize that this is an expected finding.
   2. Auscultate the thyroid area.
   3. Palpate the thyroid using a posterior approach.
   4. Refer the patient for follow-up with an endocrinologist.

3. A 24-year-old female patient has a 2-day history of clear nasal drainage. Based on these data, which question is the most logical for the nurse to ask?
   1. "Is there a foul odor coming from your nose?"
   2. "Have you recently had nosebleeds?"
   3. "Do you snore when sleeping?"
   4. "Do you have allergies?"

4. A 32-year-old woman has a 4-day history of sore throat and difficulty swallowing. The nurse observes tonsils covered with yellow patches. The tonsils are so large that they fill the entire oropharynx and appear to be touching. How does the nurse document these findings?
   1. "Tonsils yellow and edematous."
   2. "Enlarged tonsils 4+ with yellow exudate."
   3. "Strep infection to tonsils with 3+ swelling."
   4. "1+ edema of tonsils with pus."

5. A nurse is obtaining a health history from a 52-year-old male patient with a red lesion at the base of the tongue. What additional data does the nurse specifically collect about this patient?
   1. Alcohol and tobacco use
   2. Date of his last dental examination
   3. Use of dentures
   4. A history of pyorrhea

6. While talking with a patient, the nurse suspects that he has hearing loss. Which examination technique is most accurate for assessing hearing loss?
   1. Whispered voice test
   2. Rinne test
   3. Weber test
   4. Test using audioscope

7. Which data from the health history of a 42-year-old man should be evaluated further as a possible risk for hearing loss?
   1. "I watch TV in the evenings with my wife and children."
   2. "When I was younger, I wore an earring."
   3. "My primary hobby is carpentry work."
   4. "I have been an accountant for 16 years for an insurance agency."

8. The nurse examines a patient's auditory canal and tympanic membrane with an otoscope. Which finding is considered abnormal?
   1. Presence of cerumen
   2. Yellow color to the tympanic membrane
   3. Presence of a cone of light
   4. Shiny, translucent tympanic membrane

9. During an eye examination, how does a nurse recognize normal accommodation?
   1. The patient has peripheral vision of 90 degrees left and right.
   2. The patient's eyes move up and down, side to side, and obliquely.
   3. The right pupil constricts when a light is shown in the left pupil.
   4. The patient's pupils dilate when looking toward a distant object.

10. How does the nurse assess a patient's consensual reaction?
    1. By touching the cornea with a small piece of sterile cotton and observing the change in the pupil size
    2. By observing the patient's pupil size when the patient looks at an object 2 to 3 feet away and then looks at an object 6 to 8 inches away
    3. By shining a light into the patient's right eye and observing the pupillary reaction of the left eye
    4. By covering one eye with a card and observing the pupillary reaction when the card is removed

11. What are the characteristics of lymph nodes in patients who have an acute infection?
    1. They are enlarged and tender.
    2. They are round, rubbery, and mobile.
    3. They are hard, fixed, and painless.
    4. They are soft, mobile, and painless.

12. Which technique is used for palpating lymph nodes?
    1. Apply firm pressure over the nodes with the pads of the fingers.
    2. Apply gentle pressure over the nodes with the tips of the fingers.
    3. Apply firm pressure anterior to the nodes with the tips of the fingers.
    4. Apply gentle pressure over the nodes with the pads of the fingers.

Lungs and Respiratory System

evolve

http://evolve.elsevier.com/Wilson/assessment

CONCEPT OVERVIEW

The concept for this chapter is *Gas Exchange*, which represents processes that facilitate and impair the transport of oxygen to tissues and carbon dioxide from tissues. Concepts interrelated with gas exchange are shown in the illustration and include perfusion, sleep, nutrition, tissue integrity, motion, metabolism, and intracranial regulation. Understanding the interrelationships of these concepts helps the nurse recognize risk factors when conducting a health assessment.

Because adequate perfusion is necessary to deliver oxygenated blood to and remove metabolic wastes from tissues, its interrelationship is essential to all of the other concepts. Intracranial regulation supports respiratory function, and adequate gas exchange is required to support intracranial function. Metabolism, motion, tissue integrity, sleep, and nutrition all require adequate gas exchange for optimal function.

The following case provides a clinical example featuring several of these interrelated concepts.

John Armstrong is a 59-year-old man who has smoked a pack of cigarettes daily for 41 years. He has chronic obstructive pulmonary disease, which affects his lungs in two ways. Obstructed bronchi increase the work needed to get air into his lungs, and destruction of alveoli impairs diffusion of

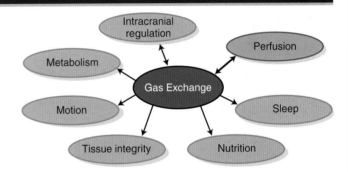

oxygen into pulmonary capillaries and leads to trapping of air. These changes in gas exchange result in hypoxemia. Low arterial oxygen causes shortness of breath (dyspnea), which limits his motion (resulting in activity intolerance), especially when he walks upstairs or any distances more than two blocks. Not only does hypoxemia reduce his appetite, but Mr. Armstrong often becomes short of breath when eating; thus he has experienced unintentional weight loss and has become malnourished. Because he becomes dyspneic when fully reclined, Mr. Armstrong props himself up with three pillows or sleeps in his recliner. He reports that he has not slept more than a few hours at a time for several months.

ANATOMY AND PHYSIOLOGY

The primary purpose of the respiratory system is to supply oxygen to cells and remove carbon dioxide using the processes of ventilation and diffusion. *Ventilation* is the process of moving gases in and out of the lungs by inspiration and expiration. *Diffusion* is the process by which oxygen and carbon dioxide move from areas of higher concentration to areas of lower concentration. For example, at the end of inspiration the concentration of oxygen is higher in the alveoli than it is in pulmonary capillaries. This concentration difference

causes oxygen to move or diffuse from alveoli across the alveolar-capillary membrane to the adjacent pulmonary capillaries, where it is carried by erythrocytes to cells. At the cellular level, oxygen diffuses into the cells; carbon dioxide diffuses from the cells into the capillaries, where it is carried by erythrocytes to alveoli. Carbon dioxide diffuses from the pulmonary capillaries to the alveoli and is exhaled. The cardiovascular system provides transportation of oxygen and carbon dioxide between alveoli and cells.

INTERNAL THORAX

There are three main structures within the thorax or chest: the mediastinum and the right and left pleural cavities. The mediastinum is positioned in the middle of the chest, and within it lie the heart, the arch of aorta, the superior vena cava, the lower esophagus, and the trachea. The pleural cavities contain the lungs. These cavities are lined with two types of serous membranes: the parietal and visceral pleurae. The interior chest wall and diaphragm are protected by the parietal pleura, and the lungs are protected by the visceral pleura. A small amount of fluid lubricates the space between the pleurae to reduce friction as the lungs move during inspiration and expiration (Fig. 11.1). The right lung has three lobes, and the left has two (Fig. 11.2). Each lung extends anteriorly approximately 1.5 inches (4 cm) above the first rib into the base of the neck in adults and posteriorly approximately to the level of T1 (first thoracic vertebra). The base or lower

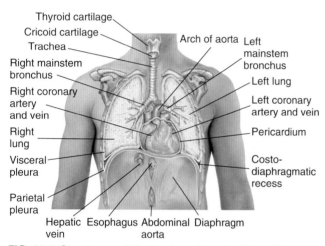

FIG. 11.1 Structures within the thoracic cavity. (From Solomon, et al., 2019.)

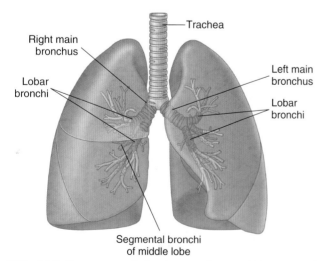

FIG. 11.2 Structures of the lower airway. Right and left lung. Notice fissures dividing lobes of the lungs. Notice structures of the lower airways. (From Drake, Vogl, and Mitchell, 2010.)

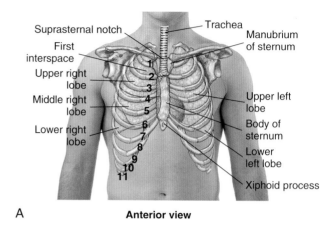

A   **Anterior view**

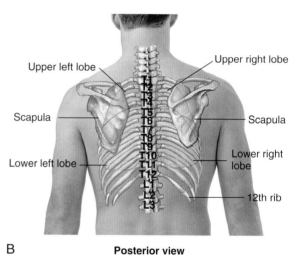

B   **Posterior view**

FIG. 11.3 Thorax and underlying structures. (A) Anterior view. (B) Posterior view.

border of each lung expands approximately down to T12 during deep inspiration and rises approximately to T9 on expiration (Fig. 11.3A and B).

EXTERNAL THORAX

Most of the respiratory system is protected by the thoracic cage, which consists of 11 thoracic vertebrae, 12 pairs of ribs, and the sternum. All the ribs are connected to the thoracic vertebrae posteriorly. The first seven ribs are also connected anteriorly to the sternum by the costal cartilages. The costal cartilages of the eighth to tenth ribs are connected immediately superior to the ribs. The eleventh and twelfth ribs are unattached anteriorly and are called *floating ribs*. The tips of the eleventh ribs are located in the lateral thorax, and those of the twelfth ribs are located in the posterior thorax (see Fig. 11.3).

The adult sternum is approximately 7 inches (17 cm) long and has three components: the manubrium, the body, and the xiphoid process. The manubrium and the body of the sternum articulate with the first seven ribs; the manubrium also supports the clavicle. The intercostal space (ICS) is the area between the ribs and is named according to the rib immediately above it. Thus the first ICS is located between the first and second ribs (Fig. 11.3A).

Topographic Markers

Surface landmarks are helpful in locating underlying structures and describing the exact location of physical findings.

Anterior Chest Wall

- Nipples
- Suprasternal notch: The depression at the anterior aspect of the neck, just above the manubrium
- Manubriosternal junction (angle of Louis): The junction between the manubrium and sternum; useful for rib identification
- Midsternal line: Imaginary vertical line through the middle of the sternum
- Costal angle: Intersection of the costal margins, usually no more than 90 degrees. The costal margins are the medial margins formed by the false ribs, from the eighth to the tenth ribs (Fig. 11.4A)
- Clavicles: Bones extending out both sides of the manubrium to the shoulder; they cover the first ribs
- Midclavicular lines: Imaginary vertical lines on the right and left sides of the chest that are "drawn" through the clavicle midpoints parallel to the midsternal line

Lateral Chest Wall

- Anterior axillary lines: Imaginary vertical lines on the right and left sides of the chest "drawn" from anterior axillary folds through the anterolateral chest, parallel to the midsternal line
- Posterior axillary lines: Imaginary vertical lines on the right and left sides of the chest "drawn" from the posterior axillary folds along the posterolateral thoracic wall with abducted lateral arm
- Midaxillary lines: Imaginary vertical lines on the right and left sides of the chest "drawn" from axillary apices; midway between and parallel to the anterior and posterior axillary lines (Fig. 11.4B).

Posterior Chest Wall

- Vertebra prominens: Spinous process of C7; visible and palpable with the head bent forward
- Vertebral line: Imaginary vertical line "drawn" along the posterior vertebral spinous processes
- Scapular lines: Imaginary vertical lines on the right and left sides of the chest "drawn" parallel to the midspinal line; they pass through inferior angles of the scapulae in the upright patient with arms at sides (Fig 11.4C).

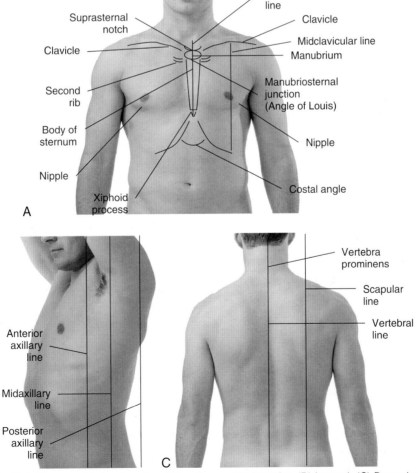

FIG. 11.4 Topographic landmarks of the thorax. (A) Anterior. (B) Lateral. (C) Posterior.

MECHANICS OF BREATHING

The diaphragm and the intercostal muscles are the primary muscles of inspiration. During inspiration, the diaphragm contracts and pushes the abdominal contents down while the intercostal muscles push the chest wall outward. These combined efforts decrease the intrathoracic pressure, which creates a negative pressure within the lungs compared with the pressure outside the lungs. This pressure difference causes the lungs to fill with air. During expiration the muscles relax, expelling the air as the intrathoracic pressure rises. Accessory muscles that may contribute to respiratory effort include, anteriorly, the sternocleidomastoid, scalenus, pectoralis minor, serratus anterior, and rectus abdominis muscles, and, posteriorly, the serratus posterior superior, transverse thoracic, and serratus posterior inferior muscles (Fig. 11-5).

During inspiration, air is drawn in through the mouth or nose and passes through the pharynx and the larynx to reach the trachea, a flexible tube approximately 4 inches (10 cm) long in the adult. These structures (i.e., the nose, pharynx, larynx, and trachea) make up the upper airway (Fig. 11.6), which has three functions in respiration: to conduct air to the lower airway; to protect the lower airway from foreign matter; and to warm, filter, and humidify inspired air. The lower airway consists of the right and left main-stem bronchi, the segmental and subsegmental bronchi, the terminal bronchioles, and alveoli (see Fig. 11.2). The trachea splits into a left and right main-stem bronchus at about the level of T4 and T5. The right bronchus is shorter, wider, and more vertical than the left bronchus. The bronchi are further subdivided into increasingly smaller bronchioles. Each bronchiole opens into an alveolar duct and terminates in multiple alveoli, where gas exchanges occur (Fig. 11.7).

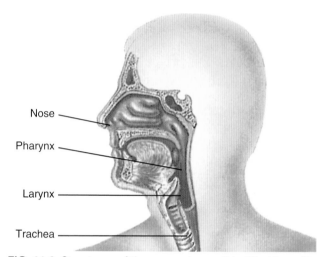

FIG. 11.6 Structures of the upper airway. (Modified from Stoy et al., 2012.)

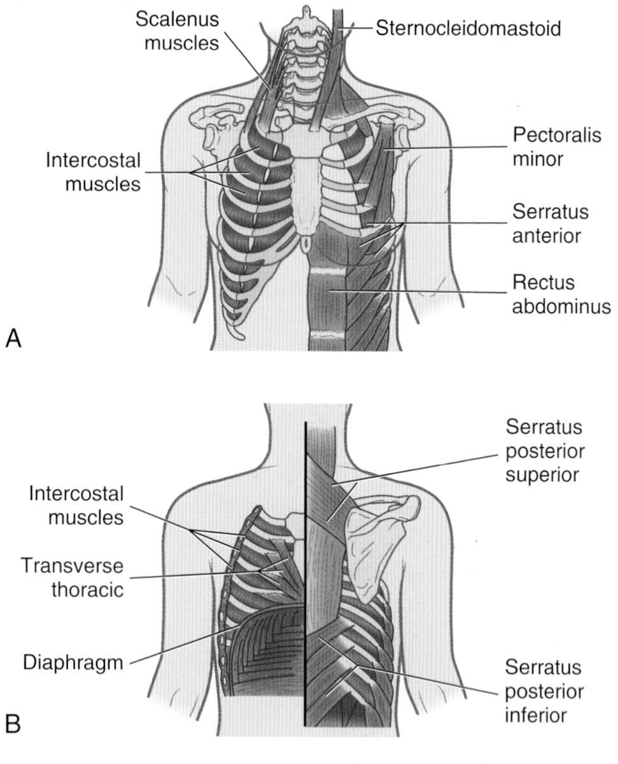

FIG. 11.5 Muscles involved in ventilation. (A) Anterior view. (B) Posterior view.

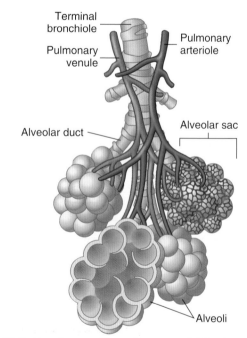

FIG. 11.7 Alveolar sac. (From Patton and Thibodeau, 2010.)

GENERAL HEALTH HISTORY

Nurses interview patients to collect subjective data about their present health status, past health history, family history, and personal and psychosocial history, which may affect the functions of their lungs and respiratory system.

GENERAL HEALTH HISTORY

Present Health Status

Do you have any chronic illnesses?
Many chronic illnesses can cause symptoms that affect the respiratory system, including heart disease or renal disease, which may cause pulmonary edema.

Do you have allergies? If so, what are you allergic to? Describe your symptoms. How frequently do you have these symptoms?
The severity of allergies can range from mild seasonal allergies to an anaphylactic allergic reaction. Respiratory symptoms can range from runny nose, nasal congestion, and cough to wheezes and dyspnea. An increased frequency of symptoms may indicate the onset of new allergies or ineffective therapy for respiratory disease.

Do you have difficulty breathing during your daily activities? If so, describe the difficulty.
Individuals who have no difficulty breathing until they are active may have pulmonary or heart disease that limits the availability of oxygen needed during exertion. Additional information may need to be collected as described under the heading "shortness of breath."

Do you have difficulty breathing when you are lying flat? Do you prop yourself up with pillows to make your breathing easier?
When the body is lying flat, the abdominal contents push against the diaphragm. Individuals with pulmonary disease may experience an increased work of breathing because of pressure of the abdominal contents against the diaphragm. They may prop themselves up with pillows, which moves the abdominal contents away from the diaphragm, to make breathing easier.

Are you currently taking any medications for a respiratory disorder? If so, which medications are you taking and how effective are they?
Medications taken to treat respiratory disorders and their effectiveness need to be documented.

Do you take any over-the-counter drugs or herbal supplements? If so, what do you take and how often? What are they for?
Nonprescription drugs and herbal supplements may be taken to improve breathing. Ginseng, turmeric, red sage, and melatonin are examples.

Do you use an inhaler? If yes, how many inhalers do you have and what medication is in each one? What is the purpose of the medication, and how often do you use the inhaler?
Individuals with asthma or chronic bronchitis may use inhalers to prevent symptoms, treat bronchial inflammation, or dilate bronchi. How frequently they use their inhalers is an indication of how well the patient's symptoms are controlled. These questions also assess the understanding of the reason for taking the medications. Individuals may report ineffective response to medications delivered by their inhaler because they are using them incorrectly.

Do you use oxygen at home? If yes, how much oxygen do you use, and how often do you use it? What situations or activities are associated with your oxygen use? Does the oxygen relieve your symptoms?
Many individuals with chronic pulmonary disease use oxygen at home. The amount, frequency, situations of use, and effect help determine the adequacy of this therapy.

Have you been exposed to anyone who has been diagnosed with an infectious respiratory disease (such as tuberculosis, flu, or COVID-19)? If yes, when did the exposure occur and did you develop symptoms?
Patients should be asked about potential exposures, particularly during times of community outbreaks and pandemics. If a potential exposure is reported, nurses may be required to conduct additional screening measures based on recommended guidelines and/or report the exposure to the local health department.

The US Preventive Services Task Forces (USPSTF) recommends screening asymptomatic adults 18 years and older at increased risk for TB. Populations at increased risk are listed in the Risk Factor box for TB and include hospital employees.[1]

Past Health History

Have you ever had any problems with your lungs or breathing? If yes, describe.
The answer to this question provides a basis for the history.

Have you ever had an injury to your chest or surgery to your chest? If yes, describe.
The incidence of injury or surgery may provide additional information about a possible respiratory or lung problem.

Family History

Is there a family history of lung disease? If yes, which family member(s) is/was affected and what was the lung condition?
Many lung conditions have a familial or genetic link. Family history may be used to determine risk for this individual.

RISK FACTORS

Lung Cancer

- *Tobacco smoking:* Smoking is the number one risk factor for lung cancer. (M)
- *Secondhand smoke:* Smoke from other people's cigarettes causes lung cancer in people and animals. (M)
- *Radon:* This naturally occurring gas comes from rocks and dirt and can get trapped in houses and buildings. It cannot be seen, tasted, or smelled. Radon causes approximately 20,000 cases of lung cancer each year, making it the second leading cause of lung cancer.
- *Asbestos:* People who work with asbestos are several times more likely to die of lung cancer. (M)
- *Environmental exposure in some workplaces:* Carcinogens include radioactive ores such as uranium; inhaled chemicals or minerals such as arsenic, beryllium, cadmium, silica, vinyl chloride, nickel compounds, chromium, coal products, mustard gas, chloromethyl ethers, and diesel exhaust. (M)
- *Air pollution:* In cities air pollution appears to raise the risk of lung cancer slightly. (M)
- *Radiation therapy to the chest:* Cancer survivors who had radiation therapy to the chest are at higher risk of lung cancer.
- *Personal and family history:* People who have lung cancer are at a higher risk of developing another lung cancer. Brothers, sisters, and children of people who have lung cancer have a slightly higher risk of lung cancer themselves. However, it is difficult to say how much of the excess risk is the result of genetic factors versus environmental tobacco smoke.

M, Modifiable risk factor.
Available at: https://www.cdc.gov/cancer/lung/basic_info/risk_factors.htm, July, 2018; https://www.cancer.org/cancer/lung-cancer/prevention-and-early-detection/risk-factors.html, February, 2016.

Personal and Psychosocial History

Do you smoke or have you been a smoker in the past? If yes, what do (did) you smoke (cigarettes, cigar, pipe, e-cigarettes)? How long have you smoked (did you smoke)? How often do you (did you) smoke? About how many cigarettes do you (did you) smoke each day? Have you ever tried to quit smoking? If yes, describe. What helped you quit? Why do you think your attempt was unsuccessful?
These questions determine the patient's smoking history and if there is an interest in quitting. If the individual is or has been a smoker, determine the number of pack-years that the individual has smoked (Box 11.1).

Home Environment

Are there environmental conditions that may affect your breathing at home? If yes, what are they and how do they affect your breathing? Common things to consider include the following:
- Air pollution (near factory, on a busy street, new construction in area)
- Possible allergens in home such as pets

RISK FACTORS

Tuberculosis

- Recent close or prolonged contact with someone with infectious TB disease
- Foreign-born person from, or recent travelers to, high-prevalence areas
- Human immunodeficiency virus (HIV) infection
- Organ transplant recipient
- Immunosuppression secondary to the use of an immunosuppressive drug, such as prednisone
- Resident or employee of a high-risk congregate setting such as a hospital, long-term care facility, prison, or homeless shelter
- Medical conditions associated with risk of progressing TB disease if infected, such as diabetes mellitus, cancer of the head or neck, leukemia, end-stage renal disease, chronic malnutrition, or gastrectomy or gastric bypass
- Cigarette smokers.(M)
- Persons who abuse drugs.(M)

Centers for Disease Control and Prevention: *Core curriculum on tuberculosis: what clinicians should know,* ed 6, Atlanta, GA, 2013. https://www.cdc.gov/tb/education/corecurr/pdf/corecurr_all.pdf
Centers for Disease Control and Prevention: *Latent tuberculosis infection: a guide for primary health care providers,* Atlanta, GA. https://www.cdc.gov/tb/pblications/ltbi/pdf/targetedltbi.pdf
M, Modifiable risk factor.

BOX 11.1 RECORDING TOBACCO USE

Cigarette use is documented by *pack-years.* A pack-year is the number of years that a person has smoked multiplied by the number of packs of cigarettes smoked each day. For example, a person who smoked one-half pack of cigarettes a day for 40 years has a 20 pack-year smoking history.
Use of pipes, cigars, marijuana, chewing tobacco, or snuff is usually recorded in the amount used daily.

- Exposure to hazards such as lead in paint, pipes, and faucets
- Water leaks associated with mold growth have been shown to increase the likelihood of asthma, coughing, and wheezing
- Hobbies: Woodworking, plants, metal work
- Inadequately vented appliances in the home may result in increased exposure to carbon monoxide.[2]
- Exposure to the smoke of others in your home[3]

A number of respiratory irritants found in or near the home may cause temporary or permanent lung damage.

Occupational Environment

Are you frequently exposed to respiratory irritants at work? Chemicals? Dust? Irritants such as asbestos? Paint fumes? Vapors? Known allergens?
Exposure to respiratory irritants in the workplace may be risk factors for pulmonary diseases.

If you are exposed to respiratory irritants, do you wear a mask or a respirator mask? Does your work area have a special ventilation system to clear out pollutants? Do you wear a monitor to evaluate exposure? Do you have periodic health examinations, pulmonary function tests, or x-ray examinations?

Individuals may not be able to alter the presence of environmental irritants in the work environment. Instead they must use protective equipment such as masks, respirators, or ventilation hoods to reduce the amount of exposure to respiratory irritants. Regulatory agencies such as the Occupational Safety and Health Administration (OSHA) have guidelines and regulations to reduce the amount of occupational exposure to respiratory irritants.

Travel

Have you recently traveled to foreign countries or areas of the United States where you may have been exposed to uncommon respiratory diseases (e.g., histoplasmosis in the sudden acute respiratory syndrome [SARS])?

Travel to other areas of the country or world may expose people to infections to which they have little or no resistance, increasing their susceptibility to infection.

PROBLEM-BASED HISTORY

Commonly reported symptoms related to the lungs are cough, shortness of breath, and chest pain with breathing. As with symptoms in all areas of health assessment, complete a symptom analysis using the mnemonic OLD CARTS, which means Onset, Location, Duration, Characteristics, Aggravating factors, Related symptoms, Treatment, and Severity (see Box 2.6).

Cough

When did you first notice the cough? Is it constant, or does it come and go?

A cough can be acute (sudden onset and usually lasting <3 weeks) or chronic (lasting longer than 8 weeks). Common causes of acute cough are viral infections, allergic rhinitis, acute asthma, acute bacterial sinusitis, or environmental irritants. Chronic cough is often caused by postnasal drip, gastroesophageal reflux disease (GERD), asthma, infections such as chronic bronchitis, and blood pressure drugs. A common adverse effect of angiotensin-converting enzyme (ACE) inhibitors such as captopril (commonly prescribed for high blood pressure and heart failure) is a chronic dry cough.[5]

Describe your cough. Is it dry? Productive? Hacking? Hoarse?

A description of the cough may provide clues to the cause. For example, viral pneumonia causes a dry cough, whereas bacterial pneumonia causes a productive cough.

How often do you cough up sputum (all of the time or periodically)? Is there a time of day when more sputum is coughed up? How much sputum do you cough up?

The frequency of sputum production and the time of day most sputum is produced should be explored. Increased sputum in the morning implies an accumulation of sputum during the night and is common with bronchitis. Sputum production with a change in position suggests lung abscess and bronchiectasis. The amount of sputum production can vary from a few teaspoons to a copious amount (a pint or more).

What is the color of the sputum?

Documenting the appearance of the sputum is important. Some conditions have characteristic sputum production; for example, white or clear sputum may occur with colds, viral infections, or bronchitis; yellow or green sputum may occur with bacterial infections; black sputum may occur with smoke or coal dust inhalation; or rust-colored sputum may occur with TB or pneumococcal pneumonia. *Hemoptysis* is the expectoration of sputum containing blood. It may vary in severity from slight streaking of blood to frank bleeding.

What is the consistency of the sputum (thick, thin, frothy)?

The consistency of sputum may be described as thin, thick, gelatinous, sticky, or frothy. Pink, frothy sputum with dyspnea is associated with pulmonary edema. Thick sputum is commonly associated with cystic fibrosis.

Have you noticed if the sputum has an odor?

Foul-smelling (fetid) sputum is typically associated with bacterial pneumonia, lung abscess, or bronchiectasis.

Are there any factors that aggravate the cough?

Avoiding aggravating factors may help relief the cough. Breathlessness during exercise and singing may aggravate cough.

Have you noticed any other symptoms accompanying the cough such as shortness of breath, chest pain or tightness with breathing, fever, stuffy nose, noisy respiration, hoarseness, or gagging? Do you feel fatigued after coughing? Does it keep you awake at night?

A cough may be a symptom of pulmonary problems, or it may exist in conjunction with other problems. Related signs and symptoms are important factors to assess when determining the underlying cause of the cough. For example, a cough associated with a fever, shortness of breath, and noisy breath sounds may indicate a lung infection; whereas tightness of the chest associated with shortness of breath and a nonproductive cough is more likely to be associated with a problem such as asthma.

What have you done to treat the cough such as medications, fluids, or a humidifier? Have these measures been effective?

Determining what has been used to relieve symptoms may help you understand the problem and may guide current treatment strategies. For example, staying hydrated, drinking warm liquids, and increasing humidity by using a humidifier or a steamy shower may help relieve a cough.

Shortness of Breath

How long have you had shortness of breath? Is the onset sudden or gradual? Are you short of breath all the time, or does it come and go?

Shortness of breath, or dyspnea, occurs when breathing becomes difficult. Some conditions such as pneumonia may cause sudden onset of shortness of breath; other conditions such as heart failure may be associated with a more gradual onset. Some people may experience shortness of breath at intervals over a period of time.

Does anything seem to trigger the shortness of breath or make it worse such as talking, activity, or environmental factors? Do you feel short of breath when you are lying flat, such as during sleep?

Determine factors that initiate dyspnea. If dyspnea occurs during activity, find out how much activity precipitates shortness of breath (e.g., number of steps climbed, blocks walked). Dyspnea that occurs during activity is called dyspnea on exertion (DOE). For example, ask the patient how many level blocks he or she can walk now before becoming short of breath compared with 6 months ago.[6] Box 11.2 describes how to document dyspnea. Positions or other conditions may also initiate dyspnea. *Orthopnea* is difficulty breathing when the individual is lying down. *Paroxysmal nocturnal dyspnea* is shortness of breath that awakens the individual in the middle of the night, usually in a panic with the feeling of suffocation. Asthma attacks may be triggered by a specific allergen, which may be external or extrinsic such as a pet or internal or intrinsic such as stress or emotions.

Have you noticed any other problems when you are short of breath? Cough? Chest pain? Breaking out in a sweat? Swelling of the feet, ankles, or legs?

Shortness of breath may be a problem of the respiratory system, or it may be a related symptom associated with the cardiovascular system such as a severe heart murmur or heart failure that may produce pulmonary edema.

BOX 11.2 DESCRIBING DYSPNEA

The severity of dyspnea can be documented either from the nurse's observations or the patient's report. When you notice the patient is dyspneic during the interview, count the words that the patient can say between breaths. Usually a person can say 10–14 words before taking a breath. A patient who has severe dyspnea may take a breath after every third word. This is documented as "three-word dyspnea." When the patient reports dyspnea when walking, ask how many level blocks the patient can walk now as opposed to 6 months ago. If the patient reports currently being able to walk one level block, that is documented as "one-block dyspnea on exertion."[6]

What relieves the shortness of breath? Do you use pillows to prop you up? Do you sleep in a recliner? Does changing your position affect the problem?

People may describe using several pillows to prop themselves up in bed to relieve the dyspnea so they can sleep. The term *three-pillow orthopnea* means that the person needs to prop up with three pillows to relieve the dyspnea. Others sleep in a reclining chair rather than use pillows. Determining what has been used successfully or unsuccessfully helps in understanding the problem and may guide current treatment strategies.

Chest Pain With Breathing

When did you first experience pain in your chest when breathing? Did it start suddenly or gradually? Where do you feel it?

Chest pain caused by respiratory disease is usually associated with disorders affecting the chest wall or parietal pleura. Prolonged coughing may cause chest pain from repeated muscle contraction of the thorax.[6] In contrast, chest pain may be caused by heart disease (see Chapter 12, Chest pain) and disorders of the gastrointestinal system (see Chapter 13, Indigestion).

How does the pain feel (viselike, tight, sharp, burning)? On a scale of 0 to 10, how would you rate the severity of the pain? Is it constant, or does it come and go?

A sudden, sharp stabbing pain felt during inspiration may be an indication of pleural lining irritation, also called *pleuritic chest pain.* It may be localized to one side, and the patient may splint the affected side to try to reduce the pain.[6] Men reporting chest pain due to heart disease such as myocardial infarction often describe viselike and tight chest pain, while women report other symptoms such as shortness of breath.[6]

When the chest pain started, was it associated with an injury to your ribs or a respiratory infection? Does it interfere with you getting enough air?

Injured ribs cause pain when the individual breathes in; as a result, the person is likely to have shallow breathing, which may lead to atelectasis (collapse of alveoli).

Is there anything that seems to make the pain worse such as movement or coughing? Is it worse with deep inspiration?

Assess for aggravating factors.

What treatment have you tried to relieve the pain, such as putting pressure over the site of pain, applying heat, or taking pain medication? How effective has the treatment been?

Assess self-care behaviors and successful treatment to relieve the pain.

HEALTH PROMOTION FOR EVIDENCE-BASED PRACTICE

Tobacco Use

Cigarette smoking is the single most preventable cause of death and disease in the United States. The majority of all cancers of the lung, trachea, bronchus, larynx, pharynx, oral cavity, and esophagus are caused by tobacco products. Smoking is a leading risk factor for cardiovascular diseases, including myocardial infarction, coronary artery disease, stroke, and peripheral vascular disease. Smoking is also an important risk factor for lung disease, including chronic obstructive pulmonary disease. During pregnancy, smoking may increase the risk for premature birth, low birth weight, stillbirth, and infant death. There is no safe tobacco alternative to cigarettes.

Environmental smoke (secondhand smoke) affects the health of nonsmokers, particularly children. Secondhand smoke can cause heart disease and lung cancer in adults and a number of health problems in infants and children, including severe asthma attacks, respiratory infections, ear infections, and sudden infant death syndrome (SIDS).

Smokeless tobacco can cause a number of serious oral health problems, including cancer of the mouth and gums, periodontitis, and tooth loss. Cigar use can cause cancer of the larynx, mouth, esophagus, and lung.

Recommendations to Reduce Risk (Primary Prevention)

NOTE: All major healthcare organizations recommend routine counseling for smoking cessation and recommend against the use of smokeless tobacco.

- Clinicians ask all adults about tobacco use and provide tobacco cessation interventions for those who use tobacco products.
- Clinicians ask all pregnant women about tobacco use and provide augmented, pregnancy-tailored counseling for those who smoke.

Tobacco use and secondhand smoke exposure: Comprehensive tobacco control programs, Guide to clinical preventive services. Systematic review August, 2014. Available at: https://www.thecommunityguide.org/content/guide-clinical-preventive-services-0. Accessed August 23, 2019. US Preventive Services Task Force: *Tobacco smoking: Cessation in adults, including pregnant women: behavioral and pharmacotherapy interventions.* Released September, 2015. Available at: https://www.uspreventiveservicestaskforce.org//uspstf/recommendations/tobacco-use-in-adults-and-pregnant-women-counseling-and-interventions

EXAMINATION

Routine techniques

- INSPECT patient's appearance, posture, and breathing effort.
- COUNT respirations and OBSERVE breathing patterns and chest expansion.
- INSPECT patient's nails, skin, and lips.
- INSPECT posterior and anterior thorax.
- AUSCULTATE posterior, lateral, and anterior thorax.

Techniques for special circumstances

- PALPATE the thoracic muscles.
- PALPATE the thoracic wall.
- PALPATE the trachea.

Techniques performed by an APRN

- PERCUSS the thorax.
- AUSCULTATE the thorax for vocal sounds.

Equipment needed

- Watch with second hand • Stethoscope

APRN, Advanced Practice Registered Nurse.

| PROCEDURES WITH EXPECTED FINDINGS | ABNORMAL FINDINGS |

ROUTINE TECHNIQUES

PERFORM hand hygiene.

INSPECT patient for appearance, posture, and breathing effort.

The patient's appearance and posture should be relaxed. The posture should be upright. Breathing should be quiet, effortless, and at a rate appropriate for the patient's age (Fig. 11.8).

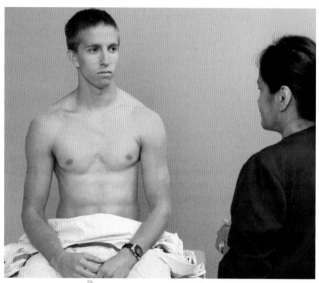

FIG. 11.8 Observing patient for breathing effort.

Indications of respiratory distress include an appearance of apprehension, restlessness, nasal flaring, supraclavicular or intercostal retractions, and use of accessory muscles. *Pursed-lip breathing* is exhalation through the mouth with the lips pursed together to slow exhalation seen in patients with chronic obstructive pulmonary disease (COPD) or asthma. It reduces respiratory rate, decreases arterial carbon dioxide, and increases oxygen saturation.[7] *Tripod position* (leaning forward with the arms braced against the knees, a chair, or a bed) also suggests respiratory distress in patients with COPD or asthma. Tripod position enhances accessory muscle use (Fig. 11.9). *Paradoxical chest wall movement* may occur after chest trauma when the chest wall moves in during inspiration and out during expiration.[8]

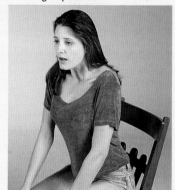

FIG. 11.9 Tripod position and use of accessory muscles. (From Shade et al., 2012.)

COUNT respirations for rate; OBSERVE breathing pattern and chest expansion.

Count the respiratory rate (each inhalation and exhalation is one breath). In the adult, passive breathing should occur at a rate of 12–20 breaths/min (this range in respiratory rate is referred to as *eupnea*) (Fig. 11.10). The pattern of breathing should be quiet and effortless, with an even respiratory depth. The chest wall should rise and expand symmetrically and then relax without effort. An expected variation is the abdominal breathing pattern. Men tend to use abdominal breathing (or diaphragmatic breathing), whereas women tend to use more thoracic breathing.[9] Signing is another expected variation observed with breathing. It is occasional deep breaths interspersed with an expected breathing pattern (see Fig. 11.10).

Common abnormal breathing patterns are described in Fig. 11.10 (bradypnea, tachypnea, hyperventilation, air trapping, Cheyne-stokes, Kussmaul, biot, ataxic). Differentiate the subjective sensation of shortness of breath (dyspnea) from the objective finding of tachypnea. A patient may be breathing rapidly while stating that he or she is not short of breath. Conversely, a patient may be breathing slowly but have dyspnea. Never assume that a patient with rapid respiratory rate is dyspneic.[6]

Chest retraction appears when intercostal muscles are drawn inward between the ribs and indicates airway obstruction that may occur during asthma attack or pneumonia.

Frequent sighing is considered an abnormal finding and may indicate fatigue or anxiety.

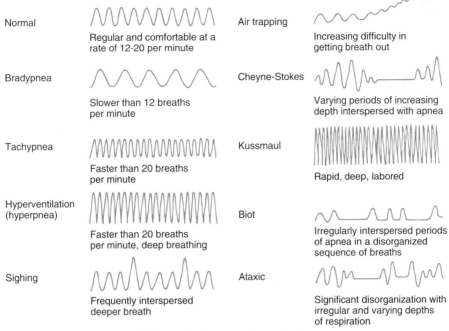

FIG. 11.10 Patterns of respiration.

PROCEDURES WITH EXPECTED FINDINGS

INSPECT patient's nails for color and angle; INSPECT skin and lips for color.

In light-skinned individuals nailbeds are pink, while individuals with darker-pigmented skin have nailbeds that are yellow or brown. The angle should be 160 degrees at the nail bed (see Fig. 9.10A). Skin and lip tones vary among individuals; therefore the general color should be consistent with the patient's race. In dark skinned patients, cyanosis is assessed by inspecting the oral mucosa and lips (see Table 9.1). If there is any question about adequate oxygenation, measure the person's oxygen saturation level using a pulse oximeter (see Chapter 3).

INSPECT the posterior thorax for shape, symmetry, and muscle development.

Move behind the individual who is seated on an examination table or on a bed with the gown removed for men or back of the gown open for women to prevent exposing the breasts.

The ribs should slope down at approximately 45 degrees relative to the spine. The thorax should be symmetric. The spinous processes should appear in a straight line. The scapulae should be bilaterally symmetric. Muscle development should be equal.

AUSCULTATE the posterior and lateral thoraxes for breath sounds.

Procedure:
- Instruct the person to sit upright and breathe deeply and slowly through the mouth. Ask the person periodically about feeling dizzy from frequent deep breaths. If dizziness is reported, wait for it to subside before proceeding.
- Clean the diaphragm of your stethoscope.
- Place the diaphragm of the stethoscope against the person's skin to auscultate breath sounds. Use a systematic pattern to listen over the posterior and lateral chest walls (Fig. 11.11). Move from the apex (above the clavicle) to the base (at the 12th rib).
- Leave the stethoscope in each location during at least one respiratory cycle so you can hear breath sounds during both inspiration and expiration. Compare one side with the other following the landmarks (Fig. 11.12A and C).
- When auscultating over the lateral thorax, ask the patient to fold the arms in front to give you better access.

ABNORMAL FINDINGS

Cyanosis or pallor of the nails, skin, or lips may be a sign of inadequate oxygenation of tissues caused by an underlying respiratory or cardiovascular condition. Yellow discoloration of the fingers maybe associated with cigarette smoking. Clubbing of the nails is associated with chronic hypoxia observed in patients with cystic fibrosis or COPD (Fig. 9.10B and C).

Notice asymmetry or unequal muscle development. Skeletal deformities such as scoliosis may limit the expansion of the chest. (see Fig. 14.17E, F, and G). Patients with emphysema may have a barrel-shaped chest due to chronic air trapping in the alveoli (Fig. 11.15).

Breath sounds can be considered abnormal if heard over areas of the lungs where they are not expected. Bronchial breath sounds are abnormal when heard anywhere over the posterior or lateral thorax and may indicate consolidation of the lung, which may be found with pneumonia. (The sound heard is loud and high pitched. It sounds as if the air source is just under the stethoscope.) Bronchovesicular breath sounds should be considered abnormal when heard over the peripheral lung areas.

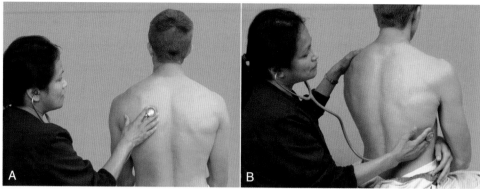

FIG. 11.11 Auscultating the posterior and lateral chest. (A) Posterior thorax. (B) Lateral thorax.

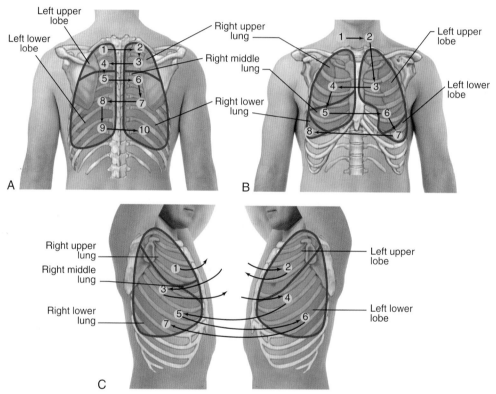

FIG. 11.12 Landmarks for chest auscultation and percussion. (A) Posterior view. (B) Anterior view. (C) Lateral view. (Modified from Ball et al., 2015.)

PROCEDURES WITH EXPECTED FINDINGS

Findings: Breath sounds should be clear over the posterior and lateral thoraxes.
Vesicular breath sounds should be heard over almost all of the posterior and lateral thoraxes. *Bronchovesicular breath sounds* are expected over the upper center area of the posterior thorax between the vertebrae between the scapulae (Fig. 11.13B and Table 11.1).

ABNORMAL FINDINGS

A decrease in breath sounds is the most common abnormality due to the patient not breathing deeply, airway blockage by a foreign body or tumor, airway narrowing from asthma or COPD, or depression of the central nervous system.[10] Adventitious breath sounds (crackles, wheezing, and rhonchi) are extraneous sounds (Table 11.2). If an adventitious sound is heard, have the patient cough; repeat the auscultation to determine if the sound has changed or disappeared (Box 11.3).

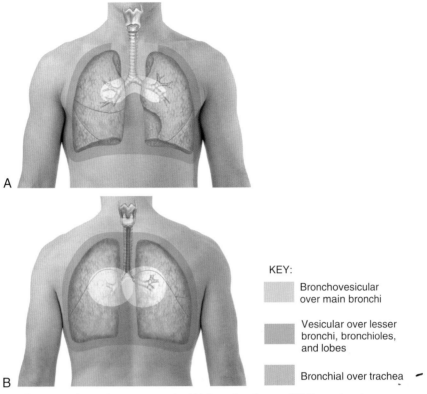

KEY:

Bronchovesicular over main bronchi

Vesicular over lesser bronchi, bronchioles, and lobes

Bronchial over trachea

FIG. 11.13 Auscultatory sounds. (A) Anterior thorax. (B) Posterior thorax.

TABLE 11.1 CHARACTERISTICS OF BREATH SOUNDS

	BRONCHIAL	BRONCHOVESICULAR	VESICULAR
Pitch	High	Moderate	Low
Intensity	Loud	Medium	Soft
Duration: Inspiration and expiration	Insp < Exp 1:2	Insp = Exp 1:1	Insp > Exp 2.5:1
Expected location	Over trachea	First and second intercostal spaces at sternal border anteriorly; posteriorly at T4 medial to scapula	Peripheral lung fields
Abnormal location	Over peripheral lung fields	Over peripheral lung fields	Not applicable

PROCEDURES WITH EXPECTED FINDINGS

BOX 11.3 FACTORS AFFECTING DETECTION OF ADVENTITIOUS SOUNDS

Before you decide that the patient has an adventitious sound, remember that the following may also be causes of sound distortion:

- If you bump the stethoscope tubing against something or if the patient touches the tubing, the sound will be distorted.
- If the patient is cold and shivering, the sound will be distorted.
- If a patient has excess chest hair, movement of the stethoscope may give a false finding of crackles or pleural friction rub.
- Extraneous environmental noises such as the rustling of a paper gown or drape might sound like crackles or pleural friction rub.

ABNORMAL FINDINGS

If the adventitious sound does not disappear, identify the type of sound, the location (i.e., right lung, left lung, or bilaterally; upper lobes or lower lobes; anterior or posterior), and the phase of breathing in which it is heard (i.e., inspiration or expiration). The term *stridor* is used to describe a harsh, high-pitched sound associated with breathing that is often caused by laryngeal or tracheal obstruction. Diminished breath sounds may be heard in patients whose alveoli have been damaged, which may occur in patients with emphysema. Diminished or absent breath sounds may be heard in patients with collapsed alveoli, which may occur in patients who have atelectasis or are having a severe asthma attack.

TABLE 11.2 CHARACTERISTICS OF ADVENTITIOUS SOUNDS

ADVENTITIOUS SOUNDS	CHARACTERISTICS	CLINICAL EXAMPLES
Crackles (previously called rales)	Fine, high-pitched crackling and popping noises (discontinuous sounds) heard during inspiration and sometimes during expiration; not cleared by cough or altered by changes in body position.	May be heard in pneumonia, heart failure, and restrictive pulmonary diseases
Wheeze (also called *sibilant wheeze*)	High-pitched, musical sound similar to a squeak; heard more commonly during expiration but may also be heard during inspiration; occurs in small airways	Heard in airway diseases when the thickness of airways increases such as asthma
Rhonchi (also called *sonorous wheeze*)	Low-pitched, coarse, loud, low snoring or moaning tone; heard primarily during expiration but may also be heard during inspiration; coughing may clear	Heard in disorders causing obstruction of the trachea or bronchus such as bronchitis or COPD
Pleural friction rub	Superficial, low-pitched, coarse rubbing or grating sound; sounds like two surfaces rubbing together; heard throughout inspiration and expiration; loudest over the lower anterolateral surface; not cleared by cough	Heard in individuals with pleurisy (inflammation of the pleural surfaces) or with pericarditis

COPD, chronic obstructive pulmonary disease.
From Bohadana A, Izbicki G, Kraman SS: Fundamentals of lung auscultation, *N Engl J Med* 370(8):744, 2014.

PROCEDURES WITH EXPECTED FINDINGS

INSPECT the anterior thorax for shape, symmetry, muscle development, and costal angle.

Move in front of the person to assess the anterior thorax.

When examining women, limit the time of breast exposure as much as possible. The ribs should slope down at approximately 45 degrees relative to the spine. The thorax should be symmetric. Muscle development should be equal. The costal angle should be less than 90 degrees (Fig. 11.14).

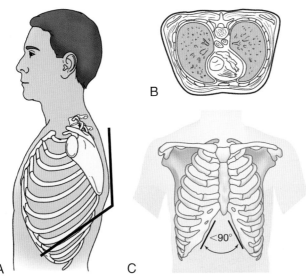

FIG. 11.14 Expected chest findings. (A) Angulation of ribs. (B) Anteroposterior diameter is approximately one half the lateral diameter. (C) Costal angle less than 90 degrees. (A from Urden, Stacy, and Lough, 2010. B from Salvo, 2009.)

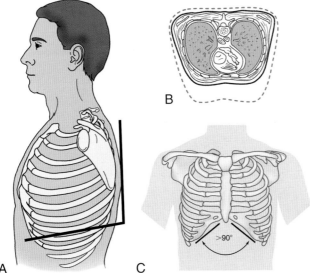

FIG. 11.15 Barrel chest. (A) Horizontal ribs. (B) Increased anteroposterior diameter. (C) Costal angle greater than 90 degrees. (A, From Urden, Stacy, and Lough, 2010. B, From Salvo, 2009.)

ABNORMAL FINDINGS

The barrel chest caused by emphysema increases the costal angle (Fig. 11.15). Other chest wall skeletal deformities include scoliosis, pectus carinatum (Fig. 11.16), and pectus excavatum (Fig. 11.17).

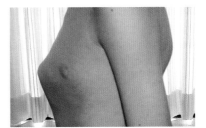

FIG. 11.16 Pectus carinatum, or pigeon chest. Notice prominent sternum. (From Townsend et al., 2008.)

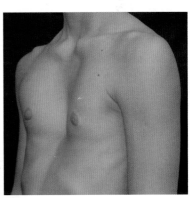

FIG. 11.17 Pectus excavatum, or funnel chest. Notice that sternum is indented above xiphoid. (From Townsend et al., 2008.)

PROCEDURES WITH EXPECTED FINDINGS

INSPECT the anterior thorax for anteroposterior to lateral diameter.

Procedure: The anteroposterior (AP) diameter can be visualized or indirectly determined by using the distance between hands as a "measure." Standing in front of the patient, place your hands on either side of his or her anterior chest, noticing the distance between your hands. Next, maintaining the distance between hands, move to the side of the patient to compare the distance from front to back with the distance between the hands.

Findings: The AP diameter of the chest should be approximately one half the lateral diameter or approximately 1:2 ratio of AP to lateral diameter. Therefore the distance from the front to the back of the chest should be half the distance from one side of the chest to the other.

AUSCULTATE the anterior thorax for breath sounds.

Procedure: Follow the same procedure as used to auscultate the posterior thorax. When examining women, you may reach under the gown with the stethoscope to auscultate while maintaining her modesty. Using the diaphragm of the stethoscope, auscultate from the apex of the lungs (above the clavicles) to the base (at the 12th rib). Compare one side to the other (see Fig. 11.12B; Fig. 11.18).

ABNORMAL FINDINGS

In disorders causing lung hyperinflation such as emphysema, the chest wall may have a barrel chest appearance because of an increased AP diameter. The ribs are more horizontal, and the chest looks as if it is held in constant inspiration.

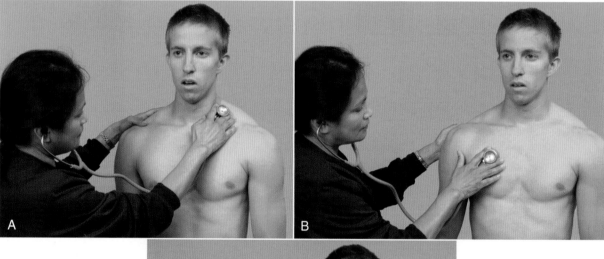

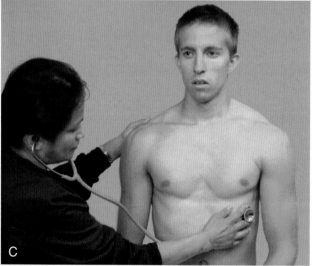

FIG. 11.18 Auscultating the anterior chest. (A) Left apex. (B) Right middle anterior thorax. (C) Left lower anterior thorax.

PROCEDURES WITH EXPECTED FINDINGS

Findings: *Vesicular breath sounds* should be heard throughout the anterior thorax, including the apex of the lungs above the clavicles. *Bronchovesicular breath sounds* are expected sounds heard over the central area of the anterior thorax around the sternal border. These sounds are heard in an area that approximates the area where the bronchi split off from the trachea. *Bronchial breath sounds* are the expected sounds heard over the trachea and the area immediately above the manubrium.

TECHNIQUES FOR SPECIAL CIRCUMSTANCES

PALPATE posterior and anterior thoracic muscles for pain and symmetry.

Perform when patient reports tenderness or when nurse notices bulges, depressions, or unusual movement of these muscles.

Procedure: With the palmar surface of your fingers, feel the texture and consistency of the skin over the chest and the alignment of vertebrae. Identify areas that the patient reports as painful. Use both hands simultaneously to compare the two sides of the posterior and anterior chest walls.

Findings: *Posterior:* The vertebrae should be straight and painless from C7 through T12. The scapulae should be symmetric, and the surrounding musculature well developed. The posterior ribs should be stable and painless. The posterior rib cage should be symmetric and firm. *Anterior:* The clavicles should be symmetric, and the surrounding musculature well developed. The anterior ribs should be stable and painless. The rib cage should be symmetric and firm. The sternum and xiphoid should be relatively inflexible.

PALPATE the posterior and anterior thoracic walls for expansion.

Perform when asymmetry suspected.

Procedure: For posterior thorax, stand behind the patient and place both thumbs on either side of the spinal processes at about the level of T9 or T10. While maintaining the thumb position, extend the fingers of both hands laterally (outward) over the posterior chest wall. Instruct the patient to take several deep breaths. Observe for lateral movement of both thumbs during the patient's inspirations (Fig. 11.19).

For anterior thorax, face the patient, place both thumbs along the costal margin and the xiphoid process with your palms against the anterolateral chest wall (Fig. 11.20). Instruct the patient to take several deep breaths. Observe for lateral movement of both thumbs during the patient's deep breaths.

Findings: Both thumbs should move apart symmetrically on the posterior and anterior chest walls with each breath.

ABNORMAL FINDINGS

Abnormal findings are the same as for the posterior thorax. When a pleural friction rub is heard, its source (lung or heart) can be determined by asking the patient to hold his or her breath. If the rub is not heard, the source is lung pleura rubbing together. If the sound persists, it is caused by pericardial pleura rubbing together.[6]

Notice any crepitus, which feels like a crackly sensation under your fingers. This finding indicates air in the subcutaneous tissue caused by an air leak from somewhere in the respiratory tree. Pleural friction rub may be felt as a coarse, grating sensation during inspiration. It occurs secondary to inflammation of the pleural surface. Muscular development that is asymmetric or an unstable chest wall may indicate a thoracic disorder such as fractured ribs.

A unilateral or unequal movement of your thumbs suggests asymmetry of expansion, which may be caused by pain or localized pulmonary disease such as fractured ribs or chest wall injury, pneumonia, and atelectasis or collapsed lung. A patient who has a barrel chest from emphysema may not have expansion due to over inflation.[6]

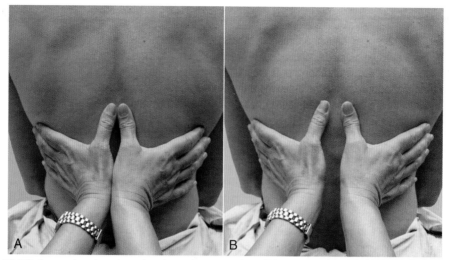

FIG. 11.19 Assessing for posterior thoracic expansion. (A) With thumbs together on either side of patient's spinal process, extend fingers and ask patient to take deep breaths through the mouth. (B) As patient takes deep breaths, observe lateral movement of both thumbs.

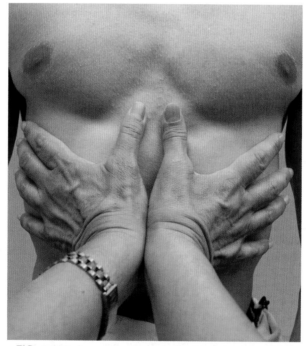

FIG. 11.20 Assessing for anterior thoracic expansion.

PROCEDURES WITH EXPECTED FINDINGS

PALPATE the posterior and anterior thoracic walls for vocal (tactile) fremitus.

Perform when congestion, obstruction, or compression of lung tissue suspected.

Procedure: Fremitus provides information about the density of underlying lung tissue and thorax.[6] Vocal fremitus is a vibration resulting from verbalizations. You can feel this vibration using the palmar surface of your hand and fingers or the ulnar surfaces of your hands. *Posterior Thorax:* Place your hands on the posterior thorax over the right and left lung fields following the landmarks shown in Fig. 11.21A. Instruct the patient to recite "one-two-three" or "ninety-nine" while you systematically palpate the chest wall from apices to bases (Fig. 11.21B).

Anterior Thorax: Place the palmar side of your hands and fingers or ulnar side of your hands on the anterior thorax over the right and left lung fields. Instruct the patient to recite "one-two-three" while you systemically palpate the chest wall following the landmarks shown in Fig. 11.22.

Findings: The fremitus should feel bilaterally equal over posterior and anterior chest walls, although the quality of the vibrations may vary from person to person because of chest wall density and relative location of the bronchi to the chest wall. Vocal fremitus is more prominent in men than in women, because men have lower-pitched voices, which conduct more easily through lung tissue than higher-pitched voices. Therefore tactile fremitus may be absent in a healthy person, especially those with high-pitched or soft voices.[7]

ABNORMAL FINDINGS

Vibrations feel unequal when comparing sides. Fremitus is asymmetrically diminished when air, fluid, or tumor pushes the lung away from the chest wall due to unilateral pneumothorax, pleural effusion, or tumor. Fremitus is asymmetrically increased when there is consolidation of the underlying lung.[7]

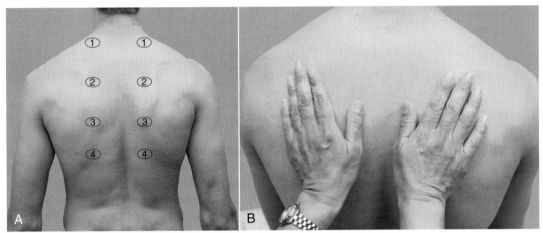

FIG. 11.21 Assessing for posterior vocal (Tactile) fremitus. (A) Hand position for assessment. (B) Position hands over both lung fields, making bilateral comparisons.

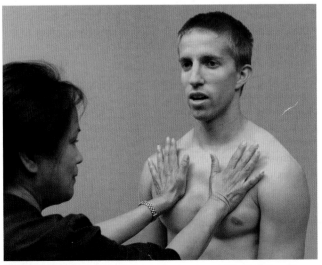

FIG. 11.22 Assessing for posterior vocal (Tactile) fremitus.

PROCEDURES WITH EXPECTED FINDINGS

PALPATE the trachea for position.

Perform this procedure when you suspect tracheal deviation.
Procedure: Stand facing the patient. Using the thumbs of both hands (or index finger and thumb of one hand), palpate the trachea on the anterior aspect of the neck by placing the thumbs on either side (Fig. 11.23).
Findings: The trachea should be palpable, midline, and slightly movable.

ABNORMAL FINDINGS

The trachea may deviate due to problems within the chest. Pulmonary fibrosis or atelectasis pull the trachea toward the affected side. Thyroid enlargement or pleural effusion may push the trachea away from the affected side. In a tension pneumothorax, pressure builds up on the side of the collapsed lung creating deviation away from the affected side; however, with a simple collapsed lung, the deviation is toward the affected side.[9]

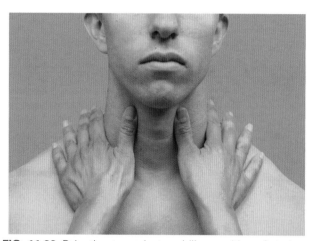

FIG. 11.23 Palpating to evaluate midline position of trachea.

TECHNIQUES PERFORMED BY AN ADVANCED PRACTICE REGISTERED NURSE

Specialty practice may require advanced techniques that are beyond the skill set of a nurse generalist. Knowing the purposes of these techniques may be helpful when caring for patients who require advanced assessment techniques.

- **Percuss the thorax for tone.** Percussion of the thorax is performed when the practitioner suspects overinflation of the lung (which may be found in a patient with emphysema) or consolidation (which may be found in a patient with pneumonia). Different percussion sounds are produced in each of these abnormalities. Percussion technique is reviewed in Chapter 3.
- **Percuss the thorax for diaphragmatic excursion.** This technique uses percussion to estimate the location of the diaphragm during inspiration and expiration. It is used when increased downward expansion is suspected (which may be found in patients with emphysema) or when decreased expansion is suspected (which may be found in patients with an enlarged liver).
- **Auscultate the thorax for vocal sounds (vocal resonance).** This technique is performed when the patient has consolidation of the lung or when there was an abnormal finding during tactile fremitus. The spoken voice vibrates and transmits sounds through the lung fields heard posteriorly

with a stethoscope. These sounds are usually muffled and cannot be understood clearly.

Three types of vocal resonance include:

1. Bronchophony is performed by asking the patient to repeat one of the following phrases: "ninety-nine," "e-e-e," or "one-two-three."
2. Whispered pectoriloquy is performed when there is a positive finding of bronchophony. The patient is asked to whisper "one-two-three."
3. Egophony evaluates the intensity of the spoken voice by asking the patient to say "e-e-e."

DOCUMENTING EXPECTED FINDINGS

Breathing quiet and effortless at 16 breaths/min. Color of skin, nails, and lips consistent with race, nail base angles 160 degrees. Thorax symmetric, with ribs sloping downward at approximately 45 degrees relative to the spine. Muscle development of the thorax equal bilaterally without tenderness. Thoracic expansion symmetric. Tactile fremitus equal anteriorly and posteriorly. Spinous processes aligned; scapulae symmetric. Anteroposterior chest diameter approximately a 1:2 ratio to lateral diameter. Trachea midline. Breath sounds clear, with vesicular breath sounds heard over most lung fields, bronchovesicular breath sounds in posterior chest over upper center area of the back and around sternal border, and bronchial breath sounds heard over the trachea.

CLINICAL JUDGMENT

Respiratory System

Case Presentation

Maki Chiba, a 52-year-old woman, is a patient on a surgical unit at a hospital. She is 12 hours post-op for a nephrectomy and has been on the surgical unit for about 10 hours. Mr. Chiba (Maki's husband) approaches his wife's primary nurse shortly after shift change and says, "Something seems to be wrong with my wife – she was fine when she got back from surgery, but she has become progressively less responsive over the last few hours."

Reflecting

The nurse reflects on Mrs. Chiba's care, clinical presentation, and this clinical encounter. She was seen by the surgeon who determined she had a medication reaction to morphine. Her pain medication was changed, and her vital signs and oxygenation status were closely monitored for the next 8 hours. This experience contributes to the nurse's expertise when encountering a similar situation.

Noticing / Recognizing Cues

The nurse reviews her notes taken at the hand-off report and notes that Mrs. Chiba's last set of vital signs were stable. Because of her experience, the nurse is aware that there are several possible complications in the postoperative period and also knows that 12 hours following a surgical procedure the patient should be more responsive than described.

The nurse immediately goes to Mrs. Chiba's room to investigate the situation. Mrs. Chiba is difficult to arouse, and her vital signs are blood pressure 100/60 mm Hg; heart rate 118/minute; temperature 97.2°F (36.2°C); respiratory rate 10/minute; SpO2 92% on 2L of oxygen. Her lungs are clear bilaterally; respirations are shallow. The nurse notices that Mrs. Chiba's skin is warm and dry; her surgical dressing is dry and intact.

Responding / Taking Action

The nurse initiates appropriate initial interventions (increases oxygen delivery and turns off the PCA device) and contacts the attending surgeon to discuss the situation, ensuring the patient receives appropriate immediate and follow-up care.

Interpreting / Analyzing Cues & Forming Hypotheses

The nurse follows the cognitive cues and recalls two possible causes associated with these findings: medication reaction or hypovolemia. To determine if either has any probability of being correct, the nurse gathers additional data:

• How much intravenous fluid has been administered?

According to the intake and output record, 950 mL of intravenous fluid infused with 620 mL of urine output recorded on the last shift.

• How much pain medication has Mrs. Chiba received?

Mrs. Chiba has a patient-controlled analgesia (PCA) device delivering morphine sulfate 1 mg every 10 minutes on demand. The PCA has delivered a total of 15 mg in the last 2 ½ hours.

The experienced nurse recognizes the adverse effects of morphine (hypotension, respiratory depression, and hypoxia as evidenced by low oxygenation saturation and changes in cognition) and interprets this information in the context of a postoperative patient 12 hours after surgery with a PCA device.

AGE-RELATED VARIATIONS

This chapter discusses assessment techniques with adult patients. These data are important to assess in individuals of all ages, but the approach and techniques used to collect the information may vary depending on the patient's age.

INFANTS, CHILDREN, AND ADOLESCENTS

Assessing the respiratory status of an infant, child, or adolescent usually follows the same sequence as for an adult, although there are a few differences worth noting. Assessing neonates and infants requires use of different equipment and an unhurried approach. Use a pediatric stethoscope when examining an infant or child. The infant must be undressed at least to the diaper to perform an adequate assessment. Keep the infant covered when you are not performing the examination to prevent exposure and cooling. Conduct the examination while the infant is calm, if possible; examination of a crying infant is difficult. By the ages of 2 or 3 years the child is usually cooperative during the respiratory examination. Before that age you need to develop a relationship with the child to improve cooperation during the examination. Chapter 19 presents further information regarding the respiratory assessment of infants, children, and adolescents.

OLDER ADULTS

Assessing the respiratory status of an older adult follows the same procedures as for an adult, although structural and functional differences may be noticed. When assessing older adults, use an unhurried approach. Expected variations from younger adults may include changes in the musculoskeletal system, which affect respiratory function. Posterior thoracic stooping or bending or kyphosis may alter the thorax wall configuration and make thoracic expansion more difficult. Chapter 21 presents further information regarding the respiratory assessment of an older adult.

COMMON PROBLEMS AND CONDITIONS

INFLAMMATION/INFECTION

Acute Bronchitis

An inflammation of the mucous membranes of the bronchial tree is called *acute bronchitis*. **Clinical Findings:** The cough is initially nonproductive, but after a few days it may become productive with yellow or green sputum. Patients may complain of sore ribs from prolonged periods of coughing and malaise.[11] Rhonchi are heard on auscultation, with wheezing heard after coughing (Fig. 11.24).

COVID-19

Coronavirus causes this contagious disease that is spread by respiratory droplets. **Clinical Findings:** A wide range of symptoms have been reported including cough, dyspnea, fever, chills, muscle pain, headache, sore throat, and loss of the sense of taste or smell. Symptoms may appear 2 to 14 days after exposure to the virus.[12]

Pneumonia

An infection of the terminal bronchioles and alveoli is referred to as *pneumonia*. **Clinical Findings:** Symptoms range from mild to severe, requiring hospitalization. Viral pneumonia tends to produce a nonproductive cough or clear sputum, whereas bacterial pneumonia causes a productive cough that may produce white, yellow, or green sputum. Changes in vital signs include fever, tachycardia, and tachypnea. Subjective data include shaking chills, malaise, and pleuritic chest pain when deep breathing and coughing.[13] Crackles or rhonchi may be heard on auscultation (Fig. 11.25).[8]

Tuberculosis

This contagious, bacterial infection caused by Mycobacterium tuberculosis is transmitted by airborne droplets. The infection primarily affects the upper airways, but kidneys, bones, lymph nodes, and meninges can also become involved. The CDC estimates up to 13 million people in the United States have latent TB and more than 85% of the US cases of TB each year are the result of reactivation infection instead of recent transmission.[14] **Clinical Findings:** The infected person is usually asymptomatic during the early stages of the disease. The initial manifestations may be fatigue, anorexia, weight loss, night sweats, and fever. For people who have a healthy immune system, the body walls off the bacteria preventing further spread, which is called latent TB. However, the immune response to TB can be detected by a skin test in 2 to

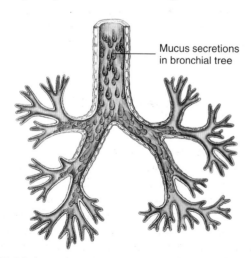

FIG. 11.24 Acute bronchitis. Irritation of the bronchi causes inflammation.

Mucus secretions in bronchial tree

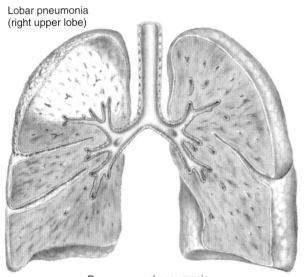

Lobar pneumonia
(right upper lobe)

Pneumococcal pneumonia

FIG. 11.25 Right upper lobe pneumonia.

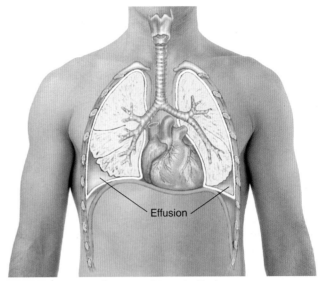

Effusion

FIG. 11.27 Pleural effusion.

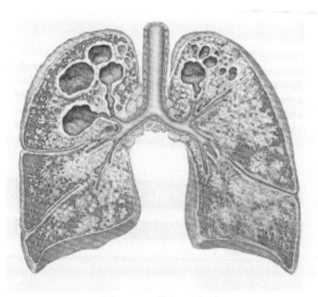

FIG. 11.26 Tuberculosis.

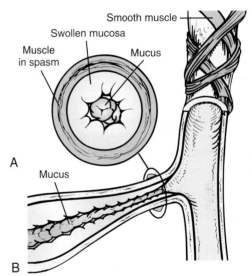

Smooth muscle

Swollen mucosa

Muscle in spasm

Mucus

A

Mucus

B

FIG. 11.28 Factors causing airway obstruction in asthma. (A) Cross-section of a bronchiole occluded by muscle spasm, mucosal edema, and mucus. (B) Longitudinal section of a bronchiole. (From Lewis et al., 2011. Redrawn from Price and Wilson, 2003.)

8 weeks after infection so that treatment can be started. Without treatment approximately 5% of people with latent TB develop active TB within 1 to 2 years (Fig. 11.26).[15]

Pleural Effusion

An accumulation of serous fluid in the pleural space between the visceral and parietal pleurae is called *pleural effusion*. **Clinical Findings:** Manifestations depend on the amount of fluid accumulation and the position of the patient. Signs may be fever, tachypnea, tachycardia, decreased fremitus, trachea shifted to the other side, and absent breath sounds on the affected side. Symptoms may include dyspnea and sharp chest pain that is worse with cough or deep breaths (Fig. 11.27).[6]

CHRONIC PULMONARY DISEASE

Asthma

Asthma is a hyperreactive airway disease characterized by bronchoconstriction, airway obstruction, and inflammation. The number of adults diagnosed with asthma in 2015 was 18,445.[16] **Clinical Findings:** Symptoms include dyspnea and tightness in the chest. Signs include tachycardia, tachypnea with prolonged expiration, audible wheeze, use of accessory muscles, and cough.[6] Expiratory and occasionally inspiratory wheeze and diminished breath sounds are common findings (Fig. 11.28).

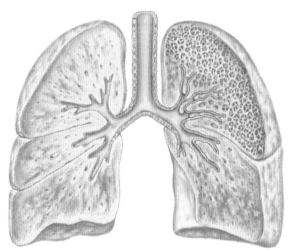

FIG. 11.29 Emphysema upper left lobe.

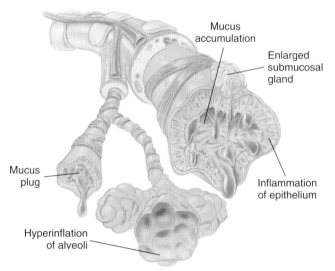

FIG. 11.30 Chronic bronchitis. (From McCance and Huether, 2002. Modified from Des Jardins and Burton, 1995.)

Emphysema

Destruction of the alveolar walls causes permanent abnormal enlargement of the air spaces in emphysema. The number of adults diagnosed with emphysema in 2016 was 3.4 million.[17] **Clinical Findings:** The classic appearance of a patient with advanced emphysema is an underweight individual with a barrel chest who becomes short of breath with minimal exertion. When the patient is short of breath, pursed-lip breathing and tripod position are frequently observed. Other signs may be diminished breath sounds, possible wheezing or crackles, clubbing of nails, and increased AP to lateral diameter (Fig. 11.29).[6]

Chronic Bronchitis

Chronic bronchitis is characterized by hypersecretion of mucus by the goblet cells of the trachea and bronchi, resulting in a productive cough for 3 months in each of 2 successive years.[18] The number of adults diagnosed with chronic bronchitis in 2016 was 8.6 million.[16] **Clinical Findings:** Symptoms include productive cough, increased mucus production, and dyspnea. Findings are rhonchi, sometimes cleared by coughing, cyanosis, and clubbing of nails (Fig. 11.30).[6]

ACUTE OR TRAUMATIC CONDITIONS

Pneumothorax

Air in the pleural spaces results in a pneumothorax. There are three types of pneumothorax: (1) closed, which may be spontaneous, traumatic, or iatrogenic (caused by illness or medical treatment); (2) open, which occurs following penetration of the chest by either injury or surgical procedure; and (3) tension, which develops when air leaks into the pleura and cannot escape. **Clinical Findings:** The signs vary, depending on the amount of lung collapse. If there is very minor collapse, the patient may be slightly short of breath, anxious, and report chest pain. If a large amount of lung collapses, the patient may experience severe respiratory distress, including

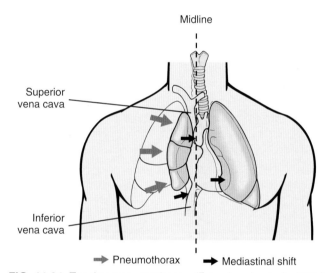

FIG. 11.31 Tension pneumothorax. (From Lewis et al., 2011.)

tachycardia, dyspnea, tachypnea, and cyanosis. Breath sounds over the affected area are absent. Decreased chest wall movement on the affected side may be noticed. The patient may also have paradoxical chest wall movement, when the chest wall moves in on inspiration and out on expiration. If severe, there may be tracheal displacement toward the unaffected side with a mediastinal shift, termed a *tension pneumothorax* (Fig. 11.31).[6]

Hemothorax

Blood in the pleural space results in hemothorax. **Clinical Findings:** Chest pain and dyspnea are common symptoms. Signs may include hypotension; cold, clammy skin; tachycardia; rapid, shallow breathing; and diminished-to-absent breath sounds over the affected lung (Fig. 11.32).[19]

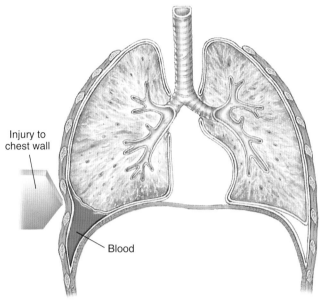

FIG. 11.32 Hemothorax.

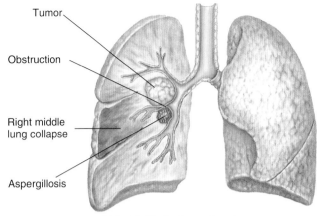

FIG. 11.33 Atelectasis.

OTHER PULMONARY CONDITIONS

Atelectasis

Atelectasis refers to collapsed alveoli caused by external pressure from a tumor, fluid, or air in the pleural space (compression atelectasis) or by lack of air from hypoventilation or obstruction by secretions (absorption atelectasis). **Clinical Findings:** The affected area has decreased fremitus and diminished or absent breath sounds.[6] The oxygen saturation may decrease to less than 90% (Fig. 11.33).

Lung Cancer

This malignancy is an uncontrolled growth of abnormal cells in one or both lungs. Lung cancer remains the leading cause of cause and cancer related deaths, with an estimated 228,820 new cases and 135,700 deaths in 2020.[20] **Clinical Findings:** Symptoms can take years to develop and may not appear until the disease is advanced. The most common initial symptom reported is a persistent cough. Other symptoms include pain in the chest, shoulder or back unrelated to pain of coughing, hemoptysis, and dyspnea. Lung sounds may be

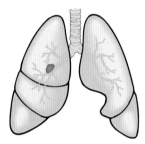

A Squamous cell carcinoma

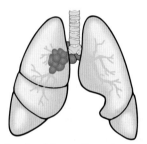

B Small cell (oat cell) carcinoma

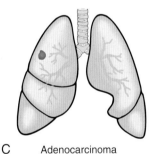

C   Adenocarcinoma

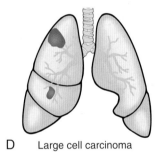

D   Large cell carcinoma

FIG. 11.34 Cancer of the lung. (From Lewis et al., 2004.)

normal or diminished over the affected area. If there is a partial obstruction of airways from the tumor, wheezes may be heard. Generalized symptoms may be loss of appetite, unexplained weight loss, and fatigue (Fig. 11.34).[21]

CLINICAL APPLICATION AND CLINICAL JUDGMENT

See Appendix B for answers to exercises in this section.

CASE STUDY

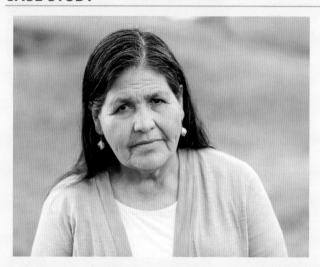

Ms. Martinez is a 66-year-old woman complaining of shortness of breath. The following initial data were collected.

Interview Data

Ms. Martinez says that she has had breathing problems "for years" but her breathing is getting worse. She tells the nurse that she gets short of breath with activity, adding that she can do things around the house for only a few minutes before she has to sit down to catch her breath. She says that she can sleep for only a couple of hours at a time. She sleeps best using two pillows to prop up, but on some nights she just sits in a chair.

Ms. Martinez does not currently use oxygen, but she thinks oxygen would help. She admits to smoking 1.5 packs of cigarettes a day. She has never quit because she says she "just can't do it."

Examination Data

*   *General survey:* Alert and slightly anxious female, sitting slightly forward, with moderately labored breathing. Skin pale with slight cyanosis around the lips and in nail beds. Slight clubbing of fingers.
*   *Chest and lungs:* Chest is round shaped and symmetric with increased AP diameter. Small muscle mass is noticed over chest; ribs protrude. Respiratory rate is 24 breaths/min and labored. Chest wall expansion with respirations is reduced but symmetric. Wheezes are heard on expiration throughout lung fields. Lung sounds are diminished in lung bases bilaterally.

Clinical Judgment

1. What cues do you recognize that suggest a deviation from expected findings, suggesting a need for further investigation?
2. For which additional information should the nurse ask or assess?
3. Based on the data, which risk factors does Ms. Martinez have for lung cancer?
4. With which health care team member would you collaborate to meet this patient's needs?

REVIEW QUESTIONS

1. A nurse suspects a viral infection or upper respiratory allergies when the patient describes the sputum as being which color?
    1. Green
    2. Clear
    3. Yellow
    4. Pink tinged

2. During inspection of the respiratory system the nurse documents which finding as abnormal?
    1. Skin color consistent with patient's race
    2. 1:2 ratio of anteroposterior to lateral diameter
    3. Respiratory rate of 20 breaths per minute
    4. Patient leaning forward with arms braced on the knees

3. A patient has an infection of the terminal bronchioles and alveoli that involves the right lower lobe of the lung. Which abnormal findings are expected?
    1. Dyspnea with diminished breath sounds bilaterally
    2. Asymmetric chest expansion and rhonchi on the right side
    3. Fever and tachypnea with crackles over the right lower lobe
    4. Prolonged expiration with an occasional wheeze in the right lower lobe

4. On auscultation of a patient's lungs, the nurse hears a low-pitched, coarse, loud, and low snoring sound. Which term does the nurse use to document this finding?
    1. Rhonchi
    2. Wheeze
    3. Crackles
    4. Pleural friction rub

5. A nurse finds the patient's AP diameter of the chest to be the same as the lateral diameter. Based on this finding, what additional data would the nurse anticipate?
    1. Bronchial breath sounds in the posterior thorax
    2. Decrease in respiratory rate
    3. Decreased breath sounds on auscultation
    4. Complaint of sharp chest pain on inspiration

6. How does the nurse palpate the chest for tenderness, bulges, and symmetry?
   1. Uses the fist of the dominant hand to gently tap the anterior, lateral, and posterior chest, comparing one side with another
   2. Uses the ulnar surface of one hand to palpate the anterior, posterior, and lateral chest, comparing one side with another
   3. Uses the tips of the fingers to palpate the skin over the chest and the alignment of vertebrae
   4. Uses the palmar surface of fingers of both hands to feel the texture of the skin over the chest and the alignment of vertebrae

7. Which breath sounds are expected over the posterior chest of an adult?
   1. Vesicular
   2. Bronchovesicular
   3. Bronchial
   4. Bronchoalveolar

8. Narrowing of the bronchi creates which adventitious sound?
   1. Wheeze
   2. Crackles
   3. Rhonchi
   4. Pleural friction rub

9. A nurse is auscultating the lungs of a healthy female patient and hears crackles on inspiration. What action can the nurse take to ensure this is an accurate finding?
   1. Make sure the bell of the stethoscope is used rather than the diaphragm.
   2. Ask the patient to cough then repeat the auscultation.
   3. Ask the patient not to talk while the nurse is listening to the lungs.
   4. Change the patient's position.

10. A nurse in the emergency department is assessing a patient with a moderate left pneumothorax. What does this nurse expect to find during the respiratory examination?
    1. Increased fremitus over the left chest
    2. Tracheal deviation to the left side
    3. Crepitus on the left chest during palpation
    4. Distant to absent breath sounds over the left chest

CHAPTER

12

Heart and Peripheral Vascular System

evolve

http://evolve.elsevier.com/Wilson/assessment

CONCEPT OVERVIEW

The concept for this chapter is *Perfusion*, which represents mechanisms that facilitate and impair circulation of oxygenated blood throughout the body. Concepts interrelated with perfusion include gas exchange, nutrition, metabolism, motion, tissue integrity, pain, elimination, and intracranial regulation, and are depicted in the illustration below. Understanding these interrelationships helps the nurse recognize risk factors when conducting a health assessment.

```
        Nutrition          Gas exchange

  Metabolism                        Pain

              Perfusion

  Motion                         Elimination

      Tissue integrity    Intracranial
                          regulation
```

Blood flow supplies oxygen and nutrients continuously to tissues so they can perform their functions. These tissues include skin, the kidneys to produce urine, the brain for intracranial regulation, the gastrointestinal tract for metabolism, and muscles and nerves for motion. Pain results when perfusion is interrupted. The following case provides a clinical example featuring several of these interrelated concepts.

Eva Schmanski is a 79-year-old woman who has heart failure resulting from long-standing hypertension. Reduced cardiac output from the left ventricle has resulted in a back-up of blood into the pulmonary vascular system. The increased pressure has caused fluid to leak out of the pulmonary capillaries into alveoli, which interferes with gas exchange. Furthermore, poor perfusion of oxygenated blood limits motion (because of activity intolerance and fatigue) and elimination (caused by poor perfusion to the kidneys), and potentially results in confusion as a result of poor perfusion to the brain.

ANATOMY AND PHYSIOLOGY

The cardiovascular system transports oxygen, nutrients, and other substances to body tissues and metabolic waste products to the kidneys and lungs. This dynamic system is able to adjust to changing demands for blood by constricting or dilating blood vessels and altering the cardiac output.

HEART AND GREAT VESSELS

The heart is a pump about the size of a fist that beats 60 to 100 times a minute without rest, responding to both external and internal demands such as exercise, temperature changes,

and stress. Each side of the heart has two chambers, an atrium and a ventricle. The right side receives blood from the superior and inferior venae cavae and pumps it through the pulmonary arteries to the pulmonary circulation; the left side receives blood from the pulmonary veins and pumps it through the aorta into the systemic circulation.

The upper part of the heart is called the *base*, and the lower left ventricle is called the *apex*. The heart lies at an angle so the right ventricle makes up most of the anterior surface and the left ventricle lies to the left and posteriorly. The right atrium forms the right border of the heart, and

214

the left atrium lies posteriorly. The pulmonary arteries and aorta are termed the *great vessels.* The aorta curves upward out of the left ventricle and bends posteriorly and downward. The pulmonary arteries emerge from the superior aspect of the right ventricle near the third intercostal space (Fig. 12.1).

Pericardium and Cardiac Muscle

The heart wall has three layers: pericardium, myocardium, and endocardium (Fig. 12.2). The heart is encased in the pericardium, which has a fibrous layer and two serous layers. The fibrous layer, termed the *fibrous pericardium* or *parietal layer,* is a fibrous sac of elastic connective tissue that shields the heart from trauma and infection. One of the serous layers lies next to the fibrous pericardium, and the other lies next to the myocardium. Between the fibrous pericardium and the serous pericardium is the pericardial space, which contains a small amount of pericardial fluid to reduce friction as the myocardium contracts and relaxes. The serous pericardium, also termed the *visceral layer* or *epicardium,* covers the heart surface and extends to the great vessels. The middle layer, or myocardium, is thick muscular

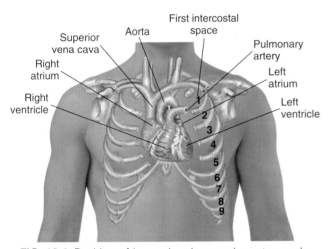

FIG. 12.1 Position of heart chambers and great vessels.

tissue that contracts to eject blood from the ventricles. The endocardium lines the inner chambers and valves. The coronary arteries supply blood to the pericardium and cardiac muscle.

Blood Flow Through the Heart

Four valves govern blood flow through the four chambers of the heart. The tricuspid valve on the right and mitral valve on the left are termed the *atrioventricular (AV)* valves because they separate the atria from the ventricles (Fig. 12.3). The aortic valve opens from the left ventricle into the aorta; the pulmonic valve opens from the right ventricle into the pulmonary artery. The aortic and pulmonic valves are termed *semilunar (SL)* valves because of their half-moon shape.

Cardiac Cycle

The sequence of events that moves blood through the heart is called the cardiac cycle, which has two phases: diastole and systole. These events are shown at the bottom of Fig. 12.4. The first heart sound, S_1, indicates the beginning of systole, while the second heart sound, S_2, indicates the beginning of diastole. The S_3 and S_4 heart sounds are abnormal; however, they are shown in Fig. 12.4 at the point in the cardiac cycle where they would be heard if present. Further discussion of abnormal heart sounds is in Table 12.2.

Diastole

During diastole, the ventricles are relaxed and fill with blood from the atria. The movement of blood from the atria into the ventricles is accomplished when the pressure of the blood in the atria becomes higher than the pressure in the ventricles. The higher atrial pressures passively open the AV valves, allowing blood to fill the ventricles (Fig. 12.5). Approximately 80% of the blood from the atria flows into relaxed ventricles. A contraction of the atria forces the remaining 20% into the ventricles. This added atrial thrust is termed the *atrial kick.* At the end of diastole the ventricles are filled with blood.

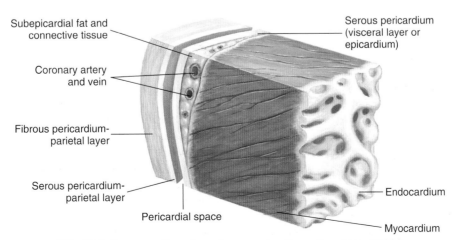

FIG. 12.2 Cross-section of cardiac muscle. (From Canobbio, 1990.)

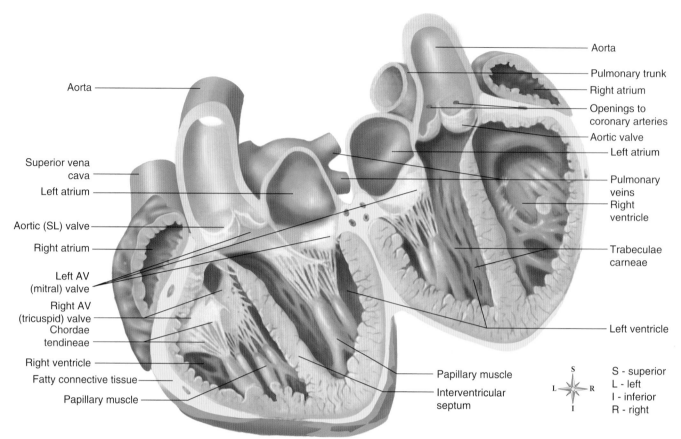

FIG. 12.3 Anterior cross section showing valves and chambers of the heart. *AV*, Atrioventricular; *SL*, semilunar. (From Patton, Thibodeau, 2012.)

Systole

During systole the ventricles contract, creating a pressure that closes the AV valves, preventing the backflow of blood into the atria. This ventricular pressure also forces the semilunar valves to open, resulting in ejection of blood into the aorta (from the left ventricle) and the pulmonary arteries (from the right ventricle) (Fig. 12.6). As blood is ejected, the ventricular pressure decreases, causing the semilunar valves to close. The ventricles relax to begin diastole.

Electric Conduction

The heart is stimulated by an electric impulse that originates in the sinoatrial (SA) node in the superior aspect of the right atrium and travels in internodal tracts to the AV node. The SA node, termed the *cardiac pacemaker*, normally discharges between 60 and 100 impulses per minute. The electric impulses stimulate contractions of both atria and then flow to the AV node in the inferior aspect of the right atrium. The impulses are then transmitted through a series of branches (bundle of His) and Purkinje fibers in the myocardium, which results in ventricular contraction (Fig. 12.7). The AV node prevents excessive atrial impulses from reaching the ventricles. If the SA node fails to discharge, the AV node can generate ventricular contraction at a slower rate, 40 to 60 impulses per minute. If both SA and AV nodes are ineffective, the bundle branches may stimulate contraction but at a very slow rate of 20 to 40 impulses per minute.

PERIPHERAL VASCULAR SYSTEM

Arteries, capillaries, and veins provide blood flow to and from tissues. The tough and tensile arteries and their smaller branches, the arterioles, are subjected to remarkable pressure generated from the myocardial contractions. They maintain blood pressure by constricting or dilating in response to stimuli. The veins and their smaller branches, the venules, are less sturdy but more expansible, enabling them to act as a reservoir for extra blood, if required, to decrease the workload on the heart. Pressure within the veins is low compared with arterial pressure. The valves in each vein keep blood flowing in a forward direction toward the heart. A comparison of the structures of arteries and veins is shown in Fig. 12.8.

LYMPH SYSTEM

The lymph system works in collaboration with the peripheral vascular system in removing fluid from the interstitial spaces. As blood flows from arterioles, oxygen and nutrient-rich fluids are forced out at the arterial end of the capillaries into the interstitial spaces and then into cells. Waste products from cells flow through the interstitial spaces to venules and then into the capillaries.

Excess fluid left in the interstitial spaces is absorbed by the lymph system and carried to lymph nodes throughout the

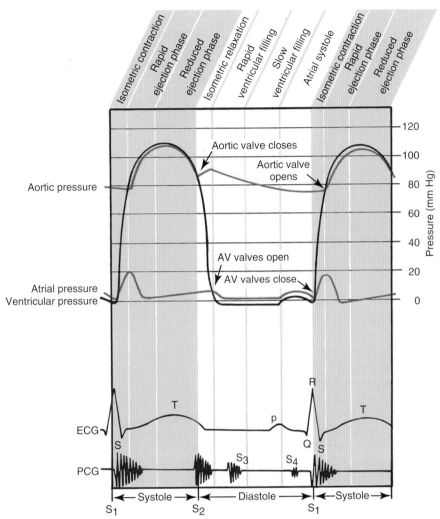

FIG. 12.4 Events of the cardiac cycle showing venous pressure waves, electrocardiograph, and heart sounds in systole and diastole. *AV,* Atrioventricular; *EKG,* electrocardiogram; *PCG,* phonocardiogram; *QRS,* QRS complex (ventricular contraction); *S1,* first heart sound; *S2,* second heart sound; *S3,* third heart sound; *S4,* fourth heart sound; *T,* T wave (ventricular repolarization).

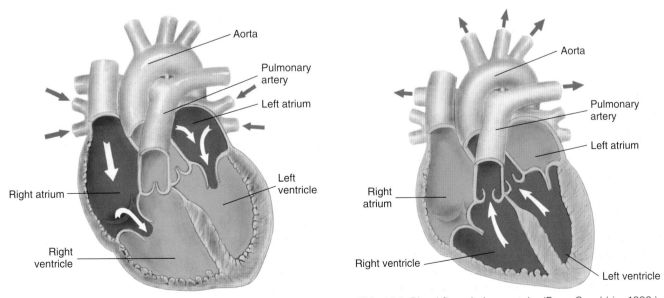

FIG. 12.5 Blood flow during diastole. (From Canobbio, 1990.)

FIG. 12.6 Blood flow during systole. (From Canobbio, 1990.)

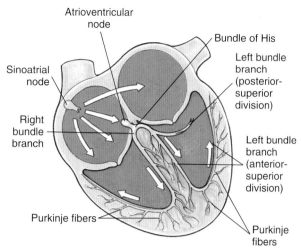

FIG. 12.7 Cardiac conduction. (From Canobbio, 1990.)

body. Lymphatic fluid is clear, composed mainly of water and a small amount of protein, mostly albumin. Lymph nodes are tiny oval clumps of lymphatic tissue, usually located in groups along blood vessels. In the peripheral vascular system, the lymph node locations of interest are the arm, groin, and leg. The brachial (axillary) nodes receive lymph drainage from the neck, chest, axilla, and arm. The epitrochlear nodes receive fluid via the radial, ulnar, and median lymph vessels. In the upper thigh the inguinal lymph nodes are superficial; they receive most of the lymph drainage from the great and small saphenous lymphatic vessels in the legs. In men, lymph from the penile and scrotal surfaces drains to the inguinal nodes, but nodes of the testes drain into the abdomen. In the posterior surface of the leg behind the knee are the popliteal nodes, which receive lymph from the medial portion of the lower leg (Fig. 12.9). Ducts from the lymph nodes empty into the subclavian veins.

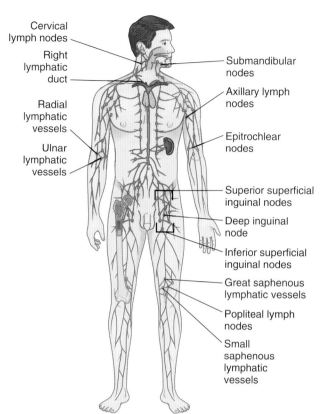

FIG. 12.9 System of deep and superficial collecting ducts carrying lymph from upper extremity to subclavian lymphatic trunk. The only peripheral lymph center is the epitrochlear, which receives some of the collecting ducts from the pathway of the ulnar and radial vessels.

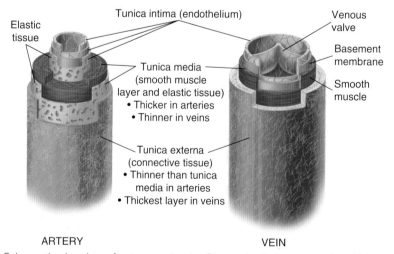

ARTERY   VEIN

FIG. 12.8 Schematic drawing of artery and vein. Shown is the comparative thickness of three layers: fibrous connective tissue (tunica externa), muscle layer (tunica media), and lining of endothelium (tunica intima). Notice that the muscle and outer coats are much thinner in the veins than in the arteries and that veins have valves. (From Thibodeau and Patton, 2010.)

HEALTH HISTORY

Nurses interview patients to collect subjective data about their present health status, past health history, family history, and personal and psychosocial history, which may affect the functions of their heart and peripheral vascular system.

GENERAL HEALTH HISTORY

Present Health Status

Do you have any chronic illnesses such as diabetes mellitus, renal failure, chronic obstructive pulmonary disease, or hypertension? If yes, describe.
Chronic illnesses can cause symptoms affecting the cardiovascular system when they increase the workload of the heart by narrowing peripheral vessels (diabetes mellitus, hypertension), increasing the fluid volume to be pumped (diabetes mellitus, renal failure), increasing the heart rate, or causing pulmonary capillary vasoconstriction (chronic obstructive pulmonary disease).

Do you take any medications? If yes, what do you take and how often? What are the medications for?
Medications may be taken to treat a cardiovascular problem, such as hypertension or a dysrhythmia. Medications taken to treat another disorder may have adverse effects on the cardiovascular system. For example, tricyclic antidepressants, phenothiazines, or lithium can cause dysrhythmias; hormonal contraceptives can cause thrombophlebitis; corticosteroids can cause sodium and fluid retention; and theophylline can cause tachycardia and dysrhythmias.

Do you take any over-the-counter drugs or herbal supplements? If yes, what do you take and how often? What are they for?
Nonprescription drugs and herbal supplements may affect the cardiovascular system. For example, decongestants containing pseudoephedrine may aggravate hypertension. Ayurvedic herbs can act as a cardiac stimulant, whereas other herbs act as a cardiac depressant.

Past Health History

Were you born with congenital heart disease or a heart defect?
Data from past medical history gives information about clinical findings to anticipate.

During childhood did you have "growing pains" (i.e., unexplained joint pains)? Recurrent tonsillitis? Rheumatic fever? Heart murmur?
These questions relate to diagnosis of rheumatic fever, which may have contributed to rheumatic heart disease.

Have you been told that you have high levels of cholesterol or elevated triglycerides?
Elevated serum lipids can build up in arteries creating deposits called plaque, which may impede blood flow to tissues and increase workload on the heart.

Have you ever had surgery on your heart or on your blood vessels? If yes, which procedure was done? When was it done? How successful was the surgery?
Knowledge of past surgical procedures may provide additional information about possible cardiovascular problems. These data also explain the presence of scars that you will observe on examination.

Have you ever had any tests on your heart? Electrocardiogram (EKG or ECG), stress EKG, or other heart tests? What did the tests reveal? What, if any, treatment did you receive?
These tests provide baseline data on the health of the patient's heart.

RISK FACTORS

Hypertension and Coronary Artery Disease

RISK FACTOR	HYPERTENSION (HTN); HIGH BLOOD PRESSURE (HBP)	CORONARY ARTERY DISEASE (CAD)
Family history	Increased risk when parents of close relatives have HTN	Increased risk when parents of close relatives have HTN
Age	Risk increases with age	Risk increases with age
Gender	Before age 64: Males > Females After age 65, risk increases for women	Men have a greater risk of acute myocardial infarction (AMI) than women and have them earlier in life
Race	African Americans highest risk	African Americans, Mexican Americans, American Indians, native Hawaiians, and some Asian Americans highest risk
Hypertension (M)	—	Yes
Lack of physical activity (M)	Yes	Yes
Unhealthy diet, especially one high in fats and sodium (M)	Yes	Yes
Overweight and Obesity (M)	Yes	Yes
Excessive alcohol consumption (M)	Yes	Yes

Continued

RISK FACTORS—cont'd

Hypertension and Coronary Artery Disease

RISK FACTOR	HYPERTENSION (HTN); HIGH BLOOD PRESSURE (HBP)	CORONARY ARTERY DISEASE (CAD)
High cholesterol (M)	Yes	Yes
Smoking and tobacco use (M)	Yes	Yes
Stress (M)	Yes	Yes

M, Modifiable risk factor.

Data from Know your risk factors for high blood pressure. Available at https://www.heart.org/en/health-topics/high-blood-pressure/why-high-blood-pressure-is-a-silent-killer/know-your-risk-factors-for-high-blood-pressure. Accessed December 31, 2017. Coronary artery disease—coronary heart disease. Available at https://www.heart.org/en/health-topics/heart-attack/understand-your-risks-to-prevent-a-heart-attack?s=q%3Drisk%2520factors%2520for%2520coronary%2520artery%2520disease%26sort%3Drelevancy.

Family History

Does anyone in your family have a history of cardiovascular disease, hyperlipidemia, or hypertension? If yes, what conditions does your family member(s) have? Which family member(s)?

These conditions are risk factors for heart disease and have familial tendencies.

Personal and Psychosocial History

Do you exercise? If yes, what kind of exercise? How often do you exercise? How much time do you spend exercising? If no, have you ever exercised? What motivated you to start in the past? What influenced you to stop exercising?

Physical inactivity is a risk factor for cardiovascular disease. The recommendations for physical activity for adults is at least 150 minutes weekly of moderate-intensity aerobic activity or 75 minutes weekly of vigorous aerobic exercise, or a combination of both, preferably spread throughout the week.[1,2] Patients who no longer exercise should be encouraged to resume an exercise program, especially women since exercise has been proved to provide greater effects for women than men.[3] Exploring reasons for stopping can begin the problem-solving process to determine what can motivate them to start again.

How would you describe your personality type? How do you deal with stress?

Stress and persistent intensity are risk factors for heart disease. (Observe the patient as he or she responds and throughout the examination to detect stress or intensity.) Patients who are frequently in stressful environments should be encouraged to use strategies to relieve stress and change their perceptions of the situations.

How often do you take time to relax? What do you do to relax? Hobbies? Sports? Meditation? Yoga? Music?

Physical relaxation can relieve stress and reduce blood pressure.

Describe your usual eating habits. Do you monitor your fat and salt intake? Do you eat whole grains each day?

The DASH diet (Dietary Approaches to Stop Hypertension) and Mediterranean diet have the highest level of evidence for cardiovascular protection.[3] Calories from fat should be limited to 20% of daily calories, with 10% limited to saturated fat. Whole grains (e.g., cereals) have been found to reduce heart disease. (Refer to Chapter 8 for dietary guidelines.)

Do you drink alcoholic beverages? What type of alcohol do you drink? How much? How often?

Excessive alcohol intake has been associated with hypertension and the development of cardiomyopathy. See Chapter 7 for alcohol use.

Do you use cocaine? Other street drugs? How often do you use these drugs?

Cocaine use has been associated with myocardial infarction and stroke.

Do you consume caffeine? In coffee? Chocolate? Soft drinks? How much caffeine do you consume? How often?

Excessive caffeine intake can cause tachycardia, which can increase the workload of the heart.

Do you smoke or have you been a smoker in the past? If yes, what forms of tobacco do (did) you use (cigarettes, cigars, pipe, e-cigarettes, marijuana, smokeless or chewing tobacco)? How often do (did) you use tobacco? Have you ever quit smoking? If yes, how did you accomplish it, and for what length of time? Are you interested in quitting smoking?

Nicotine in tobacco causes vasoconstriction, which may decrease blood flow to extremities and increase blood pressure, both of which increase the workload on the heart. Patients who previously were successful at stopping their tobacco use may be more easily convinced to repeat their success. Patients must be interested in stopping tobacco use; otherwise there is little motivation to change behavior. Perhaps educating them about the negative effects of nicotine on the cardiovascular system may provide some motivation.

PROBLEM-BASED HISTORY

Commonly reported symptoms related to the heart and peripheral vascular system are chest pain, shortness of breath, cough, urinating during the night (nocturia), fatigue, fainting (syncope), swelling of the extremities, leg pain, and enlarged lymph nodes. As with symptoms in all areas of health assessment, a symptom analysis is completed using the mnemonic OLD CARTS, which includes the *On*set, *Location*, *Duration*, *Characteristics*, *Aggravating* factors, *Related* symptoms, *Treatment*, and *Severity* (see Box 2.6).

Chest Pain

Where are you feeling the chest pain? What does it feel like? Does it radiate to any location? How severe is it on a scale of 0 to 10?
The origin of chest pain may be pulmonary, musculoskeletal, or gastrointestinal rather than cardiac. Table 12.1 describes different types of chest pain. If patients indicate that they are having active chest pain, the nurse assesses quickly to determine the need for immediate treatment. Angina is an important symptom of coronary artery disease, which indicates myocardial ischemia caused by a lack of oxygen to meet the demand of the myocardium. Typical angina is described as substernal discomfort that is precipitated by exertion, relieved with rest or nitroglycerin or both, and lasts less than 10 minutes. Many patients describe the pain as radiating to the shoulder, jaw, or inner aspect of the arm.[4] The chest discomfort may be described as uncomfortable pressure, squeezing, fullness, or pain.[5] Women report chest pain that is milder than men report as well as pain in the neck, jaw, shoulder, arms, or upper back. Women's symptoms are vague and easy to miss by both patients and health care providers.[6]

When did the pain start? Is it intermittent or constant? If intermittent, how long does it last?
These questions help distinguish different types of chest pain (see Table 12.1). Stable angina often has a gradual onset, whereas unstable angina may have a sudden onset.

Which symptoms have you noticed along with the pain? Sweating? Heart skipping beats or racing? Shortness of breath? Nausea or vomiting? Dizziness? Anxiety?
These related symptoms frequently accompany an acute myocardial infarction. Women may experience fatigue, difficulty sleeping, shortness of breath, indigestion, anxiety, and chest pressure for up to a year before having a myocardial infarction.[6]

What were you doing just prior to the onset of the pain? Exercise? Rest? Highly emotional situation? Eating? Sexual intercourse?
Angina is frequently precipitated by physical exertion.[4]

What makes the pain worse? Moving the arms or neck? Deep breathing? Lying flat? Exercise?
The chest pain from pericarditis is aggravated by deep breathing, coughing, or lying supine. Chest pain from muscle strain may be aggravated by movement of the arms.

What relieves the pain? Rest? Nitroglycerin? How many nitroglycerin tablets does it take to relieve chest pain?
These questions assess for alleviating factors. Chest pain that is relieved by nitroglycerin may be caused by myocardial

ischemia (stable angina), whereas chest pain that is not relieved by four or more nitroglycerin tablets taken 5 minutes apart may be caused by myocardial necrosis (unstable angina), which may lead to myocardial infarction.

Shortness of Breath

How long have you had shortness of breath? Do you feel short of breath now?
Dyspnea may be caused by respiratory or cardiac problems. A gradual onset may be caused by heart failure that develops slowly from backup of fluid from the left heart into the alveoli.

During which activities do you experience shortness of breath? How many pillows do you require when you lie down? Do you breathe easier when in a recliner? How often does the shortness of breath occur?
These questions determine the onset of dyspnea. Walking upstairs increases the workload of the heart. Dyspnea experienced when lying down is called *orthopnea* and may be relieved by sitting up. The number of pillows necessary to relieve the orthopnea is documented (e.g., *two-pillow orthopnea* means that the patient must elevate his or her chest with two pillows to breathe easily). Some patients use a recliner for elevation rather than using pillows.

Does the shortness of breath interfere with your daily activities? How many level blocks can you walk before you become short of breath? How many blocks could you walk 6 months ago?
Dyspnea that interferes with activities of daily living may require the patient to use supplemental oxygen. If the distance the patient can walk is decreased, it is a sign that the dyspnea is getting worse. Notice if the patient has to take a breath in the middle of sentences (see Box 11.2).

Do you have any related symptoms with the shortness of breath (e.g., a cough, chest pain, or your feet swell during the day when you are sitting or standing)?
Shortness of breath may be a symptom of the cardiovascular system such as a severe heart murmur or heart failure. Dependent edema seen in the ankles or feet may develop from retained fluid because of right-sided heart failure.

When these episodes of shortness of breath occur, what do you do to ease the symptoms?
Determine the effectiveness of the action(s) to relieve dyspnea such as stopping activity, sitting up. This information may be helpful in planning future treatment strategies.

Cough

When did your cough start? Do you cough up anything? What does it look like?
Coughing up blood (hemoptysis) is a symptom of mitral stenosis and pulmonary disorders. White, frothy sputum may be a sign of pulmonary edema that occurs with left-sided heart failure.

TABLE 12.1 DIFFERENTIATION OF CHEST PAIN

DISORDER	ONSET AND DURATION	LOCATION	CHARACTERISTICS	SEVERITY	RELATED SYMPTOMS	AGGRAVATING FACTORS	TREATMENT/ ALLEVIATING FACTORS
Stable angina	Intermittent onset; lasts only a few minutes	Usually located substernally, can radiate to left arm, neck, jaw, shoulders	Pressure, burning, heaviness, crushing	Variable, mild to severe	Dyspnea, diaphoresis, palpitations, nausea, weakness	Physical exertion, stress, cold, stimulants, e.g., cocaine	Rest, nitroglycerin, beta-blocker, calcium channel blocker, aspirin
Myocardial infarction (MI)	Sudden or gradual onset, constant pain, lasts 20 minutes or longer	Substernal, radiates to arms, neck, jaw	Heavy pressure, squeezing, crushing; burning, not relieved with rest, position change or nitrates	10 of 10 on pain scale	Dyspnea, diaphoresis, palpitations, nausea, weakness, fever	Physical exertion, stress, excitement	Beta-blocker, aspirin, heparin, oxygen.
Acute pericarditis	Onset hours to days, lasts hours to weeks	Substernal, radiates to left shoulder, neck, or arms	Constant, sharp, stabbing pain	Moderate, 4 to 6 of 10 on pain scale	Fever, dyspnea, orthopnea, anxiety	Deep inspiration, coughing, lying down	Sitting up and leaning forward, shallow breathing to reduce pain
Esophageal reflux	Spontaneous onset, often associated with eating	Midepigastric to xiphoid; radiates to neck, ear, or jaw	Burning, tight sensation, squeezing	Moderate to severe	Dysphagia, dyspnea, coughing, disturbed sleep patterns	Spicy or acidic meal, alcohol, lying supine	Weight loss, antacids, H_2 blocker, proton pump inhibitors
Costochondritis	Sudden onset, intermittent duration	Rib cage or sternum, confined to one area	Variable	Variable	None	Coughing, deep breathing, sneezing	Localized heat, analgesics, anti-inflammatory

Is your cough associated with position (more coughing when lying down), anxiety, or talking or activity? What makes it worse? Which actions do you take to relieve the cough?
Coughing more when lying down may indicate heart failure. Knowing how the patient relieves the cough may help to identify treatment strategies.

Urinating During the Night

How long have you been getting up during the night to urinate? How many times a night do you get up to urinate?
Nocturia occurs with heart failure in persons who are ambulatory during the day. Lying down at night creates a fluid shift and increases the need to urinate. Taking a diuretic before bedtime may also contribute to nocturia.

What have you done to reduce the frequency or prevent this from happening? How successful have your efforts been?
Stopping fluid intake within a few hours of bed or changing the time for taking a diuretic may help prevent nocturia. This information may guide future teaching and treatment strategies.

Fatigue

Was the onset of fatigue sudden or gradual? Is the fatigue worse in the morning or evening? Are you too tired to take part in your usual activities?
Fatigue may be experienced during daily activities such as shopping, climbing stairs, carrying groceries, or walking because the heart cannot pump enough blood to meet the body tissue needs. Fatigue from other causes (e.g., depression or anxiety) occurs all day or is worse in the morning. Fatigue from anemia lasts all day. Fatigue from anemia and heart disease occurs gradually, whereas fatigue from acute blood loss occurs more rapidly.

Do you take iron pills? Do you eat foods with iron such as green leafy vegetables and liver? For women: Do you have a heavy menstrual flow?
These questions relate to iron deficiency anemia, which can cause fatigue. Women may have iron deficiency from monthly blood loss.

Have you had any related symptoms with the fatigue such as shortness of breath with activity, rapid heart rate, headache, pale skin, sore tongue or lips, or changes in your nails?
Fatigue and exertional dyspnea are manifestations of mild anemia and heart failure. Additional signs of tachycardia, headache, pallor, brittle, spoon-shaped nails, glossitis (inflammation of the tongue), and cheilitis (inflammation of the lips) occur with moderate-to-severe anemia.

Have you noticed any unusual feelings in your feet and hands, muscle weakness, or trouble thinking?
Neurologic symptoms in addition to those described previously may indicate anemia from vitamin B_{12} deficiency.

Fainting

What were you doing just before you fainted? Did you feel dizzy? Did you lose consciousness?
A brief lapse of consciousness is termed *syncope*. When syncope occurs with activity or position changes and causes dizziness, it may be the result of hypotension or inadequate blood flow to the brain.

Has this happened to you before? How often has this occurred?
These questions determine frequency of syncope.

Was fainting preceded by any other symptoms? Nausea? Chest pain? Headache? Sweating? Rapid heart rate? Confusion? Numbness? Hunger? Ringing in your ears?
These questions attempt to determine whether the cause of fainting is a cardiovascular, a neurologic, or an inner ear problem. It may be caused by small emboli in the cerebral circulation. Emboli may be the result of atrial fibrillation, valvular disease, or cardiac dysrhythmias. Cerebral emboli may cause a stroke, resulting in reports of headache, confusion, and numbness. Fluid or infection of the inner ear can cause vertigo, which may be described as fainting (see Box 10.2).

Swelling of Extremities

Where is the swelling located? Arms or legs? Unilateral or bilateral?
Edema of both legs may be caused by fluid overload from systemic disease (e.g., heart failure, renal failure, or liver disease). Unilateral edema of an extremity may be lymphedema caused by occlusion of lymph channels (e.g., elephantiasis or trauma) or surgical removal of lymph channels (e.g., after mastectomy). Localized edema of one leg may be caused by venous insufficiency from varicosities or thrombophlebitis.

Is there anything you do to reduce the swelling or make it go away? Does elevating your arms or feet reduce the swelling? Does the swelling disappear after a night's sleep?
Edema that increases during the day and decreases at night or with elevation may be related to venous stasis, which may occur with right-sided heart failure. Compression garments for the arms or legs may reduce lymphedema or venous insufficiency.

Are there any related symptoms associated with the swelling? Shortness of breath? Weight gain? Warmth? Discoloration?
Dyspnea may be caused by heart failure. Weight gain occurs anytime there is fluid retention, regardless of cause. Warmth and redness of the legs may indicate an inflammatory process, whereas discoloration and ulceration may indicate ischemia.

For women: Is the swelling associated with your menstrual period?

Hormonal contraceptives may be associated with thrombophlebitis, which may cause unilateral leg edema. Changes in estrogen and progesterone blood levels can contribute to fluid retention, resulting in dependent edema.

Leg Cramps or Pain

Describe the pain and its location. Calf? Thighs? Buttocks? When does the pain occur?

Leg pain that occurs while walking and that is relieved within 10 minutes or less with rest is termed *intermittent claudication.* This occurs when the artery is approximately 50% occluded. Calf claudication indicates femoral or popliteal artery involvement, while pain in the buttocks and thighs indicates iliac artery involvement. Arterial insufficiency produces pain that worsens with activity, especially prolonged walking. As the insufficiency becomes worse, the patient reports pain when walking that is not relieved after rest. This is termed *rest pain.*[7]

What makes the leg pain worse? What relieves it?

Leg pain caused by arterial insufficiency is worse when legs are elevated and improves when they are in a dependent position. By contrast, pain caused by venous insufficiency intensifies with prolonged standing or sitting in one position. Pain is worse when legs are in a dependent position and is relieved when they are elevated. Discomfort increases throughout the day, being worse at the end of the day.[7]

Have you noticed any changes in the skin of your legs such as coldness, pallor, hair loss, sores, redness or warmth over the veins, or visible veins?

These signs may indicate arterial insufficiency of the legs.

HEALTH PROMOTION FOR EVIDENCED-BASED PRACTICE

Cardiovascular Disease

Cardiovascular disease is the leading cause of death and a major cause of disability in the United States, contributing to increases in health care costs. These diseases include coronary artery disease and myocardial infarction, stroke, hypertension, hyperlipidemia, and peripheral vascular diseases.

Recommendations to Reduce Risk (Primary Prevention)

Smoking cessation (see Health Promotion: Tobacco Use in Chapter 11)

Nutrition: Plant-based or Mediterranean-like diet high in vegetables, fruits, nuts, whole grains, lean vegetable or animal protein (preferably fish) and vegetable fiber

Blood lipid management: Total cholesterol less than 190 mg/dL

Weight: Achieve and maintain a desirable body weight (body mass index [BMI] between 18.5 and 24.9)

Physical activity: At least 150 min a week of at least moderate-intensity physical activity such as brisk walking

Screening Recommendations (Secondary Prevention)
U.S. Preventive Services Task Force
Blood Pressure Screening

Screening for high blood pressure is recommended for all adults age 18 and older. Annual screening is recommended for adults aged 40 and older and for those who are at increased risk for high blood pressure. Persons at increased risk include those who have elevated blood pressure (120 to 129/>80 mm Hg), those who are overweight or obese, and African Americans. Adults aged 18–39 years with normal blood pressure (<120/<80 mm Hg) who do not have other risk factors should be rescreened every 3–5 years.

Lipid-level Screening

Screening for lipid disorders is strongly recommended for men age 35 and older and women age 45 and older.

Screening for lipid disorders is recommended for younger adults (men ages 20–35 years and women ages 20–45 years) if they have other risk factors for heart disease (family history of cardiovascular disease before age 50 in male relatives or age 60 in female relatives, family history of hyperlipidemia, diabetes mellitus, and multiple other risk factors, including tobacco use, hypertension).

Arnett DK, Blumenthal RS, Albert MA, et al: 2019 ACC/AHA Guidelines on the Primary Prevention of Cardiovascular Disease: A Report of the American College of Cardiology/American Heart Association Task Force on Clinical Practice Guidelines. *J Am Coll Cardiol* March 17, 2019. Retrieved from https://www.acc.org/latest-in-cardiology/ten-points-to-remember/2019/03/07/16/00/2019-acc-aha-guideline-on-primary-prevention-gl-prevention; U.S. Preventive Services Task Force: Final recommendation statement: High blood pressure in Adults, Screening. Retrieved from https://www.uspreventiveservicestaskforce.org/Page/Document/RecommendationStatementFinal/high-blood-pressure-in-adults-screening. Current as of October, 2015; Whelton PK, Carey RM, Aronow WS, et al: ACC/AHA/AAPA/ABC/ACPM/AGS/APhA/ASH/ASPC/NMA/PCNA Guideline for the Prevention, Detection, Evaluation, and Management of High Blood Pressure in Adults: A Report of the American College of Cardiology/American Heart Association Task Force on Clinical Practice Guidelines. *J Am Coll Cardiol* 2018;71:e127–e248; and Retrieved from www.uspreventiveservicestaskforce.org/Page/Document/UpdateSummaryFinal/lipid-disorders-in-adults-cholesterol-dyslipidemia-screening. Current as of July, 2015.

EXAMINATION

Routine Techniques

General Appearance
- INSPECT for general appearance, skin color, and breathing effort.

Heart
- INSPECT the anterior chest wall.
- PALPATE the apical pulse.
- AUSCULTATE the apical pulse.
- AUSCULTATE the heart.
- CALCULATE the pulse deficit.
- INTERPRET the electrocardiogram.

Peripheral Vascular System
- PALPATE temporal and carotid pulses.
- INSPECT the jugular veins.
- MEASURE the blood pressure.
- INSPECT the upper extremities
- PALPATE the upper extremities.
- PALPATE upper-extremity pulses.
- INSPECT the lower extremities.
- PALPATE the lower extremities.
- PALPATE lower-extremity pulses.

Techniques for Special Circumstances

Peripheral Vascular System
- AUSCULTATE the temporal and carotid arteries.
- PALPATE the epitrochlear lymph nodes.
- PALPATE inguinal lymph nodes.
- MEASURE leg circumferences.
- CALCULATE the ankle-brachial indexes.

Techniques Performed by an APRN
- PALPATE the precordium.
- ESTIMATE jugular vein pressure.
- ASSESS for varicose veins.

Equipment needed

- Penlight • Watch or clock with second hand • Stethoscope • Sphygmomanometer • Tape measure • Marker • Doppler • Ultrasonic gel

APRN, Advanced Practice Registered Nurse.

PROCEDURES WITH EXPECTED FINDINGS

ROUTINE TECHNIQUES: GENERAL APPEARANCE

PERFORM hand hygiene.

INSPECT the patient for general appearance, skin color, and breathing effort.

Observe the patient. He or she should appear at ease and relaxed with skin color appropriate for race and regular, unlabored respirations.

ROUTINE TECHNIQUES: HEART

INSPECT the anterior chest wall for contour and retractions.

Procedure: Provide modesty and privacy while inspecting the female patient's unclothed chest. Use a penlight to create tangential light to inspect the patient's chest at eye level. Box 12.1 has abbreviations of topographic landmarks. Box 12.2 describes a technique for locating intercostal spaces for inspecting, palpating, and auscultating the heart. Look for a slight retraction of the apical pulse at the fourth or fifth intercostal space (ICS), medial to the left midclavicular line (LMCL).
Findings: The chest should be rounded. The apical pulse is located at 5th ICS LMCL.

ABNORMAL FINDINGS

Dyspnea, cyanosis, pallor, and use of accessory muscles to breathe may require further evaluation.

Marked retraction of apical space may indicate pericardial disease or right ventricular hypertrophy.

BOX 12.1 ABBREVIATIONS FOR TOPOGRAPHIC LANDMARKS

ICS	Intercostal space	LSB	Left sternal border
RICS	Right intercostal space	MCL	Midclavicular line
LICS	Left intercostal space	RMCL	Right midclavicular line
SB	Sternal border	LMCL	Left midclavicular line
RSB	Right sternal border		

BOX 12.2 TECHNIQUE FOR LOCATING INTERCOSTAL SPACES FOR AUSCULTATION OF THE HEART

- A systematic approach is required for this assessment. Some nurses begin at the apex and proceed upward toward the base of the heart, whereas others begin at the base and proceed downward toward the apex. The sequence is irrelevant as long as the assessment is systematic. Listen first with the diaphragm to hear high-pitched sounds and then with the bell to hear low-pitched sounds.
- When auscultating from base to apex, begin by locating the right sternal border (RSB) by palpating the right sternoclavicular joint (where the right clavicle joins the sternum).
- Next, palpate the first rib and then move down to palpate the space between the first and second ribs: this is the first right intercostal space (1st RICS).
- Continue palpating downward to the space between the second and third ribs. This is the second ICS at the right sternal border (RSB), the auscultatory site for the aortic

valve area, shown as 2nd RICS below. This is not the anatomic site of the aortic valve, but the site on the chest wall where sounds produced by the valve are heard best.
- Move your stethoscope to the left side of the sternum at the second ICS. This is the area for auscultating the pulmonic valve, shown as 2nd LICS below.
- Remain at the left sternal border (LSB), move the stethoscope down to the third ICS, which is called Erb's point, an area to which pulmonic or aortic sounds frequently radiate, shown as 3rd LICS below.
- The fourth ICS, the LSB is over the tricuspid valve area, shown as 4th LICS below.
- At the fifth ICS, move the stethoscope laterally to the left midclavicular line (LMCL), where the mitral valve area is located, shown 5th LMCL below.

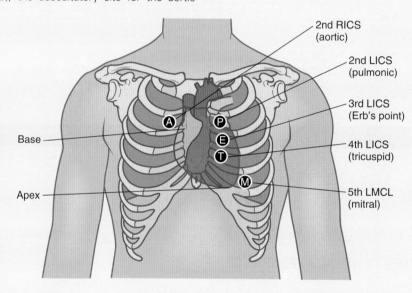

PROCEDURES WITH EXPECTED FINDINGS

PALPATE the apical pulse for location.

Procedure: Use fingertips to palpate over the apex of the heart at the fifth intercostal space, left midclavicular line (5th ICS, LMCL) shown in Fig. 12.10. This is the point of maximal impulse (PMI) that corresponds to the left ventricular apex. If the PMI cannot be palpated, place the patient in lying position, turned to the left side. This position places the left ventricle closer to the chest wall. **Findings:** The apical pulse or PMI is expected in the 5th ICS, LMCL.

AUSCULTATE the apical pulse for rate and rhythm.

Procedure:
- Clean the bell and diaphragm of your stethoscope.
- Place the diaphragm of the stethoscope on the anterior chest and listen carefully for the two distinct sounds of the heartbeat.
- Count the number of heartbeats heard for 1 min, and note the rhythm (the spacing between heartbeats).

Findings: The heart rate should be between 60 and 100 beats/min. Spacing between each heartbeat should be equal, indicating a regular rhythm.

ABNORMAL FINDINGS

If the patient has left ventricular hypertrophy, the myocardium is enlarged, which may move the PMI laterally. Patients who have COPD have overinflated lungs, which displaces the PMI downward and to the right.[8]

Rates greater than 100 or less than 60 beats/min are abnormal. Irregular rhythm, sporadic, or extra beats, or occasional slight pauses between heartbeats are considered abnormal and may require further evaluation.

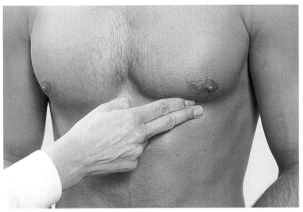

FIG. 12.10 Palpating apical pulse at fourth or fifth intercostal space, left midclavicular line.

PROCEDURES WITH EXPECTED FINDINGS	ABNORMAL FINDINGS

AUSCULTATE the heart for sounds, pitch, and splitting.

Heart sounds are auscultated using a stethoscope and requires a quiet room, knowing where to place the stethoscope on the chest and knowing which sounds to identify. Heart sounds are generated by the closing of heart valves and are best heard where blood flows away from the valve (instead of directly over the valve area) (Fig. 12.11). Auscultation occurs in five areas on the anterior chest, corresponding to the projection of sound for each heart valve (see Box 12.2).

Procedure:

- Place the patient in an upright sitting position, leaning slightly forward (which brings the heart closer to the chest wall).
- Start by using the diaphragm of the stethoscope, which is best for hearing high-pitched sounds. Using firm pressure, place the diaphragm on the chest to listen for heart sounds over the aortic valve area located at the 2nd ICS, RSB (see Box 12.1 for abbreviations) (Fig. 12.12A). Next, move the stethoscope across the sternum to the pulmonic valve area (2nd ICS, LSB) (Fig. 12.12B), then Erb's point (3rd ICS, LSB) Fig. 12.12C), then the tricuspid valve area (4th ICS, LSB) (Fig. 12.12D), and finally the mitral valve area/apical pulse (5th ICS, LMCL) (Fig. 12.12E).
- Box 12.3 shows two different mnemonics to help you remember which valve you are hearing. Repeat the auscultation of the five areas using the bell of the stethoscope, which is best for hearing low-pitched sounds. As a reminder, light pressure is applied when using the bell of the stethoscope.
- When heart sounds are difficult to hear, ask the patient to hold the breath in expiration to eliminate lung sounds. Closing your eyes to concentrate on each sound (i.e., selective listening) may also help.

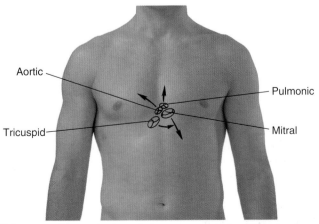

FIG. 12.11 Transmission of closure sounds from heart valves.

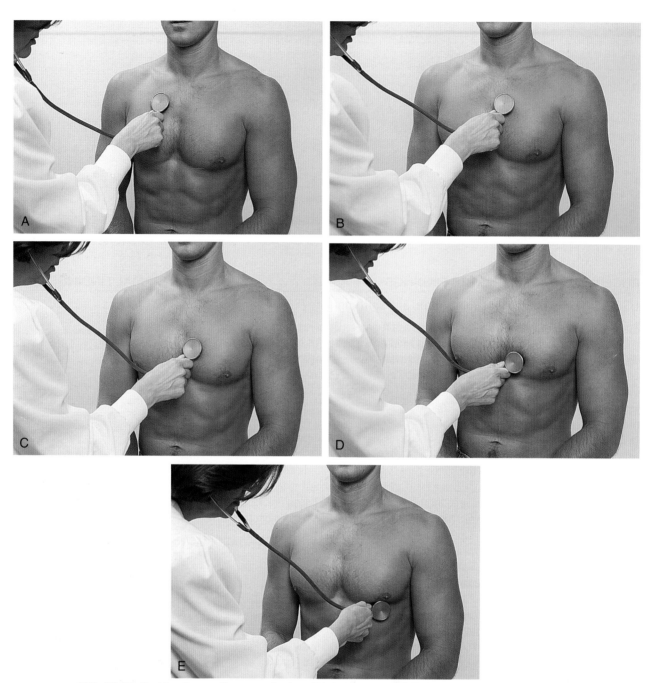

FIG. 12.12 Position for cardiac auscultation. (A) Aortic area. (B) Pulmonic area. (C) Erb's point. (D) Tricuspid area. (E) Mitral area.

BOX 12.3 **AUSCULTATING HEART VALVES**

Use the mnemonics below to help you remember which valve you are listening to (aortic, pulmonic, tricuspid, or mitral),

APARTMENT M OR APT M:	APE TO MAN:
Aortic	**A**ortic
Pulmonic	**P**ulmonic
	Erb's point
Tricuspid	**T**ricuspid
Mitral	**M**itral

PROCEDURES WITH EXPECTED FINDINGS

Findings. Two distinct heart sounds should be heard. The first heart sound is S_1 (or "*lubb*") and is made by the simultaneous closing of the mitral and tricuspid valves. S_1 indicates the beginning of systole. The second heart sound is S_2 (or "*dubb*") and is made by the simultaneous closing of the aortic and pulmonic valves and indicates the beginning of diastole. S_1 is louder at the apex, and S_2 is louder at the base. Heart sounds are typically low-pitched sounds and low in intensity. S_1 heart sounds tend to be slightly higher in pitch compared to S_2 heart sounds.

ABNORMAL FINDINGS

Abnormal heart sounds may include splitting, S_3 and S_4 sounds, rubs, or murmurs.

Splitting occurs when the mitral and tricuspid valves do not close at the same time (referred to as an S_1 split) or when the pulmonic and aortic values do not close at the same time (referred to as an S_2 split), therefore creating two sounds instead of one.

S_3 and S_4 heart sounds are described in Table 12.2. Abnormal heart sounds are shown in the bottom of Fig. 12.4. These sounds may indicate cardiac pathology such as heart failure, cardiomyopathy, valvular regurgitation, or stenosis.

Pericardial friction rub is a low-pitched coarse rubbing or grating sound caused by fluid accumulation in the pericardial sac. (See Table 12.2)

Murmurs are usually a result of turbulent blood flow, which produces prolonged extra sounds heard during systole or diastole. Murmurs are described by timing in the cardiac cycle, pitch, quality, intensity, and location in Table 12.3. Murmurs caused by valvular defects are presented in Table 12.4.

TABLE 12.2 ABNORMAL HEART SOUNDS

Friction rubs are extracardiac sounds of short duration that sound like scratching on sandpaper. Rubs may result from irritation of the pleura or pericardium. The source (lung or heart) can be determined by having the patient hold his or her breath. If the sound is not heard, it is a pleura rub. If the sound persists, it is a pericardial, usually present in both diastole and systole and best heard over the 3rd LICS.[9]

Abnormal heart sounds are described by where they occur in the cardiac cycle. The normal sequence of events in the cardiac cycle can be diagrammed as follows:

$S_1 \rightarrow$ systole $\rightarrow S_2 \rightarrow$ diastole $\rightarrow S_1$ etc.

To determine if an abnormal sound occurs in systole or diastole, determine if the sound occurs after S_1 or after S_2.

- During diastole, when 80% of the blood in the atria rapidly fills the ventricles, a third heart sound may be heard (S_3). It is often heard at the apex. An S_3 occurs just after the S_2 and lasts approximately the same time as it takes to say "me too." The "me" is the S_2, and the "too" is the S_3. An S_3 is normal in children and young adults; however, when an S_3 is heard in adults over 30 years of age, it signifies fluid volume overload to the ventricle that may be caused by heart failure or mitral or tricuspid regurgitation.[8]

- At the end of diastole, when atrial contraction completes the filling of the ventricle, a fourth heart sound may be heard (S_4). An S_4 occurs just before the S_1 and lasts approximately the same time as it takes to say "middle." The "mi" is the S_4, and the "ddle" is the S_1. An S_4 is normal in children and young adults; however, when an S_4 is heard in adults over 30 years of age, it signifies a noncompliant or "stiff" ventricle.

One way to remember the cadence of the S_3 and S_4 heart sounds is to use the words "Kentucky" and "Tennessee."

Ken-tuck-y	Ken-tuck-y	Ken-tuck-y
S_1 S_2 S_3	S_1 S_2 S_3	S_1 S_2 S_3
Ten-ness-ee	Ten-ness-ee	Ten-ness-ee
S_4 S_1 S_2	S_4 S_1 S_2	S_4 S_1 S_2

TABLE 12.3 LISTENING TO MURMURS

When you identify a heart murmur, consider the following variables for documentation:

Timing and duration	At what part of the cycle is the murmur heard? Is it associated with S_1 or S_2, or is it continuous?
Pitch	Is it a low or high pitch? Low pitches are best heard with the bell of the stethoscope.
Quality	Quality refers to the type of sound, including a harsh sound; a raspy, machine-like sound; or a vibratory, musical, or blowing sound.
Intensity	Murmur intensity refers to how loud the murmur is: • Grade I is barely audible in a quiet room. • Grade II is quiet but clearly audible. • Grade III is moderately loud. • Grade IV is loud and associated with a thrill. • Grade V is very loud, and a thrill is easily palpable. • Grade VI is very loud, and a thrill is palpable and visible.
Location	Where is the sound heard loudest? Most often it is over one of the five anatomic landmarks used to auscultate heart sounds.
Example of documentation	S_1, grade II, low-pitch murmur auscultated at 5th ICS, MCL. No thrill palpable.

ICS, Intercostal space; *MCL,* midclavicular line.

TABLE 12.4 MURMURS CAUSED BY VALVULAR DEFECTS

TYPE		DETECTION	QUALITY/PITCH
Systolic Ejection Murmur			
Aortic valve stenosis		Use the bell over aortic valve area; ejection sound at second right intercostal border Radiates to neck, down left sternal border	Medium pitch, coarse, with crescendo-decrescendo pattern Pitch low
Pulmonic valve stenosis		Use the bell over pulmonic valve; radiates left to neck; thrill at second and third left intercostal spaces	Same as for aortic valve stenosis Pitch medium
Diastolic Regurgitant Murmur			
Aortic valve regurgitation		Use the diaphragm, patient sitting and leaning forward; second right intercostal space radiates to left sternal border	Blowing in early diastole Pitch high

TABLE 12.4 MURMURS CAUSED BY VALVULAR DEFECTS—cont'd

TYPE		DETECTION	QUALITY/PITCH
Pulmonic valve regurgitation		Use the diaphragm, patient sitting or leaning forward; third and fourth left intercostal spaces	Blowing Pitch high or low
Diastolic Murmur	Systole Diastole		
Mitral valve stenosis		Use the bell at apex with patient on the left side	Low rumble more intense in early and late diastole Pitch low
Tricuspid valve stenosis		Use the bell over tricuspid area	Similar to mitral valve stenosis but louder on inspiration Pitch low
Holosystolic Murmur	Systole Diastole		
Mitral valve regurgitation		Use the diaphragm at apex, radiates to left axilla or base	Harsh blowing quality Pitch high
Tricuspid valve regurgitation		Use the diaphragm at fifth intercostal space, left lower sternal border	Blowing Pitch high

Murmurs are created by turbulent blood flow. *Stenosis* is a term that describes a heart valve that does not open completely. *Regurgitation* describes a valve that does not close completely. A *holosystolic* murmur occupies all of systole.

PROCEDURES WITH EXPECTED FINDINGS

CALCULATE the pulse deficit.

Procedure: The pulse deficit is the difference in the apical rate and the peripheral pulse rates. It is determined by auscultating the apical pulse and palpating the radial pulse rates simultaneously.

Findings: The apical and radial pulse rates should be equal.

ABNORMAL FINDINGS

The apical rate may be faster than the radial rate when the patient has a cardiac dysrhythmia, commonly atrial fibrillation.

PROCEDURES WITH EXPECTED FINDINGS

INTERPRET the EKG of the conduction of the heart.

The electrical conduction of the heart can be seen on an EKG to assess rate and rhythm. When spoken, the abbreviation for this assessment tool is called an EKG rather than an ECG to avoid errors because the sound of ECG is similar to that of EEG (electroencephalogram). Fig. 12.13A shows the EKG reflections of one cardiac cycle. The P wave represents the atrial contraction or depolarization. The QRS complex represents the ventricular contraction or depolarization. The atrial repolarization occurs at the same time but is overshadowed by the ventricular contraction. The T wave represents the repolarization of the ventricle. Fig. 12.13B shows the time intervals of each part of the cardiac cycle. Fig. 12.13C shows which part of the heart is represented by the wave or complex.

ABNORMAL FINDINGS

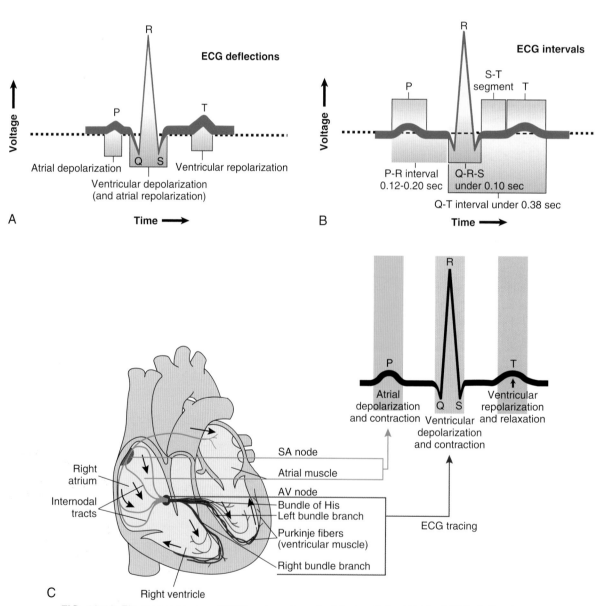

FIG. 12.13 Electrocardiogram (ECG) and cardiac electrical activity. (A) Ideal EKG deflections represent depolarization and repolarization of cardiac muscle tissue. (B) Principal EKG interval among *P*, *QRS*, and *T* waves. Notice that the *P-R* interval is measured from the start of the P wave to the end of the Q wave. (C) Schematic representation of EKG and its relationship to the cardiac electrical activity. *AV*, Atrioventricular; *LA*, left atrium; *LBB*, left bundle branch; *LV*, left ventricle; *RA*, right atrium; *RBB*, right bundle branch; *RV*, right ventricular; *SA*, sinoatrial. (A and B, From Patton and Thibodeau, 2010. C, From Gould and Dyer, 2011.)

PROCEDURES WITH EXPECTED FINDINGS	ABNORMAL FINDINGS

ROUTINE TECHNIQUES: PERIPHERAL VASCULAR SYSTEM

PALPATE temporal and carotid pulses for amplitude.

Procedure: For the temporal pulse, palpate over the temporal bone on each side of the head lateral to each eyebrow to assess amplitude and pain (Figs. 12.14 and 12.15). For the carotid pulse, palpate along the medial edge of the sternocleidomastoid muscle in the lower third of the neck to assess amplitude. Palpate one carotid pulse at a time to avoid reducing blood flow to the brain (Figs. 12.16 and 12.17).

Findings: Pulses have regular rhythm, smooth contour with 2+ amplitude. Expected findings for pulses are described in the left column of Box 12.4.

Abnormalities for the temporal arteries may include pain and edema. For the carotid arteries notice irregular rhythm and weak or bounding upstroke. See right column of Box 12.4 for other abnormal findings.

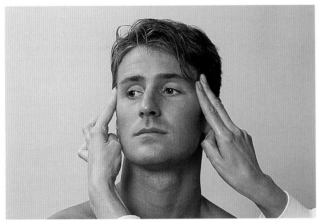

FIG. 12.14 Palpating temporal pulses lateral to each eyebrow.

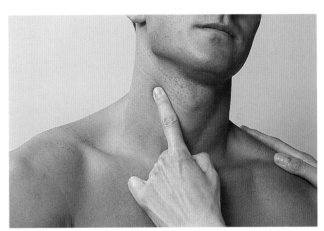

FIG. 12.16 Palpating carotid pulse in lower third of the neck.

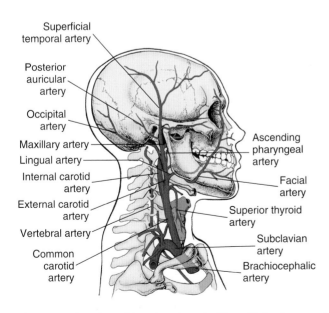

FIG. 12.15 Arteries of head and neck. (From Thibodeau and Patton, 1999.)

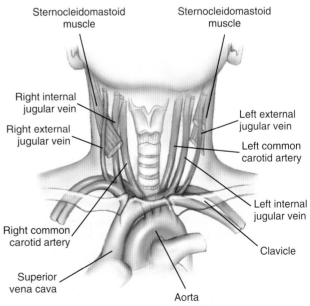

FIG. 12.17 Right and left common carotid arteries that are palpated. (From Barkauskas et al., 2002.)

BOX 12.4 PALPATING PULSES

Palpate arteries using the finger pads of the first two fingers and applying light pressure. If you press too hard, you obscure the pulse. Notice the rate, rhythm, amplitude, and contour of each pulse. Comparing pulses on each side of the body is customary. When you are unable to palpate a pulse, use a Doppler to amplify the sounds of the pulse (see Fig. 3.22).

EXPECTED FINDINGS	ABNORMAL FINDINGS
Rate 60–100 beats/min (athletes may be as low as 50 beats/min). Pulse rates in women tend to be 5–10 beats/min faster than men.	Rates above 100 beats/min (tachycardia) or below 60 beats/min (bradycardia) are typically abnormal, although recent exertion, smoking, or anxiety elevate the rate.
Rhythm Regular (i.e., equal spacing between beats).	Irregular rhythms without any pattern should be documented. Coupled beats (two beats that occur close together) are abnormal also. When you palpate an irregular pulse rhythm, notice whether there is a pattern to the irregularity. For example, pulses of patients who have premature ventricular contractions may have a pattern to the irregularity such as an extra beat every third heartbeat. This is documented as a *regular irregularity*. By contrast, pulses of patients who have atrial fibrillation may not have any pattern to the irregularity. This is documented as an *irregular irregularity*.
Amplitude (Force) Easily palpable, smooth upstroke. Compare the strength of upper-extremity with lower-extremity pulses and the left with the right. Rating 2+ normal.	Notice any exaggerated or bounding upstroke or, conversely, pulses that are weak, small, or thready or when the peak is prolonged. Upstrokes should not vary (seen in pulsus alternans). The force of the beat should not be reduced during inspiration (paradoxical pulse). Ratings 0+ Absent 1+ Diminished, barely palpable 3+ Full volume 4+ Full volume, bounding hyperkinetic
Contour (Outline or shape of the pulse that is felt) Compare the outline of upper-extremity with lower-extremity pulses and the left with the right. Smooth and rounded, a series of unvaried, symmetric pulse strokes	Varied strokes or asymmetry between left and right extremities suggests impaired circulation.

PROCEDURES WITH EXPECTED FINDINGS

INSPECT the jugular veins for pulsations.

The external jugular veins reflect the right atrial pressure.

Procedure: With the patient in supine position, elevate the head of the bed until venous pulsation in the external jugular vein is seen above the clavicle, close to the insertion of the sternocleidomastoid muscles. The angle may be 30 to 45 degrees or as high as 90 degrees if venous pressure is elevated. Elevate the patient's chin slightly and tilt the head away from the side being examined. Use a penlight to create tangential light across the jugular veins and observe for pulsations (Fig. 12.18). Examine the other side.
Findings: Pulsations of the veins are visible, but not the veins themselves.

ABNORMAL FINDINGS

Notice any fluttering or oscillating of the pulsations. Notice irregular rhythms or unusually prominent waves (Fig. 12.19). These may indicate right-sided heart failure.

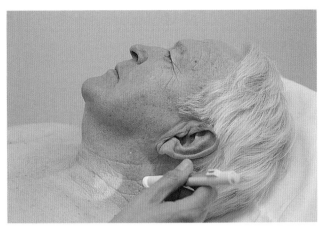

FIG. 12.18 Inspection of jugular venous pulsations. (From Monahan et al., 2007.)

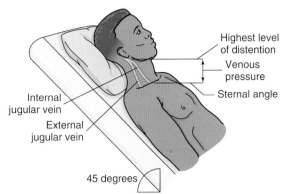

FIG. 12.19 Neck vein distention. (From Swartz, 2010.)

PROCEDURES WITH EXPECTED FINDINGS

MEASURE the blood pressure.

(See Chapter 4 for procedure.) The blood pressure is frequently taken in both arms during an initial visit to compare the readings. Blood pressure varies with gender, body weight, and time of day; but the upper limits for adults are less than 120 mm Hg systolic, less than 80 mm Hg diastolic. The *pulse pressure* is the difference between systolic and diastolic pressures and is normally between 30 and 40 mm Hg. The blood pressure normally varies between 5 to 10 mm Hg between arms. Fig. 12.20 shows assessment of blood pressure and Box 12.5 shows normal blood pressure values.

If the patient offers a history of dizziness or is taking antihypertensive medications, measure the blood pressure and heart rate while he or she is supine, sitting, and standing. The blood pressure is usually lower in the supine position than sitting. The blood pressure taken when standing may be lower than it is when sitting by 10 to 15 mm Hg systolic and 5 mm Hg diastolic.

ABNORMAL FINDINGS

Notice elevated systolic or diastolic pressures (hypertension) and lowered systolic or diastolic pressures (hypotension). Also notice significant discrepancies in measurements between the two arms. See Box 12.5 for values for elevated blood pressure, stage 1 hypertension, and stage 2 hypertension.

A decrease in systolic blood pressure of at least 20 mm Hg and/or diastolic blood pressure of at least 10 mm Hg within 3 min of standing indicates orthostatic (postural) hypotension. This may be caused by a fluid volume deficit, several classes of drugs (e.g., antihypertensives), or prolonged bed rest.[10]

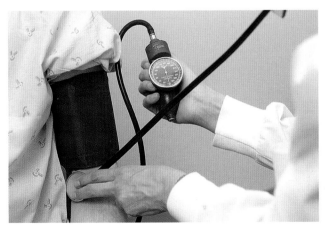

FIG. 12.20 Assessing blood pressure.

BOX 12.5 CLASSIFICATION OF BLOOD PRESSURE FOR ADULTS AGE 18 AND OLDER

CATEGORY*	SYSTOLIC (MM HG)		DIASTOLIC (MM HG)
Normal	<120	And	<80
Elevated	120–129	And	< 80
Stage 1 hypertension	130–139	Or	80–89
Stage 2 hypertension	140 or higher	Or	90 or higher
Hypertensive crisis	>180	And/or	>120

*Whelton PK, Carey RM, Aronow WS, et al: ACC/AHA/AAPA/ABC/ACPM/AGS/APhA/ASH/ASPC/NMA/PCNA Guideline for the Prevention, Detection, Evaluation, and Management of High Blood Pressure in Adults: A Report of the American College of Cardiology/American Heart Association Task Force on Clinical Practice Guidelines. *J Am Coll Cardiol* 2018;71:e127–e248.

PROCEDURES WITH EXPECTED FINDINGS

INSPECT the upper extremities for symmetry, skin integrity, and color, and nail beds for color and angle

Procedure: Compare one side with the other.

Findings: The arms should appear symmetric, with skin intact and color consistent with race. Nail beds should be consistent with patient's race, with an angle of 160 degrees at the nail bed (see Fig. 9.10A).

PALPATE the upper extremities for temperature, turgor, and capillary refill.

Procedure: Use the back of your hand to assess skin temperature (Fig. 12.21). Pinch an area of the skin between your finger and thumb and release the skin to assess turgor (see Fig. 9.4). Assess capillary refill by gently squeezing pads of fingers or nails until they blanch. Release pressure and observe capillary refill (i.e., how many seconds it takes for the original color to appear) (Fig. 12.22).

Findings: The skin should feel warm bilaterally. Skin should immediately fall back into place indicating elastic turgor. Capillary refill should be 2 seconds or less.

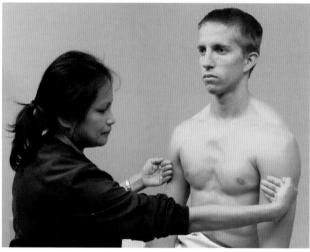

FIG. 12.21 Assess for skin temperature comparing sides using the back of the hand.

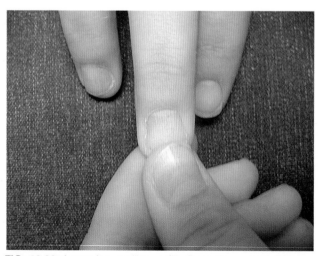

FIG. 12.22 Assessing capillary refill. (From Cummings, Stanley-Green, and Higgs, 2009.)

ABNORMAL FINDINGS

When one arm appears larger, use a tape measure to determine the circumference of each arm. Lymphedema may be the cause of the enlargement. Thickening skin, skin tears, and ulceration are abnormal findings. Marked pallor or mottling when the extremity is elevated or any ulcerated fingertips may require further evaluation.

Arterial insufficiency may cause cold extremities in a warm environment and is abnormal. When edema is found, notice if it is unilateral or bilateral; the consistency is soft, firm, or hard; or whether there is pain. When one arm is larger in circumference than the other, it may be caused by lymphedema. When skin does not immediately fall back in place, the finding is called *tenting* and indicates reduced fluid in the interstitial space from fluid volume deficit (see Fig. 9.5). A capillary refill greater than 2 seconds indicates poor perfusion. Clubbing of fingers (angle of nails greater than 160 degrees) indicates chronic hypoxia (Fig. 12.23 and see Fig. 9.10B and C).

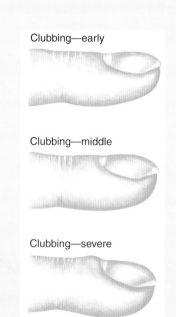

Clubbing—early

Clubbing—middle

Clubbing—severe

FIG. 12.23 Clubbing of fingers. (From Canobbio, 1990.)

PROCEDURES WITH EXPECTED FINDINGS

PALPATE brachial and radial pulses for rate, rhythm, amplitude, and contour. When indicated, palpate ulnar pulses.

Procedure: Recall from Chapter 4 that pulses are palpated with the pads of the index and second fingers using pressure that is firm but not so hard as to occlude the pulsations. For the brachial pulse palpate in the groove between the biceps and triceps muscle just medial to the biceps tendon at the antecubital fossa (in the bend of the elbow) (Figs. 12.24 and 12.26). For the radial pulses palpate at the radial or thumb sides of the forearm at the wrist. Often both radial pulses are palpated at the same time to assess for equality (Fig. 12.25; see Fig. 12.26).

When palpating the radial artery is difficult or it has been injured, palpate the ulnar pulses located on the medial side of the forearm (Fig. 12.27).

Findings: A rate between 60 and 100 beats/min, regular rhythm, and smooth contour with 2+ amplitude are expected. See the left column of Box 12.4.

ABNORMAL FINDINGS

Abnormalities include an irregular rhythm and weak or bounding upstroke. See the right column of Box 12.4 for abnormal findings. Patients who take certain medications such as beta-adrenergic antagonists or digoxin may have slow pulse rates because of the medication.

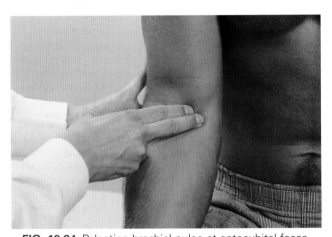

FIG. 12.24 Palpating brachial pulse at antecubital fossa.

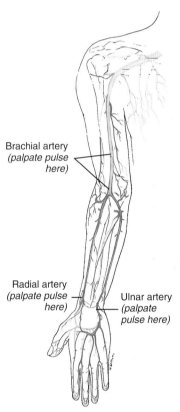

FIG. 12.26 Arteries of upper extremity that are palpated. (Modified from Francis and Martin, 1975.)

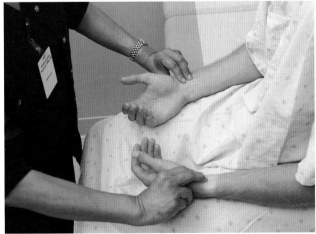

FIG. 12.25 Palpating radial pulse on thumb side of forearm at the wrist. Often both radial pulses are palpated at the same time to assess for equality.

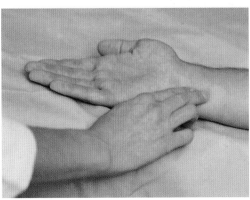

FIG. 12.27 Palpating ulnar pulse on medial side of forearm. (From Potter et al., 2013.)

PROCEDURES WITH EXPECTED FINDINGS

INSPECT the lower extremities for symmetry, skin integrity, color, hair distribution, and superficial veins.

Procedure: Follow the same procedures performed on the upper extremities for assessment of the lower extremities. Observe the hair distribution. Some women shave leg hair, while others do not. With the patient's legs dependent, observe for superficial veins that appear dilated.

Findings: The legs should appear symmetric. The skin should be intact, with color appropriate for race. Women who do not shave their legs and men should have hair evenly distributed. Superficial veins should not be visible.

PALPATE the lower extremities for temperature, skin turgor, capillary refill, pain, numbness, edema, and angle of nail beds.

Procedure: Follow the same procedures performed on the upper extremities for assessment of the lower extremities.

Findings: The skin should feel warm. Skin turgor is elastic. Capillary refill should be 2 s or less. Sensation of the legs should be present without pain or numbness. No edema should be found. Nails should be consistent with patient's race, with an angle of 160 degrees at the nail bed.

ABNORMAL FINDINGS

Thickening skin, skin tears, and ulceration are abnormal findings. Marked pallor or mottling when the extremity is elevated or any ulcerated toes may require further evaluation. Arterial insufficiency may cause a decrease in, or lack of, hair peripherally or skin that appears thin, shiny, and taut. Varicose veins appear as dilated, often tortuous veins when legs are in a dependent position.

Abnormalities of temperature, turgor, capillary refill, and nail color and angle are similar to those described for the upper extremities. When the indentation of the thumb or finger remains in the skin, it is termed *pitting edema* and is an indication of excess fluid in the interstitial space (Fig. 12.28). Refer to Table 12.5 for an interpretation of edema. Pitting edema is seen in venous thromboembolism (VTE) and venous insufficiency.[11] Abnormalities include pain on palpation or the sensation of "stocking anesthesia," wherein legs feel numb in a pattern resembling stockings.

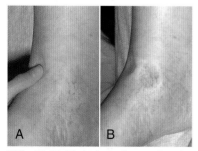

FIG. 12.28 Technique for testing for pitting edema. (A) The nurse presses into the ankle area. (B) An indentation remains after the fingers are lifted when pitting edema is present. (From Forbes and Jackson, 2003.)

TABLE 12.5 PITTING EDEMA SCALE

SCALE	DESCRIPTION	DEPTH OF EDEMA
1+	Barely perceptible pit	2 mm ($3/32$ in)
2+	Deeper pit, rebounds in a few seconds	4 mm ($5/32$ in)
3+	Deep pit, rebounds in 10–20 seconds	6 mm (¼ in)
4+	Deeper pit, rebounds in >30 seconds	8 mm ($5/32$ in)

Description column data from Kirton C: Assessing edema, *Nursing 96* 26(7):54, 1996.
Illustration from Seidel et al: *Mosby's guide to physical examination*, ed 7, St Louis, 2011, Mosby.

PROCEDURES WITH EXPECTED FINDINGS

PALPATE femoral, popliteal, posterior tibial, and dorsalis pedis pulses for amplitude bilaterally.

Procedure:

- To locate the *femoral pulses*, palpate below the inguinal ligament, midway between the symphysis pubis and anterior superior iliac crest, and move your fingers inward toward the pubic hair. You can locate the anatomy using the mnemonic NAVEL: *N,* nerve; *A,* artery; *V,* vein; *E,* empty space; *L,* lymph. Firm compression may be required for obese patients (Fig. 12.29; see Fig. 12.33).
- For the *popliteal pulses,* palpate the popliteal artery behind the knee in the popliteal fossa (Fig. 12.30; see Fig. 12.33). This pulse may be difficult to find. Having the patient in the prone position and flexing the leg slightly may help to locate it.
- For the *posterior tibial pulses,* palpate on the inner aspect of the ankle below and slightly behind the medial malleolus (ankle bone) (Fig. 12.31; see Fig. 12.33).
- For the *dorsalis pedis pulse,* palpate lightly over the dorsum of the foot between the extension tendons of the first and second toes (Fig. 12.32; see Fig. 12.33). Often both dorsalis pedis pulses are palpated at the same time to assess for equality.

Findings: Pulses have regular rhythm, smooth contour with 2+ amplitude. See left column of Box 12.4.

ABNORMAL FINDINGS

Abnormalities include irregular rhythm and weak or bounding upstroke. See right column of Box 12.4. Impaired peripheral pulses may indicate arterial insufficiency.

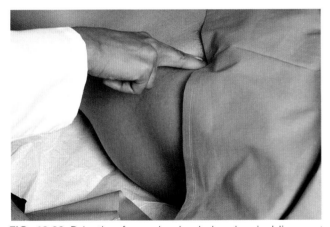

FIG. 12.29 Palpating femoral pulse below inguinal ligament between symphysis pubis and anterior-superior Iliac crest. (From Canobbio, 1990.)

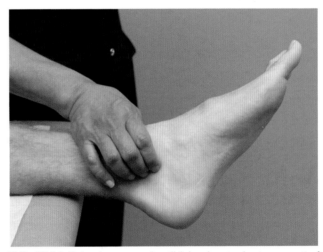

FIG. 12.31 Palpating posterior tibial pulse on inner aspect of the ankle.

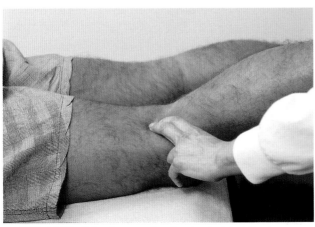

FIG. 12.30 Palpating popliteal pulse behind the knee.

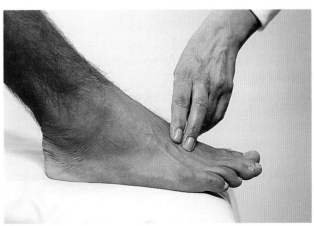

FIG. 12.32 Palpating dorsalis pedis pulse on top of foot between first and second toes.

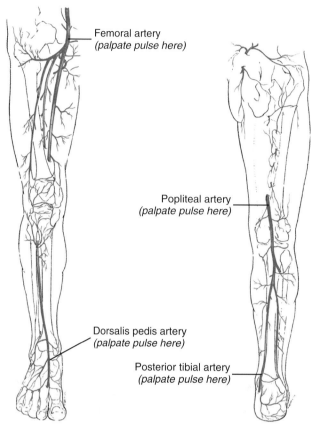

Femoral artery
(palpate pulse here)

Popliteal artery
(palpate pulse here)

Dorsalis pedis artery
(palpate pulse here)

Posterior tibial artery
(palpate pulse here)

FIG. 12.33 Arteries of leg that are palpated. (From Francis and Martin, 1975.)

PROCEDURES WITH EXPECTED FINDINGS

SPECIAL CIRCUMSTANCES: PERIPHERAL VASCULAR SYSTEM

AUSCULTATE the temporal and carotid arteries for bruits.

Perform when the patient has a history of atherosclerosis or reports dizziness or syncope.

Procedure:. Listen for bruits using the bell of the stethoscope to auscultate each temporal and each carotid artery. Ask the patient to hold his or her breath while you listen so that breath sounds will not interfere (Fig. 12.34).[9]

Finding: No sound should be heard over these arteries.

PALPATE epitrochlear lymph nodes for size, consistency, mobility, tenderness, and warmth.

Palpate these lymph nodes when the patient has an acute infection of the ulnar aspect of the arm or a malignancy such as non-Hodgkin lymphoma.[9]

Procedure: Flex the patient's arm to a 90-degree angle and palpate below the elbow posterior to the medial condyle of the humerus (Fig. 12.35). Compare the sizes of the upper and lower arms for symmetry.

Findings: The arms should be symmetric with no palpable lymph nodes.

ABNORMAL FINDINGS

Bruits are low-pitched blowing sounds usually heard during systole that indicates turbulent blood flow from an occlusion of the vessel. Occlusion of a temporal or carotid artery may impair perfusion of the brain and increase the risk for transient ischemic attack (TIA).

Enlarged, firm, movable, tender, and warm nodes may be associated with infection of the ulnar aspect of the forearm and the fourth and fifth fingers. When one arm is larger in circumference than the other, it could be caused by lymphedema.

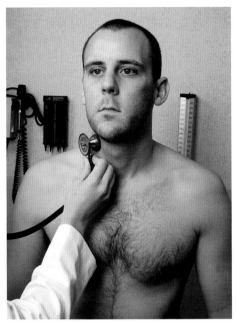

FIG. 12.34 Auscultating carotid artery. (From Harkreader, Hogan, and Thobaben, 2007.)

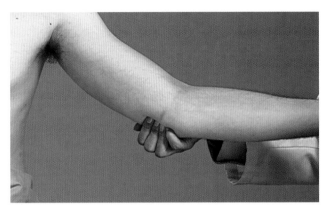

FIG. 12.35 Palpation for epitrochlear lymph nodes is performed in the depression above and posterior to the medial condyle of the humerus. (From Ball et al, 2015.)

PROCEDURES WITH EXPECTED FINDINGS

PALPATE inguinal lymph nodes for size, consistency, mobility, tenderness, and warmth bilaterally.

Palpate these nodes when an inflammatory process is suspected or the patient complains of pain.

Procedure: With the patient in the supine position, lightly palpate with finger pads in a circular motion in the area just below the inguinal ligament and on the inner aspect of the thigh at the groin (Fig. 12.36; see Fig. 12.9 to review anatomic location of inguinal nodes). Moving inward toward the genitalia, you can locate the anatomy using the mnemonic NAVEL: *N*, nerve; *A*, artery; *V,* vein; *E,* empty space; *L,* lymph nodes. The superior superficial inguinal nodes are close to the surface over the inguinal canals. The inferior superior inguinal nodes lie deeper in the groin.

Findings: The inguinal nodes may not be palpated at all; however, if felt, the nodes are small, soft, mobile, and nontender.

ABNORMAL FINDINGS

Enlarged, firm, non-mobile, tender, and warm nodes indicate an inflammatory process distal to these nodes such as in the leg, vulva, penis, or scrotum. When one leg is larger in circumference than the other, it could be caused by lymphedema.

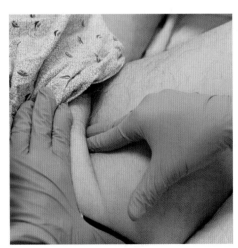

FIG. 12.36 Palpation of inferior superficial inguinal (femoral) lymph nodes. (From Yoost and Crawford, 2016.)

PROCEDURES WITH EXPECTED FINDINGS

MEASURE each leg circumference to assess for symmetry.

When one of the patient's thighs or calves looks bigger than the other or the patient complains of pain in these areas, place the patient in a supine position and measure the circumferences of the affected area and the other leg to compare values.

Procedure: Place a tape measure around the enlarged area (in the thigh or calf) and notice the circumference (Fig. 12.37A and B). To measure the other leg in the same location, measure the distance from the end of the patella to the affected area. Notice the distance and measure the same distance from the end of the patella on the other leg; at that location measure the circumference and compare. To ensure consistent location for measurement, you can use a marker to indicate the area measured on the affected leg.

Findings: The circumferences of both legs should be the same.

ABNORMAL FINDINGS

Although signs and symptoms of venous thromboses are often silent, an increase in thigh or calf circumference indicating edema may be an early indicator of a venous blood clot. Calf asymmetry of more than 1.5 cm is abnormal, indicating significant edema of the larger leg. Other signs may be differences in the color or temperature of the legs. Some patients report pain at the site.[4] Chronic venous stasis may produce increases in circumferences bilaterally.

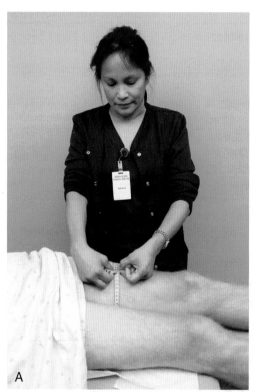
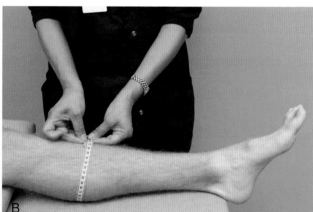

FIG. 12.37 (A) Measurement of thigh. (B) Measurement of calf circumference.

PROCEDURES WITH EXPECTED FINDINGS

CALCULATE the ankle-brachial indexes (ABIs) to estimate arterial occlusion. (Also known as the arm-to-ankle index, AAI.)

Calculate the ABI when the patient has peripheral arterial disease.

Procedure: The ABI is calculated by dividing the ankle systolic blood pressure by the brachial systolic blood pressure. With the patient in a supine position, take the brachial systolic blood pressure in both arms using Doppler sound (Fig. 12.38). Apply the blood pressure cuff above the ankle to measure the systolic blood pressure of the posterior tibialis or dorsalis pedis pulses using the Doppler. Divide the posterior tibial or dorsalis pedis (ankle) systolic blood pressure by the brachial systolic blood pressure for each side.

Findings: Calculate the values using the website http://www.sononet.us/abiscore/abiscore.htm. The expected value of ABI is greater than 1.0–1.4.

ABNORMAL FINDINGS

The patient who has peripheral artery disease (PAD) has impaired peripheral perfusion that is reflected in a lower systolic pressure in the leg than the arm, which reveals an ABI less than normal.

- 0.91–0.99 indicates some narrowing of arteries (borderline PAD).
- Less than 0.90 indicates PAD.[12]

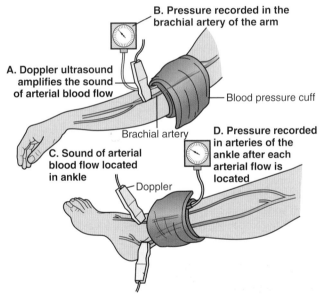

FIG. 12.38 Measuring systolic pressures in arms and legs for ankle-brachial index. (From Roberts and Hedges, 2009.)

A. Doppler ultrasound amplifies the sound of arterial blood flow

B. Pressure recorded in the brachial artery of the arm

Blood pressure cuff

Brachial artery

C. Sound of arterial blood flow located in ankle

D. Pressure recorded in arteries of the ankle after each arterial flow is located

Doppler

Thrills may occur with a murmur from a disorder of the aortic or pulmonic valve. Lifts and heaves may indicate ventricular hypertrophy.

- **ESTIMATE jugular venous pressure.** Jugular venous pressure estimates the pressure in the right side of the heart. This advanced practice technique is performed when the patient has fluid retention or right-sided heart failure, which increases the jugular venous pressure. The APRN identifies the highest level at which jugular vein pulsations are visible and measures to estimate jugular venous pressure.
- **ASSESS for varicose veins.** The Trendelenburg's test evaluates the competence of venous valves and is performed on patients who have varicose veins. With the patient lying supine, the APRN lifts one leg to allow veins to empty and then helps the patient to stand. The procedure is repeated with the other leg. Competent veins fill slowly, while those with varicosities fill rapidly.

TECHNIQUES PERFORMED BY AN ADVANCED PRACTICE REGISTERED NURSE

Specialty practice may require advanced techniques that are beyond the skill set of a nurse generalist. Knowing the purposes of these techniques may be helpful when caring for patients who require advanced assessment techniques.

- **PALPATE the precordium.** The APRN palpates the base, left sternal border (LSB), and apex for pulsations, thrills, lifts, and heaves. Pulsations may indicate an aortic aneurysm.

DOCUMENTING EXPECTED FINDINGS

Patient sitting in a relaxed position. BP 120/68, pulse 70 beats/min. Chest rounded and symmetric. PMI at 5th ICS, MCL, S_1 low-pitched, louder at the apex; and S_2 high-pitched, louder at the base, regular rate and rhythm without splitting. No temporal or carotid bruit. Jugular pulsations visible without distention; extremities symmetric in size; skin intact with elastic turgor, warm with color appropriate for patient; pulses regular rhythm, smooth contour with pulse amplitude 2+; capillary refill <2 in all extremities; nail beds pink with angle 160 degrees. Hair distribution even on upper and lower legs (unless purposefully removed). No lymph nodes palpated. Thigh circumferences equal. ABI=1.2.

Cardiovascular System

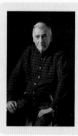

Case Presentation
Steve Fisher, a 68-year-old man with a long-standing history of emphysema and hypertension, presents to the emergency department with shortness of breath, productive cough, fatigue, and reduced appetite that have progressed over the last 2 days. His vital signs, taken at triage, were blood pressure 128/92 mm Hg; heart rate 122/minute; respiratory rate 26/minute; SpO2 91% on room air; temperature 99.2°F (37.3°C).

Reflecting
The nurse reflects on Mr. Fisher's clinical presentation and this clinical encounter; he was subsequently diagnosed with heart failure and admitted to an inpatient unit. This experience contributes to the nurse's expertise when encountering a similar situation.

Noticing / Recognizing Cues
Based on the presenting information, the experienced nurse recognizes the emergent nature of Mr. Fisher's condition. The nurse would not be surprised if a patient with advanced emphysema reported dyspnea with exertion and a periodic cough. However, Mr. Fisher's symptoms have become worse, and his cough is productive – both of which are a change from his baseline health status. Furthermore, the respiratory rate and oxygen saturation are consistent with respiratory compromise. The nurse notices that Mr. Fisher's skin is warm and slightly diaphoretic.

Responding / Taking Action
The emergency department nurse initiates appropriate initial interventions (oxygen delivery and obtaining intravenous access) and notifies the emergency department physician of the situation, ensuring that the patient receives prompt medical care.

Interpreting / Analyzing Cues & Forming Hypotheses
Early in the encounter, the nurse recalls two possible causes of these findings: pneumonia, heart failure, or both. To determine if either has any probability of being correct, the nurse gathers additional data:
• What is the color and character of the sputum?
Mr. Fisher tells the nurse it is whitish in color – kind of bubbly.
• Is there evidence of excessive fluid?
The nurse examines Mr. Fisher's feet and notes 2+ edema in his legs and feet; and he is wearing house slippers. When asked about this, Mr. Fisher tells the nurse he couldn't get his shoes on because of the swelling in his feet.
• Does he have abnormal breath and/or heart sounds?
The nurse auscultates Mr. Fisher's heart and lungs. His lungs have crackles bilaterally, and an S_3 heart sound is auscultated.
The experienced nurse not only recognizes the abnormal clinical findings (productive cough with white sputum, fatigue, fluid retention, crackles, and S_3 heart sound) but also interprets this information in the context of an older adult with underlying emphysema and hypertension.

AGE-RELATED VARIATIONS

This chapter discusses assessment techniques with adult patients. These data are important to assess for individuals of all ages, but the approach and techniques used to collect the information may vary depending on the patient's age.

INFANTS, CHILDREN, AND ADOLESCENTS

There are several differences in the assessment of the cardiovascular system for infants and young children. For example, the equipment used to measure blood pressure is smaller, the sequence of the examination may be different, and findings may differ based on anatomic differences. Assessment of the older child and adolescent follows the same procedures as an adult and reveals similar expected findings. One exception in the examination is the EKG, which is not typically performed. Chapter 19 presents further information regarding the cardiovascular assessment of infants, children, and adolescents.

OLDER ADULTS

Assessing the cardiovascular status of an older adult usually follows the same procedures as for an adult. Expected variations may be found in heart rate and blood pressure. Chapter 21 presents further information regarding the cardiovascular assessment of an older adult.

COMMON PROBLEMS AND CONDITIONS

CARDIAC DISORDERS

Valvular Heart Disease

An acquired or congenital disorder of a heart valve can result in *valvular heart disease (VHD)*. It can be characterized by a heart valve that does not either open completely (stenotic valve) or close completely (incompetent valve). Rheumatic fever and endocarditis account for most cases of acquired VHD. **Clinical Findings:** See Table 12.4 for murmurs associated with VHD. The symptom in common with all patients with any VHD is dyspnea on exertion.

Angina Pectoris

Chest pain that is caused by ischemia of the myocardium is called *angina pectoris,* or *stable angina.* Angina can occur during activity, stress, or exposure to intense cold because of an increased demand on the heart. It can also occur during rest as a result of spasms of the coronary arteries. From 2009 to 2012, there were an average 3.4 million people in the United States each year with angina. The large majority (72%) of individuals with angina were ages 40 to 64 years, and the large majority (61%) were women.[13] **Clinical Findings:** Men with stable angina describe the pain as a pressure in the chest, often a squeezing, suffocating, fullness or pain that may be felt in one or both arms, the back, jaw, or stomach.[5] Women report chest pain that is milder than men report as well as pain in the neck, jaw, shoulder, arms, or upper back.[6]

Acute Coronary Syndrome

This syndrome refers to a spectrum of myocardial conditions from unstable angina to acute myocardial infarction.[5]

Unstable Angina

Unstable angina is chest pain described as a new onset, experienced at rest, or a worsening pattern than previously experienced. The pain occurs with increasing frequency and is easily provoked by minimal or no exertion during sleep or at rest. **Clinical findings:** Patients describe their chest pain as occurring with increased frequency, with increased intensity, without a precipitating event, or at rest. Women's symptoms continue to be under-recognized as heart related. Fatigue is the most prominent symptom followed by shortness of breath, indigestion, and anxiety for women.[5]

Acute Myocardial Infarction

Sustained myocardial ischemia results in death of myocardial cells (necrosis) and acute myocardial infarction. The left ventricle is more commonly affected, but the right ventricle may also be affected. Every year approximately 790,000 Americans have an AMI. Of these, 580,000 are the first AMI and 210,000 are among those experiencing a reoccurrence.[14]

Clinical Findings: Patients describe the pain as the worst chest pain ever experienced, a pain that lasts longer than 5 minutes. It may radiate to the left shoulder, jaw, arm, or other areas of the chest, and it is not relieved by rest or nitroglycerin. Dysrhythmias are common. Heart sounds may be distant with a thready pulse.

Heart Failure

When either ventricle fails to pump blood efficiently into the aorta or pulmonary arteries, the condition is termed *heart failure*, which may occur in the left or right ventricle or both. Approximately 5 to 7 million adults in the United States have heart failure, and about half of these people will die within 5 years of initial diagnosis.[15]

Left Ventricular Failure

This cardiac condition is caused by (1) increased resistance to blood flow that occurs with aortic stenosis or hypertension when the ventricle can no longer contract effectively due to the increased workload, or (2) weakening of the left ventricular contraction that occurs after a myocardial infarction when the death of myocardial cells causes an ineffective contraction. Because the left ventricle cannot pump sufficient blood forward, some of the blood backs up into the left atrium and eventually into the pulmonary capillaries, causing pulmonary edema. **Clinical Findings:** The patient complains of fatigue and shortness of breath, including orthopnea, dyspnea on exertion, and paroxysmal nocturnal dyspnea. Findings may reveal displaced apical pulse and palpable thrill, S_3 heart sound, and systolic murmur at apex. In the acute phase, the patient usually has crackles bilaterally from pulmonary edema.

Right Ventricular Failure

This cardiac condition is caused by hypertrophy of the ventricle from pulmonary hypertension or necrosis from a myocardial infarction. The failure of the right ventricle to pump blood into the pulmonary arteries causes a backflow of blood into the inferior and superior venae cavae. Right ventricular failure caused by pulmonary disease is termed *cor pulmonale.* **Clinical Findings:** Findings may include dependent peripheral edema, S_3 heart sound at lower left sternal border, systolic murmur, and weight gain.

Pericarditis

Inflammation of the pericardium is termed *pericarditis.* **Clinical Findings:** A friction rub is best heard with the stethoscope at the lower left sternal border with the patient leaning forward moving the heart closer to the chest wall. The sound is described as a scratching, grating, high-pitched sound believed to result from friction between the roughened pericardium and epicardial surfaces and is louder during inspiration. The chest pain is described as a severe, sharp pain that is aggravated by deep breathing, lying flat, or coughing, and is relieved by sitting up and leaning forward.[16]

PERIPHERAL VASCULAR DISEASES

Hypertension

A diagnosis of hypertension is based on the mean of two or more properly measured seated blood pressure readings on each of two or more occasions that are above 120/80 mm Hg in an adult over 18 years of age. The American Heart Association estimates that 46% or 103 million adults have high blood pressure.[17] **Clinical Findings:** Expected blood pressure values are less than 120 mm Hg systolic and less than 80 mm Hg diastolic. Criteria for hypertension are shown in Box 12.5. Since there are no specific symptoms of hypertension, periodic screening is important.

Venous Thromboembolism and Thrombophlebitis

Venous thromboembolism includes both deep vein thrombosis (DVT) and pulmonary embolism (PE). When a thrombus (clot) develops within a vein, it is called a deep vein thrombosis (DVT). In contrast, thrombophlebitis is inflammation of a vein that may or may not be accompanied by a clot. DVT typically forms in deep veins of the lower leg, thigh, pelvis, or arm. If the thrombus dislodges, it can travel to the lungs causing pulmonary embolus (PE).[18] The precise number of people affected by DVT is unknown, although as many as 900,000 people could be affected (1 to 2 per 1000) each year in the United States.[19] **Clinical Findings:** Thromboses are sometimes recognized by dilated superficial veins, edema and redness of the involved extremity, and increased circumference of the involved leg. In the upper extremity, venous thrombosis and thrombophlebitis may occur in superficial veins and are recognized by redness, warmth, and tenderness over the affected area.[8] Veins may be visible and palpable.

Peripheral Artery and Venous Insufficiencies

Peripheral arterial disease (PAD) develops from arterial insufficiency. Approximately 8.5 million people in the United States have PAD, including 12% to 20% of individuals older than age 60.[20] Chronic venous insufficiency (CVI) results from incompetent valves due to either congenital defects or changes in the venous wall pathology or due to a precipitating event such as a DVT. Each year, approximately 150,000 new patients are diagnosed with CVI. Studies have suggested that in the general population, as many as 17% of men and 40% of women may experience CVI.[21] **Clinical Findings:** A comparison of the clinical findings is found in Table 12.6. Vascular insufficiencies may produce ulcers, which appear as circumscribed, craterlike lesions of the skin. An arterial leg ulcer is shown in Fig. 12.39, and a venous leg ulcer is shown in Fig. 12.40.

TABLE 12.6 COMPARISON OF PERIPHERAL ARTERIAL AND VENOUS DISEASE		
CHARACTERISTIC	**PERIPHERAL ARTERY DISEASE**	**PERIPHERAL VENOUS DISEASE**
Peripheral pulses	Decreased or absent	Present; may be difficult to palpate with edema
Capillary refill	>3 seconds	<3 seconds
Ankle-brachial index	<0.90	>0.90
Edema	Absent unless leg constantly in dependent position	Lower leg edema
Hair	Loss of hair on legs, feet, toes	Hair may be present or absent
Ulcer		
Location	Tips of toes, foot, or lateral malleolus	Near medial malleolus
Margin	Rounded, smooth, looks "punched out"	Irregularly shaped
Drainage	Minimal	Moderate-to-large amount
Tissue	Black eschar or pale pink granulation	Yellow slough or dark red, "ruddy" granulation
Pain	Intermittent claudication or rest pain in foot; ulcer may or may not be painful	Dull ache or heaviness in calf or thigh; ulcer often painful
Nails	Thickened; brittle	Normal or thickened
Skin color	Dependent rubor; elevation pallor	Bronze-brown pigmentation; varicose veins may be visible
Skin texture	Thin, shiny, taut	Skin thick, hardened, and indurated
Skin temperature	Cool, temperature gradient down the leg	Warm, no temperature gradient
Dermatitis	Rarely occurs	Frequently occurs
Pruritus	Rarely occurs	Frequently occurs

(From Wipke-Tevis D, Rich K: Vascular disorders. In Lewis S, et al: *Medical-surgical nursing: assessment and management of clinical problems,* ed 10, St Louis, 2017, Elsevier.)

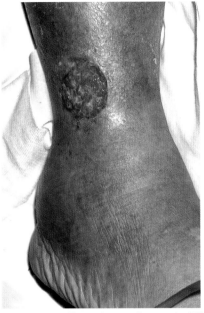

FIG. 12.39 Arterial ulcer. (From James, Berger, and Elston, 2011.)

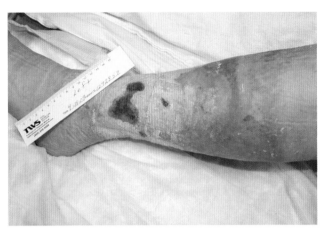

FIG. 12.40 Venous stasis ulcer. (From Townsend et al., 2012.)

CLINICAL APPLICATION AND CLINICAL JUDGMENT

See Appendix B for answers to exercises in this section.

CASE STUDY

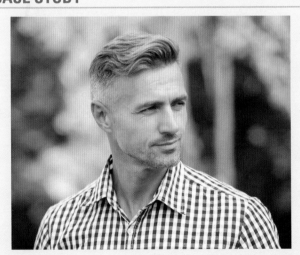

Mr. Cox is a 56-year-old man complaining of difficulty breathing. The following initial data are collected.

Interview Data

Mr. Cox does not know exactly when his breathing difficulty started, but it has become noticeably worse during the last couple of days. His father died of a heart attack at age 60. Mr. Cox plays golf twice a week; however, he tells the nurse that this last week he has "just felt too tired to do anything." He says that he has not been able to sleep very well at night because of his breathing difficulty. He adds, "I keep coughing out this bubbly-looking phlegm." He denies taking any medications. He says that he does not smoke or drink alcoholic beverages.

Examination Data

- *General survey:* Alert, anxious, cooperative, well-groomed male. Appears stated age. Breathing labored.
- *Vital signs:* BP, 142/112 mm Hg, right arm; 144/110 mm Hg, left arm; temperature, 98.8°F (37.1°C); pulse, 120 beats/min; respiration, 26 breaths/min.
- *Pulses:* All pulses palpable 2+. No carotid bruits bilaterally.
- *Neck:* Jugular distention and pulsation noticed with patient in supine position.
- *Lower extremities:* Skin warm and dry, without cyanosis. Even hair distribution. 2+ pitting edema noticed bilaterally. No lesions present.

Clinical Judgment

1. What cues do you recognize that suggest a deviation from expected findings, suggesting a need for further investigation?
2. For which additional information should the nurse ask or assess?
3. Based on these data, which risk factors for coronary artery disease does Mr. Cox have?
4. With which health care team member would you collaborate to meet this patient's needs?

REVIEW QUESTIONS

1. The nurse is listening to the patient's heart at the 2nd LSB. Which area is being auscultated?
   1. Erb's point
   2. Mitral area
   3. Aortic area
   4. Pulmonic area

2. A patient complains of pain in the calf when walking. Which question should the nurse ask for further data?
   1. "Does your calf also swell when this pain occurs?"
   2. "Does the pain go away when you stop walking?"
   3. "Do you become short of breath when you're walking?"
   4. "Do you feel dizzy when the pain occurs?"

3. A nurse who is auscultating a patient's heart hears a harsh sound, a raspy machine-like blowing sound, after S1 and before S2. How does this nurse document this finding?
   1. An opening snap
   2. A diastolic murmur
   3. A systolic murmur
   4. A pericardial friction rub

4. When a patient complains of chest pain, which question is pertinent to ask to gain additional data?
   1. "What were you doing when the pain first occurred?"
   2. "What does the pain feel like?"
   3. "Do you have shortness of breath?"
   4. "Has anyone in your family ever had a similar pain?"

5. How does a nurse determine jugular vein pulsations?
   1. Raises the head of the bed about 90 degrees and looks for the jugular vein pulsation parallel to the sterno-cleidomastoid muscle as the bed is slowly lowered
   2. Looks for jugular vein pulsations at the jaw line as the patient turns from supine to a side-lying position
   3. Elevates the head of the bed until the external jugular vein pulsation is seen above the clavicle
   4. Positions the patient supine and asks him or her to cough; inspects for jugular vein pulsations during the cough

6. Where does a nurse palpate the posterior tibial pulse?
   1. Behind the knee in the popliteal fossa
   2. The inner aspect of the ankle below and slightly behind the medial malleolus
   3. Over the dorsum of the foot between the tendons of the first and second toes
   4. The outer side of the ankle below and slightly behind the lateral malleolus

7. Which finding does the nurse expect during auscultation of the heart?
   1. A low-pitched blowing sound is heard over the apex of the heart.
   2. A high-pitched vibration is heard over the base of the heart.
   3. The S1 heart sound is louder at the apex of the heart.
   4. The S3 heart sound sounds like "Ken-tuck-y."

8. What is the most accurate technique for detecting a venous thrombosis at the bedside?
   1. Measure the thigh circumference to detect an increase from the baseline.
   2. Dorsiflex the calf and notice if the patient complains of pain.
   3. Elevate one leg above the level of the heart to determine if the veins empty.
   4. Palpate the pulses distal to the areas of the suspected thrombosis.

9. Each patient has had consistent blood pressure readings during the last three clinic visits. Which patient has a blood pressure consistent with expected findings?
   1. Ms. J, whose blood pressure has been 140/90
   2. Mr. Q, whose blood pressure has been 130/76
   3. Ms. Y, whose blood pressure has been 120/80
   4. Mr. P, whose blood pressure has been 110/78

10. While inspecting the legs of a male patient, the nurse notices that the skin is shiny and taut with little hair growth. Which additional data would the nurse find to indicate that this patient has peripheral arterial disease?
    1. Pitting edema of one or both feet or legs
    2. Increased circumference in the thighs bilaterally
    3. Pale, cool legs with diminished-to-absent dorsalis pedis pulses
    4. Pain when legs are dependent that is relieved when legs are elevated

CHAPTER

13

Abdomen and Gastrointestinal System

evolve

http://evolve.elsevier.com/Wilson/assessment

CONCEPT OVERVIEW

The concept for this chapter is *Elimination*, which represents mechanisms that facilitate the excretion of waste products from the body. Waste is removed from the body by many systems including the respiratory system, skin, and gastrointestinal and urinary systems. This concept focuses on the elimination of waste in the form of stool and urine. Many concepts associated with elimination are represented in the adjacent illustration. Understanding the interrelationships of these concepts helps the nurse recognize risk factors when conducting a health assessment. Elimination has a close relationship with nutrition, specifically food and fluids consumed. Normal elimination of urine and stool requires precise hormonal regulation as part of the digestive process and the process of urine formation. Adequate fluid and electrolyte balances affect elimination processes, and impaired elimination can disrupt fluid and electrolyte imbalances as well as acid-base balance.

The following case provides a clinical example featuring several of these interrelated concepts.

Cameron Sullivan is a 34-year-old man who has Crohn disease. He was diagnosed 6 years ago and, until a few months ago, experienced relatively mild symptoms. However, in the past 2 months he has experienced an

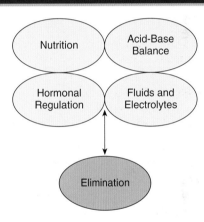

exacerbation of his condition including abdominal pain and cramping, diarrhea, reduced appetite, weight loss, and fatigue. Without intervention, Cameron is at risk for dehydration, electrolyte imbalance, and acid-base disturbance. Inflammation of the intestine causes diarrhea, which reduces water reabsorption in the colon. The pain and loss of appetite lead to reduced food and fluid intake. Compensatory mechanisms include the secretion of several hormones to maintain adequate blood glucose levels, to conserve fluid, and to make adjustments to electrolytes.

ANATOMY AND PHYSIOLOGY

The abdominal cavity, the largest cavity in the human body, contains the stomach, small and large intestines, liver, gallbladder, pancreas, spleen, kidneys, ureters, bladder, adrenal glands, and major vessels (Figs. 13.1 and 13.2). In women the uterus, fallopian tubes, and ovaries are also located within the abdominal cavity. Lying outside the abdominal cavity, but a vital part of the gastrointestinal (GI) system, is the esophagus.

PERITONEUM, MUSCULATURE, AND CONNECTIVE TISSUE

The abdominal lining, called the *peritoneum*, is a serous membrane forming a protective cover. It is divided into two layers: the parietal peritoneum and the visceral peritoneum. The parietal peritoneum lines the abdominal wall, and the

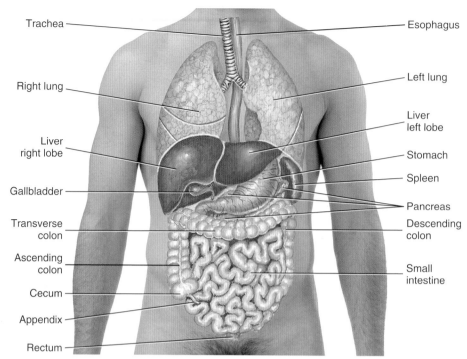

FIG. 13.1 Anatomy of the gastrointestinal system.

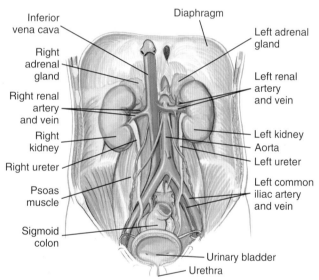

FIG. 13.2 Anatomy of the urinary system and major vessels of the abdominal cavity. (From Lewis et al., 2014.)

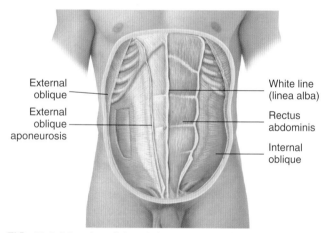

FIG. 13.3 Muscles of the abdomen. (From Seidel et al., 2011.)

visceral peritoneum covers organs. The space between the parietal peritoneum and visceral peritoneum is the peritoneal cavity. It usually contains a small amount of serous fluid to reduce friction between abdominal organs.

The rectus abdominis muscles form the anterior border of the abdomen, and the vertebral column and lumbar muscles form the posterior border. Lateral support is provided by the internal and external oblique muscles. The transverses abdominis is one of a pair of transverse abdominal muscles that lie immediately under the internal oblique muscles. The external oblique aponeurosis is a strong membrane that covers the entire ventral surface of the abdomen and lies superficial to the rectus abdominis. Fibers from both sides of the aponeurosis interlace in the midline to form the linea alba, a tendinous band that protects the midline of the abdomen between the rectus abdominis muscles. This band extends from the xiphoid process to the symphysis pubis. The abdomen is bordered superiorly by the diaphragm and inferiorly by the superior aperture of the lesser pelvis (Fig. 13.3).

ALIMENTARY TRACT

From the mouth to the anus, the adult alimentary tract extends 27 feet (8.2 m) and includes the mouth, esophagus, stomach, small intestine, large intestine, rectum, and anal canal (see Figs. 10.8 and 13.1). Its main functions are to ingest and digest food; absorb nutrients, electrolytes, and water; and excrete waste products. Products of digestion are moved along the digestive tract by peristalsis, under the control of the autonomic nervous system.

Mouth

Teeth chew food that is mixed with saliva from three pairs of salivary glands, beginning the breakdown of carbohydrates.

Esophagus

Connecting the pharynx to the stomach is the esophagus, a tube approximately 10 inches (25.4 cm) long and extending just posterior to the trachea through the mediastinal cavity and diaphragm. The usual pH of the esophagus is between 6.0 and 8.0.

Stomach

The stomach is a hollow, flask-shaped, muscular organ located directly below the diaphragm in the left upper quadrant. Contents from the esophagus enter the stomach through the lower esophageal sphincter and mix with digestive enzymes and hydrochloric acid to break down proteins and fats as well as continue the digestion of carbohydrates. The stomach also liquefies food into chyme and propels it into the duodenum of the small intestine. The usual pH of the stomach ranges from 2.0 to 4.0. The pyloric sphincter regulates the outflow of chyme into the duodenum. Movement of air and fluid through the stomach and small and large intestines produces bowel sounds heard on auscultation.

Small Intestine

The longest section of the alimentary tract, the small intestine, is approximately 21 feet (6.4 m) long, beginning at the pyloric orifice and joining the large intestine at the ileocecal valve. The small intestine is divided into three segments: the duodenum, jejunum, and ileum. The duodenum occupies the first 1 foot (30 cm) of the small intestine and forms a C-shaped curve around the head of the pancreas. The usual pH of the small intestine ranges from 6.0 to 7.4. Absorption occurs through the intestinal villi of the duodenum, jejunum (8 feet [2.4 m] long), and ileum (12 feet [3.6 m] long). The ileocecal valve between the ileum and the large intestine prevents backward flow of fecal material (see Fig. 13.1).

Large Intestine (Colon) and Rectum

The large intestine is approximately 5 feet (1.5 m) long, consisting of cecum, appendix, colon, rectum, and anal canal. The ileal contents empty into the cecum through the ileocecal valve; the appendix extends from the base of the cecum. The colon is divided into three parts: ascending, transverse, and descending. The end of the descending colon turns medially and inferiorly to form the S-shaped sigmoid colon. The rectum extends from the sigmoid colon to the pelvic floor, where it continues as the anal canal, terminating at the anus. The usual pH of the rectum is 6.7. The large intestine absorbs water and electrolytes. Stool is formed in the large intestine and held until defecation (see Fig. 13.1). While the rectum and anus are the terminal structures of the gastrointestinal system, their assessment is described in Chapter 17, because they are usually examined in conjunction with the reproductive system.

ACCESSORY ORGANS

The salivary glands, liver, gallbladder, and pancreas are the accessory organs of the GI tract. Salivary glands are described in Chapter 10.

Liver

The largest organ in the body is the liver, weighing approximately 3.5 pounds (1.6 kg). It lies under the right diaphragm, spanning the upper quadrant of the abdomen from the fifth intercostal space to slightly below the costal margin (see Fig. 13.1). The rib cage covers a substantial portion of the liver; only the lower margin is exposed beneath it. The liver is divided into right and left lobes.

This complex organ has a variety of functions, including bile production and secretion for the digestion and absorption of fats and fat-soluble vitamins, production of clotting factors and fibrinogen, synthesis of most plasma proteins (albumin and globulin), and detoxification of a variety of substances, including drugs and alcohol.

Gallbladder

Attached to the inferior surface of the liver is the gallbladder, a pear-shaped sac 3 inches (7.6 cm) long, (see Fig. 13.1). It concentrates and stores bile produced in the liver. The cystic duct combines with the hepatic duct to form the common bile duct, which drains bile into the duodenum. Bile contained in stool creates the characteristic brown color.

Pancreas

The pancreas lies in the upper left abdominal cavity, immediately under the left lobe of the liver, behind the stomach (see Fig. 13.1). It has both endocrine and exocrine functions. Endocrine secretions include the release of insulin, glucagon, somatostatin, and gastrin for carbohydrate metabolism. Exocrine secretions contain bicarbonate and pancreatic enzymes that flow into the duodenum. Lipase breaks down fats, amylase breaks down carbohydrates, and protease breaks down proteins for absorption.

Spleen

The spleen is a highly vascular, concave, encapsulated organ approximately the size of a fist, situated in the upper left quadrant of the abdomen between the stomach and diaphragm. It is composed of two systems: the white pulp (consisting of lymphatic nodules and diffuse lymphatic tissue) and the red pulp (consisting of venous sinusoids) (see Fig. 13.1). Its functions include removal of old or agglutinated erythrocytes and platelets and activation of B and T lymphocytes.

URINARY TRACT

The urinary tract includes the kidneys, ureters, urinary bladder, and urethra. Together they remove water-soluble waste materials.

Kidneys

The kidneys are located in the posterior abdominal cavity on either side at the spinal levels T12 through L3, where they are covered by the peritoneum and attached to the posterior abdominal wall. Each kidney is partially protected by the ribs and a cushion of fat and fascia. The right kidney is slightly lower than the left because of displacement by the liver (see Fig. 13.2). Kidney functions include secretion of erythropoietin to stimulate red blood cell production and production of a biologically active form of vitamin D. The nephron regulates fluid and electrolyte balance through an elaborate microscopic filter and pressure system that eventually produces urine.

Ureters

The urine formed in the nephrons flows from the distal tubes and collecting ducts into the ureters and on into the bladder through peristaltic waves. Each ureter is composed of long, intertwining muscle bundles that extend for approximately 12 inches (30 cm) to insertion points at the base of the bladder (see Fig. 13.2).

Bladder

The bladder, a sac of smooth muscle fibers, is located behind the symphysis pubis in the anterior half of the pelvis (see Fig. 13.2). It contains an internal sphincter, which relaxes in response to a full bladder. Generally, when the urine volume of the bladder reaches approximately 300 mL, moderate distention is felt; a level of 450 mL causes discomfort. For voiding to occur, the external sphincter relaxes voluntarily; and urine exits through the urethra, which extends out of the base of the bladder to the external meatus.

VASCULATURE OF THE ABDOMEN

The descending aorta travels through the diaphragm just to the left of midline until it branches into the two common iliac arteries, approximately at the level of the umbilicus. Perfusion of the kidneys is provided by the right and left renal arteries, which branch off the descending aorta. Blood is returned to the right side of the heart from the abdomen in the inferior vena cava, which parallels the abdominal aorta (see Fig. 13.2). Several veins empty into the inferior vena cava. These include the hepatic portal system, which is composed of veins that drain the intestines, pancreas, stomach, and gallbladder; and the renal veins, which drain the kidneys and ureters.

HEALTH HISTORY

Nurses interview patients to collect subjective data about their present health status, past health history, family history, and personal and psychosocial history, which may affect the functions of the abdomen, GI system, and urinary tract. Questions regarding the patient's nutrition and eating habits are asked in the health history in Chapter 8.

GENERAL HEALTH HISTORY

Present Health Status

Do you have any chronic diseases? If yes, describe.
Some chronic diseases such as diabetes mellitus may affect the GI or urinary systems. Diseases such as chronic hepatitis or cirrhosis may impair the ability of the liver to metabolize nutrients and drugs.

Do you take any medications? If yes, what do you take and how often? What are the medications for?
Medications may be taken periodically to relieve symptoms such as heartburn, diarrhea, or constipation. Other medications may cause adverse GI effects. Because drugs are metabolized in the liver, they may not be metabolized well in patients with liver diseases, which causes increased blood levels of these drugs.

Do you take any over-the-counter drugs or herbal supplements? If so, what do you take and how often? What are they for?

Nonprescription drugs and herbal supplements may affect the gastrointestinal system. For example, probiotics resemble good bacteria to help digestion, antacids relieve heartburn, and laxatives relieve constipation.

How often do you have a bowel movement? When was your last bowel movement? Describe the color and consistency of the stool.
Frequency of bowel movements is individual for each person. The frequency, color, and consistency of stool are documented as baseline data. These questions also give the patient an opportunity to describe disorders of the colon such as diarrhea, constipation, dark or light stools, or blood in stool.

What is your usual pattern of urination? When was the last time you urinated? Describe the color of the urine. Do you have any difficulty urinating?
Frequency of urination is individual for each person. The color is documented as baseline data. These questions also give the patient an opportunity to describe disorders of urination such as painful urination, dark color, presence of blood, or for men, difficulty starting the urine stream or sensation of incomplete bladder emptying.

Past Health History

Have you had problems with your abdomen or digestive system in the past? Esophagus? Stomach? Intestines? Liver? Gallbladder? Pancreas? Spleen? If yes, describe.

History of GI disorders may provide insight into anticipated findings at this examination. These data give clues to a patient's education needs about reducing risk for other diseases such as cancers.

Have you had problems with your urinary tract in the past? If yes, describe.

History of urinary disorders may provide insight into anticipated findings at this examination. These data also give clues

to patient's education needs about reducing risk for other diseases such as urinary tract infection and cancers.

Have you ever experienced the leaking of urine? When did this occur? Have you ever used pads, tissues, or cloth in your underwear to absorb urine?

Many patients do not report incontinence unless asked about it, often because of embarrassment. *Stress incontinence* is the most common type and is characterized by involuntary loss of small amounts of urine during physical exertion such as coughing, sneezing, jogging, and lifting. It may begin around the time of menopause. *Urge incontinence* is associated with a sudden strong urge to void and may occur in people with

RISK FACTORS

Esophageal, Stomach, and Colon Cancers

Esophageal Cancer

- *Age:* Risk increases with age. Less than 15% of cases are found in people younger than 55 years.
- *Gender:* Men have a rate higher than women.
- *Gastroesophageal reflux disease (GERD):* People with reflux of gastric acid into the lower esophagus have a slightly higher risk of getting adenocarcinoma of the esophagus. (M)
- *Barrett esophagus:* This condition is associated with long-term esophageal reflux and results in a higher risk of esophageal cancer. (M)
- *Tobacco use:* The longer a person uses tobacco products (cigarettes, cigars, pipes, and chewing tobacco), the greater the risk. (M)
- *Alcohol use:* The more alcohol someone drinks, the higher the risk. Alcohol and smoking together raise a person's risk more than using either alone. (M)
- *Obesity:* The risk of this cancer is higher in people who are obese because obesity increases the risk of esophageal reflux. (M)
- *Diet:* A diet high in processed meats and low in fruits and vegetables may increase the risk. (M)
- *Workplace exposures:* Exposures to chemical fumes such as solvents used by dry cleaners might lead to a greater risk. (M)
- *Injury to the esophagus:* Lye is a chemical found in drain cleaners that is a corrosive agent. Accidentally drinking from a lye-based cleaner bottle can cause severe chemical burn in the esophagus and strictures that can increase risk of cancer. (M)

Stomach Cancer

- *Age:* There is a sharp increase after age 50. Most people are diagnosed between their late 60s and 80.
- *Gender:* Disease is more common in men.
- *Race:* Rates are higher in Hispanic Americans, African Americans, and Asian/Pacific Islanders than in non-Hispanic whites.

- *Geography:* Worldwide, stomach cancer is more common in Japan, China, Southern and Eastern Europe, and South and Central America.
- *Infection: Helicobacter pylori* infection is a major cause of this cancer. (M)
- *Diet:* Eating large amounts of smoked foods, salted fish and meat, and pickled vegetables increases risk. (M)
- *Smoking:* The rate of proximal stomach cancer is approximately double in smokers. (M)
- *Previous stomach surgery:* Risk is higher in those who have had surgery to treat noncancerous disease such as ulcers.
- *Blood type:* For unknown reasons, people with blood type A have a greater risk.
- *Family history:* Risk is higher in those with a first-degree family member (parents, siblings, or children) with stomach cancer.

Colorectal Cancer

- *Age:* Commonly diagnosed in people over 50 years old.
- *Diet:* A diet high in red and/or processed meats increases risk. (M)
- *Physical activity:* Lack of regular physical exercise increases risk. (M)
- *Weight:* Being overweight or obese increases risk, with a stronger association observed in men than in women. (M)
- *Smoking:* Long-term smokers are more likely than non-smokers to develop and die from colorectal cancer. (M)
- *Alcohol use:* Heavy use of alcohol increases risk. (M)
- *Personal history of colorectal polyps or colorectal cancer:* A history of adenomatous polyps increases risk. Even though colorectal cancer was removed, people are more likely to develop cancers in other areas of the colon and rectum.
- *Personal history of chronic inflammatory bowel disease (IBD):* IBD includes Crohn disease or ulcerative colitis.
- *Family history:* Having a first-degree relative (parents, siblings, or children) with colorectal cancer increases risk.
- *Inherited syndrome:* Approximately 5% of people who develop colorectal cancer have inherited gene defects (mutations).

M, Modifiable risk factor.

Data from www.cancer.org/cancer/esophagus-cancer/causes-risks-prevention/risk-factors.html. Last revised 6/14/17.
www.cancer.org/cancer/stomach-cancer/causes-risks-prevention/risk-factors.html. Last revised 12/14/17.
www.cancer.org/cancer/colon-rectal-cancer/causes-risks-prevention/risk-factors.html. Last revised 2/21/2018.

diabetes mellitus, Parkinson disease, multiple sclerosis, or stroke. *Overflow incontinence* occurs when urine leaks from a bladder that is always full, which may occur in a man with an enlarged prostate gland. *Functional incontinence* occurs in people with normal bladder function who have difficulty getting to the toilet because of arthritis or other disorders that impair mobility.[1]

Have you had surgery involving your abdomen or urinary tract? If yes, describe. Did the surgery require that you change any of your former routines such as the food you eat or bowel or urinary elimination? How have you adjusted to the effects of these surgeries?
Patients who have had bariatric procedures for weight loss or gastrectomies may have changed the foods they eat and the amount and frequency of meals. Patients may have a colostomy or an ileostomy after surgery for such disorders as colon cancer or ulcerative colitis. Patients who have had bladder cancer may have an ileal conduit as an alternative route for urine excretion. Any of these surgeries requires that the patient change an appliance over the stoma. These questions convey concern about their adjustment to this change in their body.

Family History

In your family, is there a history of diseases of the GI system such as gastroesophageal reflux disease (GERD), peptic ulcer disease, Crohn disease, ulcerative colitis, or colon cancer?
Family history may be used to determine a patients' risk factors for GI disorders. Twin and family studies revealed approximately 31% inheritability of GERD.[2] Genetic factors play a role in the acquisition of *Helicobacter pylori* infection causing peptic ulcer disease.[3] Crohn disease tends to cluster in families with approximately 15% of affected people having a first-degree relative (such as a parent or sibling) with the disorder.[4] Even though the inheritance pattern of ulcerative colitis is unclear, having a family member with it increases the risk of developing the condition.[5] People with a history of colorectal cancer in a first-degree relative are at increased risk, with the risk even higher if that relative was diagnosed with cancer when younger than age 45, or if more than one first-degree relative is affected.[6]

In your family, is there a history of diseases of the urinary tract such as kidney stones, kidney cancer, or bladder cancer?
The risk of developing kidney stones is greater when a person has a close relative (such as parent or sibling) with kidney stones.[7] People with a strong family history of renal cell cancer have a higher chance of developing this cancer. This risk

is highest for people who have a brother or sister with the cancer.[8] People who have family members with bladder cancer have a higher risk of this type of cancer.[9]

Personal and Psychosocial History

Do you drink alcohol? If so, how much and how often? When was your last drink (of alcohol)?
Alcohol is a risk factor for peptic ulcer disease, pancreatitis, cirrhosis and cancers of the esophagus, stomach, and colon. Alcoholism may damage the liver, the organ that metabolizes alcohol.

Do you smoke? If so, how much and for how long? Have you considered stopping or cutting down?
Cigarette smoking is a risk factor for peptic ulcer disease and cancers of the colon, pancreas, liver, kidney, and bladder.[6,8,9]

PROBLEM-BASED HISTORY

Specific areas of assessment of the abdomen, GI system, and urinary tract include abdominal pain, nausea and vomiting, indigestion, abdominal distention, change in bowel habits, jaundice, and problems with urination. As with symptoms in all areas of health assessment, a symptom analysis is completed using the mnemonic OLD CARTS, which includes the *Onset, Location, Duration, Characteristics, Aggravating* factors, *Related* symptoms, *Treatment,* and *Severity* (see Box 2.6).

Abdominal Pain

How long have you had abdominal pain? Where is it located? When did you first feel it?
The onset and location of pain may help determine the cause. Box 13.1 shows the quadrants where organs are located. For example, right upper quadrant pain is associated with disorders of the gallbladder, colon, liver, lung, and kidney, whereas left upper quadrant pain may occur with cardiac, pancreatic, gastric, renal, or vascular disorders. Both right and left lower quadrant pain may accompany colonic, gynecologic, or renal disorders.[10] Sudden, severe pain that awakens the patient may be related to acute perforation, inflammation, or torsion of an abdominal organ.

Describe the pain. What does it feel like? Is it constant or does it come and go? Have you had episodes of this pain before? Did it start suddenly?
Table 13.1 differentiates various types of abdominal pain. Pain description is helpful in determining its cause. Intense pain may be caused by a stone in the biliary tract or ureter,

TABLE 13.1 DIFFERENTIATION OF ABDOMINAL PAIN

DISORDER	PATIENT DESCRIPTIONS	LOCATION	CHARACTERISTICS	AGGRAVATING FACTORS	RELATED SYMPTOMS	TREATMENT OR ALLEVIATING FACTORS	EXAM FINDINGS
Gastro-esophageal reflux	Any age	Mid-epigastric. May radiate to jaw	Heartburn, regurgitation, angina relieved by antacids	Recumbency, bending, stooping	Weight loss	Antacids, sitting up, food	
Gastro-enteritis	Any age	Diffuse	Cramping	Food	Nausea, vomiting, fever, diarrhea	Some relief with vomiting or diarrhea	Hyperactive BS
Gastritis	Alcoholism	Epigastric	Constant, burning	Alcohol, food, salicylates	Hemorrhage, nausea, vomiting, anorexia	Antacids	Epigastric tenderness
Peptic ulcer	30–50 years; more men than women	Epigastrium. Gastric: 1–2 h after meals. Duodenal: 2–4 h after meals, pain in back	Burning, cramping	Gastric: food if perforated. Duodenal: empty stomach	Nausea, vomiting, weight loss, can precipitate asthma attack	Gastric: antacids. Duodenal: antacids, food	Epigastric tenderness
Pancreatitis	Alcoholism, cholelithiasis	LUQ, epigastric; radiates to back	Sudden onset, steady, severe, knifelike	Food, lying supine	Nausea, vomiting, diarrhea, diaphoresis, fever	In a knee-chest position	Abdominal distension, ↓ BS, LUQ tenderness
Appendicitis	Any age: peak 10–20 years	Umbilical moving to RLQ	Colicky	Moving, coughing, sneezing, deep inhalation	Nausea, vomiting, fever	Lying still with right leg flexed	Muscle guarding, tenderness in RLQ
Cholecystitis or cholelithiasis	Adults; more women than men	RUQ or epigastric radiates to R shoulder	Severe, progressing to constant	Fatty foods, alcohol	Fever, anorexia, jaundice		RUQ tenderness, palpable gallbladder, +Murphy sign
Ectopic pregnancy	History of menstrual irregularities	Lower quadrants referred to shoulder	Sudden onset, persistent pain		Vaginal bleeding		Palpable mass on affected side
Irritable bowel syndrome	Young women	LLQ	Cramping, recurrent, sharp, burning		Bloating, excess gas, diarrhea, constipation, mucus in stool	Defecation	
Intestinal obstruction	Older adults; those with prior abdominal surgery	Referred to epigastrium, umbilicus	Sudden onset, severe, colicky		Vomiting, constipation. Abdominal distention		Absent or hyperactive BS depending on cause, visible peristalsis

LLQ, Left lower quadrant; *LUQ,* left upper quadrant; *RLQ,* right lower quadrant; *RUQ,* right upper quadrant; *BS,* bowel sounds.

the rupture of a fallopian tube from an ectopic pregnancy, or inflammation such as peritonitis following perforation of a gastric ulcer.

Do you feel it in any other parts of your body?

Radiation of the pain is an important component of the history. Pain from acute appendicitis starts around the umbilicus and radiates to the right lower quadrant (RLQ), whereas back pain may occur with duodenal ulcers or pancreatitis. Pain from gallbladder disease may be felt in the right shoulder[10] and pain from GERD may radiate to the jaw or neck.

Is the pain worse when your stomach is empty? Is it affected by eating? Is it worse at night or during the day?

Determine aggravating factors. For example, the pain of a duodenal ulcer may awaken the patient from sleep. Pain in gastroenteritis and irritable bowel disease is worse in the presence of food because peristalsis is stimulated, which causes pain.

What relieves the pain? Is there any particular position that relieves it? Is the pain relieved after a bowel movement?

A particular position may relieve abdominal pain. For example, pain from pancreatitis may be relieved in the knee-chest position, whereas pain from appendicitis is relieved by lying very still. Pain relieved after a bowel movement may indicate diverticulitis.

Is the pain related to other symptoms? (Suggest stress, fatigue, nausea and vomiting, gas, fever, chills, constipation, diarrhea, rectal bleeding, frequent urination, or vaginal or penile discharge as possible other symptoms.)

Identifying symptoms related to pain may assist in determining the cause. For example, constipation is the symptom with the highest positive predictive value for diagnosing bowel obstruction.[10]

For females: Is the pain associated with your menstrual period? When was your last menstrual period? Could you be pregnant?

Dysmenorrhea (pain associated with menstruation) may cause lower abdominal pain and vomiting because of the increase in prostaglandin. An ectopic pregnancy may cause abdominal pain.

Nausea and Vomiting

How long have you been experiencing nausea or vomiting? How often does this occur?

Learning additional details helps to determine the cause. Vomiting that precedes the onset of abdominal pain may suggest infection as a possible cause. However, abdominal pain that precedes vomiting may indicate appendicitis.[11]

How much do you vomit? What does the vomitus look like? Does it contain blood? Does it have an odor?

The characteristics of the vomitus may help determine its cause. Acute gastritis leads to vomiting of stomach contents; obstruction of the bile duct results in greenish-yellow vomitus; and an intestinal obstruction may have a fecal odor to the

vomitus. Gastric or duodenal ulcers may cause blood in vomitus (hematemesis).

For females: Could you be pregnant?

Pregnancy should be ruled out as a cause of nausea and vomiting. Pregnant women have high serum levels of chorionic gonadotropin, which stimulates vomiting.

Do you have nausea without vomiting?

Nausea without vomiting is a common symptom of pregnant patients or those with metastatic disease.

Which foods have you eaten in the last 24 hours? Where did you eat? How long after you ate did you vomit? Has anyone else who ate with you had these symptoms over the same time period?

These questions are asked to detect food poisoning or stomach influenza.

Do you have other symptoms with the nausea or vomiting? Pain? Constipation? Diarrhea? Change in color of stools? Change in color of urine? Fever or chills?

Knowing related symptoms may help determine the cause of nausea and vomiting. For example, liver disease may change stool color from brown to tan and an infection such as hepatitis may cause fever and chills.

Indigestion or Heartburn

How long after eating do you have indigestion or heartburn? Where do you feel the discomfort? In your stomach? Chest? How long has this been happening? How often does this occur?

Heartburn felt in the chest, over the esophagus, or in the stomach that occurs after eating may indicate GERD.

What makes the symptoms worse? Does a change in position such as lying down affect your indigestion?

Heartburn caused by GERD or hiatal hernia is often worse when the patient lies down because the gastric acids move by gravity toward the esophagus.

What relieves these symptoms?

When acid-reducing drugs relieve the indigestion, excessive acid may be the cause.

Are there other symptoms that occur with the heartburn? Radiating pain? Sweating? Light-headedness?

Knowing related symptoms may help determine the cause of indigestion. Angina or myocardial infarction may be the cause of the "indigestion-like" symptoms that are not relieved by taking antacids. Questions about radiating pain to the arms or jaw, along with other questions, are asked with these cardiovascular disorders in mind.

Abdominal Distention

How long has your abdomen been distended? Does it come and go? Is it related to eating? What relieves the distention?

Answers to these questions may help determine the cause of the distention. Constipation contributes to distention and develops slowly but is not relieved without bowel movement. Distention caused by ascites is a progressive process and increases abdominal girth.

Are other symptoms related to the abdominal distention? Vomiting? Loss of appetite? Weight loss? Change in bowel habits? Shortness of breath? Abdominal pain?

Vomiting may indicate intestinal obstruction as a cause of distention. Loss of appetite occurs with cirrhosis and malignancy. Shortness of breath is associated with heart failure and with ascites that occur with chronic liver disease.

Change in Bowel Habits

Describe the change in your bowel movements. Change in frequency? Change in consistency of stool (feces)?

Changes in bowel habits can be related to a number of factors, including changes in diet, activity, stress, and medications. A change in bowel habits is one of the seven warning signs of cancer.

When did you first notice the change? What does the stool look like: bloody, mucoid, fatty, watery?

Answers to these questions may help determine the cause of the change in bowel function.

Watery diarrhea containing blood, mucus, and pus may indicate ulcerative colitis, whereas a greater-than-expected amount of fat in the stool (steatorrhea) may indicate pancreatitis.

Are there related symptoms such as increased gas, pain, fever, nausea, vomiting, abdominal cramping, or diarrhea? Is there a time of day when the change occurs, such as after eating or at night?

Knowing related symptoms may help determine the cause of the change in bowel function. Some foods cause increased gas, fever suggests inflammation or infection, and abdominal cramping with diarrhea may indicate gastroenteritis.

Yellow Discoloration of Eyes or Skin (Jaundice)

When did you first notice the yellow discoloration of your skin or eyes?

Jaundice indicates elevated serum bilirubin that can be caused by liver disease or obstruction of bile flow from gallstones.

Is the yellow discoloration of your skin or eyes associated with abdominal pain, loss of appetite, nausea, vomiting, or fever?

Fever, nausea, vomiting, and loss of appetite are signs and symptoms of hepatitis.

In the last year, have you had a blood transfusion or tattoos? Are you using any intravenous drugs?

These are possible sources of transmission of the hepatitis B and C viruses.

RISK FACTORS

Liver and Pancreatic Cancers

Liver Cancer
- *Gender:* Men develop this cancer more often than women.
- *Race:* In the United States Asian Americans and Pacific Islanders have the highest rate of this cancer.
- *Liver disease:* Hepatitis B and C infections or cirrhosis increase the risk. (M)
- *Heavy alcohol use:* Alcohol abuse is a leading cause of cirrhosis in the United States, which, in turn, is linked with an increased risk of liver cancer. (M)
- *Obesity:* Risk probably increases because obesity can result in fatty liver disease and cirrhosis. (M)
- *Type 2 diabetes mellitus:* Risk increases in combination with other risk factors such as heavy alcohol use and/or chronic hepatitis. There is additional risk when people with type 2 diabetes are overweight or obese, which can cause liver problems.
- *Smoking:* The risk increases with smoking. (M)

Pancreatic Cancer
- *Smoking:* One of the most important risk factors is smoking. (M)
- *Obesity:* Obese people are approximately 20% more likely to develop this cancer. (M)
- *Workplace exposure to certain chemicals:* Heavy exposure to certain pesticides, dyes, and chemicals used in metal refining may increase the risk. (M)
- *Age:* The average age of diagnosis is 70 years.
- *Gender:* Men are slightly more likely to develop this cancer due in part to higher tobacco use.
- *Race:* African Americans are slightly more likely to develop this cancer than whites partly because of higher rates of smoking, obesity, and type 2 diabetes.
- *Family history:* While pancreatic cancer seems to occur in some families, most people who develop it do not have a family history.
- *Genetic syndromes:* Inherited gene changes (mutations) can be passed from parent to child. These abnormal genes may cause as many as 10% of this cancer.
- *Type 2 Diabetes mellitus:* Pancreatic cancer is more common in people who have diabetes. The reason is not known.

M, Modifiable risk factor.
Data from https://www.cancer.org/cancer/bladder-cancer/causes-risks-prevention/risk-factors.html. Last revised 1/30/19.

Do you eat raw shellfish (e.g., oysters)? Have you traveled abroad in the last year? Where? Did you drink unclean water?

These are possible sources of transmission of the hepatitis A virus.

Has the color of your urine or stools changed?

Urine changing color from amber to brown and stools changing color from brown to tan suggest high serum bilirubin, which occurs with liver disease or obstruction of the common bile duct.

RISK FACTORS

Bladder Cancer

- *Smoking:* The greatest risk factor for this cancer is smoking. (M)
- *Workplace exposures:* Chemicals sometimes used in the dye industry called aromatic amines, such as benzidine and beta-naphthylamine, can cause this cancer. *(M)*
- *Not drinking enough fluids:* People who drink a lot of fluid daily have a low rate of bladder cancer. This is thought to be because they empty their bladders often to keep chemicals from lingering in their bodies. (M)
- *Race:* Whites are 2 times more likely to develop this cancer than African Americans and Hispanic Americans.
- *Age:* Risk increases with age. Approximately 9 out of 10 people with this cancer are older than 55.
- *Gender:* Men get this cancer more often than women.
- *Chronic bladder irritation and inflammation:* Urinary tract infections, kidney and bladder stones, and bladder catheters left in place a long time are linked to this cancer.
- *Genetics and family history:* People who have family members with this cancer have an increased risk.

M, Modifiable risk factor.
American Cancer Society: Can colorectal cancer be prevented? Retrieved from https://www.cancer.org/cancer/colon-rectal-cancer/causes-risks-prevention/prevention.html. Last revised 5/30/18. Centers for Disease Control and Prevention: Colorectal cancer screening tests. Retrieved from: https://www.cdc.gov/cancer/colorectal/basic_info/screening/tests.htm. Last reviewed 2/4/19.

Problems with Urination

Describe the change in your urination. Have you felt any pain or burning when urinating? Are you urinating frequently in small amounts (frequency) or feeling you cannot wait to urinate (urgency)? If yes, when did this begin?
Pain, burning, or frequency may indicate a bladder infection. Loss of muscle tone may cause incontinence, particularly in women. Men who have an enlarged prostate may have difficulty initiating or maintaining their urinary stream (see Chapter 17).

Have you had any related signs or symptoms such as fever, chills, and back pain?
These signs and symptoms may indicate a kidney disorder such as pyelonephritis or kidney stones.

Describe the color of the urine. Is there blood in the urine?
Dark amber urine may occur with kidney or liver disease. Blood in the urine is associated with menstrual periods in women or with kidney disease.

Have you had an unexplained weight gain? Have you noticed swelling in your ankles at the end of the day or shortness of breath? Are you urinating less?
These clinical manifestations may indicate renal failure when kidney dysfunction causes fluid retention.

HEALTH PROMOTION FOR EVIDENCE–BASED PRACTICE

Colorectal Cancer

Recommendations to Reduce Risk of Colorectal Cancer (Primary Prevention)
An individual can lower the risk of developing colorectal cancer by managing controllable risk factors such as diet and physical activity. Information to share with patients includes the following:
- Consume diet high in fruits, vegetables, and whole-grain foods; limit intake of high-fat foods.
- Participate in moderate-to-vigorous activity for 30 minutes 5 days or more a week.
- Attain and maintain a healthy weight.
- Do not smoke.
- Limit alcohol to no more than 2 drinks per day for men and one drink per day for women.

Screening Recommendations (Secondary Prevention)
Men and women of average risk should be screened from ages 45 to 75. Adults aged 76–85 should consult their care provider about screening. Screening tests can be used to find polyps or colorectal cancer. The care provider can determine which of the following tests is appropriate for each person:
- Fecal occult blood test (FOBT) annually
- Flexible sigmoidoscopy every 5 years
- Colonoscopy every 10 years
- Computed tomography (CT) colonoscopy (virtual colonoscopy) every 5 years
- For individuals with higher risk, screening should begin earlier.

Data from uspreventiveservicestaskforce.org/uspstf/draft-recommemdation/coloractal-cancer-screening3, 2020; cancer.org/cancer/colon-rectal-cancer.html, 2020.

EXAMINATION

Routine techniques

- OBSERVE patient's general appearance, behavior, and position.
- INSPECT the abdomen.
- AUSCULTATE the abdomen.
- PALPATE the abdomen lightly.
- PALPATE the abdomen deeply.

Techniques for special circumstances

- PERCUSS the abdomen.
- PERCUSS the liver.
- PERCUSS the spleen.
- PALPATE the liver.
- PALPATE the gallbladder.
- PALPATE the spleen.
- PALPATE the kidneys.
- PERCUSS the kidneys.

Techniques Performed by an APRN

- ASSESS the abdomen for fluid.
- ASSESS for abdominal pain caused by inflammation.
- ASSESS the abdomen for a floating mass.

Equipment Needed

- Stethoscope • Penlight • Tape measure • Marking pen • Centimeter ruler

APRN, Advanced Practice Registered Nurse.

PROCEDURES WITH EXPECTED FINDINGS

ROUTINE TECHNIQUES: ABDOMEN

PERFORM hand hygiene.

OBSERVE patient's general appearance, behavior, and position.

The patient should appear well-nourished, lying supine quietly with slow, even respirations, and skin tone appropriate for race.

INSPECT the abdomen for skin color, surface characteristics, and venous patterns.

Skin color may be paler than other parts of the skin because of lack of exposure.

ABNORMAL FINDINGS

Findings such as emaciation, obesity, distended abdomen, marked restlessness, a rigid posture, knees drawn up, facial grimacing, and rapid respirations may require further evaluation. Patients with gallstones or ureteral stones may be restless, those with peritonitis or appendicitis may lie very still, patients with pancreatitis may prefer the knee-chest position, and those with intestinal obstruction may have rapid respirations[12] Jaundice skin tone may suggest liver disease or obstructed bile duct.

Jaundice may indicate liver disease, erythema may indicate inflammation, bruises may indicate trauma or low platelet count, and striae may indicate abdominal distention.

PROCEDURES WITH EXPECTED FINDINGS

Surface characteristics should be smooth. Silver-white striae, scars, and a very faint, fine vascular network may be present. The umbilicus should be centrally located (Fig. 13.4). The pattern of veins of the abdomen is usually barely visible.

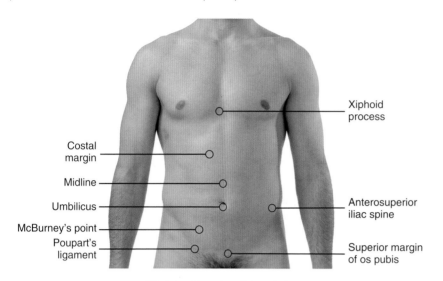

Xiphoid process

Costal margin

Midline

Umbilicus

McBurney's point

Poupart's ligament

Anterosuperior iliac spine

Superior margin of os pubis

FIG. 13.4 Landmarks of the abdomen.

INSPECT the abdomen for contour.

Contour is the view of the abdomen from the rib margin to the pelvis, viewed on a horizontal plane, which requires use of several procedures.

Adjusting the light source to form shadows may highlight small changes in the contour.
Procedure: Evaluate symmetry by viewing the abdomen from two additional angles: standing behind the patient's head and squatting at the side to view the abdomen at eye level.
Findings: Expected contours may be described as flat, rounded, or scaphoid. A flat contour is found in muscular, athletic adults. A rounded contour is a result of subcutaneous fat or poor muscle tone. A scaphoid contour is seen in thin adults.[11]

Procedure: Ask the patient to take a deep breath and hold it. This maneuver lowers the diaphragm and compresses the organs of the abdominal cavity.
Findings: The contour of the abdomen should remain smooth and symmetric.

Procedure and findings: Ask the patient to raise his or her head. This contracts the rectus abdominis muscles, which reveals a muscle prominence in thin or athletic adults.

Procedure and findings: When abdominal distention is noticed, place a measuring tape around the abdomen at the level of the superior iliac crests to measure the abdominal girth (circumference). This provides an objective measure to assess the increase or decrease in abdominal distention.

INSPECT the abdomen for surface movements.

Peristalsis is usually not visible, but an upper midline pulsation may be visible in thin individuals. The abdomen should move smoothly and evenly with respirations. Generally, females exhibit thoracic movements during inhalation, whereas males exhibit abdominal movements. Areas of bulges are considered expected variations in pregnancy and marked obesity.

ABNORMAL FINDINGS

The umbilicus should not be displaced upward, downward, or laterally; nor should a hernia be visible around or slightly above the umbilicus. An inverted umbilicus is often a sign of increased abdominal pressure, usually from ascites or a large mass. Glistening or taut appearance is associated with ascites. Notice prominent venous patterns or engorgement of the veins around the umbilicus. In patients with portal hypertension, the veins are dilated and appear to radiate from the umbilicus.[12]

Generalized distention may occur as a result of obesity, enlarged organs, or fluid or gas. Check for marked concavity, which is associated with general wasting signs or anteroposterior rib expansion.

This maneuver may cause previously unseen bulges or masses to appear. Superficial abdominal wall masses may become visible. If a hernia is present, the increased abdominal pressure may cause it to protrude.[12] Abdominal distention may result from the "seven Fs": fat (obesity), fetus (pregnancy), fluid (ascites), flatulence (gas), feces (stool) (constipation), fibroid tumor, or fatal tumor. Notice any bulges or masses, particularly of the liver or spleen. Abdominal or incisional hernias can also create bulges of the abdomen.

Notice visible peristalsis or marked pulsations. The area of pulsation observed is not palpated because it may indicate an abdominal aneurysm (i.e., a weakening in the wall of the abdominal aorta). Grunting or labored movements or restricted abdominal movements with respirations should be evaluated.

PROCEDURES WITH EXPECTED FINDINGS

AUSCULTATE the abdomen for bowel sounds.

Auscultate *before* palpating the abdomen so the presence or absence of bowel sounds or pain is not altered. A quiet environment may be necessary. The value of bowel sounds has been questioned. This assessment was found not to be useful in clinical practice in differentiating patients with normal versus pathologic bowel sounds (post-operative ileus or bowel obstruction).[13,14]

Procedure: Clean the diaphragm and bell of your stethoscope. Use the diaphragm of the stethoscope and press lightly. Listening in all four quadrants of the abdomen is not necessary, because a bowel sound heard in the one quadrant may originate in another quadrant.[15]

Findings: Notice the presence of bowel sounds. They may vary from moment to moment; there may be no bowel sounds for up to 4 minutes or more than 30 discrete sounds per minute.[15] The sounds are high-pitched gurgles or clicks, although this varies greatly.

Report absence of sound after listening for several minutes. Decreased or absent bowel sounds occur with mechanical obstruction or paralytic ileus and with peritonitis and bowel obstruction. Audible sounds produced by hyperactive peristalsis are termed *borborygmi* and create rumbling, gurgling, and high-pitched tinkling sounds.

AUSCULTATE the abdomen for arterial and venous vascular sounds.

Procedure: Listen with the bell of the stethoscope. For arterial vascular sounds, listen over aorta and renal, iliac, and femoral arteries for bruits. They make "swishing" sounds, during systole, and are continuous, regardless of the patient's position (Fig. 13.5). For venous vascular sounds, listen over the epigastric region and around the umbilicus for a venous hum (i.e., a soft, low-pitched, and continuous sound).[16]

Findings: Normally vascular sounds are not heard. Bruits occur in 4%–20% of healthy people.[15]

A bruit indicates a turbulent blood flow caused by narrowing of a blood vessel. Bruits over the aorta suggest an aneurysm. Venous hums are soft, low pitched, and continuous. They are associated with portal hypertension and cirrhosis.[16]

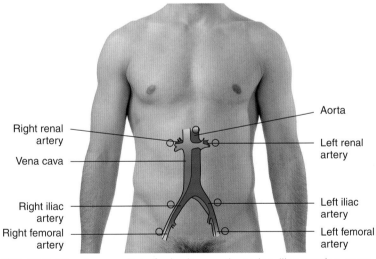

Right renal artery
Vena cava
Right iliac artery
Right femoral artery
Aorta
Left renal artery
Left iliac artery
Left femoral artery

FIG. 13.5 Sites to auscultate for bruits: renal arteries, iliac arteries, aorta, and femoral arteries.

PALPATE the abdomen lightly for tenderness and muscle tone.

Procedure: Before palpation warm your hands. Some nurses ask patients to bend their knees to relax the abdominal muscles. Palpate all quadrants of the abdomen. Fig. 13.6 shows the quarters of the abdomen, and Box 13.1 lists the anatomic correlates of the quarters of the abdomen. Use the pads of the fingertips to depress the abdomen 1 cm (0.4 inches) (Fig. 13.7). Keep the fingers together and lift the hand from one area to another instead of sliding over the abdominal wall.[12] When the patient has reported abdominal pain, palpate over the area of pain last. Some nurses reduce ticklishness by sliding their hands into each palpation position to maintain contact with the patient's skin. Another approach is to have the patient place his or her hand atop the nurse's hand as all quadrants are palpated.

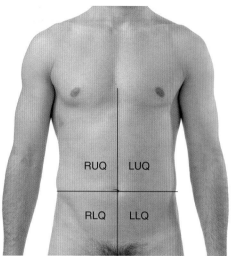

FIG. 13.6 Quadrants of the abdomen. *LLQ*, Left lower quadrant; *LUQ*, left upper quadrant; *RLQ*, right lower quadrant; *RUQ*, right upper quadrant.

BOX 13.1 ANATOMIC CORRELATES OF THE QUADRANTS OF THE ABDOMEN

Right Upper Quadrant
Liver and gallbladder
Pylorus
Duodenum
Head of pancreas
Right adrenal gland
Portion of right kidney
Portions of ascending and
    transverse colon

Left Upper Quadrant
Left lobe of liver
Spleen
Stomach
Body of pancreas
Left adrenal gland
Portion of left kidney
Portions of transverse and
    descending colon

Right Lower Quadrant
Lower pole of right kidney
Cecum and appendix
Portion of ascending colon
Bladder (if distended)
Right ureter
Right ovary and salpinx
Uterus (if enlarged)
Right spermatic cord

Left Lower Quadrant
Lower pole of left kidney
Sigmoid colon
Portion of descending colon
Bladder (if distended)
Left ureter
Left ovary and salpinx
Uterus (if enlarged)
Left spermatic cord

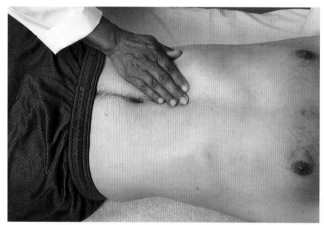

FIG. 13.7 Light palpation of the abdomen.

PROCEDURES WITH EXPECTED FINDINGS

Findings: No tenderness should be present, and the abdominal muscles should be relaxed, although anxious patients may have some muscle resistance on palpation.

PALPATE the abdomen deeply for pain, masses, and aortic pulsation.

Procedure: Palpate all quadrants. Use either the distal flat portions of the finger pads (Fig. 13.8) and press gradually and deeply (4–6 cm, or 1.6–2.4 inches) into the palpation area, or use a bimanual technique with the lower hand resting lightly on the surface and the upper hand exerting pressure for deep palpation (Fig. 13.9). When the patient has abdominal pain, palpate over the area of pain last. Observe for facial grimaces during palpation that may indicate areas of pain. Ask the patient to breathe slowly through the mouth to facilitate muscle relaxation.

ABNORMAL FINDINGS

Notice any cutaneous tenderness or hypersensitivity. Superficial masses or localized areas of rigidity or increased tension may require further evaluation. Rigidity is associated with peritoneal irritation and may be diffuse or localized.

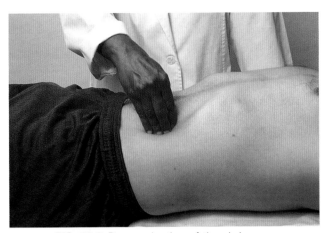

FIG. 13.8 Deep palpation of the abdomen.

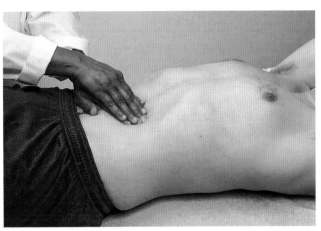

FIG. 13.9 Deep bimanual palpation.

PROCEDURES WITH EXPECTED FINDINGS

Findings: No pain or masses are expected during deep palpation. The aorta is often palpable at the epigastrium and above and slightly to the left of the umbilicus (Fig. 13.10). The borders of the rectus abdominis muscles can be felt, as can the sacral promontory and stool in the ascending or descending colon.

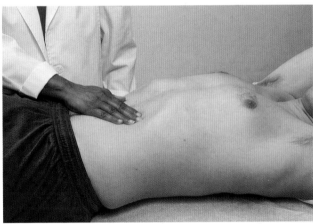

FIG. 13.10 Palpating the aorta.

Techniques for Special Circumstances: Abdomen
PERCUSS the abdomen for tones.

Percuss the abdomen when distention, fluid, or solid masses is suspected or when patient reports pain in the abdomen.

Procedure: See Chapter 3 for the procedures for percussion. Using a clockwise pattern, percuss all quadrants for tones, using indirect percussion to assess density of abdominal contents. Percuss in each quadrant for tympany and dullness.

Findings: Tympany is the most common percussion tone heard and is caused by the presence of gas. The suprapubic area may be dull when the urinary bladder is distended.

ABNORMAL FINDINGS

The patient may respond to pain by muscle guarding (tensing abdominal muscles during palpation), facial grimaces, or pulling away from the nurse. Abnormal findings include masses that descend during inspiration, lateral pulsatile masses (abdominal aortic aneurysm), laterally mobile masses, and fixed masses.

Any marked dullness in a localized area may indicate distention, fluid, or an abdominal mass.

PROCEDURES WITH EXPECTED FINDINGS	ABNORMAL FINDINGS

PERCUSS the liver to determine span and descent.

Percuss the liver when enlargement is suspected.

Procedure:

1. Beginning below the level of the umbilicus at the right midclavicular line (RMCL), percuss upward until the tone changes from a tympany to a dull percussion tone, indicating the liver border. Mark the border with a pen. The lower border is usually at the costal margin or slightly below it (Fig. 13.11A).
2. Beginning over the lung in the RMCL, percuss the intercostal spaces downward until the tone changes from resonant to dull, indicating the upper liver border. Mark the location with a pen. The upper border usually begins in the fifth to seventh intercostal space (Fig. 13.11B).
3. Measure the span between the two lines using a ruler or tape measure to estimate the midclavicular liver span.
4. To assess the liver descent, ask the patient to take a deep breath and hold it; then percuss upward from the stomach to the RMCL. The percussed liver span is dependent on the nurse's technique; the heavier the nurse's percussion stroke, the smaller the measured span and the greater the error in underestimating actual liver size.[15]

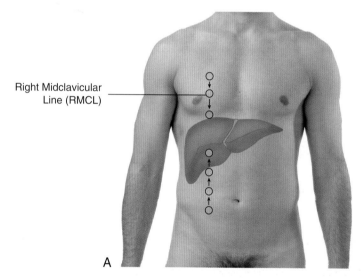

Right Midclavicular
Line (RMCL)

A

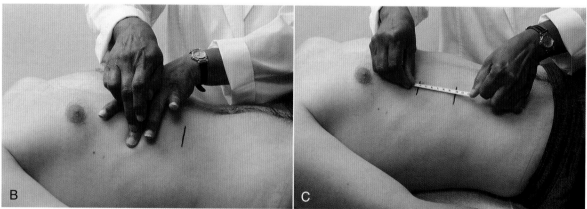

B

C

FIG. 13.11 (A) Liver percussion route. (B) Percussion method of estimating size of liver in the midclavicular line. (C) Distance between the two marks measured in estimating the liver span in midclavicular line is usually 6 to 12 cm.

PROCEDURES WITH EXPECTED FINDINGS

Findings: The midclavicular liver span is expected to be 6–12 cm (approximately 2.5–5 inches) (Fig. 13.11C). Liver span correlates with body size and gender, with large people and men tending to have larger spans. The lower border of the liver is expected to descend downward 0.4–0.8 inch (2–3 cm).

PERCUSS the spleen for size.

Perform this procedure when enlargement is suspected.

Procedure: With the patient lying supine, percuss in the lowest intercostal space just posterior to the left midaxillary line (LMAL) (Fig. 13.12). Try to outline the spleen by percussing in several directions from dullness to resonance or tympany. Percuss the lowest intercostal space in the left anterior axillary line before and after the patient takes a deep breath. Notice whether the tympany changes to dullness on inspiration.

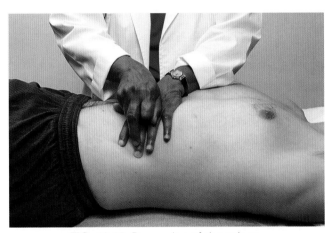

FIG. 13.12 Percussion of the spleen.

Findings: Normally, the spleen cannot be percussed, or you may hear a small area of splenic dullness at the sixth to the tenth intercostal spaces. A full stomach or stool in the transverse or descending colon may mimic dullness of splenic enlargement. The area is usually tympanic during inspiration and expiration.

PALPATE the liver for lower border and pain.

Perform this procedure when liver enlargement is suspected.

Procedure: Two techniques may be used to palpate the liver.

1. Begin by placing the left hand under the eleventh and twelfth ribs to lift the liver closer to the abdominal wall. Place your right hand parallel to the right costal margin and press down and under the costal margin (Fig. 13.13A and B) (see Fig. 13.4 for costal margin location). Ask the patient to take deep breaths. Try to feel the liver edge as the diaphragm pushes it down to meet your fingertips.[16]

2. Another technique is called the *hooking technique.* Stand on the patient's right side facing the feet. Place your hands side by side at the right costal margin and curve your fingers to "hook" them under the costal margin. Ask the patient to take a deep breath (Fig. 13.13C).

ABNORMAL FINDINGS

An enlarged liver (hepatomegaly) is indicated when the lower border of the liver exceeds 2–3 cm (0.75–1 inch) below the costal margin. This enlargement may be associated with cirrhosis and hepatitis. In addition, patients with chronic obstructive pulmonary disease may have a flat diaphragm, which makes percussion of the upper border of the liver difficult. Obesity can also make percussion difficult.

An enlarged spleen is brought forward on inspiration to produce a dull percussion tone.

Common causes of an enlarged spleen are hepatic disease (e.g., portal hypertension), hematologic disorders (e.g., leukemia or lymphomas), infectious disease (e.g., human immunodeficiency virus (HIV) infection), or primary splenic disorders (e.g., splenic infarction or hematoma).[15]

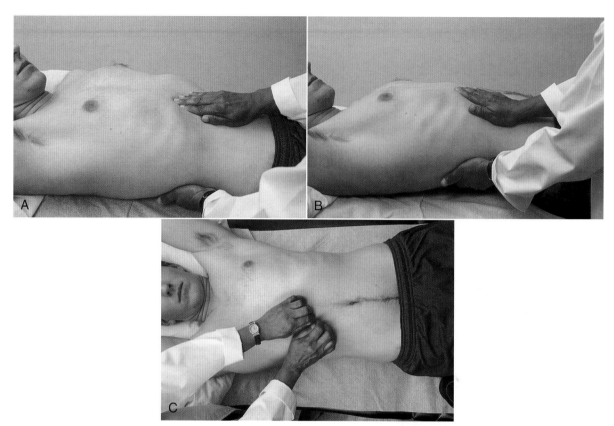

FIG. 13.13 Methods of palpating the liver. (A) Fingers are extended, with tips on right midclavicular line below the level of liver tenderness and pointing toward the head. (B) Fingers parallel to the costal margin. (C) Fingers hooked over the costal margin.

PROCEDURES WITH EXPECTED FINDINGS

Findings: You may feel the liver "bump" against your fingers when the patient takes a deep breath. The border of the liver should feel smooth; however, the border and contour of the liver often are not palpable. No pain should be present.

PALPATE the gallbladder for pain.

Perform this procedure when right upper quadrant (RUQ) pain or enlargement is suspected.
Procedure: Palpate below the liver margin at the right lateral border of the rectus abdominis muscle for the gallbladder.
Findings: A healthy gallbladder is not palpable.

ABNORMAL FINDINGS

A very enlarged liver may lie under your hand as it extends downward into the abdominal cavity. Notice any irregular surfaces or edges and any tenderness. The patient may complain of pain when taking a deep breath during this assessment.

A palpable, painful gallbladder may indicate cholecystitis. Test for cholecystitis by asking the patient to take a deep breath during deep palpation of the RUQ. If the patient experiences pain and abruptly stops inhaling during palpation, then cholecystitis is suspected. This test is called Murphy sign. A nontender, enlarged gallbladder suggests common bile duct obstruction.[15,16]

PROCEDURES WITH EXPECTED FINDINGS

PALPATE the spleen for border and pain.

Palpate the spleen when pain or enlargement is suspected.

Procedure: Standing at the patient's right side, reach across the patient to place the palmar surface of your left hand under his or her left flank at the costovertebral angle and exert pressure upward to elevate the left rib cage and move the spleen anteriorly. Press the palmar surface of your right hand gently under the left anterior costal margin (Fig. 13.14). Press your fingertips inward toward the spleen as the patient takes a deep breath. Try to feel the tip of the spleen as it descends during inspiration.

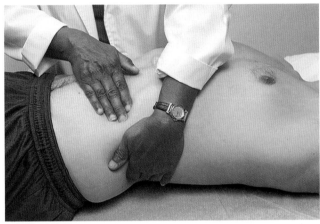

FIG. 13.14 Palpation of the spleen.

An alternative strategy for spleen palpation is to perform the procedure with the patient lying on the right side with the legs and knees flexed. Stand on the patient's right and place your left hand over his or her left costovertebral angle while pressing your right hand under the left anterior costal margin.

Findings: The spleen is normally not palpable.

A palpable spleen feels like a firm mass that bumps against your fingers. Spleen pain may indicate infection or trauma.

PALPATE the kidneys for contour and pain.

Perform this procedure when the patient reports pain in back (flank pain).

Procedure:

Left kidney: Stand to the patient's right side with the patient in a supine position. Place the left hand at the left posterior costal angle (left flank) and the right hand at the patient's left anterior costal margin (see Fig. 13.4). Ask the patient to take a deep breath, elevate his or her left flank with your left hand, and palpate deeply with your right hand (Fig. 13.15).

Right kidney: Repeat the same maneuver on the right side, which is easier to palpate because the right kidney lies lower than the left kidney.

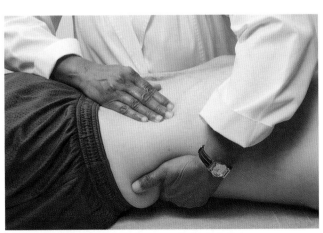

FIG. 13.15 Palpation of the left kidney.

PROCEDURES WITH EXPECTED FINDINGS

Findings: Normally, the kidney is not palpable. Occasionally, the lower pole of the kidney can be felt during inhalation in thin patients but rarely in the average patient. The contour should be smooth with no pain.

PERCUSS the kidneys for costovertebral angle pain.

Perform this procedure when the patient reports pain in back (flank pain).

Procedure: Approach the patient from behind as he or she is seated. One method for percussion is the direct approach. Use direct percussion to tap each costovertebral angle (CVA) with the ulnar surface of the dominant fist (Fig. 13.16A). An alternative method is to use indirect percussion. Place the palmar surface of the nondominant hand over the CVA and tap the dorsum of that hand with the dominant fist (Fig. 13.16B).

Fig. 13.17 shows the underlying anatomy of the kidney in relation to the CVA or the flank.

Findings: The patient should report a thud but no pain.

ABNORMAL FINDINGS

Pain is associated with kidney trauma or infection (e.g., pyelonephritis or glomerulonephritis).

CVA pain may indicate pyelonephritis, glomerulonephritis, or nephrolithiasis (kidney stones).

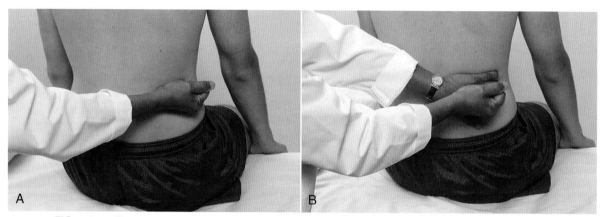

FIG. 13.16 Fist percussion of costovertebral angle for kidney tenderness. (A) Direct percussion. (B) Indirect percussion.

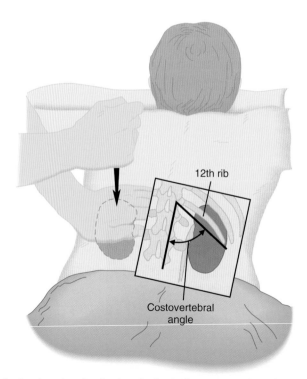

FIG. 13.17 Anatomic drawing showing landmarks for indirect percussion of the costovertebral angle. (From Black and Hawks, 2005.)

TECHNIQUES PERFORMED BY AN ADVANCED PRACTICE REGISTERED NURSE

Specialty practice may require advanced techniques that are beyond the skill set of a nurse generalist. Knowing the purposes of these techniques may be helpful when caring for patients who require advanced assessment techniques.

- **Assess the abdomen for fluid.** Assess for *shifting dullness* when fluid in the peritoneal cavity (ascites) is suspected. Assess for *fluid wave* when ascites is confirmed and the fluid wave resembles fluid moving within the abdomen from one side to the other.
- **Assess the abdomen for pain caused by inflammation.** The following techniques are performed if the patient has abdominal pain that may be caused by inflammation:
  - Test for *rebound tenderness.* Rebound tenderness is present if the patient experiences more pain when pressure applied to the abdomen is released than when pressure is exerted, indicating peritoneal inflammation.
  - **Iliopsoas muscle test.** This technique is performed when appendicitis is suspected. When the patient reports RLQ pain to pressure against the raised leg, his or her iliopsoas muscle is irritated, indicating an inflamed appendix.
  - **Obturator muscle test.** When a ruptured appendix or pelvic abscess is suspected, this technique is performed. Pain in the hypogastric region when the right leg is rotated is a positive sign indicating irritation of the obturator muscle.
- **Assess the abdomen for a floating mass.** Ballottement is a palpation technique used to determine a floating mass, which may be an abnormal growth or a fetal head.

DOCUMENTING EXPECTED FINDINGS

Abdomen smooth, flat, and lighter color than extremities, with smooth, symmetric contour and no visible peristalsis. Umbilicus midline and rectus abdominis muscles prominent when head raised. Bowel sounds present with no vascular sounds. No tenderness, masses, or aortic pulsations to light or deep abdominal palpation. Umbilical ring feels round with no irregularities or bulges. Tympany in all quadrants. Liver span 3 inches. Unable to percuss spleen. Liver border smooth. Gallbladder, spleen, and kidneys not palpable.

CLINICAL JUDGMENT

Gastrointestinal System

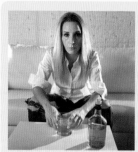

Case Presentation

Carla Wise, a 46-year-old female with a long-standing history of alcoholism, presents to the emergency department (ED) with severe abdominal pain that has been constant for the last 12 hours and several episodes of vomiting. She is screaming in pain and demanding pain medication. Her vital signs taken at triage were blood pressure 102/58 mm Hg; heart rate 120/minute; respiratory rate 24/minute; SpO2 99% on room air; temperature 100.0°F (37.7°C).

Reflecting

The nurse reflects on Ms. Wise's clinical presentation and this clinical encounter; she was subsequently diagnosed with acute pancreatitis and admitted to an inpatient unit. This experience contributes to the nurse's expertise when encountering a similar situation.

Noticing / Recognizing Cues

Based on the presenting information, the experienced nurse recognizes the emergent nature of Ms. Wise's condition. The nurse knows that patients with a long-standing history of alcoholism are at risk for gastrointestinal (GI) inflammation, bleeding, and liver disorders such as cirrhosis. The nurse also knows that inflammatory disorders can cause extreme pain. The ED nurse examines Ms. Wise's abdomen, noting that bowel sounds are hypoactive and the abdomen is distended, firm, and very tender with palpation. Her skin is warm and slightly diaphoretic.

Responding / Taking Action

The ED nurse initiates appropriate initial interventions (oxygen delivery, obtaining intravenous access) and notifies the ED physician of the situation, ensuring that Ms. Wise receives prompt medical care and pain relief.

Interpreting / Analyzing Cues & Forming Hypotheses

The nurse follows the cognitive cues, recalling that two gastrointestinal inflammatory disorders can cause extreme pain that often present in this way: pancreatitis and gastritis. To determine if either has any probability of being correct, the nurse gathers additional data:
- How is the pain described?
  Ms. Wise describes the pain as "…like sharp knives cutting me inside, and it goes into my back."
- What is the color and character of the emesis and of the stool?
  Ms. Wise describes her emesis as "yellowish green," but often she just has "dry heaves." She tells the nurse the stool from her last bowel movement was brown and formed.
- Are there any factors that aggravate or alleviate her symptoms?
  Ms. Wise indicates that nothing is helping – and any movement makes it worse.
The ED nurse not only recognizes pancreatitis by the clinical sign (severe unrelieved knife-like pain that radiates to the back) and symptoms (nausea, vomiting), but also interprets this information in the context of an adult with a history of alcohol misuse.

AGE-RELATED VARIATIONS

This chapter discusses assessment techniques with adult patients. These data are important to assess for individuals of all ages, but the approach and techniques used to collect the information may vary depending on the patient's age.

INFANTS, CHILDREN, AND ADOLESCENTS

Assessment techniques are the same for infants, children, and adolescents. There are several differences in the assessment findings in infants based on anatomic differences. Children and

adolescents may resist abdominal palpation because they are ticklish. Chapter 19 presents further information for assessing the GI and renal systems of infants, children, and adolescents.

OLDER ADULTS

Procedures and techniques for assessing an older adult are the same as for the younger adult. Chapter 21 presents further information regarding the assessments of these systems for this age group.

COMMON PROBLEMS AND CONDITIONS

ALIMENTARY TRACT

Gastroesophageal Reflux Disease

When acidic gastric secretions (with a pH 2–4) flow into the lower esophagus (with a pH 6–8), the mucosa is damaged. When this reflux of gastric secretion becomes chronic, GERD results. Fig 13.18A shows the lower esophageal sphincter in relation to the esophagus and stomach. Approximately 10% to 20% of people in the United States experience GERD symptoms at least once a week.[17] **Clinical Findings:** Patients complain of heartburn occurring more than twice weekly, regurgitation, and dysphagia (difficulty swallowing), which may interrupt sleep. GERD-related chest pain described as squeezing or radiating to the back, neck, jaw, or arms can mimic chest pain. However, when chest pain is relieved with antacids, angina is unlikely. Respiratory symptoms such as wheezing, coughing, and dyspnea may be reported.[17] Symptoms are aggravated by lying down, bending, and stooping and relieved by sitting up, antacids, and eating.

Hiatal Hernia

A protrusion of the stomach through the esophageal hiatus of the diaphragm into the mediastinal cavity is termed *hiatal hernia* (see Fig. 13.18). It is common in older adults and occurs more often in women. **Clinical Findings:** Clinical manifestations are the same as those of GERD: heartburn, regurgitation, and dysphagia.[17]

Peptic Ulcer Disease

An ulcer in the lower end of the esophagus, in the stomach, or in the duodenum is termed *peptic ulcer*. Approximately 500,000 new cases are diagnosed every year and 4 million cases of ulcer recurrence.[17] Duodenal ulcer is the more common form (Fig. 13.19). **Clinical Findings:** Patients with gastric ulcers complain of burning pain high in the epigastric area 1 to 2 hours after eating, often relieved with antacids. Patients with duodenal ulcers complain of burning pain in the mid-epigastric area and back 2 to 4 hours after eating and in the middle of the night; pain relief may occur after taking antacids or eating. The most common exam finding is epigastric pain during palpation.[17]

Crohn Disease

This chronic inflammatory bowel disease (IBD) is also called *regional enteritis* or *regional ileitis* (Fig. 13.20). The prevalence in the United States is 201 per 100,000 adults and is more common in women than men.[18] Inflammation may occur from mouth to anus, but it commonly affects the terminal ileum and colon. Affected mucosa is ulcerated, with presence of fistulas, fissures, and abscesses that may form adjacent to healthy bowel segments. **Clinical Findings:** This disorder is characterized by unpredictable periods of remission with relapses. While Crohn disease cannot be cured, it can be treated. Patients complain of severe abdominal cramping, diarrhea, and weight loss.[19]

Ulcerative Colitis

This chronic IBD starts in the rectum and progresses through the large intestine (Fig. 13.21). The prevalence in the United States is 238 per 100,000 adults and is more common in men

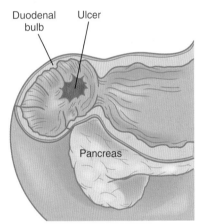

FIG. 13.19 Duodenal peptic ulcer. (From Lewis et al., 2014.)

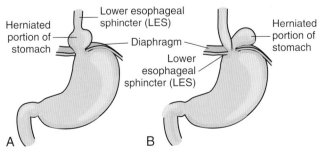

FIG. 13.18 Hiatal hernia. (A) Sliding hernia. (B) Paraesophageal. (From Monahan, 2007.)

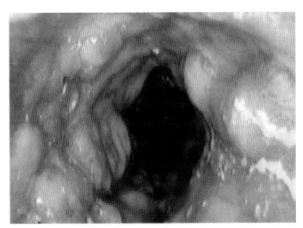

FIG. 13.20 Typical findings of advanced crohn disease showing erythema, edema, and a cobblestone appearance. (From Feldman, et al., 2020.)

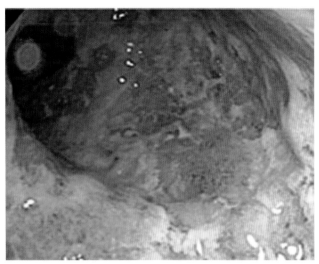

FIG. 13.21 Ulcerative colitis showing mucosal edema and inflammation with ulcerations. (From Parasothy, Kamm, Kaakoush, et al., 2017.)

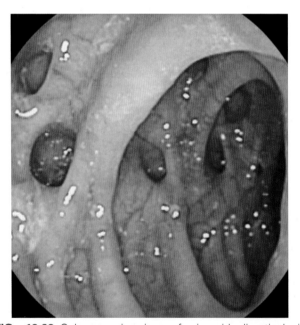

FIG. 13.22 Colonoscopic view of sigmoid diverticulosis showing herniations through the muscular wall of the colon. (From Ferri's Clinical Advisor 2019)

than women.[18] **Clinical Findings:** Ulcerative colitis is characterized by unpredictable periods of remission with relapses. Patients complain of severe, constant abdominal pain, fever during acute attacks, and rectal bleeding. The patient experiences profuse watery diarrhea of blood, mucus, and pus.[19]

Diverticulitis

Inflammation of diverticula is termed *diverticulitis*. Diverticula are herniations through the muscular wall in the colon (Fig. 13.22). Presence of fecal material through the thin-walled diverticula causes inflammation and abscesses.

Clinical Findings: Patients complain of pain in the LLQ; nausea; vomiting; and altered bowel habits, usually constipation. Examination findings include fever, decreased bowel sounds, with LLQ pain on palpation, palpable mass, and tympany to percussion.[16,19]

Colorectal Cancer

Malignant tumors arising in the mucosa of the rectum or colon are collectively referred to as colorectal cancer. An estimated 148,000 new cases of colorectal cancer were diagnosed in 2020; and over 53,000 people died from these cancers in 2020, making it the third leading cause of cancer-related deaths. **Clinical Findings:** Most cases of colorectal cancer are diagnosed through screening among asymptomatic patients. Symptoms of advanced disease depend on the location and size of the malignancy but may include blood in the stool, a change in the bowel habits (constipation), changes in consistency of stool, abdominal pain or bloating, fatigue, and weight loss.[20]

HEPATOBILIARY SYSTEM

Viral Hepatitis

The most common types of viral infection of the liver are hepatitis A (HAV), hepatitis B (HBV), and hepatitis C (HCV). In 2014 there were an estimated 2500 new cases of HAV. In that same year there were an estimated 19,200 new cases of acute HBV and 850,000 to 2.2 million cases of chronic HBV, and 30,500 new cases of acute HCV and 2.7 to 3.9 million cases of chronic HCV. **Clinical Findings:** Common symptoms of all types of hepatitis are anorexia, abdominal pain, nausea, vomiting, fatigue, and fever. Jaundice, tan-colored stools, and dark urine may also be reported.[21] An enlarged liver may be also be detected on palpation.[16]

Cirrhosis

Cirrhosis is characterized by diffuse destruction of liver cells that are replaced by fibrotic scar tissue and regenerative nodules. Fig. 13.23 illustrates the cobblestone appearance of the cirrhotic liver that results in impaired liver function and blood flow. Cirrhosis is an end-stage liver disease seen in patients with diseases such as chronic hepatitis or alcoholic liver disease.[22] From 1999 to 2016, the United States annual deaths from cirrhosis increased 65% to 34,174. During this period

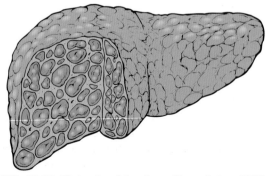

FIG. 13.23 Cirrhosis of the liver. (From Salvo, 2009.)

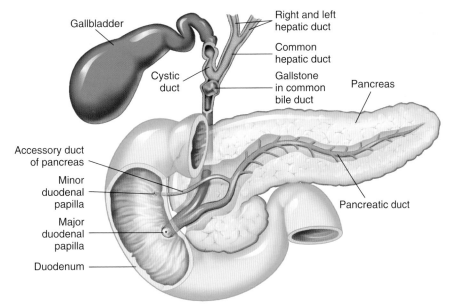

FIG. 13.24 The gallstone in the common bile duct. (Courtesy Kissane, 1990. From Thibodeau and Patton, 2003.)

people aged 25 to 34 years had the highest annual increase in deaths from cirrhosis driven by alcohol-rated liver disease.[23] **Clinical Findings:** Indications in the early stages are enlarged liver and fatigue. In the later stages, jaundice with dark urine and tan-colored stool and ascites develop as well as spider angiomas. Portal hypertension contributes to spleen enlargement, which results in thrombocytopenia, anemia, and leukopenia.[22]

Cholecystitis With Cholelithiasis

Inflammation of the gallbladder is termed *cholecystitis* and is usually associated with gallstones, a condition termed *cholelithiasis* (Fig. 13.24). The bile duct becomes obstructed by either edema from inflammation or gallstones. An estimated 10% of Americans have cholecystitis caused by cholelithiasis. **Clinical Findings:** The primary symptom is pain in the RUQ in the abdomen that may radiate the right shoulder or scapula. Related symptoms may include nausea, vomiting, restlessness, and diaphoresis. Other indications include indigestion and mild transient jaundice. Abdominal rigidity, RUQ tenderness, palpable gallbladder, and positive Murphy sign may be found during examination.[12, 22]

PANCREAS

Pancreatitis

Acute or chronic inflammation of the pancreas is called *pancreatitis*; see Fig. 13.24 for how the location of gallstones could move to obstruct the flow of digestive enzymes from the pancreas. The annual incidence of acute pancreatitis ranges from 13 to 45/100,000 persons and of chronic pancreatitis is approximately 50/100,000. The prevalence of chronic pancreatitis is approximately 50/1000 persons.[24] **Clinical Findings:** Patients complain of sudden onset of severe pain, described as steady, boring, dull, or sharp, that radiates to the

back. Pain becomes worse with intake of food. Patients prefer knee-chest position. Related symptoms include nausea and vomiting. Vital signs indicate fever, tachycardia, and hypotension. Findings on examination include ascites, jaundice, decreased-to-absent bowel sounds, and abdominal tenderness with guarding.[22]

URINARY SYSTEM

Urinary Tract Infections

These infections may involve the urethra (urethritis), urinary bladder (cystitis), or renal pelvis (pyelonephritis). Most urinary tract infections (UTIs) originate from the patient's own intestinal tract and ascend through the urethra to the bladder. UTIs cause more than 8 million visits to health care providers annually. Approximately 40% of women and 12% of men will have symptoms of at least one UTI during their lifetime.[25] **Clinical Findings:** Symptoms of cystitis include dysuria, frequency (more than every 2 hours), urgency, and suprapubic pain. The urine may contain blood or sediment, creating a cloudy appearance. By contrast, older adults report nonlocalized abdominal discomfort and may have cognitive impairment. Symptoms of acute pyelonephritis vary from fatigue to sudden onset of fever, chills, vomiting, and flank pain.[26]

Urinary Tract Calculi (Stones)

Urinary tract stones form in a kidney and may enlarge in a ureter or the bladder. The process of stone formation is termed *nephrolithiasis*. Calculi may be found in various locations in the urinary tract including within the kidney, ureter, or bladder (Fig. 13.25).[27] The prevalence of kidney stones is 8.8% (10.6% among men and 7.1% among women).[28] Urinary stasis and infection are important variables in the development of stones. **Clinical Findings:** Tiny stones may not cause any symptoms since they are not obstructing urine flow.

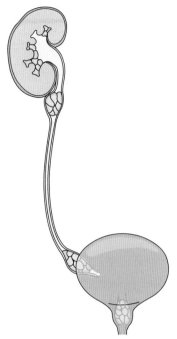

The first symptom of a kidney stone is usually a sudden onset of severe pain felt in the flank area, back, or lower abdomen. Nausea and vomiting may occur due to the severe pain.[26] When bladder stones irritate the bladder wall or block the flow of urine, they may cause symptoms of lower abdominal pain, burning during urination, frequency, or hematuria.[29]

FIG. 13.25 Most common locations of renal calculi formation. (From Monahan et al., 2007.)

CLINICAL APPLICATION AND CLINICAL JUDGMENT

See Appendix B for answers to exercises in this section.

CASE STUDY

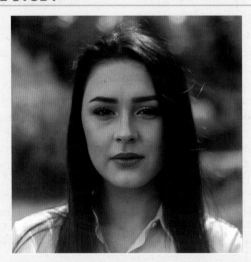

Fatima Khan is a 22-year-old woman complaining of abdominal pain. The following data are collected by the nurse during an interview and examination.

Interview Data

Ms. Khan tells the nurse that the pain started yesterday evening and has become progressively worse. She describes the pain as constant, "really bad," and located in her right lower abdomen, toward her umbilicus. She says that it feels a little better if she stays curled up and does not move. She tells the

nurse that she is in good health and that she has never had a problem with her stomach. Ms. Khan indicates that normally she has a good appetite and can eat anything—until now. She says that she ate breakfast and lunch yesterday but by dinnertime she was nauseated and had no appetite. She has not eaten anything since. She has had no recent weight changes, but she would like to weigh approximately 5 lbs (2.5 kg) less than she currently does. Ms. Khan smokes a half pack of cigarettes daily, she does not drink alcoholic beverages, and she takes no medication. She denies discomfort or problems with urination, describing her urine as "usual looking."

Examination Data

- *General survey:* Alert and anxious female in moderate distress lying in a fetal position on the examination table, with her eyes closed. Appears well nourished. Her skin is hot.
- *Inspection:* Abdomen is flat and symmetric. No lesions or scars are noticed. No surface movements are seen except for breathing.
- *Auscultation:* Bowel sounds are absent.
- *Percussion:* Tympany is noticed over most of the abdominal surface; dullness over the liver. Midclavicular liver span is 4 inches (10 cm).
- *Light palpation:* Demonstrates pain and guarding in RLQ. Unable to palpate deep structures because of excessive abdominal discomfort.

Clinical Judgment

1. What cues do you recognize that suggest deviations from expected findings, suggesting a need for further investigation?

2. For which additional information should the nurse ask or assess?

3. Based on these data, which risk factors for cancers in the abdomen does Ms. Khan have?

4. With which team members can the nurse collaborate to meet this patient's needs?

REVIEW QUESTIONS

1. A patient reports severe abdominal pain and pain in the right shoulder that gets worse after eating fried foods. What question does the nurse ask to gather more data about the possibility of cholelithiasis?
   1. "Has your abdomen been distended?"
   2. "Have you experienced fever, chills, or sweating?"
   3. "Have you vomited up any blood in the last 24 hours?"
   4. "Has the color of your urine or stools changed?"

2. The nurse is interviewing a patient with a history of flank pain, fever, and chills. Which examination technique is most appropriate for this patient?
   1. Percussion of the costovertebral angle
   2. Deep palpation of the lower abdomen
   3. Palpation of the kidney for contour
   4. Auscultation of the lower quadrants of the abdomen

3. A patient reports a gnawing, burning pain in the midepigastric area that is aggravated by bending over or lying down. Which additional question does the nurse ask as part of a symptom analysis?
   1. "Do you have a family history of this type of pain?"
   2. "How long ago did you eat?"
   3. "Is the pain worse after eating or when your stomach is empty?"
   4. "Have you noticed any yellow coloring in your eyes or on your skin?"

4. Which organs is the nurse assessing during palpation of the right upper quadrant of the abdomen?
   1. Liver and gallbladder
   2. Stomach and spleen
   3. Uterus, if enlarged, and right ovary
   4. Right ureter and ascending colon

5. Using deep palpation of a patient's epigastrium, a nurse feels a rhythmic pulsation of the aorta. Based on this finding, what is the nurse's most appropriate response?
   1. Auscultate this area using the bell of the stethoscope.
   2. Percuss the area for tones.
   3. Document this as an expected finding.
   4. Ask the patient if there is pain in this area.

6. When assessing an adult's liver, the nurse percusses the lower border and finds it to be 5 cm below the costal margin. What is the nurse's appropriate action at this time?
   1. Document this as an expected finding for this adult
   2. Palpate the upper liver border on deep inspiration
   3. Palpate the gallbladder for tenderness
   4. Use the hooking technique to palpate the lower border of the liver

7. Which is an abnormal sound the nurse would detect when auscultating the abdomen using the bell of the stethoscope?
   1. High-pitched gurgles
   2. Borborygmi
   3. Venous hum
   4. Absent bowel sounds

8. Which technique does the nurse use to palpate a patient's abdomen?
   1. Asks the patient to breath slowly though the mouth
   2. Uses the heel of the hand to perform deep palpation
   3. Uses the left hand to lift the rib cage away from the abdominal organs
   4. Uses the pads of the fingertips to depress the abdomen.

9. A nurse inspects the abdomen for skin color, surface characteristics, and surface movement. What part of the abdominal assessment does the nurse perform next?
   1. Palpate lightly for tenderness and muscle tone
   2. Auscultate for bowel sounds
   3. Palpate deeply for masses or aortic pulsation
   4. Percuss for tones

10. A patient reports having abdominal fullness and having vomited several times yesterday and today. What question is appropriate for the nurse to ask in response to this information?
    1. "Has there been a change in the amount of the distention?"
    2. "Did you have heartburn before the vomiting?"
    3. "What did the vomitus look like?"
    4. "Have you noticed a change in the color of your urine or stools?"

14

Musculoskeletal System

CONCEPT OVERVIEW

The concept for this chapter is *Mobility*, which represents mechanisms that facilitate and impair body movement. Several concepts are interrelated with mobility, including gas exchange, perfusion, intracranial regulation, tactile perception, pain, nutrition, tissue integrity, and elimination. Understanding the interrelationships of these concepts helps the nurse recognize risk factors when conducting a health assessment. These interrelationships are depicted in the following illustration.

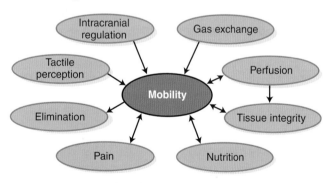

Motion depends on the delivery of oxygenated blood to tissues and coordination of movement regulated by the brain,

spinal cord, and peripheral nerves. Pain that occurs with movement can impair mobility. Just as adequate nutrition is required for mobility, so mobility is needed to purchase and prepare food. Impaired mobility can lead to impaired elimination as well as skin breakdown and impaired tissue integrity. As an example, over time, excessive body weight damages the joints, causing pain with movement. This pain may limit the walking that a person does, which may limit such activities as exercise and shopping for food. Others who have limited mobility may develop constipation. Skin breakdown may develop because of extended pressure on tissue. The following case provides a clinical example featuring several of these interrelated concepts.

> *Mrs. Wilcox is a 92-year-old widow who lives alone. One afternoon she fell in her driveway and suffered a hip fracture requiring a surgical repair. After the surgical procedure, Mrs. Wilcox experienced significant pain and delirium, and was unable to actively participate in physical therapy. Her lack of mobility contributed to her poor nutritional intake, constipation, and skin breakdown on her sacrum.*

ANATOMY AND PHYSIOLOGY

The musculoskeletal system provides both support and mobility for the body and protection for internal organs. This system also produces blood cells and stores minerals such as calcium and phosphorus. Connective tissue, which functions to protect, support, and integrate of all parts of the body, includes bones, ligament, tendons, cartilage, and bursae. Muscle is another type of tissue used for support, mobility, and protection of internal organs.

BONES, MUSCLES, AND CONNECTIVE TISSUE

Bones

The functions of bones include support for soft tissues and organs, protection of organs such as the brain and spinal cord, body movement, and hematopoiesis. Bones are continually remodeling and changing the collagen and mineral composition to accommodate stress placed on them.

The function of each bone dictates its shape and surface features. For example, long bones act as levers; they have a flat surface for the attachment of muscles, with grooves at the end for passage of tendons or nerves. Examples of long bones are the humerus, femur, fibula, and phalanges. Short bones such as carpal and tarsal bones are cube shaped. Flat bones make up the cranium, ribs, and scapula. The vertebrae are irregularly shaped bones.

Skeletal Muscles

Skeletal muscles are composed of muscle fibers that attach to bones to facilitate movement. Although some skeletal muscles move by reflex, all are controlled voluntarily. Skeletal muscle fibers are arranged parallel to the long axis of the bones they attach to, or they are attached obliquely. Muscles attach to a bone, ligament, tendon, or fascia.

Joints

Joints are articulations where two or more bones come together. They hold the bones firmly while allowing movement between them.

Joints are classified in two ways: by the type of material between them (fibrous, cartilaginous, or synovial) and by their degree of movement. Immovable joints are synarthrodial (e.g., the suture of the skull); slightly movable joints are amphiarthrodial (e.g., the symphysis pubis); and freely movable joints are diarthrodial (e.g., the knee and the distal interphalangeal [DIP] joint of the distal fingers).

Diarthrodial joints are further classified by their type of movement; they are the only joints that have one or more ranges of motion. Hinge joints (e.g., the knee, elbow, and fingers) permit extension and flexion, and some hinge joints allow hyperextension. There is, however, variability among individuals; not all hinge joints are able to hyperextend. Pivot joints permit movement of one bone articulating with a ring or notch of another bone, such as the head of the radius, which articulates with the radial notch of the ulna. The ends of saddle-shaped bones articulate with one another: the base of the thumb is the only example. Condyloid or ellipsoidal joints consist of the condyle of one bone that fits into the elliptically shaped portion of its articulating bone (e.g., the distal end of the radius articulates with three wrist bones). Ball-and-socket joints are made of a ball-shaped bone that fits into a concave area of its articulating bone (e.g., the head of the femur fits into the acetabulum within the pelvis). Gliding joints permit movement along various axes through relatively flat articulating surfaces, such as joints between two vertebrae.

Diarthrodial joints are synovial joints because they are lined with synovial fluid (Fig. 14.1). Synovial fluid lubricates the joint to facilitate its movement in various directions. Some synovial joints, such as the knee, also have a disk called the *meniscus,* which is a pad of cartilage that cushions the joint. These joints have a covering surrounding them called the *joint capsule,* which is an extension of the periosteum of the articulating bone. Ligaments also encase the capsule to add strength.

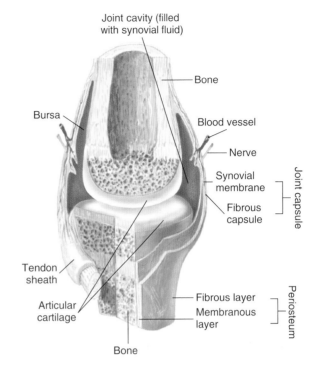

FIG. 14.1 Structures of a synovial joint (the Knee). (From Mourad, 1991.)

Ligaments and Tendons

The difference between ligaments and tendons is more functional than structural. Ligaments are strong, dense, flexible bands of connective tissue that hold bones to bones. They can provide support in several ways: by encircling the joint, gripping it obliquely, or lying parallel to the bone ends across the joint. They can simultaneously allow some movements while restricting others. For an example, see Fig. 14.9, which shows the pubofemoral ligament holding the pubis bone to the femur.

Conversely, tendons are strong, nonelastic cords of collagen located at the ends of muscles to attach them to bones. Tendons support bone movement in response to skeletal muscle contractions, transmitting remarkable force at times from the contracting muscles to the bone without sustaining injury themselves. For an example, see Fig. 14.8, which shows the tendon of the rectus femoris attaching the rectus femoris to the patella.

Cartilage and Bursae

Cartilage is a semi-smooth, gel-like tissue that is strong and able to support weight. The upper seven pairs of ribs are connected directly to the sternum by costal cartilage. The flexibility of the cartilage allows the thorax to move when the lungs expand and contract. Cartilage also reinforces respiratory passages such as the nose, larynx, trachea, and bronchi. It forms a cap over the ends of long bones, providing a smooth surface for articulation (see Fig. 14.1). Because cartilage contains no blood vessels, it receives nutrition from the synovial fluid forced into it during movement and weight-bearing activities. For this reason, weight-bearing activity and joint movement are essential to maintaining cartilage health.

Bursae are small sacs in the connective tissues adjacent to selected joints such as the shoulders (the glenohumeral joint) and knees. Each bursa is lined with synovial membrane containing synovial fluid, which acts as a lubricant to reduce friction when a muscle or tendon rubs against another muscle, tendon, or bone (see Fig. 14.1).

SKELETON AND SUPPORTING STRUCTURES BY BODY AREA

The human skeleton has two major divisions: the axial and appendicular skeletons. The axial skeleton includes the facial bones, auditory ossicles, vertebrae, ribs, sternum, and hyoid bone; the appendicular skeleton includes the scapula, clavicle, bones of the shoulders and arms, and bones of the pelvis and legs.

Skull and Neck

The six bones of the cranium (one frontal, two parietals, two temporals, and one occipital) are fused together. The face consists of 14 bones that protect facial structures. Like the skull, these bones are immobile and are fused at sutures, with the exception of the mandible. The mandible articulates with the temporal bone of the skull at the temporomandibular joint, allowing for movement of the jaw up, down, in, out, and from side to side (see Fig. 10.1A and B). The neck is supported by the cervical vertebrae, ligaments,

and the sternocleidomastoid and trapezius muscles, with its greatest mobility at the level of C4–C5 or C5–C6.

Trunk and Pelvis

The trunk is formed by the vertebrae, ribs, and sternum of the axial skeleton, and the scapula and clavicle of the appendicular skeleton. The pelvis is part of the appendicular skeleton. Fig. 14.2 shows the bones of the trunk and pelvis, and Fig. 14.3 shows the muscles. The spine is composed of 7 cervical, 12 thoracic, 5 lumbar, and 5 sacral vertebrae (see Fig. 15.6). The cervical, thoracic, and lumbar vertebrae are separated from each other by fibrocartilaginous disks, whereas the sacral vertebrae are fused. The vertebral joints, separated by disks, glide slightly over the surfaces of one another.

Upper Extremities

The bones of the upper extremities are shown in Fig. 14.4, and the muscles are shown in Fig. 14.5.

Shoulder and Upper Arm

The shoulder joint, also called the *glenohumeral joint,* consists of the point where the humerus and the glenoid fossa of the scapula articulate (Fig. 14.6). The acromial and coracoid processes (see Fig. 14.2) and surrounding ligaments protect this ball-and-socket joint. Besides the glenohumeral joint, two other joints contribute to shoulder movement: the acromioclavicular joint (between the acromial process and the clavicle) and the sternoclavicular joint (between the sternal manubrium and the clavicle).

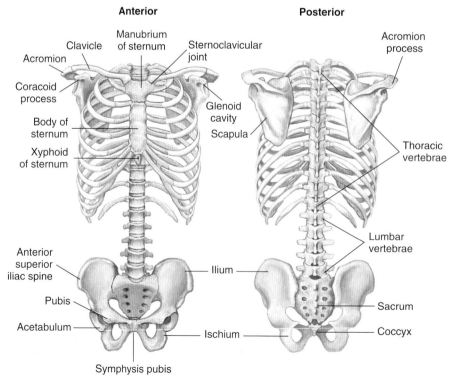

FIG. 14.2 Bones of the trunk and pelvis. (From Mourad, 1991.)

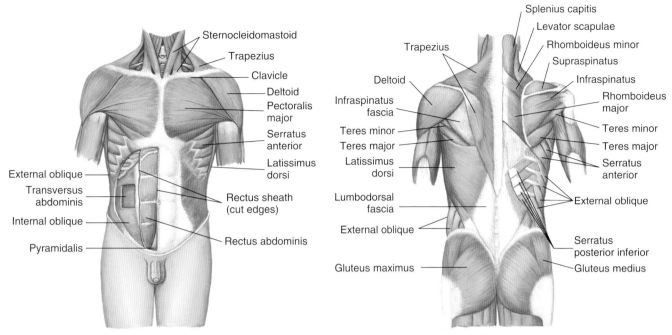

FIG. 14.3 Muscles of the trunk and pelvis. (From Mourad, 1991.)

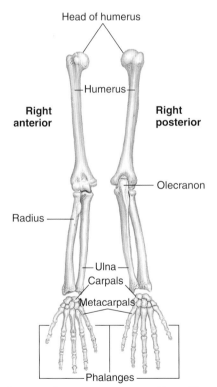

FIG. 14.4 Bones of the upper extremities. (From Mourad, 1991.)

Elbow, Forearm, and Wrist

The elbow joint is a hinge joint that consists of the humerus, radius, and ulna (see Fig. 14.4) enclosed in a single synovial cavity protected by ligaments and a bursa between the olecranon and the skin. The wrist joins the radius and the carpal bones with articular disks of the wrist, ligaments, and a fibrous capsule to form a condyloid joint.

Hand

There are small, subtle movements or articulations within the hand between the carpals and metacarpals, between the metacarpals and proximal phalanges, and between the middle and distal phalanges (see Fig. 14.4). Ligaments protect the diarthrotic joints.

The names of joints in the hands describe their location. For example, the distal joint of the fingers is called the *distal interphalangeal (DIP) joint*; the middle joint of each finger is called the *proximal interphalangeal (PIP) joint*; and the joint that attaches the metacarpal to the carpal is called the *metacarpophalangeal (MCP) joint.*

Lower Extremities

The bones of the lower extremities are shown in Fig. 14.7, and the muscles are shown in Fig. 14.8.

Hip and Thigh

The acetabulum and femur form the hip joint, protected by a fibrous capsule and three bursae. Three ligaments help stabilize the head of the femur in the joint capsule (Fig. 14.9).

Knee and Lower Leg

The knee is a hinge joint that serves as the point of articulation between the femur, the tibia, and the patella (see Fig. 14.7). The knee has medial and lateral menisci (disk-shaped fibrous cartilage) that cushion the tibia and the femur and connect to the articulated capsule. Ligaments

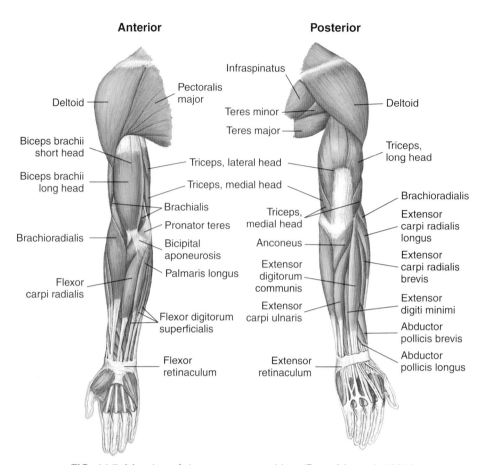

FIG. 14.5 Muscles of the upper extremities. (From Mourad, 1991.)

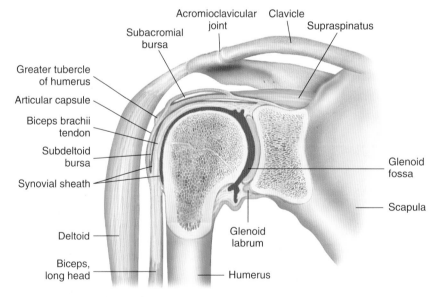

FIG. 14.6 Structures of the glenohumeral and acromioclavicular joint of the shoulder.

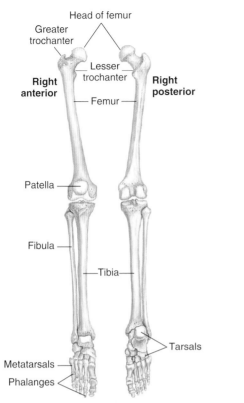

Head of femur
Greater trochanter
Lesser trochanter
Right anterior
Right posterior
Femur
Patella
Fibula
Tibia
Tarsals
Metatarsals
Phalanges

FIG. 14.7 Bones of the lower extremities. (From Mourad, 1991.)

provide stability; the bursae reduce friction on movement between the femur and the tibia.

Ankle and Foot

The ankle joint, or tibiotalar joint, forms a hinge joint that permits flexion, called *dorsiflexion,* and extension in one plane, called *plantar flexion.* Protective medial and lateral ligaments join the tibia, fibula, and talus to form the tibiotalar joint. These joints are the subtalar (talocalcaneal) and the talonavicular (transverse tarsal) joints (Fig. 14.10).

Five metatarsal bones form the sole of the foot. Like the names of joints in the hands, the names of joints in the feet describe their location. For example, the joint between the distal and proximal phalanges is called the *interphalangeal joint;* the joint between the proximal phalanx and the first metatarsal is called the *metatarsophalangeal joint;* and the joint that attaches the first metatarsal to the tarsals is called the *tarsometatarsal joint* (see Fig. 14.10).

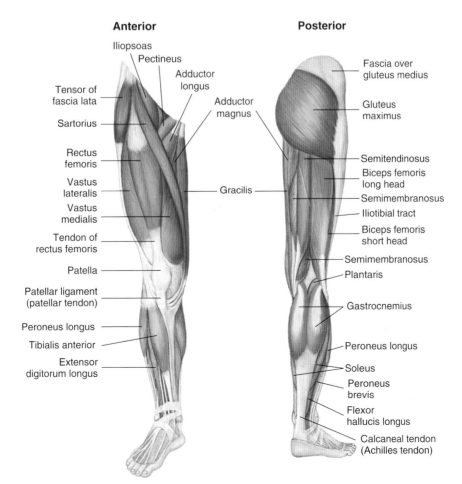

Anterior
Iliopsoas
Pectineus
Adductor longus
Adductor magnus
Tensor of fascia lata
Sartorius
Rectus femoris
Vastus lateralis
Vastus medialis
Gracilis
Tendon of rectus femoris
Patella
Patellar ligament (patellar tendon)
Peroneus longus
Tibialis anterior
Extensor digitorum longus

Posterior
Fascia over gluteus medius
Gluteus maximus
Semitendinosus
Biceps femoris long head
Semimembranosus
Iliotibial tract
Biceps femoris short head
Semimembranosus
Plantaris
Gastrocnemius
Peroneus longus
Soleus
Peroneus brevis
Flexor hallucis longus
Calcaneal tendon (Achilles tendon)

FIG. 14.8 Muscles of the lower extremities. (From Mourad, 1991.)

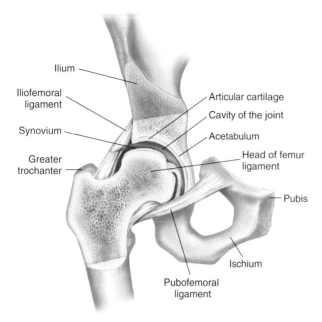

FIG. 14.9 Structures of the hip. (Modified from Thompson et al., 2002.)

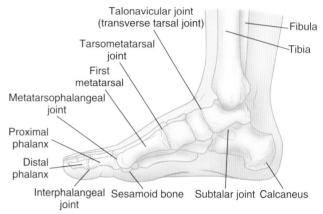

FIG. 14.10 Bones and joints of the ankle and foot.

HEALTH HISTORY

Nurses interview patients to collect subjective data about their present health status, past health history, family history, and personal and psychosocial history, which may affect the functions of the musculoskeletal system.

GENERAL HEALTH HISTORY

Present Health Status

Do you have any chronic diseases? Loss of bone density or osteoporosis?
Chronic diseases may affect mobility and activities of daily living. Reduction in weight-bearing activities contributes to loss of bone density and osteoporosis.

Do you take any medications? If yes, what do you take and how often? What are the medications for?
Patients may not report musculoskeletal problems if they are being treated successfully with medications.

Do you take any over-the-counter drugs or herbal supplements? If yes, what do you take and how often? What are they for?
Nonprescription drugs and herbal supplements may affect the musculoskeletal system. For example, calcium, magnesium, and vitamin D may strengthen bones and reduce the risk of osteoporosis. Aloe vera may be applied topically to reduce joint pain, and ginger or green tea may reduce joint inflammation.

Have you noticed any changes in your ability to move around or participate in your usual activities? Have you noticed any changes in your muscle strength? If there are changes, how do you adapt?

If there are changes, they can be diagnosed and treated promptly, or they can generate a discussion about how to prevent further changes. The health care provider needs to determine how the patient is adapting to these changes to determine their impact on his or her quality of life.

RISK FACTORS

Osteoporosis

- *Age:* Being more than 50 years.
- *Gender:* Women are at greater risk.
- *Race:* Caucasian and Asian women are at highest risk.
- *Body size:* Small-boned and thin women are at greater risk.
- *Family history:* A family history of osteoporosis increases risk.
- *Lifestyle:* Cigarette smoking, excessive alcohol intake, consuming inadequate calcium and vitamin D, and performing inadequate weight-bearing exercises increase the risk. (M)
- *Medications to treat chronic diseases:* Some medications have adverse effects that lead to osteoporosis, including glucocorticoids and some anticonvulsants. (M)
- *Sex hormones:* Estrogen deficiency from menopause or surgical removal of ovaries (oophorectomy) increases risk in women. Low levels of testosterone and estrogen increase risk in men. (M)
- *Eating disorder:* Anorexia nervosa is characterized by an irrational fear of weight gain, which increases risk. (M)

M, Modifiable risk factor.

From Centers for Disease Control and Prevention: Osteoarthritis. Available at: http:// www.cdc.gov/arthritis/basics/osteoarthritis.htm. Last reviewed January 10, 2019; National Osteoporosis Foundation: Are you at risk? Available at: http://www.nof.org/preventing-fractures/general-facts/bone-basics/are-you-at-risk/. www.bones.nih.gov/health-info/bone/osteoporosis/overview. Last reviewed October, 2018.

Past Health History

Have you ever had any accidents or trauma that affected the bones or joints, including fractures, strains of the joints, sprains, and dislocations? If yes, when? Have you noticed any continuing problems or difficulties that seem related to this previous incident?

Previous injury can leave residual problems such as muscle weakness, decreased range of motion (ROM), or impaired mobility.

Have you ever had surgery on any bones, joints, or muscles? If yes, describe the procedure(s), when it (they) occurred, and what the outcome was.

The incidence of surgery may provide additional information about possible musculoskeletal problems and the findings to anticipate during assessment.

Family History

In your family, is there a history of curvature of the spine or back problems? If yes, describe.

Family history may be used to determine a patient's risk for vertebral disorders.

Is there a history of arthritis in your family (i.e., rheumatoid arthritis, osteoarthritis, or gout)?

Family history is a risk factor for rheumatoid arthritis, osteoarthritis, and gout.[1]

Personal and Psychosocial History

What do you do for exercise? How often do you exercise and for what period of time?

Regular exercise increases bone strength to prevent osteoporosis,[2] strengthens muscles, and facilitates weight loss.

Do you smoke cigarettes or e-cigarettes? If yes, how many and how often?

Nicotine reduces blood supply to tissues, leading to hypoxia, which ultimately decreases bone mineral density. Smoking is also a risk factor for osteoarthritis.[3]

Do you drink alcohol? If yes, how much and how often?

More than two alcoholic drinks per day is a risk factor for osteoporosis.[4] Excessive alcohol use causes hyperuricemia, which contributes to gout.[5]

Do you play sports? If yes, which ones and how often? How do you protect yourself from injury while exercising or playing sports?

These questions assess for risk for injury. Adults should protect themselves from injury (e.g., stretching before running, wearing a bike helmet, and wearing elbow pads and wrist guards for in-line skating).

Do you lift, push, or pull items or bend or stoop frequently as a part of your daily routine either at home or at work? How do you protect yourself from muscle strain or injury?

Many musculoskeletal injuries are caused by heavy lifting and repetitive and forceful motions that may be prevented with proper body mechanics, appropriate help when lifting, and use of protective equipment.

PROBLEM-BASED HISTORY

Commonly reported symptoms related to the musculoskeletal system are pain, problems with movement, and problems with daily activities. As with symptoms in all areas of health assessment, a symptom analysis is completed using the mnemonic OLD CARTS, which includes the Onset, Location, Duration, Characteristics, Aggravating factors, Related symptoms, Treatment, and Severity (see Box 2.6).

Pain

Where do you feel the pain? Describe how it feels. How severe is the pain on a scale of 0 to 10, with 10 being the worst pain possible?

Back pain is the most common musculoskeletal complaint followed by knee pain and shoulder pain.[6] Pain felt in and around the joint and accompanied by edema, warmth, and erythema indicates inflammation. Bone pain typically is described as "deep," "dull," "boring," or "intense." Pain in the joints is often described as "achy." Muscle pain may be described as "cramping."[7]

Does the pain move? Can you show me where it moves?

Muscle pain is usually localized, whereas nerve pain may radiate. Some disorders cause migratory arthritis, in which pain moves among joints (e.g., acute rheumatic fever, leukemia, or juvenile arthritis).

When did you first notice the pain? Did the pain occur suddenly? Were you ill before the onset of pain?

Sudden onset of pain and erythema in the great toe, ankle, and lower leg suggests gout (also called *gouty arthritis*).[5] Viral illnesses can cause muscle aches and pain (myalgia).

Is the pain constant, or does it come and go? Was there an injury, strain, or overuse of any of your muscles or joints? Is it related to movement? Is there a pattern to when you experience pain?

Individuals with arthritis often have pain that comes and goes. Pain associated with a traumatic injury is usually constant. Joint and back pain are frequently related to movement. Pain from rheumatoid arthritis may disturb sleep.[1] Patients with osteoarthritis report stiffness upon awakening that lasts approximately 30 minutes and decreases with movement. Pain experienced during the day in weight-bearing joints is relieved by rest.[8]

What makes the pain worse? Does it change according to the weather?

Learning what makes the pain worse may help to diagnose the disorder. Arthritis pain may become worse with changes in the barometric pressure. Movement often makes joint pain worse except in rheumatoid arthritis, in which movement may reduce pain.

What have you done to relieve the pain? How effective has it been?

Many individuals with musculoskeletal pain use analgesic and heat to help alleviate pain. Rest or a specific body position may help relieve pain.

RISK FACTORS

Osteoarthritis

- *Age:* Risk increases with age.
- *Gender:* Women are more likely to develop osteoarthritis (OA) than men, especially after age 50.
- *Obesity:* Extra weight puts stress on joints, especially weight-bearing joints such as hips and knees. (M)
- *Joint injury or overuse:* Injury or overuse, such as knee bending and repetitive stress on a joint, can damage the joint and increase risk of OA to that joint. (M)
- *Genetics:* People who have family members with OA are more likely to develop it.

M, Modifiable risk factor.
U.S. Preventive Services Task Force: Draft Recommendation Statement: Osteoporosis to Prevent Fractures: Screening. Available at:https://www.uspreventiveservicestaskforce.org/Page/Document/draft-recommendation-statement/osteoporosis-screening1. Last reviewed November 2017.

Problems With Movement

How long have you had problems with movement? Is the movement in your joints limited? Are your joints swollen, red, or hot to the touch?

Decreased ROM occurs with injury to the cartilage or capsule, or with muscle contracture or edema. Acute inflammation such as arthritis or gout produces edema, erythema, and warmth.

Have your joints felt as if they are locked and will not move? If yes, when does it occur? How often does it occur? What relieves the locking? What makes it worse?

Locked joints may indicate joint instability, which may occur from chronic inflammation or joint trauma. Safety must be a concern of the patient when a joint gives way.

Do you feel any weakness in your muscles? If yes, which muscles? How long have you had this weakness? Does it become worse as the day progresses?

Muscle weakness may be caused by altered nerve innervation or muscle contraction disorder. Atrophied muscles may be the result of prolonged lack of use (e.g., atrophy occurs from disuse when an extremity is casted). Proximal muscle weakness is usually a myopathy, whereas distal weakness is usually a neuropathy.

Have you noticed your knees or ankles giving way when you put pressure on them? If yes, when does it occur? How often does it occur?

This may indicate joint instability that may occur from chronic inflammation or joint trauma. Safety must be a concern of the patient when a joint gives way.

Problems With Daily Activities

Which activities are limited? To what extent are your daily activities limited? How do you compensate for this limitation? Any impaired mobility or function may interfere with the person's ability to perform self-care activities.

- Bathing (getting in and out of the tub, turning faucets on or off)?
- Toileting (urinating, defecating, ability to raise or lower yourself onto or off of the commode)?
- Dressing (buttoning, zipping, fastening openings behind your neck, hooking your brassiere, pulling a dress or shirt over your head, pulling up your pants, tying shoes, having shoes fit your feet)?
- Grooming (shaving, brushing teeth, brushing or combing hair, washing and drying hair, applying makeup)?
- Eating (preparing meals, pouring, holding utensils, cutting food, bringing food to your mouth, drinking)?
- Moving around (walking, going up or down stairs, getting in or out of bed, getting out of the house)?
- Moving into and out of bed, moving in bed?
- Communicating (writing, talking, using the phone)?

For patients who have chronic disability or a crippling disease: How has your illness affected your ability to visit with your family and/or friends?

Assess for disturbance of self-esteem, body image, or role performance; loss of independence; or social isolation. Maintaining social relationships is an important aspect of therapy.

HEALTH PROMOTION FOR EVIDENCE-BASED PRACTICE

Arthritis and Osteoporosis

Arthritis and osteoporosis affect the quality of life, the ability to work, and activities of daily living.

Approximately half of all postmenopausal women will have an osteoporosis-related fracture during their lives. The risk for fracture increases as bone density decreases.

Recommendations to Reduce Risk (Primary Prevention)

- Counsel patients to eat a balanced diet rich in calcium and vitamin D. Calcium intake should be between 1000 and 1300 mg/day; vitamin D intake should be between 400 and 800 IU/day.
- Encourage patients to engage in weight-bearing exercise.
- Encourage patients to avoid smoking and excessive alcohol use.

Screening Recommendations (Secondary Prevention)

- For women age 65 and older, screening for osteoporosis with bone measurement testing is recommended to prevent osteoporotic fractures.
- Screening is recommended for postmenopausal women younger than age 65 years who are at increased risk of osteoporosis, as determined by a formal clinical assessment tool.

EXAMINIATION

Routine Techniques

- INSPECT skeleton and extremities.
- PALPATE muscles.
- PALPATE bones and joints.
- ASSESS range of motion of each joint.
- ASSESS muscle tone.
- ASSESS muscle strength and compare sides.

Techniques for Special Circumstances

- ASSESS for nerve root compression.

Techniques Performed by an APRN

- ASSESS for carpal tunnel syndrome.
- ASSESS for rotator cuff damage.
- ASSESS knee effusion.
- ASSESS for knee stability.
- ASSESS for meniscal damage or tear.
- ASSESS for hip flexion contractures.

Equipment needed

- Goniometer • Tape measure with centimeter markings

APRN, Advanced Practice Registered Nurse

PROCEDURES WITH EXPECTED FINDINGS

In each specific musculoskeletal region, the nurse performs the same skills: inspects the skeleton and muscles; palpates bones, joints, and muscles; assesses ROM, muscle tone, and muscle strength. Muscle strength is graded from no voluntary contraction (1/5) to full muscle strength (5/5), using the criteria in Table 14.1.

ROUTINE TECHNIQUES

PERFORM hand hygiene.
INSPECT skeleton and extremities for alignment and symmetry.

While the patient is standing, inspect the alignment and symmetry from the front, back, and sides (Fig. 14.11). The patient should stand erect. The body appears relatively symmetric when one side is compared with the other. The spine should be straight with expected curvatures (cervical concave, thoracic convex, lumbar concave) (see Fig. 14.11C). The knees should be in a straight line between the hips and ankles, and the feet should be flat on the floor and pointing directly forward.

ABNORMAL FINDINGS

Irregular posture or any asymmetry or misalignment warrants further assessment.

TABLE 14.1 CRITERIA FOR GRADING AND RECORDING MUSCLE STRENGTH

FUNCTIONAL LEVEL	GRADE
No evidence of contractility	0
Evidence of slight contractility	1
Complete range of motion with gravity eliminated	2
Complete range of motion with gravity	3
Complete range of motion against gravity with some resistance	4
Complete range of motion against gravity with full resistance	5

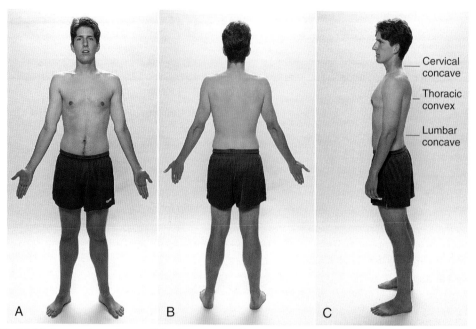

Cervical concave

Thoracic convex

Lumbar concave

A   B   C

FIG. 14.11 Inspection of overall body posture. Note the even contour of the shoulders, level scapulae and iliac crests, alignment of the head over the gluteal folds, and symmetry and alignment of extremities. (A) Anterior view. (B) Posterior view. (C) Lateral view showing normal cervical concave, thoracic convex, and lumbar concave curves of the spine.

PROCEDURES WITH EXPECTED FINDINGS

OBSERVE gait for conformity, rhythm, and symmetry.

Ask the patient to walk across the room and back. Expected findings are conformity (ability to follow gait sequencing of both stance and swing); regular smooth rhythm; symmetry in length of leg swing; smooth swaying; and smooth, symmetric arm swing. When unequal leg length is suspected, measure the leg from the anterior superior iliac spine to the medial malleolus, crossing the knee on the medial side with the patient in supine position (Fig. 14.12). (For the anterior superior iliac location, see Fig. 14.2.) The medial malleolus is the rounded bony process on the inside of the ankle formed by the lower end of the tibia (see Fig. 14.10).

ABNORMAL FINDINGS

An unstable or exaggerated gait, limp, irregular stride length, arm swing that is unrelated to gait, or any other inability to maintain straight posture or asymmetry of body parts requires further assessment. Pain, immobile joints, and muscle weakness are usually unilateral and cause asymmetric abnormalities in gait. Disorders of the neurologic system such as rigidity or cerebellar diseases cause symmetric abnormalities in gait.[7]

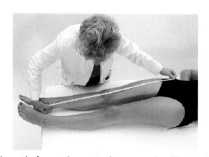

FIG. 14.12 Measure limb length from the anterior superior iliac spine to the medial malleolus.

PROCEDURES WITH EXPECTED FINDINGS

PALPATE each temporomandibular joint for movement, pain, and sounds.

With the patient in a seated position, use the pads of the first two fingers in front of the tragus of each ear to palpate the temporomandibular joint (TMJ) with the mouth closed and open. The mandible should move smoothly and painlessly. An audible or palpable snapping or clicking in the absence of other symptoms is not unusual (Fig. 14.13A).

Pain or crepitus of the TMJ with locking or popping may require further evaluation.[1]

ASSESS temporomandibular joint for range of motion.

Ask the patient to open and close the mouth. It should open between 3 and 6 cm between upper and lower teeth. Ask the patient to move the mandible side to side; it should move 1 to 2 cm in each direction (Fig. 14.13B). Motion should be smooth and without pain. Finally, the patient should be able to protrude and retract the mandible without difficulty or pain.

Difficulty opening the mouth or limited range of motion may result from injury or arthritic changes. Pain in the TMJ may indicate malocclusion of teeth or arthritic changes.

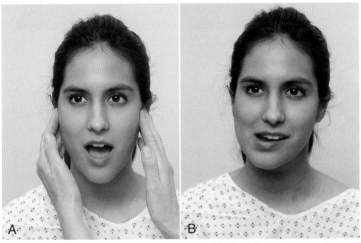

FIG. 14.13 (A) Palpation of temporomandibular joint. (B) Lateral range of motion in the temporomandibular joint.

INSPECT the neck for symmetry and PALPATE the neck muscles for tone.

The neck should be symmetric. Use the pads of thumbs and fingers to palpate the sternocleidomastoid and trapezius muscles, which should feel firm without spasms or pain.

Asymmetric neck muscles may indicate previous injury. Pain on palpation may indicate inflammation of the muscle (myositis). Neck spasm may indicate nerve compression or stress.

ASSESS the cervical spine for range of motion.

Ask the patient to flex the chin to the chest; the cervical spine should move to a point 45 degrees from midline. Ask the patient to hyperextend the head if possible; the cervical spine should reach 55 degrees from midline (Fig. 14.14A). Have the patient laterally bend his or her head to the right and the left. Range should be 40 degrees from midline in each direction (Fig. 14.14B). Have the patient rotate the chin to the shoulders, first to the right and then to the left. It should reach 70 degrees from midline (Fig. 14.14C).

ROM may be impaired by pain or muscle spasms. Hyperextension and flexion may be limited because of cervical vertebral disk herniation, degeneration, or osteoarthritic changes. Pain, numbness, or tingling reported during ROM may indicate compression of cervical spinal root nerves.

ASSESS the neck muscles for strength.

Ask the patient to rotate the head against resistance of your hand to assess strength of the sternocleidomastoid muscles (Fig. 14.15A). (See Fig. 14.3 for location of sternocleidomastoid muscles.) The patient should be able to rotate the neck to withstand your resistance. Use criteria in Table 14.1 to grade the muscle strength from 1/5 to 5/5. Ask the patient to flex the chin to the chest and maintain that position while you palpate the sternocleidomastoid muscles and try to manually force the head upright (Fig. 14.15B). The sternocleidomastoid muscle should contract, and the patient should be able to flex the neck to withstand your resistance.

If you can prevent the patient's rotation before the anticipated point, the patient has muscle weakness.

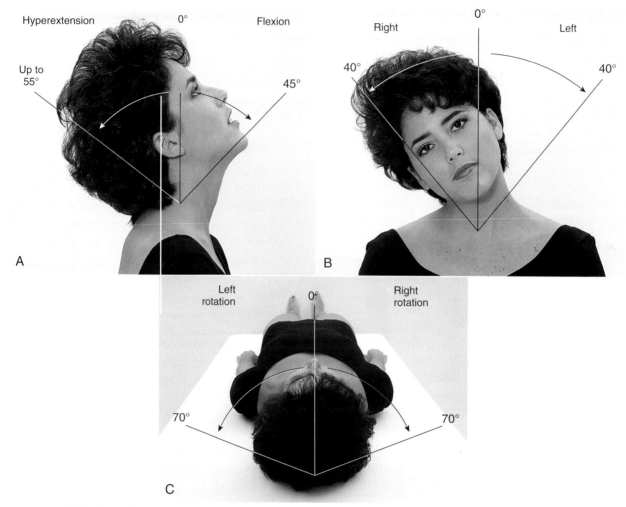

FIG. 14.14 Range of motion of the cervical spine. (A) Flexion and hyperextension. (B) Lateral bending. (C) Rotation.

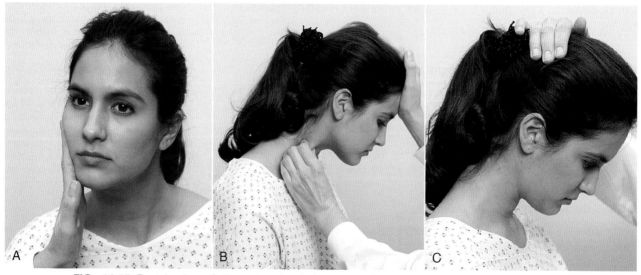

FIG. 14.15 Examination of the strength of the sternocleidomastoid and trapezius muscles. (A) Rotation against resistance. (B) Flexion with palpation of the sternocleidomastoid muscle. (C) Extension against resistance.

PROCEDURES WITH EXPECTED FINDINGS

Have the patient extend the head and maintain position while you try to manually force the head upright to assess the trapezius muscle strength (Fig. 14.15C). (See Fig. 14.3 for location of trapezius muscles.) The patient should be able to extend the head to withstand your resistance.

INSPECT the shoulders and cervical, thoracic, and lumbar spine for alignment and symmetry.

Procedure: Ask the patient to stand while you stand to his or her side to inspect the cervical concave, the thoracic convex, and the lumbar concave curves (see Fig. 14.11C). Notice the landmarks on the back: spinous processes protruding slightly at C7 and T1, paravertebral muscles, and the alignment across the iliac crests at L4 and the posterior superior iliac spine at S2 (Fig. 14.16). Ask the patient to touch the toes. Move behind the patient to inspect the spine.

Findings: Expected concave and convex curves should be present (Fig. 14.17A). Vertebrae should be aligned, indicating a straight spine (Fig. 14.17D). Shoulders should be level or at equal heights, indicating symmetry. Posterior thoraces should be symmetric when patient touches his or her toes.

ABNORMAL FINDINGS

Notice deviation of the spine or asymmetry of shoulder or iliac height. *Kyphosis* is a posterior curvature (convexity) of the thoracic spine (Fig. 14.17B); lordosis is an anterior curvature (concavity) of the spine (Fig. 14.17C); and *scoliosis* is a lateral curvature of the spine (Fig. 14.17E, F, and G). Curvature of the spine may create asymmetry of the shoulders.

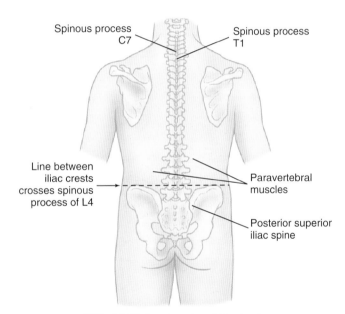

FIG. 14.16 Landmarks of the back.

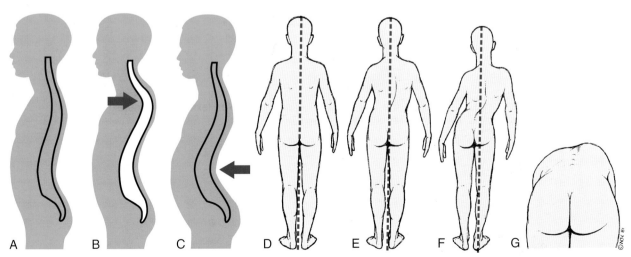

FIG. 14.17 Defects of the spinal column. (A) Normal spine. (B) Kyphosis. (C) Lordosis. (D) Normal spine in balance. (E) Mild scoliosis. (F) Severe scoliosis, not in balance. (G) Rib hump and flank asymmetry seen in flexion. (Modified from Hilt and Schmitt, 1975. In Hockenberry et al., 2011.)

PROCEDURES WITH EXPECTED FINDINGS

ASSESS range of motion of the thoracic and lumbar spine.

Flexion

Ask the patient to bend forward and touch the toes. The patient should be able to reach 75 degrees of flexion while touching his or her toes (Fig. 14.18A). Document how close the patient gets to the floor by measuring from fingertips to the floor (e.g., 15 cm from the floor). Some patients are unable to touch the floor because of tight hamstrings and leg muscles or obesity. These are considered expected variations.

Hyperextension

Ask the patient to lean backward from the waist to hyperextend the spine, which should reach 30 degrees back from the neutral position (extension) (Fig. 14.18B).

Flexion

Ask the patient to bend laterally right and left. (NOTE: You may need to stabilize the patient's hips.) He or she should be able to reach 35 degrees of flexion both directions from midline (Fig. 14.18C).

Rotation

Have the patient rotate the upper trunk (you may need to stabilize the pelvis) to the right and left; he or she should achieve 30 degrees of rotation in both directions from a directly forward position (Fig. 14.18D).

PALPATE the posterior neck, spinal processes, and paravertebral muscles for alignment and pain.

ABNORMAL FINDINGS

Flexion less than 75 degrees with pain or muscle spasm may require further evaluation.

Impaired ROM during hyperextension or lateral flexion may be caused by pain from muscle strain or spasms or a herniated vertebral disk.

Impaired ROM during rotation may be caused by pain from muscle strain or spasms.

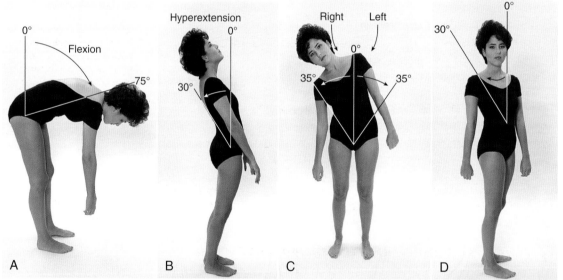

FIG. 14.18 Range of motion of the thoracic and lumbar spine. (A) Flexion. (B) Hyperextension. (C) Lateral bending. (D) Rotation of the upper trunk.

PROCEDURES WITH EXPECTED FINDINGS

Stand behind the patient who is seated. Use the pads of the thumbs and fingers for palpation. The posterior neck and spine should be straight and painless. (NOTE: Having the patient hunch his or her shoulders forward and slightly flex the neck may help your palpation (Fig. 14.19).

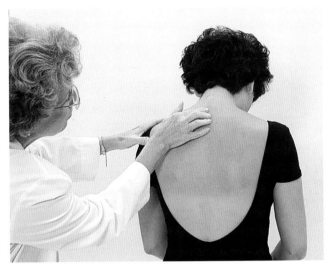

FIG. 14.19 Palpation of the spinal processes of the vertebrae.

TAP the spinal processes for pain.

First tap each process with one finger and then lightly tap each side of the spine with the ulnar surface of your fist. No pain should be noted.

INSPECT the shoulders and shoulder girdle for equality of height, symmetry, and contour.

Procedure: Facing the patient, who is in a seated position, inspect scapulae, clavicles, and the acromioclavicular junctions for equality of height and symmetry. (See Fig. 14.6 for review of location of the acromioclavicular joint.)

Findings: Right and left shoulders should be level, symmetric, and rounded, with smooth contour and no bony prominences. Each shoulder should be equidistant from the vertebral column.

PALPATE the shoulders and upper arms for firmness, fullness, symmetry, and pain.

Procedure: Use the pads of the thumbs and fingers to palpate the acromioclavicular joint; humerus; and trapezius, biceps, triceps, and deltoid muscles (see Figs. 14.5 and 14.6). Compare one side with the other side.

Findings: The shoulders should feel firm, full, and bilaterally symmetric without pain. The muscles of the dominant arm may be slightly larger.

ABNORMAL FINDINGS

Misalignment may be caused by muscle weakness. Pain may be caused by inflammation such as myositis or herniated vertebral disk.

Pain may be caused by compression fracture, infection, inflammation, or tumor. Muscle spasm caused by muscle strain may cause pain on percussion.

Shoulder joints may have some deformity from trauma, arthritic changes, or scoliosis.

Pain may be caused by inflammation of the muscles, overwork of unconditioned muscles, or sports injuries.

PROCEDURES WITH EXPECTED FINDINGS

ASSESS the trapezius muscles for strength.

Ask the patient to shrug the shoulders while you attempt to push them down (Fig. 14.20). This also assesses function of cranial nerve (CN) XI; spinal accessory.

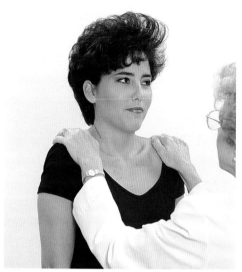

FIG. 14.20 Assess strength of the trapezius muscle with the shrugged shoulder movement.

ASSESS the shoulders for range of motion and symmetry.

The patient may be seated or standing. If needed, use a goniometer to measure the degree of flexion and extension as shown in Fig. 14.21 (See Box 14.1 also).

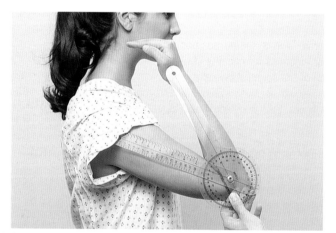

FIG. 14.21 Use of goniometer to measure joint range of motion.

ABNORMAL FINDINGS

Weakness of the trapezius muscles may indicate compressed spinal nerve root or compression of spinal accessory CN XI.

BOX 14.1 HOW TO USE A GONIOMETER

A goniometer looks like a protractor with two long arms (see Fig. 14.21). Place the 0 setting of the goniometer over the middle of a joint that is in neutral position. The middle of one arm of the goniometer is aligned with the extremity proximal to that joint, and the other arm is aligned with the middle of the distal joint. Keeping the 0 at the middle of the joint, move the distal joint through its range of motion and notice the degrees of flexion, extension, or hyperextension on the goniometer.

PROCEDURES WITH EXPECTED FINDINGS

Flexion and hyperextension

Ask the patient to raise the arms straight up beside the ears. The arms should reach 180 degrees from resting neutral position, be bilaterally equal, and cause no pain (Fig. 14.22A). Ask the patient to hyperextend the arms backward. They should reach 50 degrees, be bilaterally equal, and cause no discomfort.

Abduction and adduction

Ask the patient to lift both arms laterally over his or her head. Expected shoulder abduction is 180 degrees. Then ask the patient to swing each arm across the front of the body. Expected adduction is 50 degrees, with symmetric movement without pain (Fig. 14.22B).

External rotation

Ask the patient to place the hands behind the head with elbows out. External rotation of 90 degrees is expected; movement should be bilaterally equal and without pain (Fig. 14.22C).

Internal rotation

Ask the patient to place the hands at the small of the back. Internal rotation of 90 degrees is expected, with movements bilaterally equal and without pain (Fig. 14.22D).

ASSESS arms for muscle tone.

Procedure: Muscle tone is assessed by feeling the resistance to passive stretch.[1] Ask the patient to relax the arms. Hold one hand with yours and support the elbow while you passively flex and extend the fingers, wrists, and elbow, and put the shoulder through ROM.[9] Repeat the procedure with the other arm. **Findings:** Muscle should have slight tension or resistance during passive movement.[1]

ABNORMAL FINDINGS

Limited ROM, pain with movement, crepitation, and asymmetry may require further evaluation. Degenerative joint changes or sports injuries may impair ROM.

Crepitation or tenderness may indicate joint inflammation. A decrease in tone is documented as hypotonia or flaccidity, which may indicate peripheral neuropathy. By contrast, an increase in tone is documented as hypertonia, which may indicate spasticity or rigidity from central nervous system disorders.[9]

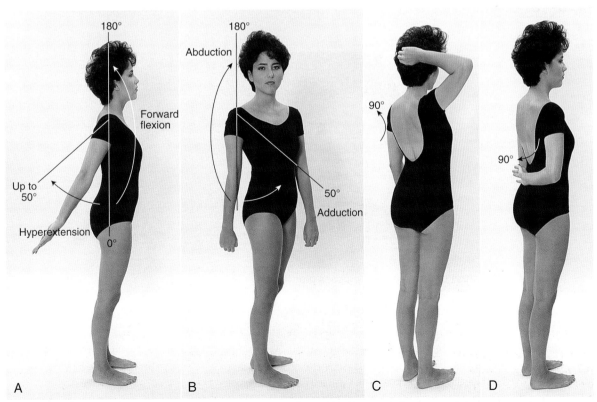

FIG. 14.22 Range of motion of the shoulders. (A) Forward flexion and hyperextension. (B) Abduction and adduction. (C) External rotation. (D) Internal rotation.

PROCEDURES WITH EXPECTED FINDINGS	ABNORMAL FINDINGS

ASSESS the arms for muscle strength.

To assess the deltoid muscle strength, have the patient hold the arms up while you try to push them down. Remember to compare one side with the other. They should be strong bilaterally, preventing you from moving them out of position. Use criteria in Table 14.1 for grading.

To assess triceps muscle strength, ask the patient to extend the arm while you resist by pushing it to a flexed position (Fig. 14.23A). Expected muscle strength is recorded as 5/5. To assess biceps strength, have the patient try to flex the arm while you try to extend his or her forearm. You should be unable to move the arm out of position, and strength should be equal bilaterally, documented as 5/5 (Fig. 14.23B).

Unequal response, weak response, muscular spasm, and pain may be caused by joint or muscle inflammation, trauma, or injuries.

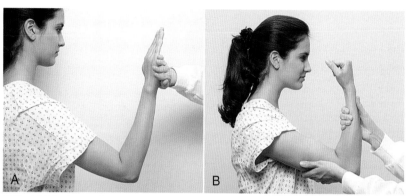

FIG. 14.23 Assessing muscle strength of arms. (A) Assessing triceps muscle strength. (B) Assessing biceps muscle strength.

PALPATE the elbows for pain, edema, temperature, and nodules.

With the patient in a sitting position, hold the patient's lower arm in your nondominant hand while using the pads of the thumb and fingers of the dominant hand to palpate the olecranon process and lateral epicondyle (Fig. 14.24). Repeat the procedure on the other side. The elbows should have no pain, edema, heat, or nodules.

Edema, nodules, point tenderness, and heat may occur in rheumatoid arthritis. Point tenderness is pain felt when pressure is applied to one location.

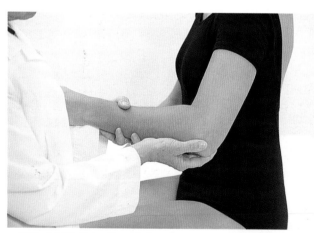

FIG. 14.24 Palpation of the olecranon process grooves.

ASSESS the elbows for range of motion.

Ask the patient to flex and extend the elbow; 160 degrees of full movement should be present bilaterally without pain (Fig. 14.25A). Assess pronation and supination of the elbow by having the patient rotate the hands palms up (supinate) and palms down (pronate) while keeping the elbow flexed 90 degrees. The expected ROM is 90 degrees in each direction, with movements bilaterally equal and without pain (Fig. 14.25B).

Limitation of motion, asymmetry of movement, or pain at the elbow may require further evaluation.

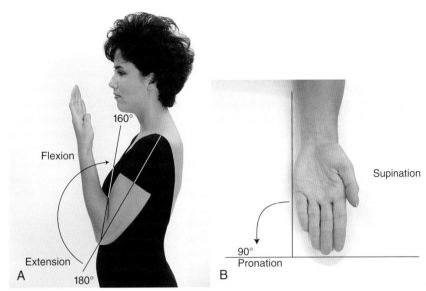

FIG. 14.25 Range of motion of the elbow. (A) Flexion and extension. (B) Palm up, supination; palm down, pronation.

PROCEDURES WITH EXPECTED FINDINGS

INSPECT the joints of the wrists and hands for symmetry, alignment, and number of digits.

Compare the right wrist and hand with the left. They should be symmetric. The hand with five digits is aligned with the wrist, and fingers are aligned with wrist and forearm (Fig. 14.26).

ABNORMAL FINDINGS

Missing fingers are recorded. Osteoarthritis may cause Bouchard nodes in the PIP joints, whereas Heberden nodes form in the DIP joints (Fig. 14.27). Swan-neck and boutonniere deformities of interphalangeal joints may be related to rheumatoid arthritis (Fig. 14.28).[6]

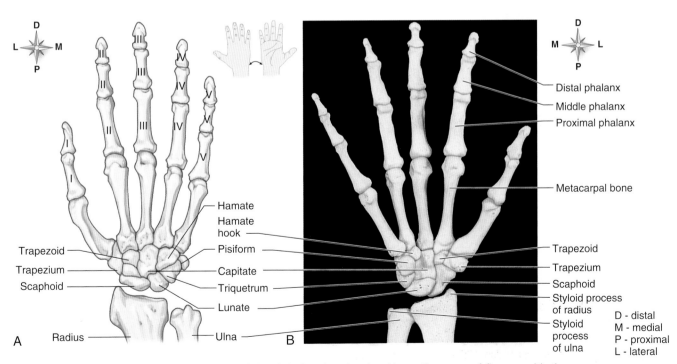

FIG. 14.26 (A) Bony structures of the right hand and wrist. Note alignment of fingers with the radius. (B) Palmar aspect of right hand. (From Patton and Thibodeau, 2012.)

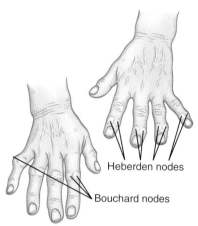

FIG. 14.27 Osteoarthritis. (From Huether and McCance, 2008.)

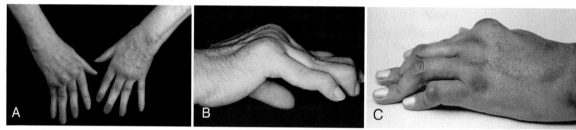

FIG. 14.28 (A) Ulnar deviation and subluxation of metacarpophalangeal Joints. (B) Swan-neck deformity. (C) Boutonniere deformity. (A, From Firestein, et al., 2021. B, From Chung, 2018. C, From Seidel et al., 2011.)

PROCEDURES WITH EXPECTED FINDINGS

PALPATE each joint of the hand and wrist for surface characteristics and pain.

Palpate the interphalangeal joints with your thumb and index finger. Palpate the metacarpophalangeal joints with both thumbs. Palpate the wrist and radiocarpal groove with your thumbs on the dorsal surface and your fingers on the palmar surface. (See Fig. 14.4 for a review of the hand anatomy.) Joint surfaces should feel smooth, without pain (Fig. 14.29).

ABNORMAL FINDINGS

Painful, edematous DIP or PIP joints are found in osteoarthritis. A firm nodule over the dorsum of the wrist may be a ganglion. Rheumatoid arthritis may cause wrists and PIP joints to appear hot, painful, deformed, and edematous.[6]

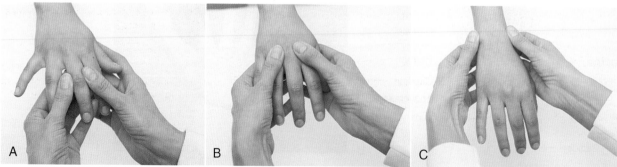

FIG. 14.29 Palpation of joints of the hand and wrist. (A) Interphalangeal joints. (B) Metacarpophalangeal joints. (C) Radiocarpal groove.

PROCEDURES WITH EXPECTED FINDINGS

ASSESS for muscle strength of hands and fingers.

First, ask the patient to extend and spread the fingers (both hands) while you attempt to push them together (Fig. 14.30A). The response should be symmetric to full flexion and extension, without discomfort and with sufficient muscle strength to overcome the resistance you apply.

Next, have the patient grip your first two fingers on each hand. The response should be bilaterally equal, and the grip tight and full flexion (Fig. 14.30B). Some nurses cross their hands for the patient to grip the fingers so the patient's right hand is gripping the nurse's right hand. This maneuver helps the nurse remember on which side the patient may have deficits.

Muscle weakness or impaired ROM may be caused by rheumatoid arthritis and osteoarthritis. Fractures of metatarsals or phalanges may weaken the muscle strength.

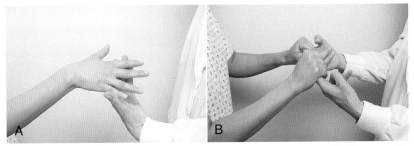

FIG. 14.30 (A) Assessment of finger strength. (B) Assessment of grip strength.

ASSESS range of motion of wrists and hands.

Procedure and Findings: Ask the patient to:

- Bend the hand up at the wrist; hyperextension to 70 degrees is expected. Bend the hand down at the wrist; palmar flexion of 90 degrees is expected (Fig. 14.31A).
- Flex the fingers up and down at the metacarpophalangeal joints; flexion of 90 degrees and hyperextension of 30 degrees are expected (Fig. 14.31B).
- Place palms flat on the table and turn them outward and inward; ulnar deviation of 50 to 60 degrees and radial deviation of 20 degrees are expected (Fig. 14.31C).
- Spread the fingers apart; abduction is expected (Fig. 14.31D). Bring fingers back together; adduction is expected.
- Make a fist; flexion of all fingers is expected (Fig. 14.31E).
- Straighten fingers; extension of all fingers is expected.
- Touch the thumb to the tip of each finger to demonstrate opposition and to the base of the fifth finger for flexion (Fig. 14.31F).
- Move thumb away from hand to demonstrate extension.

Unequal response, weak response, muscular spasm, and pain may be caused by joint or muscle inflammation.

INSPECT the hips for symmetry.

Ask the patient to stand. Inspect the symmetry of the hips anteriorly and posteriorly. The hips should be the same height and symmetric. You may need to move the patient's clothing aside to visualize the hips.

Asymmetric hips may occur from curvature of the spine, hip deformities, or unequal leg length.

PALPATE the hips for stability and pain.

Assist the patient to a supine position. Use the iliac crests as landmarks (see Fig. 14.16). Palpate iliac crests to determine if they are symmetric. Findings should be bilaterally symmetric hips that are stable and painless.

Osteoarthritis or hip dislocation may cause pain and hip instability.

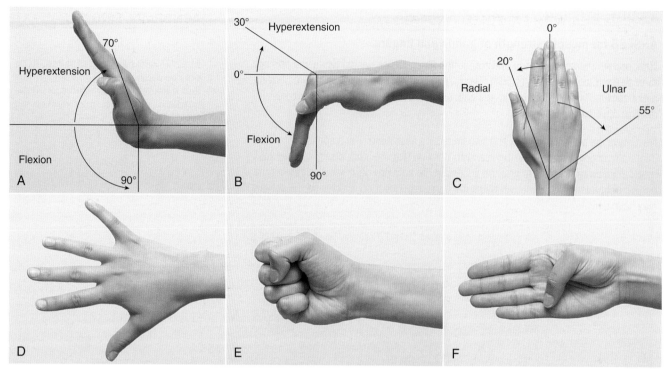

FIG. 14.31 Range of motion of hand and wrist. (A) Wrist flexion and hyperextension. (B) Metacarpophalangeal flexion and hyperextension. (C) Wrist radial and ulnar deviation. (D) Finger abduction. (E) Finger flexion: fist formation. (F) Finger extension: thumb to each fingertip and to base of little finger.

PROCEDURES WITH EXPECTED FINDINGS

ASSESS range of motion of hips.

Hip flexion with knee flexed

Ask the patient to alternately pull each knee up to the chest. The patient should achieve 120-degree flexion from the straight, extended position (Fig. 14.32A).

Hip flexion with leg extended

Next have the patient raise the leg to flex the hip as far as possible without bending the knee. Repeat the procedure with the other leg. Results should be 90 degrees from the straight, extended position (Fig. 14.32B).

External rotation

Ask the patient to place the heel of one foot on the opposite patella. Apply gentle pressure to the medial aspect of the flexed knee as the patient externally rotates the hip until the knee or lateral thigh touches the examination table. Repeat the procedure with the other hip. Rotation should reach 45 degrees from the straight, midline position (Fig. 14.32C).

Internal rotation

Ask the patient to flex the knee and turn medially (inward) as you pull the heel laterally (outward). Repeat the procedure with the other hip. Rotation should reach 40 degrees from the straight, midline position (Fig. 14.32D).

Abduction and adduction

Ask the patient to move one leg laterally with the knee straight to assess abduction and medially to assess adduction. Repeat the procedure with the other leg. The expected range for abduction is up to 45 degrees; the expected range for adduction is up to 30 degrees (Fig. 14.32E).

ABNORMAL FINDINGS

Osteoarthritis or hip dislocation impair hip ROM. Vertebral compression of spinal nerves may cause back or leg pain during hip flexion with leg extension.

PROCEDURES WITH EXPECTED FINDINGS

Hyperextension

With patient prone or standing, assess hyperextension of the hip by raising the leg upward with the knee straight (if prone) or swinging straight leg behind the body without arching back (if standing). Repeat the procedure with the other leg. The expected range of movement is up to 30 degrees (Fig. 14.32F).

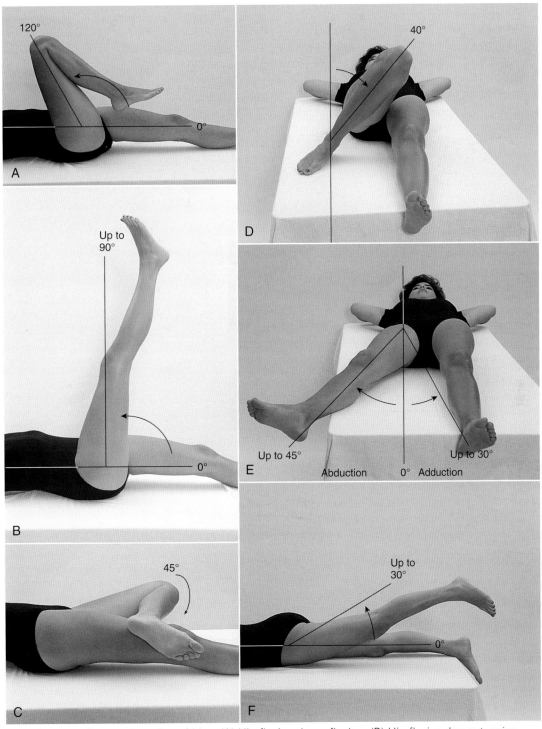

FIG. 14.32 Range of motion of hips. (A) Hip flexion, knee flexion. (B) Hip flexion, leg extension. (C) External rotation of hip. (D) Internal rotation of hip. (E) Abduction and adduction of hip. (F) Hyperextension of hip, leg extension.

PROCEDURES WITH EXPECTED FINDINGS	ABNORMAL FINDINGS

ASSESS the hips for muscle strength.

Assist the patient to a supine position. Ask him or her to attempt to raise the legs while you try to hold them down. Evaluate one leg at a time, noting if the response is bilaterally strong and if you are unable to interfere with the movement. Use the criteria from Table 14.1 for grading muscle strength. It should be 5/5 or normal bilaterally.

An unequal response, weak response, muscular spasm, or pain may be caused by joint or muscle inflammation, trauma, or injuries.

INSPECT leg muscles for symmetry and size.

Procedure: Muscle circumference can be measured with a cloth or paper tape measure to provide a baseline for future comparisons and make side-to-side comparisons. To ensure consistency of measurement, record the number of centimeters above or below the joint where the muscle was measured, or include a diagram such as the one shown in Fig. 14.33.

Findings: Muscles should appear relatively symmetric bilaterally. (No person has exact side-to-side symmetry.) The dominant side is usually slightly larger than the nondominant side. Measurement differences less than 1 cm are usually not significant.

Atrophy of muscle mass bilaterally may indicate lack of nerve stimulation, such as a spinal cord injury or malnutrition. Unilateral muscle atrophy may be from disuse, from pain on movement, or after removal of a cast. Fasciculations (muscle twitching of a single muscle group) may be caused by adverse effects of drugs. Fasciculations are localized, whereas spasms (involuntary muscle contractions) tend to be more generalized.

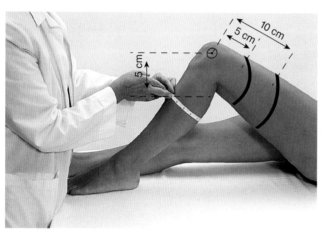

FIG. 14.33 Measurement of the lower leg circumference at 5 cm below the patella, and the upper leg at 5 and 10 cm above the patella. Exact location of measurement should be noted for future comparison.

ASSESS legs for muscle tone.

Procedure: With the patient in supine position, support the patient's thigh with one hand and grasp the foot with the other. Flex and extend the patient's ankle and knee and put the hip through ROM.[9] Repeat the procedure with the other leg. **Findings:** Muscles should have slight tension or resistance during passive movement.[1]

Crepitation or tenderness may indicate joint inflammation. A decrease in tone is documented as hypotonia or flaccidity, which may indicate peripheral neuropathy. By contrast, an increase in tone is documented as hypertonia, which may be spasticity from a central nervous system disorder.[9]

ASSESS the leg muscles for strength.

Procedure: To assess the quadriceps with the patient sitting, have the patient extend the legs at the knee while you attempt to flex the knee. To evaluate the hamstrings with the patient sitting, have the patient attempt to bend his or her knee while you attempt to straighten it.

Findings: For quadriceps and hamstring, strength should be bilaterally equal, and you should be unable to flex the knee (Fig. 14.34). Use criteria from Table 14.1 for grading muscle strength, which should be 5/5 or normal bilaterally.

An unequal response, weak response, muscular spasm, or pain may be caused by joint or muscle inflammation, trauma, or injuries.

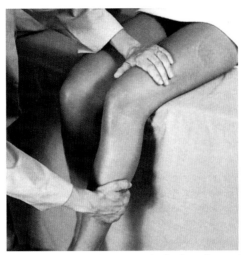

FIG. 14.34 Assessment of hamstring muscle strength. Patient flexes knee while examiner tries to straighten it. (From Barkauskas et al., 2002.)

PROCEDURES WITH EXPECTED FINDINGS	ABNORMAL FINDINGS

INSPECT the knees for symmetry and alignment.

The patient resumes a supine position. The knees should be lined up with the tibia and ankle and symmetric without medial or lateral deviation.

Knees that appear bowlegged (genu varum) or knock-kneed (genu valgum) are abnormal.

PALPATE the knees for contour.

First, palpate the suprapatellar pouch on each side of the quadriceps with the thumb and fingers of one or both hands. Compare one side with the other. The knees should feel smooth. Next, with the knee flexed to 90 degrees, palpate over the medial and lateral aspects of the tibiofemoral joint space. Palpate the popliteal space. The joint should feel firm and smooth.

Edema, heat, or pain may occur from rheumatoid arthritis, osteoarthritis, or bursitis.

ASSESS the knees for range of motion.

Evaluate the ROM by having the patient flex the knees (Fig. 14.35). Flexion should reach 130 degrees from the straight, extended position without discomfort or difficulty. If the knee is able to hyperextend, it should reach 15 degrees from the extended position (midline).

A decrease in the ROM may occur as a result of arthritis, trauma, or ligament, tendon, or meniscus injury.

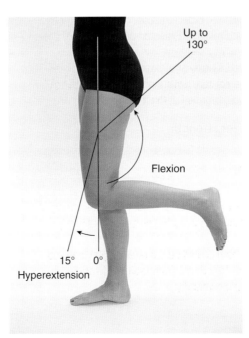

Up to 130°

Flexion

15°　0°
Hyperextension

FIG. 14.35 Flexion and hyperextension of knee.

PROCEDURES WITH EXPECTED FINDINGS

INSPECT the ankles and feet for contour, number of toes, alignment, or deformity.

The ankles should be smooth, with no deformity. The feet are in straight position aligned with the long axis of the lower leg with five toes that are extended and straight on each foot.

PALPATE the ankles and feet for contour.

Use the pads of the thumbs and fingers to palpate the ankle and heel; use both hands to palpate one foot at a time. These structures should feel firm and smooth.

ASSESS the ankles and feet for range of motion.

Procedure and Findings: Ask the patient to stand and:
- Dorsiflex the ankle by pointing the toes toward the face. Dorsiflexion should reach 20 degrees from midline.
- Plantar flex the ankle by pointing the toes toward the floor. Plantar flexion should reach 45 degrees from midline (Fig. 14.37A).
- Evert the foot by rotating it outward. (Note: You may need to stabilize the heel during these maneuvers.) Eversion should be 20 degrees.
- Invert the foot by rotating it inward. Inversion should be 30 degrees from midline position (Fig. 14.37B).
- Abduct the foot by turning it away from midline. Expected abduction is 10 degrees.
- Adduct the foot by turning it inward toward midline. Expected adduction is 20 degrees (Fig. 14.37C).
- Flex toes by curling them downward. Extend toes by straightening them
- Abduct toes by spreading them apart. Adduct toes by bringing them together. All movements should be bilaterally equal and performed without pain.

ASSESS the ankle and feet muscles for strength.

Have the patient maintain dorsiflexion and then plantar flexion while you apply opposing force to evaluate muscle strength.

ABNORMAL FINDINGS

Misalignment of the feet with the ankle or leg or amputation or deformity of toes may require further evaluation. Medial deviation of the toes, hallux valgus (Fig. 14.36), claw toes, hammer toes, and calluses are abnormal.

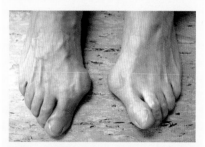

FIG. 14.36 Hallux valgus. (From Jachmann-Jahn, 2009.)

Heat, redness, edema, and pain are signs of an inflamed joint due to rheumatoid arthritis, gout, fracture, or tendonitis.[1]

Limitations in ROM, pain, and asymmetry may require further evaluation. Nerve damage or prolonged immobility may cause foot drop, which prevents the patient from dorsiflexing the foot, causing it to remain in plantar flexion.

An unequal response, weak response, muscular spasm, or pain may be caused by joint or muscle inflammation, trauma, or sports injuries.

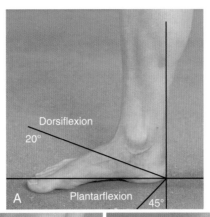
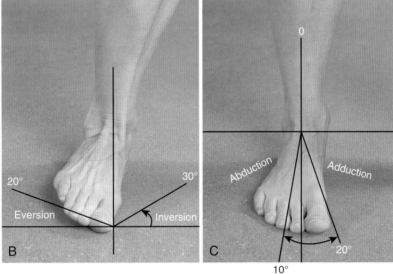

FIG. 14.37 Range of motion of the ankle. (A) Dorsiflexion and plantar flexion. (B) Inversion and eversion. (C) Abduction and adduction. (From Evans, 2009.)

PROCEDURES WITH EXPECTED FINDINGS	ABNORMAL FINDINGS

TECHNIQUES FOR SPECIAL CIRCUMSTANCES

ASSESS for nerve root compression.

Perform this technique when the patient reports numbness or radiating pain in the affected buttock or leg.

To evaluate for nerve root irritation or lumbar disk herniation, perform *straight leg raises*. With the patient supine, raise one leg, keeping the knee straight.

Tightness of the hamstring may be reported, but no pain should be felt (Fig. 14.38).

Pain in the back of the leg with 30 to 60 degrees of elevation indicates pressure on a peripheral nerve by an intervertebral disk.[6]

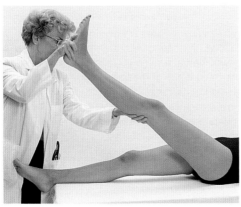

FIG. 14.38 Straight leg raising test.

TECHNIQUES PERFORMED BY AN ADVANCED PRACTICE REGISTERED NURSE

Specialty practice may require advanced techniques that are beyond the skill set of a nurse generalist. Knowing the purposes of these techniques may be helpful when caring for patients who require advanced assessment techniques.

- **Assess for carpal tunnel syndrome.** When patients report numbness, tingling, or pain over the palmar surface of the hands, the first three fingers and part of the fourth finger, they are assessed for carpal tunnel syndrome by pressing the dorsal surfaces of the hands together for 1 minute. Numbness and paresthesia are suggestive of carpal tunnel.
- **Assess for rotator cuff damage.** When the patient complains of shoulder pain, the APRN adducts the patient's affected arm and asks the patient to lower the arm slowly.
- **Assess for knee effusion.** When fluid in the knee joint is suspected, the APRN palpates the knee joint to determine presence of a small or large amount of fluid.
- **Assess knee stability.** This assessment is performed when trauma to the knee is suspected. The APRN adducts the lower leg to detect abnormal movement of the collateral and cruciate ligaments. The affected knee is manipulated forward and backward to assess for abnormal movement of the anterior and posterior cruciate ligaments.
- **Meniscal damage or tear.** With the patient in a supine position, assessment for damage of the meniscus is performed by rotating the knee to determine pain, audible clicks, or locking of the knee. Assessment of a meniscal tear is performed when the patient is unable to bear weight on or flex the knee.
- **Assess for hip flexion contracture.** With the patient lying supine with one leg extended, the APRN flexes the other knee to the chest and watches the movement of the extended leg. If the extended leg lifts off the exam table, the patient has a hip flexion contracture.

DOCUMENTING EXPECTED FINDINGS

Coordinated smooth gait, full ROM in all joints without pain, muscles symmetric and firm with 5/5 strength bilaterally, and adequate muscle tone. Vertebral column straight, shoulders are symmetric, and knees are aligned with hips and ankles.

? CLINICAL JUDGMENT

Musculoskeletal System

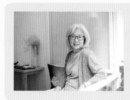

Case Presentation
Cynthia Yung, a 61-year-old female presents to an urgent care clinic with severe pain to her right wrist following a 4-foot fall from a ladder. She states she is unable to move her right hand or wrist.

Reflecting
The nurse reflects on Ms. Yung's clinical presentation and this clinical encounter; she was subsequently diagnosed with right wrist fracture and sent home with a referral to an orthopedic surgeon the following day. This experience contributes to the nurse's expertise when encountering a similar situation.

Noticing / Recognizing Cues
Based on the presenting information, the experienced nurse recognizes the emergent nature of Ms. Yung's condition. The nurse knows that a 4-foot fall can potentially result in significant injury – particularly for an older adult. The nurse observes Ms. Yung sitting upright, holding her arm against her abdomen under a pillow, and recognizes this is a common protective posture with upper-extremity trauma. The nurse learns that Ms. Yung is in good health but has a history of osteoporosis for which she takes alendronate (Fosamax). The nurse knows that Ms. Yung's age and medical history are risk factors for musculoskeletal injury.

Responding / Taking Action
The nurse initiates appropriate initial interventions (protection of the joint, ice, pain relief, and monitoring of perfusion distal to the injury site) and notifies the nurse practitioner of the situation, ensuring that Ms. Yung receives prompt medical care, and also provides the nurse practitioner with the name of the orthopedic physician on call.

Interpreting / Analyzing Cues & Forming Hypotheses
The nurse follows the cognitive cues, recalling several possible causes for Ms. Yung's pain: hematoma, muscle sprain, fracture, or a combination of these. To determine if any of these have any probability of being correct, the nurse gathers additional data:
- What is the appearance of the right wrist joint?
  There is moderate edema to the wrist and forearm.
- Is there evidence of joint instability?
  The nurse notes crepitus and increased pain to the right wrist with palpation. The experienced nurse not only recognizes a fracture by the clinical signs (edema and crepitus) and symptoms (pain, loss of motion), but also interprets this information in the context of an older adult with osteoporosis who has fallen.

AGE-RELATED VARIATIONS

This chapter discusses assessment techniques with adult patients. These data are important to assess for individuals of all ages, but the approach and techniques used to collect the information may vary depending on the patient's age.

INFANTS, CHILDREN, AND ADOLESCENTS

There are several differences in the assessment of the system for infants and young children. Infants' movement is assessed during voluntary movement, and hip joints and feet are assessed for abnormalities. Children's motor development is compared with standardized tables of normal age and sequences described in Chapter 18. Further information regarding musculoskeletal assessment of infants, children, and adolescents is presented in Chapter 19.

OLDER ADULTS

Assessing the musculoskeletal system of an older adult usually follows the same procedures as for an adult. The pace of the examination is individualized to accommodate their mobility. Older adults may be slower at performing ROM, and their muscle strength may be less than that of a younger adult. They may also need assistance to maintain balance when performing procedures while standing. Chapter 21 presents further information regarding the musculoskeletal assessment of older adults.

COMMON PROBLEMS AND CONDITIONS

BONES

Fracture

A partial or complete break in the continuity of a bone is a fracture. The skin remains intact in a closed fracture and is broken in an open fracture (Fig. 14.39). Fractures occur when the bone is subjected to excessive force, such as a crushing injury or direct blow, or when the bone has insufficient integrity causing a pathologic or spontaneous fracture. In the United States, the incidence of fractures has been increasing, in part due to increases in lifespan, urbanization, and trauma. Six million fractures occur on an annual basis.[10] Fractures are a common injury at any age but are more likely to occur in children and older adults. **Clinical Findings:** The most pronounced symptom is pain, which can be associated with the trauma to the bone and surrounding tissues or caused from muscle spasm. Deformity and loss of function are caused by the shortening of tissue around the bone and localized edema. Diminished function and pain that increases with movement develop along with localized edema and discoloration.[10]

Osteoporosis

Loss of bone density (osteopenia) and decreased bone formation result in osteoporosis. Approximately 54 million Americans have low bone mass, increasing their risk for osteoporosis. Approximately one in two women and up to one in four men age 50 years and older will have a fracture associated with osteoporosis.[11] **Clinical Findings:** Osteoporosis is referred to as a *silent disease* because bone loss occurs without signs or symptoms. Patients may not know they have osteoporosis until they discover a loss of height, experience a spontaneous fracture (pathologic fracture) from brittle bones, or develop kyphosis (convex curvature of the thoracic spine) (Fig. 14.40).[11]

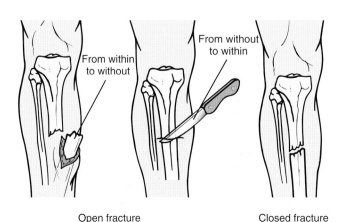

Open fracture   Closed fracture

FIG. 14.39 Open and closed fractures. (From Lewis et al., 2007.)

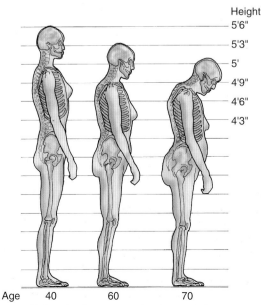

FIG. 14.40 Hallmark of osteoporosis: dowager's hump (kyphosis). (From Ignatavicius and Workman, 2010.)

JOINTS

Rheumatoid Arthritis

This form of arthritis is a chronic, systemic autoimmune disease involving inflammation and degeneration of joints.[12] Approximately 1.3 million of the Unites States' adult population have rheumatoid arthritis.[13] As the disease progresses, the synovial lining of joints becomes inflamed, leading to deterioration of cartilage and erosion of surfaces, causing bone spurs. Ligaments and tendons around inflamed joints become fibrotic and shortened, causing contractures and subluxation (partial dislocation) of joints.[12] **Clinical Findings:** Joint involvement is usually bilateral. Localized symptoms are pain; edema; and stiffness of the fingers, wrists, ankles, feet, and knees. Patients report pain and stiffness after awakening in the morning that lasts more than 30 minutes. Systemic symptoms caused by the autoimmune response include low-grade fever and fatigue. As the disease process continues, ulnar deviation, swan-neck deformity, and boutonniere deformity may be observed (see Fig. 14.28).[13]

Osteoarthritis

Degenerative joint disease is another name for this form of arthritis, which results in progressive breakdown and loss of cartilage in one or more joints. It affects weight-bearing joints such as vertebrae, hips, knees, and ankles, but it also affects fingers. Osteoarthritis affects more than 30 million adults in the Unites States.[14] **Clinical Findings:** Patients report edema and aching, with diffuse pain during movement. Also, they report stiffness after awakening in the morning that lasts less than 30 minutes and decreases with movement.[8] Joint deformities of fingers develop (Heberden nodes in DIP joints and Bouchard nodes in PIP joints) (see Fig. 14.27).[1]

Bursitis

Bursa become inflamed by constant repetitive motions or positions that put pressure on the joints they surround (see Figs. 14.1 and 14.41). The shoulder, elbow, and hip are commonly affected, but bursitis also occurs in the knee, heel, and base of the great toe. **Clinical Findings:** Edema, point tenderness, and erythema of the affected joint are common. Patients may report sudden inability to move the joint. Pain may be described as aching or a sharp or shooting pain with exercise.[15]

Gout

Gout is a form of arthritis that develops from an increase in serum uric acid. In acute gout, crystals of uric acid deposit in one or more joints. The great toe is the most common initial joint affected, but other joints include wrists, knees, and ankles. Chronic gout is characterized by multiple joint involvement with visible deposits of sodium urate crystals called tophi. In the United States, gout affects approximately 8 million people, with men being affected three times as often as women. **Clinical Findings:** Patients report sudden and progressively severe onset of pain and

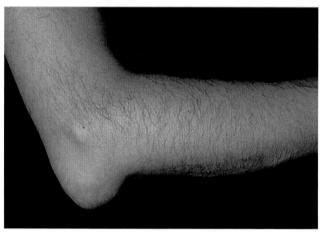

FIG. 14.41 Olecranon bursitis. (Reprinted from the Clinical slide collection of the rheumatic diseases, copyright 1991, 1995, 1997. Used with permission of the American College of Rheumatology.)

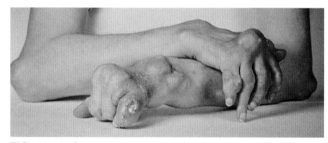

FIG. 14.42 Gout with many tophi present on the hands, on the wrists, and in both olecranon bursae. (Reprinted from the clinical slide collection of the rheumatic diseases, copyright 1991, 1995, 1997. Used with permission of the American College of Rheumatology.)

edema in the affected joint triggered by trauma, surgery, alcohol ingestion, or systemic infection. The onset of symptoms is often at night and persists 2 to 10 days with or without treatment. Affected joints appear cyanotic and are extremely tender. Tophi seen in chronic gout are round, pea-like deposits of uric acid in ear cartilage or large, irregularly shaped deposits in subcutaneous tissue or other joints (Fig. 14.42). Kidney stones from uric acid crystals can cause manifestations of flank pain and costovertebral angle pain.[5]

SPINE

Herniated Nucleus Pulposus

The intervertebral disk provides a cushion between two vertebrae and contains a nucleus pulposus encased in fibrocartilage. When the fibrocartilage surrounding an intervertebral disk is damaged, the nucleus pulposus is displaced and compresses adjacent spinal nerves (Fig. 14.43). *Herniated disk* and *slipped disk* are other names for this disorder.

Common sites of herniation are lumbosacral disks at L4–L5 and L5–S1 and cervical disks at C5–C6 and C6–C7.[4] **Clinical Findings:** Symptoms depend on the location of the herniated disk. For example, when L4 is affected, the patient reports pain along the front of the leg, sensory loss around the knee, and loss of knee-jerk reflex. However, when L5 is affected, the patient reports pain along the side of the leg, sensory loss in the web of the big toe, and no loss of reflexes. (Refer to the dermatome map shown in Fig. 15.8 to see the areas of the leg that are innervated by the spinal nerves.) The patient may complain of numbness and radiating pain in the affected extremity from a herniated lumbar disk. Straight leg raises cause pain in the involved leg by putting pressure on the spinal nerve. Cervical herniated nucleus pulposus causes arm pain and paresthesia. Deep tendon reflexes may be depressed or absent, depending on the spinal nerve root involved.

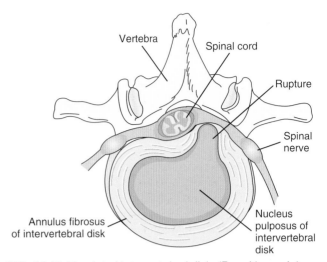

FIG. 14.43 Herniated intervertebral disk. (From Young-Adams and Proctor, 2011.)

CLINICAL APPLICATION AND CLINICAL JUDGMENT

See Appendix B for answers to exercises in this section.

CASE STUDY

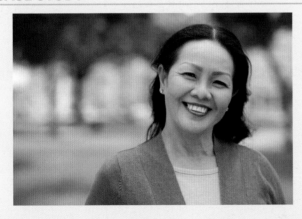

Mrs. Soto is a 46-year-old Asian woman with rheumatoid arthritis (RA). The following data are collected by the nurse during an interview and examination.

Interview Data

Mrs. Soto was diagnosed with RA at age 30. Her mother and grandmother had osteoporosis. She has been taking oral medication to treat her RA. She complains of a great deal of pain in her joints, particularly in her hands, and says that she has "just learned to live with the pain because it will always be there." She states that the stiffness and pain in her joints are always worse in the morning or if she sits for too long. She denies muscle weakness other than the fact that her stiffness and soreness prevent her from doing much activity. Mrs. Soto reports that the RA is progressing to the point at which she is having difficulty doing things requiring fine-motor dexterity, such as changing clothes, holding eating utensils, and cutting up her food. She had different faucet handles installed in her home so she could turn the water on and off. Mrs. Soto says that she rarely goes out because she feels ugly.

Examination Data

The patient is able to stand, but standing erect is not possible. Gait is slow, steady, and purposeful. Significant edema and pain are noted on palpation of wrists, hands, knees, and ankles bilaterally. Hand grips are weak bilaterally. Subcutaneous nodules are noted at ulnar surface of elbows bilaterally.

Clinical Judgment

1. Which cues do you recognize that suggest deviations from expected findings, suggesting a need for further investigation?
2. For which additional information should the nurse ask or assess?
3. Based on the data, which risk factors for RA does Mrs. Soto have?
4. With which team members would the nurse collaborate to meet this patient's needs?

REVIEW QUESTIONS

1. Which patient's description of pain is consistent with injury to a bone?
   1. "Deep, dull, and boring"
   2. "Cramping even when not moving"
   3. "Intermittent, sharp, and radiating"
   4. "Tingling with pins and needles sensation with movement"

2. How does the nurse determine if a patient's musculoskeletal examination is normal?
   1. By reading the examination findings documented in the patient's chart
   2. By comparing findings from other patients in the same age group
   3. By reading descriptions in health assessment books
   4. By comparing the patient's left side with the right side

3. While assessing a patient's bicep muscle strength, the nurse applies resistance and asks the patient to perform which motion?
   1. Extension of the arm
   2. Flexion of the arm
   3. Adduction of the arm
   4. Abduction of the arm

4. The nurse assessing the patient's muscle strength finds that the patient has full resistance to opposition. Using Table 14.1, how would this finding be documented?
   1. Poor or 2/5
   2. Fair or 3/5
   3. Good or 4/5
   4. Normal or 5/5

5. While assessing the range of motion of the patient's knee, the nurse expects the patient to be able to perform which movements?
   1. Flexion, extension, and hyperextension
   2. Circumduction, internal rotation, and external rotation
   3. Adduction, abduction, and rotation
   4. Flexion, pronation, and supination

6. A patient reports joint pain interfering with sleep and morning joint stiffness for the first hour after getting out of bed. Considering this report, what abnormal findings does the nurse anticipate during the examination?
   1. Hot, painful, deformed, and edematous wrists and peripheral interphalangeal joints bilaterally
   2. Decreased range of motion of one hip and knee, with pain on flexion and crepitus during movement of these joints

   3. Erythema in one great toe, ankle, and lower leg that is painful to the touch
   4. Abrupt onset of local tenderness, edema, and decreased range of motion of the shoulder and hip bilaterally

7. The nurse is comparing the right and left legs of a patient and notices that they are asymmetric. Which additional data does the nurse collect at this time?
   1. Passively moves each leg through range of motion and compares the findings
   2. Observes the patient's gait and legs as he or she walks across the room
   3. Measures the length of each leg and compares the findings
   4. Palpates the joints and muscles of each leg and compares the findings

8. A patient complains of her jaw popping when chewing. Which examination techniques are appropriate for the nurse to use with this patient?
   1. Inspecting the musculature of the face and neck for symmetry
   2. Observing the range of motion of and palpating each temporomandibular joint for movement, sounds, and pain
   3. Asking the patient to move her chin to her chest, hyperextend her head, and move her head from the right side to the left side
   4. Asking the patient to open her mouth as widely as possible and inspecting the lower jaw for redness, edema, or broken teeth

9. When a nurse asks a patient to place the right arm behind the head, the nurse is assessing for which range of motion?
   1. Flexion of the elbow
   2. Hyperextension of the shoulder
   3. Internal rotation and adduction of the shoulder
   4. External rotation and abduction of the shoulder

10. With the patient in a supine position, how does a nurse assess the external rotation of the patient's right hip?
    1. Asking the patient to move the right leg laterally with the right knee straight
    2. Asking the patient to flex the right knee and turn medially toward the left side (inward)
    3. Asking the patient to place the right heel on the left patella
    4. Asking the patient to raise the right leg straight up and perpendicular to the body

Neurologic System

evolve

http://evolve.elsevier.com/Wilson/assessment

CONCEPT OVERVIEW

The concept for this chapter is *Intracranial Regulation*, representing mechanisms that facilitate or impair neurologic function. Because brain function requires perfusion of oxygenated blood and because the respiratory and cardiovascular systems are impacted by neurologic control, strong bidirectional interrelationships exist among these concepts as shown in the figure. Both motion and perception (sensory and tactile) are extensions of neurologic function that impact other concepts, such as nutrition, development, pain, and elimination. Understanding the interrelationships of these concepts helps the nurse recognize risk factors when conducting a health assessment.

The following case provides a clinical example featuring several of these interrelated concepts.

Rose Montoya is a 77-year-old female who suffered a stroke (cerebrovascular accident) in the right hemisphere of the brain 2 months ago. The stroke has resulted in left hemiplegia (meaning that she has no sensation or movement on the left side of her body). She is no longer able to walk and is now confined to a wheelchair or bed. Mrs. Montoya has developed a pressure ulcer on her left foot because of a loss of tactile perception and motion. She can chew and swallow but with difficulty; thus she has experienced weight loss. She is unable to meet basic care needs (dressing, bathing, and toileting), making her dependent on others. This previously independent woman is now experiencing depression as a result of her current health status.

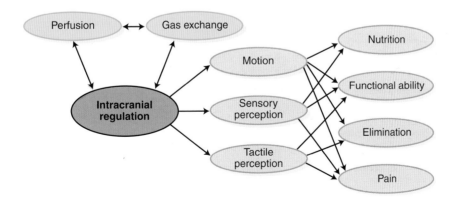

ANATOMY AND PHYSIOLOGY

The nervous system controls body functions through voluntary and autonomic responses to external and internal stimuli. Structural divisions of the nervous system are the central nervous system (CNS), which consists of the brain and spinal cord; the peripheral nervous system; and the autonomic nervous system (ANS).

CENTRAL NERVOUS SYSTEM

Protective Structures

The skull protects the brain. At the base of the skull in the occipital bone is a large oval opening termed the *foramen magnum*, through which the spinal cord extends from the medulla oblongata. There are other openings (foramina) at this base for the entrance and exit of paired cranial nerves and cerebral blood vessels.

Between the skull and the brain are three layers, termed *meninges*. The outer layer is a fibrous layer, termed the *dura mater*. The middle meningeal layer, the *arachnoid*, is a two-layer, fibrous, elastic membrane that covers the folds and fissures of the brain. The inner meningeal layer, the *pia mater*, contains small vessels that supply blood to the brain. Between the arachnoid and the pia mater is the subarachnoid space, where the cerebrospinal fluid (CSF) circulates. A fold of dura mater termed the *falx cerebri* separates the two cerebral hemispheres. Another fold of dura mater, the *tentorium cerebelli*, supports the temporal and occipital lobes and separates the cerebral hemispheres from the cerebellum. Structures above the tentorium cerebelli are referred to as *supratentorial*, and those below it are referred to as *infratentorial* (Fig. 15.1).

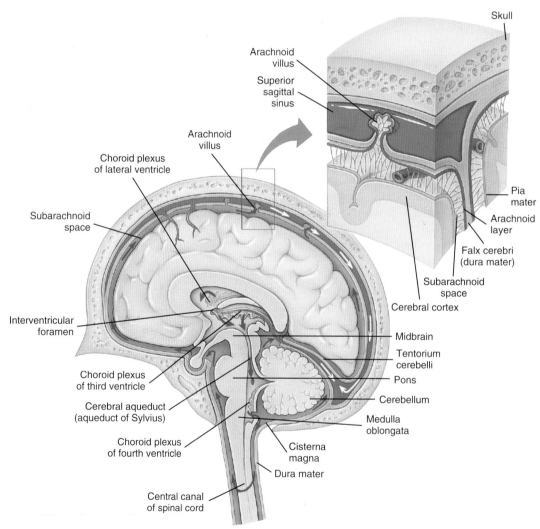

FIG. 15.1 Structures of the brainstem and cerebrospinal fluid (CSF) circulation. Red arrows represent the route of the CSF. White arrows represent the route of blood flow. Cerebrospinal fluid is produced in the ventricles, exits the fourth ventricle, and returns to the venous circulation in the superior sagittal sinus. The inset depicts the arachnoid granulations in the superior sagittal sinus, where the CSF enters the circulation. (Modified from Thibodeau and Patton, 1999.)

Cerebrospinal Fluid and Cerebral Ventricular System

CSF is a colorless, odorless fluid made in the choroid plexus of ventricles, which contains glucose, electrolytes, oxygen, water, carbon dioxide, protein, and leukocytes. It circulates around the brain and spinal cord to provide a cushion, maintain normal intracranial pressure, provide nutrition, and remove metabolic wastes.

The cerebral ventricular system consists of four interconnecting chambers or ventricles that produce and circulate CSF (see Fig. 15.1). There is one lateral ventricle in each hemisphere, with a third ventricle adjacent to the thalamus and a fourth adjacent to the brainstem. The CSF circulates from the lateral ventricles through the interventricular foramen to the third ventricle and through the aqueduct of Sylvius to the fourth ventricle and into the cisterna magna, which is a small reservoir for CSF. From the cisterna magna, the CSF flows within the subarachnoid space up around the brain and down around the spinal cord. The CSF is absorbed through arachnoid villi that extend into the subarachnoid space and is returned to the venous system.

Brain

The brain, consisting of the cerebrum, diencephalon, basal ganglia, brainstem, and cerebellum, is made up of gray matter (unmyelinated cell bodies) and white matter (myelinated nerve fibers). The carotid arteries supply most of the blood to the brain and branch off into the posterior cerebral, middle cerebral, and anterior cerebral arteries (see Figs. 12.15 and 12.17). The remaining blood flows through two vertebral arteries and into the posterior and anterior communicating arteries that supply blood through the circle of Willis. Blood leaves the brain through venous sinuses that empty into the jugular veins.

Cerebrum

The cerebrum is the largest part of the brain and is composed of two hemispheres. Each hemisphere is divided into four lobes: frontal, parietal, temporal, and occipital (Fig. 15.2).

The frontal lobes control intellectual function, awareness of self, personality, and autonomic responses related to emotion. The left frontal lobe contains Broca's area, which is involved in the formulation of words (see Fig. 15.2). The frontal lobes contain the primary motor cortex and are also responsible for functions related to voluntary motor activity. The distribution of the nerves that provide movement to specific parts of the body is shown in Fig. 15.3A. Nerves from the motor cortex cross over in the medulla oblongata, so that nerves on the right side of the frontal lobe control movement on the left side of the body and nerves on the left side of the frontal lobe control movement on the right side of the body.

The parietal lobes contain the primary somesthetic (sensory) cortex. One of its major functions is to receive sensory input such as position sense, touch, shape, and texture of objects. The distribution of the nerves that receive sensations from specific parts of the body is adjacent to the motor cortex

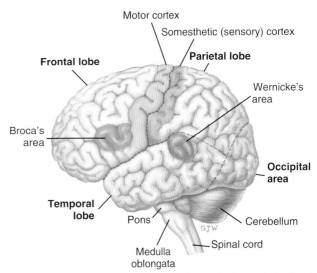

FIG. 15.2 Cerebral hemispheres. Lateral view of the brain. The motor cortex in the frontal lobes is depicted in pink, and the somesthetic cortex in the parietal lobes is depicted in blue. (Modified from Chipps, Clanin, and Campbell, 1992.)

and is shown in Fig. 15.3B. Like the frontal lobe, the sensory nerves from the body cross over in the medulla, so that nerve impulses from the right side of the body are received in the left side of the parietal lobe and impulses from the left side are received in the right side of the parietal lobe.

The temporal lobes contain the primary auditory cortex. Wernicke's area (see Fig. 15.2), located in the left temporal lobe, is responsible for comprehension of spoken and written language. The temporal lobe also interprets auditory, visual, and somatic sensory inputs that are stored in thought and memory.

The occipital lobes contain the primary visual cortex and are responsible for receiving and interpreting visual information.

Diencephalon

The thalamus, hypothalamus, epithalamus, and subthalamus make up the diencephalon. The thalamus is a relay and integration station from the spinal cord to the cerebral cortex and other parts of the brain. The hypothalamus has several important functions in maintaining homeostasis. Some of these functions include regulation of body temperature, hunger, and thirst; formation of ANS responses; and storage and secretion of hormones from the pituitary gland. The epithalamus contains the pineal gland, which causes sleepiness and helps regulate some endocrine function. The subthalamus is part of the basal ganglia.

Basal Ganglia

Between the cerebral cortex and midbrain and adjacent to the diencephalon lie the structures that form the basal ganglia (Fig. 15.4). These structures include the putamen, caudate nucleus, globus pallidus, thalamus, red nucleus, and substantia nigra. The function of the basal ganglia is to create smooth, coordinated voluntary movement by balancing the production of two neurotransmitters: acetylcholine and dopamine.

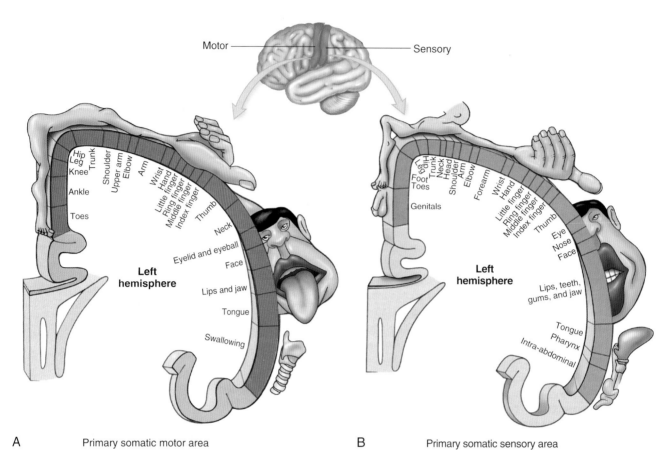

FIG. 15.3 Topography of the somesthetic and motor cortex. Cerebral cortex is seen in coronal section on the left side of the brain. The figure of the body (homunculus) depicts the relative nerve distributions; the size indicates the relative number of nerves in the distribution. Each cortex occurs on both sides of the brain but appears only on one side in this illustration. The inset shows the motor and somesthetic regions of the left hemisphere. (A) Primary somatic motor area. (B) Primary somatic sensory area. (From Patton and Thibodeau, 2010.)

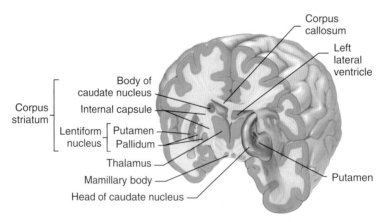

FIG. 15.4 Frontal section of the brain shows nuclei that make up the basal ganglia. (From Patton and Thibodeau, 2010.)

Brainstem

The midbrain, pons, and medulla oblongata make up the brainstem (see Fig. 15.1). A network of neurons throughout the brainstem called the reticular activating system (RAS) controls arousal and awareness. Ten of the 12 cranial nerves originate from the brainstem (Fig. 15.5). The major function of the midbrain is to relay stimuli concerning muscle movement to other brain structures. It contains part of the motor tract pathways that control reflex motor movements in response to visual and auditory stimuli. The oculomotor nerve (CN III) and trochlear nerve (CN IV) originate in the midbrain.

The pons relays impulses to the brain centers and lower spinal nerves. The cranial nerves that originate in the pons

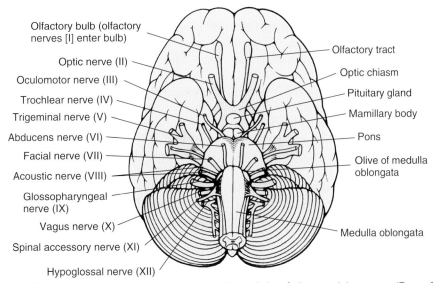

FIG. 15.5 Inferior surface of the brain showing the origin of the cranial nerves. (From Seeley, Stephens, and Tate, 1995.)

are trigeminal (CN V), abducens (CN VI), facial (CN VII), and acoustic (CN VIII).

The medulla oblongata contains reflex centers for controlling involuntary functions such as breathing, sneezing, swallowing, coughing, vomiting, and vasoconstriction. Motor and sensory tracts from the frontal and parietal lobes cross from one side to the other in the medulla, resulting in lesions on the right side of the brain creating abnormal movement and sensation on the left side and vice versa. The cranial nerves that originate in the medulla are glossopharyngeal (CN IX), vagus (CN X), spinal accessory (CN XI), and hypoglossal (CN XII).

Cerebellum

The cerebellum is separated from the cerebral cortex by the tentorium cerebelli (see Fig. 15.1). Functions of the cerebellum include coordinating movement, equilibrium, muscle tone, and proprioception. Each of the cerebellar hemispheres controls movement for the same (ipsilateral) side of the body.

PERIPHERAL NERVOUS SYSTEM

Spinal Cord

The spinal cord is a continuation of the medulla oblongata that begins at the foramen magnum and ends at the first and second lumbar (L1 and L2) vertebrae. At L1 and L2 the spinal cord branches into lumbar and sacral nerve roots termed the *cauda equina.* The spinal cord consists of 31 segments, each giving rise to a pair of spinal nerves (Fig. 15.6). Nerve fibers, grouped into tracts, run through the spinal cord transmitting sensory, motor, and autonomic impulses between the brain and the body. Myelinated nerves form the white matter of the spinal cord and contain ascending and descending tracts of nerve fibers. The descending, or motor, tracts (e.g., anterior and lateral corticospinal or pyramidal tracts) carry impulses from the frontal lobe to muscles for voluntary movement. They also play a role in muscle tone and posture.

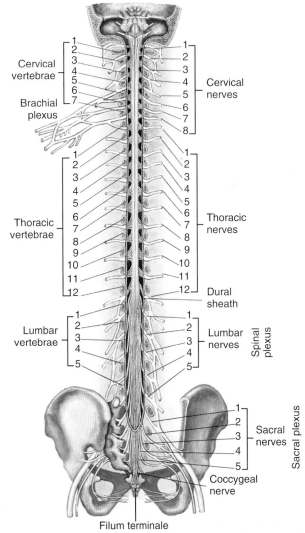

FIG. 15.6 View of the spinal column showing vertebrae, spinal cord, and spinal nerves exiting. (From Chipps, Clanin, and Campbell, 1992.)

The ascending, or sensory, tracts carry sensory information from the body through the thalamus to the parietal lobe. The fasciculus gracilis track travels in the posterior (dorsal) column carrying sensations of touch, deep pressure, vibration, the position of joints, stereognosis, and two-point discrimination. The lateral spinothalamic tract carries fibers for sensations of light touch, pressure, temperature, and pain. The gray matter, which contains the nerve cell bodies, is arranged in a butterfly shape with anterior and posterior horns (Fig 15.7).

Cranial Nerves

Of the 12 pairs of cranial nerves, some have only motor fibers (five pairs) or only sensory fibers (three pairs), whereas others have both motor and sensory fibers (four pairs). Each cranial nerve controls movement or sensation for the same (ipsilateral) side of the body.

Table 15.1 lists the 12 cranial nerves and their functions. Box 15.1 describes ways to remember the names and functions of the cranial nerves. See Fig. 15.5 for the locations of the cranial nerves on the inferior surface of the brain.

Spinal Nerves

The 31 pairs of spinal nerves emerge from different segments of the spinal cord: 8 pairs of cervical, 12 pairs of thoracic, 5 pairs of lumbar, 5 pairs of sacral, and 1 pair of coccygeal nerves. The first seven cervical nerves exit above their corresponding vertebrae. There are eight cervical nerves but seven cervical vertebrae. The remaining spinal nerves exit below the corresponding vertebrae (see Fig. 15.6).

Each pair of spinal nerves is formed by the union of an efferent or motor (ventral) root and an afferent or sensory (dorsal) root. The motor fibers carry impulses from the brain (frontal lobe) through the spinal cord to muscles and glands, whereas sensory fibers carry impulses from the sensory receptors of the body through the spinal cord to the brain (parietal lobe). Each pair of spinal nerves and its corresponding part of the spinal cord make up a spinal segment and innervate specific body segments. The dorsal root of each spinal nerve supplies the sensory innervation to a segment of the skin known as a *dermatome*. Refer to the dermatome map to determine the spinal nerve that corresponds to the area where the patient reports sensory alteration (Fig. 15.8). For example, if the patient complains of pain with numbness and

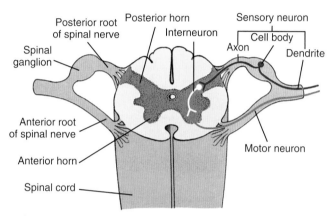

FIG. 15.7 Cross-section of the spinal cord showing three-neuron reflex arc. (From Chipps, Clanin, and Campbell, 1992.)

TABLE 15.1 THE CRANIAL NERVES AND THEIR FUNCTIONS

CRANIAL NERVES	FUNCTION
Olfactory (I)	Sensory: Smell reception and interpretation
Optic (II)	Sensory: Visual acuity and visual fields
Oculomotor (III)	Motor: Raise eyelids, most extraocular movements
	Parasympathetic: Pupillary constriction, change lens shape
Trochlear (IV)	Motor: Downward, inward eye movement
Trigeminal (V)	Motor: Jaw opening and clenching, chewing and mastication
	Sensory: Sensation to cornea, iris, lacrimal glands, conjunctiva, eyelids, forehead, nose, nasal and mouth mucosa, teeth, tongue, ear, facial skin
Abducens (VI)	Motor: Lateral eye movement
Facial (VII)	Motor: Movement of facial expression muscles except jaw, close eyes, labial speech sounds (b, m, w, and rounded vowels)
	Sensory: Taste on the anterior two-thirds of tongue, sensation to pharynx
	Parasympathetic: Secretion of saliva and tears
Acoustic or vestibulocochlear (VIII)	Sensory: Hearing and equilibrium
Glossopharyngeal (IX)	Motor: Voluntary muscles for swallowing and phonation (guttural speech sounds)
	Sensory: Sensation of nasopharynx, gag reflex, taste on the posterior one-third of tongue
	Parasympathetic: Secretion of salivary glands, carotid reflex
Vagus (X)	Motor: Voluntary muscles of swallowing and phonation
	Sensory: Sensation behind ear and part of external ear canal
	Parasympathetic: Secretion of digestive enzymes; peristalsis; carotid reflex; involuntary action of heart, lungs, and digestive tract
Spinal accessory (XI)	Motor: Turn head, shrug shoulders, some actions for phonation
Hypoglossal (XII)	Motor: Tongue movement for speech sound articulation (l, t, n) and swallowing

From Ball J, Dains J, Flynn J, et al: *Seidel's guide to physical examination*, ed 8, St. Louis, 2015, Mosby.

BOX 15.1 HOW TO REMEMBER NAMES AND NERVE TYPE OF CRANIAL NERVES

MEMORY WORD	CN NUMBER	CN NAME	TYPE	MEMORY WORD
On	CN I	Olfactory	Sensory	Some
Old	CN II	Optic	Sensory	Say
Olympus	CN III	Oculomotor	Motor	Marry
Towering	CN IV	Trochlear	Motor	Money
Top	CN V	Trigeminal	Both	But
A	CN VI	Abducens	Motor	My
Finn	CN VII	Facial	Both	Brother
And	CN VIII	Acoustic (vestibulocochlear)	Sensory	Says
German	CN IX	Glossopharyngeal	Both	Bad
Viewed	CN X	Vagus	Both	Business to
Some	CN XI	Spinal accessory	Motor	Marry
Hops	CN XII	Hypoglossal	Motor	Money

Read the words in the column on the left from top to bottom. The first letter of each word is the same as the first letter in the name of the cranial nerve (CN). The fourth column gives the type of impulses carried by the nerves (i.e., sensory, motor, or both sensory and motor). The last column is a phrase to remember the type of nerve for each cranial nerve.

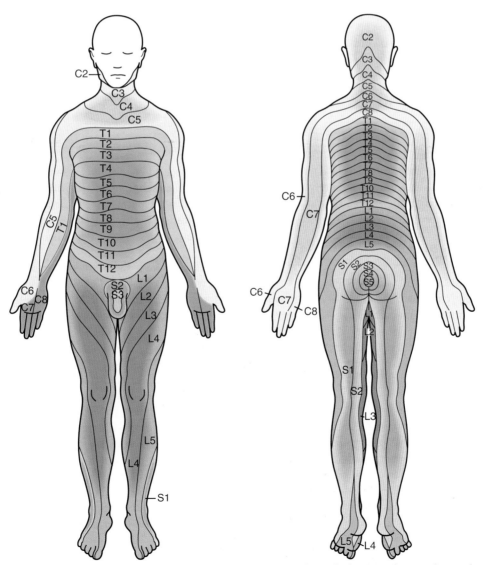

FIG. 15.8 Dermatome map. Letters and numbers indicate the spinal nerves innervating a given region of skin. (From Marx, Hockberger, and Walls, 2010.)

tingling across the right knee, the nurse knows that the fourth lumbar spinal segment is involved, and perhaps compressed.

Reflex Arc

Reflex arcs are assessed by observing muscle movement in response to sensory stimuli. Deep tendon reflexes are responses to stimulation of a tendon that stretches the neuromuscular spindles of a muscle group. Striking a deep tendon stimulates a sensory neuron that travels to the spinal cord, where it stimulates an interneuron that stimulates a motor neuron to create movement (see Fig. 15.7). Superficial reflexes are assessed in the same manner. Each reflex corresponds to a specific spinal segment. Table 15.2 shows the deep tendon and superficial reflexes and the segments of the spinal cord that innervate each reflex.

AUTONOMIC NERVOUS SYSTEM

The ANS regulates the internal environment of the body in conjunction with the endocrine system. It has two components: the sympathetic nervous system (SNS) and the parasympathetic nervous system (PNS). The SNS arises from the thoracolumbar segments of the spinal cord and is activated during stress (the fight-or-flight response). The SNS actions include increasing blood pressure and heart rate, vasoconstricting peripheral blood vessels, inhibiting gastrointestinal peristalsis, and dilating bronchi. By contrast, the PNS arises from craniosacral segments of the spinal cord and controls vegetative functions (breed and feed). The PNS actions are involved in functions associated with conserving energy, such as decreasing heart rate and force of myocardial contraction, decreasing blood pressure and respiration, and stimulating gastrointestinal peristalsis.

TABLE 15.2 SUPERFICIAL AND DEEP TENDON REFLEXES

REFLEX	SPINAL LEVEL
Superficial	
Upper abdominal	T8, T9, and T10
Lower abdominal	T10, T11, and T12
Cremasteric	T12, L1, and L2
Plantar	L5, S1, and S2
Deep	
Biceps	C5 and C6
Brachioradial	C5 and C6
Triceps	C6, C7, and C8
Patellar	L2, L3, and L4
Achilles	S1 and S2

Modified from Ball J, Dains J, Flynn J, et al: *Seidel's guide to physical examination*, ed 8, St. Louis, 2015, Mosby.

HEALTH HISTORY

Nurses interview patients to collect subjective data about their present health status, past health history, family history, and personal and psychosocial history, which may affect the functions of the nervous system.

GENERAL HEALTH HISTORY

Present Health Status

Have you noticed any changes in your ability to move around or participate in your usual activities?
The patient's perception of his or her functioning is the primary source of data. Difficulty moving because of weakness, flaccidity, or spasticity may indicate a neuromuscular problem. Often patients can identify that they are experiencing difficulty performing their usual activities, but they may not associate this with a neurologic disorder.

Do you have any chronic diseases that affect your brain, spine, or nerves? If yes, describe. How long have you had the disease?
There are a number of chronic diseases associated with the neurologic system, including Parkinson disease (PD), multiple sclerosis (MS), stroke, and seizures, to name a few. These questions may help identify risks for injury, opportunities for teaching, and needs for additional resources.

Do you take any medications? If yes, which medications do you take and how often? What are they for?

Adverse effects of medications may influence the nervous system. Drugs (prescription or street drugs) or alcohol may interfere with the functioning of the nervous system. Anticonvulsant medications, antitremor drugs, antivertigo agents, or pain medications could alter a patient's neurologic examination.

Do you take any over-the-counter drugs or herbal supplements? If yes, what do you take and how often? What are they for?
Nonprescription drugs and herbal supplements may affect the nervous system. For example, stimulants found in weight-loss drugs can affect the CNS.

Past Health History

Have you ever experienced an injury to your head or spinal cord? If yes, describe how and when this happened. What residual changes have you experienced since the injury?
Previous injury to the CNS may leave residual deficits such as weakness or spasticity that you can anticipate during the examination. Injury to the frontal lobe can cause changes in memory and cognition.

Have you ever had surgery on your brain, spinal cord, or any of your nerves? If yes, describe. What was the outcome of the surgery?
A history of surgery may provide additional information about possible neurologic problems and the findings to anticipate during the examination.

Have you ever had a stroke? If yes, describe when and what residual changes you have as a result of the stroke.

Previous stroke (cerebrovascular accident [CVA]) may leave residual deficits such as aphasia that affect your subjective data collection or hemiparesis, which you will assess further during the examination.

RISK FACTORS
Cerebrovascular Accident (Stroke)

Biographic data and family history
- *Age:* Older adults are at greater risk. The chance of having a stroke about doubles every ten years after age 55.
- *Gender:* Stroke is more common in women than men, and women of all ages are more likely than men to die from stroke.
- *Genetics and family history:* Risk is greater if parent, grandparent, or sibling had a CVA.
- *Race:* Blacks, Hispanics, American Indians, and Alaska Natives may be more likely have to a stroke than non-Hispanic whites or Asians.

Behaviors
- *Tobacco use:* Cigarette smoking can damage the heart and blood vessels, increasing the risk. (M)
- *Alcohol:* Excessive alcohol intake increases blood pressure and increases triglycerides that can harden arteries. (M)
- *Unhealthy Diet:* A diet high in saturated fat, trans fats, and cholesterol have been linked to stroke and related conditions such as heart disease. Also getting to much salt (sodium) in the diet can raise blood pressure. (M)
- *Physical Inactivity:* Not getting enough physical activity can lead to other health conditions that can increase risk, such as obesity, high blood pressure, high cholesterol, and diabetes mellitus. (M)

Conditions
- *High blood pressure:* A blood pressure (>120/80 mm Hg) is a leading cause of stroke. It occurs when the pressure in blood vessels is too high. (M)
- *High blood cholesterol:* Cholesterol is a waxy fat-like substance made in the liver and found in certain foods. If we take in more cholesterol than the body can use, the extra cholesterol can build up in arteries, including those in the brain.
- *Diabetes mellitus:* Inadequate insulin causes an increase in blood glucose and prevents oxygen and nutrients from reaching various parts of the body, including the brain. High blood pressure is also common in people with diabetes.
- *Obesity:* Obesity is excess body fat, which can lead to high blood pressure and diabetes mellitus. It is also linked to high cholesterol and triglycerides. (M)
- *Previous CVA or transient ischemic attack (TIA):* Having any of these conditions increases the risk.
- *Heart disease:* Common heart disorders increase the risk. These include coronary artery disease, heart valve defects, irregular heartbeats such as atrial fibrillation, and enlarged heart chambers.
- *Sickle cell disease:* This genetic disorder is linked to ischemic strokes that affect mainly black and Hispanic children.

M, Modifiable risk factor.
Data from: National Institutes of Health, National Heart, Lung, and Blood Institute: Stroke. https://www.nhlbi.nih.gov/health-topics/stroke. February 2020.

Family History

In your family, has anyone ever had a stroke,[1] seizures,[2] or brain tumor?[3]

Family history may be used to determine the patient's risk for these conditions.

Personal and Psychosocial History

Have you experienced any changes in your ability to perform your personal care or daily activities? If yes, when did you first notice these changes? Describe the changes you have experienced.

Disorders of the neurologic system such as PD, MS, or myasthenia gravis may interfere with the patient's completion of functional abilities.

How much alcohol do you drink per week? Do you use or have you ever used substances such as marijuana, cocaine, barbiturates, tranquilizers, or any other mood-altering drugs?

Use of these substances may alter the patient's cognitive or neuromuscular function. In addition, the actions of these substances may interfere with the actions of medications.

Do you use a seat belt when riding in a car? If you ride a bicycle, motorcycle, or all-terrain vehicle, do you wear a helmet?

Brain injury can be prevented by using seat belts and wearing helmets when indicated (see the Health Promotion box).

PROBLEM-BASED HISTORY

Commonly reported problems related to the neurologic system are headache; seizures; loss of consciousness; changes in movement (tremors, weakness, or incoordination); changes in sensations (numbness or tingling); difficulty swallowing; or difficulty communicating, such as the inability to understand speech or the inability to speak. As with symptoms in all areas of health assessment, a symptom analysis is completed using the mnemonic OLD CARTS, which includes the Onset, Location, Duration, Characteristics, Aggravating factors, Related symptoms, Treatment, and Severity (see Box 2.6).

Headache

Describe your headaches. What do they feel like? Where do you feel the pain? How long do they last? How often do you have them?

These questions analyze the symptoms of headaches to help determine the cause. Headaches may be related to compression from tumors or increased intracranial pressure or ischemia from impaired circulation within the brain. (Also see Chapter 10 for a description of migraine, cluster, and tension headache symptoms.)

Have you had any recent surgeries or medical procedures such as spinal anesthesia or lumbar puncture?

A transient headache can occur after some diagnostic tests, such as a lumbar puncture. When the patient is in an upright position, the loss of CSF creates tension on the meninges, causing a headache.

Seizures

Have you had a seizure or convulsion? How often do seizures occur? When was your last seizure? What was it like? Did you become unconscious?

Knowing the characteristics of the seizures may indicate whether the patient has focal (partial) or generalized seizures.

Do any factors seem to trigger seizures, such as sleep deprivation, poor nutrition, dehydration, photic stimulation, stress, or alcohol or drug use or withdrawal?[4]

Answers to these questions help plan prevention strategies for seizures.

Do you have any warning signs before the seizure starts? Describe what happens.

An aura can precede a seizure; it can involve auditory, gustatory, olfactory, visual, or motor sensations. The area in the brain that corresponds to the aura provides information about seizure origin.

Which drug(s) do you take to treat seizures and how often? When was your last blood drug level drawn, and what were the results?

Patients who take medications to prevent seizures need to have a blood level of the drug tested periodically to ensure the level is high enough to prevent seizures.

If the patient loses consciousness during the seizure, refer the following questions to people who observed the seizure. Describe the seizure movements that you observed. Did you notice any other signs, such as a change in color of the face or lips or loss of consciousness (and for what length of time)? Did the patient urinate or have a bowel movement during the seizure? After the seizure, how long did it take him or her to return to the preseizure level of consciousness?

Responses to these questions help identify the areas of the brain involved in the seizure activity. Fig. 15.3A is helpful for understanding the path that a seizure may follow. For example, if the seizure begins in the wrist and travels to the head, neck, and trunk, its path moves along the motor cortex. This is an example of a simple seizure in which the patient maintains consciousness.

How do you feel after the seizure? Are you confused? Do you have a headache or aching muscles? Do you sleep more than usual?

Affirmative answers to these questions may indicate the expected recovery phase of a generalized seizure. Patients may be weak, confused, or sleepy after a seizure because the brain's glucose supply was used during the seizure and must be restored.

How have the seizures affected your life? Your occupation? Do you wear any identification to indicate that you have seizures?

Seizures can be a chronic disease that affects patients' driving, personal relationships, and employment. Thus, the nurse needs to learn how seizures have affected the patient's life and if he or she has adapted. Carrying identification about seizures helps those who may assist a patient who is having a seizure.

Loss of Consciousness

When did you lose consciousness? Did the change occur gradually or suddenly? Can you describe what happened to you just before you lost consciousness? Were there other symptoms related to the change of consciousness?

Loss of consciousness may be caused by neurologic disorders or cardiovascular disorders, which tend to cause symptoms more rapidly. It is also associated with drugs; psychiatric illness; or metabolic diseases such as hypoxia, liver or kidney failure, or diabetes mellitus.

Changes in Movement

How long have you had changes in your movement? Describe the change. Is it continuous or intermittent?

The patient's description helps guide subsequent questions for the symptom analysis.

Have you noticed any tremors or shaking of the hands or face? When did they start? What makes the tremors worse? What relieves the tremors: rest, activity, or alcohol? Do they affect your performance of daily activities?

Answers to these questions may help identify the cause of the altered mobility. For example, PD causes tremor at rest, whereas cerebellar disorders cause tremor with intentional movement.

Have you felt any sense of weakness in or difficulty moving parts of your body? Is this confined to one area or generalized? Is it associated with anything in particular (e.g., activity)?

Decreased circulation to the brain can cause these symptoms. Some type of transient ischemic attack (TIA) or CVA may have occurred.

Do you have problems with coordination? Do you have difficulty keeping your balance when you walk? Do you lean to one side or fall? Which direction? Do your legs suddenly give way?

A CVA may be the cause, but dysfunction of the cerebellum or inner ear should be considered when balance is impaired. Multiple sclerosis, PD, or brain tumor may also be causes. If a patient reports falls in one direction, such as to the right, this may indicate that muscle weakness is caused by impaired nerve function on the left side of the brain.

Changes in Sensation

Describe the change(s) in your sensation and its location(s). How does it feel? Is it associated with any activity?

These questions relate to some types of CNS disorders (e.g., MS or CVA), peripheral nerve disorder (e.g., diabetes mellitus may cause peripheral neuropathy), peripheral vascular disease, or anemia (vitamin B_{12} deficiency anemia causes paresthesia). Paresthesias often fluctuate with posture, activity, rest, edema, or underlying disease. Hypoesthesia is decreased sensation that may indicate a sensory problem from impaired circulation or nerve compression. Identifying the location of the abnormal sensation may help identify its cause.

Difficulty Swallowing (Dysphagia)

How long have you had problems swallowing? Do these problems involve liquids or solids? Both? Do you have excessive saliva or drooling? Do you cough or choke when trying to swallow?
These questions are part of a dysphagia screening tool.[5] Dysphagia may be caused by impaired cognitive function, stroke, PD, MS, or muscular disease.[6]

Difficulty Communicating

How long have you had problems speaking? Are you having difficulty forming words or finding the right words? Have you had difficulty understanding things that are said to you? When did this difficulty begin?
PD may create difficulty forming words because of bradykinesia (slow movement) of facial muscles. *Aphasia* is the term for defective or absent language function, whereas *dysphasia* is an impairment of speech not as severe as aphasia. The inability to comprehend the speech of others and of oneself is termed *receptive aphasia* or *fluent aphasia*, and is associated with lesions in the Wernicke's area in the temporal lobe (see Fig. 15.2). The inability to spontaneously communicate or translate ideas into meaningful speech or writing is termed *expressive aphasia* or *nonfluent aphasia*, and is associated with lesions in the Broca's area in the frontal lobe. NOTE: These questions may need to be asked of the person accompanying the patient when the patient is unable to respond.

HEALTH PROMOTION FOR EVIDENCE-BASED PRACTICE

Traumatic Brain Injury

TBI results from a bump, blow, or jolt to the head or a penetrating head injury. The severity of injury may range from mild to severe. TBI accounted for approximately 2.5 million ED visits, hospitalizations, and deaths in the United States in a year. Of these persons, approximately 87% (2,213,826) were treated and released from the ED, another 11% (283,630) were hospitalized and discharged, and approximately 2% (52,844) died. This estimate does not account for those treated in an outpatient or office-based visit nor does it count those treated in federal facilities, such as those serving in the US military or those seeking care from a Veterans Affairs hospital. Those most likely to have TBI are children 0–4 years, adolescents 15–19 years, and adults aged 75 years and older.

The leading causes of non-fatal TBI are falls (35%), motor vehicle-related injuries (17%), and strikes or blows to the head from or against an object (17%), such as sports injuries. The leading causes of TBI-related deaths are motor vehicle crashes, suicides, and falls.

Recommendations to Reduce Risk (Primary Prevention)

- Counsel individuals to use lap/shoulder belts while in a car. Children should ride in an appropriate-size child safety seat, in accordance with the manufacturer's instructions, in the middle of the rear seat.
- Advise individuals against riding in the back of pickup trucks or in cargo areas of vehicles unless equipped with seat belts.
- Distracted driving (such as using a cell phone, texting, and eating while driving) increases the chance of a motor vehicle crash.
- Advise individuals against driving while under the influence of drugs or alcohol or riding as a passenger with an impaired driver.
- Advise individuals to wear approved safety helmets for activities such as riding bicycles, motorcycles, all-terrain vehicles, skateboards, scooters, playing contact sports, skiing or snowboarding, or riding horses.
- Review risk for falls.
- Increase safety of homes and play areas for children by using safety gates at the top and bottom of stairs, installation of window guards, and placement of soft material (mulch or sand) around playground equipment.

Data from Centers for Disease Control and Prevention. (2015). Report to Congress on Traumatic Brain Injury in the United States: Epidemiology and Rehabilitation. National Center for Injury Prevention and Control; Division of Unintentional Injury Prevention. Atlanta, GA. Available at: https://www.cdc.gov/traumaticbraininjury/pdf/TBI_Report_to_Congress_Epi_and_Rehab-a.pdf.

EXAMINATION

Routine techniques

- ASSESS mental status and level of consciousness.
- ASSESS speech.
- NOTICE cranial nerve functions.
- OBSERVE gait.
- ASSESS extremities for muscle strength and tone.

Techniques for special circumstances

- ASSESS cranial nerves.
- ASSESS cerebellum.
- ASSESS sensory function.
- ASSESS deep tendon reflexes.
- ASSESS altered level of consciousness.

Equipment needed

Aromatic materials • Penlight • Tuning fork (200 to 400 Hz) • Cotton-tipped applicator • Tongue blade • Examination gloves • Reshaped paper clip • Cotton ball • Percussion hammer • Monofilament

PROCEDURES WITH EXPECTED FINDINGS	ABNORMAL FINDINGS

ROUTINE TECHNIQUES

PERFORM hand hygiene.

ASSESS mental status and level of consciousness.

Greet the patient and notice the response. The patient is expected to turn toward you and respond appropriately. Ask the patient his or her preferred name, his or her current location, and the date to assess knowledge of person, place, and time. While taking the patient's history, you gather data about his or her mental status. More detail is provided on this assessment in Chapter 7. The patient should be alert and oriented to person, place, and time.

Patients who do not know their name or location are disoriented. Patients may be awake (aroused) but not aware (unable to respond to questions). For example, patients in a persistent vegetative state are awake but unable to speak or respond to any requests. Those who require excessive stimulation or even painful stimuli to respond have a decrease in level of consciousness. A change in level of consciousness is the first sign of impaired cerebral function.[7]

ASSESS speech for articulation and voice quality and conversation for comprehension of verbal communication.

The patient's speech is coherent with sufficient volume. His or her responses indicate an understanding of what is said.

Findings requiring further assessment include errors in choice of words or syllables, difficulty in articulation, slurred speech, poorly coordinated or irregular speech, monotone or weak voice; nasal tone, rasping, or hoarseness; whispering voice; and stuttering.

NOTICE cranial nerve functions.

Assessing cranial nerves is not performed during a routine examination. They are assessed when you suspect an abnormal finding of one or more of the cranial nerves. However, you collect data about the expected cranial nerve functions during the interview. If you notice the following expected findings, you would document "CN II-CN XII grossly intact."

- The olfactory nerves (CN I) are frequently not assessed; however, if the patient mentions altered taste, this may indicate a need to assess for smell.

- The patient's ability to enter the exam room and sit down without difficulty indicates function of the optic nerves (CN II).

- Observe the patient's eye movements during the interview. The patient's eyes moving equally from side to side, up and down, and obliquely indicates oculomotor (CN III), trochlear (CN IV), and abducens nerves (CN VI) are intact.

- The patient's eyelids blinking indicate the ophthalmic branches of the trigeminal nerves (CN V) are intact.

- The patient's facial symmetry when talking indicates the facial nerves (CN VII) are intact.

- The patient's ability to hear you indicates the acoustic or vestibulocochlear nerves (CN VIII) are intact.

- The patient's ability to swallow indicates the glossopharyngeal nerves (CN IX) and vagus nerves (X) are intact.

- Hearing the patient's guttural speech sounds (e.g., k or g) indicates another function of the vagus nerves (CN X).

- The patient shrugging the shoulders or turning the head during the interview indicates the spinal accessory nerves (XI) are intact.

- The patient's ability to enunciate words indicates the hypoglossal nerves (CN XII) are intact.

Patient reports an absence of smell or lack of taste of food and drink.

If the patient bumps into furniture, squints, or needs assistance to locate a chair, it may indicate a vision problem. Notice a lack of eye movement or eyes moving in opposite directions.

Lack of blinking is abnormal.

Asymmetry of the patient's face is abnormal.
Indications of hearing loss include the patient asking you to repeat yourself; repeatedly misunderstanding questions asked; leaning forward or placing the hands behind his or her ears to screen out environmental noises.
An inability to swallow saliva may need further evaluation.

An absence of guttural sounds or nasal speech may indicate a vagus nerve abnormality.
An absence or difficulty in turning the head may indicate a CN XI abnormality.

Speech that is not clearly articulated may indicate an abnormality with the tongue.

PROCEDURES WITH EXPECTED FINDINGS

OBSERVE gait for balance and symmetry.

When the patient walks into the room, notice the gait and its symmetry. The patient should be able to maintain upright posture, walk unaided, maintain balance, and use opposing arm swing. Equilibrium indicates the function of acoustic or vestibular (CN VIII) nerves.

ASSESS extremities for muscle strength and tone.

Assess muscle strength and tone using procedures outlined in Chapter 14. Muscle strength may be part of the musculoskeletal or neurologic system assessment. Ask the patient to flex the muscles being evaluated and then resist when you apply opposing force against the muscles. Expect muscle strength to be 5/5, bilaterally symmetric, with full resistance to opposition.[9] Assess muscle tone by feeling the resistance to passive muscle stretch.[10]

TECHNIQUES FOR SPECIAL CIRCUMSTANCES

ASSESS cranial nerves.

Assess these nerves when an abnormality is noticed during the routine exam.

ASSESS nose for smell.

Evaluate the olfactory cranial nerves (CN I). Have the patient close his or her eyes and mouth. Occlude one nostril while assessing the other. Ask the patient to identify common aromatic substances held under the nose. Examples include coffee, toothpaste, orange, or peppermint (Fig. 15.9). Assess the other nostril using a different aroma.
The patient should be able to identify aromas from each nostril.

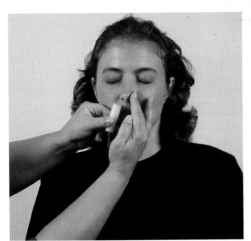

FIG. 15.9 Examination of the olfactory cranial nerve (CN I). (From Chipps, Clanin, and Campbell, 1992.)

ASSESS eyes for visual acuity.

Assess the optic nerves (CN II) for visual acuity using a Snellen chart and an ophthalmoscopic examination of the eye (see Chapter 10).

ABNORMAL FINDINGS

Disorders of the neurologic system, such as rigidity or cerebellar diseases, cause symmetric abnormalities in gait.[8] Poor posture, ataxia, unsteady gait, rigid or absent arm movements, wide-based gait, trunk and head held tight, lurching or reeling, scissors gait, or parkinsonian gait (stooped posture; flexion at hips, elbows, and knees) may require further evaluation (see Fig. 15.24).

Notice muscle weakness (less than 5/5). Paralysis is a lack of voluntary movement or movement that is spastic or flaccid. Spastic paralysis indicates increased tone and occurs after a spinal cord injury or CVA. Flaccid paralysis is the lack of muscle tone and deep tendon reflexes; an example is found in those with spina bifida.[10]

An inability to smell anything or incorrect identification of odors may require further evaluation. Nasal allergies can impair the ability to smell. Loss of smell may be caused by an olfactory tract lesion. *Anosmia* is the term used for loss of or impaired sense of smell.

Refer the patient to an ophthalmologist for further evaluation of vision and eye function when abnormalities are suspected.

PROCEDURES WITH EXPECTED FINDINGS

ASSESS eyes for peripheral vision.

See Chapter 10 for the confrontation test. The presence of peripheral vision indicates the function of the optic nerves (CN II).

Lesions in the central nervous system (e.g., tumors) may cause peripheral visual defects such as loss of vision in one half or one quarter of the visual field, either medially or laterally.

INSPECT eyes for extraocular muscle movement.

The oculomotor (CN III), trochlear (CN IV), and abducens (CN VI) nerves are assessed together because they control muscles that provide eye movement (see Chapter 10).
There will be parallel tracking of an object with both eyes.

Eye movements that are not parallel indicate extraocular muscle weakness or dysfunction of CN III, CN IV, or CN VI.

INSPECT eyes for pupillary size, shape, equality, constriction, and accommodation.

Pupils should appear equal, round, and reactive to light and accommodation. See Chapter 10 for this assessment technique.

Dilated pupil in one or both eyes may indicate increased intracranial pressure on CN III.

ASSESS face for movement and sensation.

- Assess the trigeminal nerves (CN V) for facial movement and sensation. Assess motor function by having the patient clench his or her teeth; then palpate the temporal and masseter muscles for muscle mass and strength. There should be bilaterally strong muscle contractions (Fig. 15.10A).

Notice an inequality in muscle contractions, pain, twitching, or asymmetry. Disorders of the pons (e.g., a tumor) may cause altered function of CN V or CN VII. A tic or mimic spasm is an involuntary movement of small muscles, usually of the face. Occasional tics may have psychogenic causes aggravated by anxiety or stress.

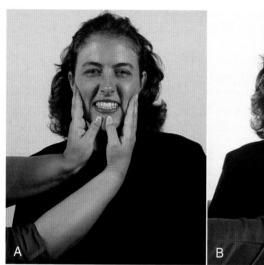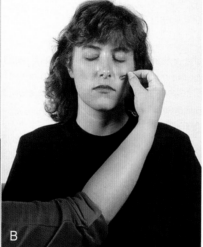

FIG. 15.10 Examination of the trigeminal nerve (CN V) for motor function (A) and sensory function (B). (From Chipps, Clanin, and Campbell, 1992.)

- To assess sensation of light touch, have the patient close his or her eyes while you wipe cotton lightly over the anterior scalp (ophthalmic branch), paranasal sinuses (maxillary branch), and jaw (mandibular branch). A tickle sensation should be reported equally over the three areas touched. Repeat the procedure on the other side of the face.
- To assess deep sensation, use alternating blunt and sharp ends of a paper clip over the patient's forehead, paranasal sinuses, and jaw. The patient should be able to feel pressure and pain equally throughout these areas and differentiate between sharp and dull (Fig. 15.10B). Repeat the procedure on the other side of the face.
- Assess the ophthalmic branch (sensory) of CN V and motor function of CN VII by assessing for the corneal reflex. *This assessment may be omitted when the patient is alert and blinking naturally.* Ask the patient to remove contact lenses if applicable and to look up and away from you. Approach the patient from the side and lightly touch the cornea with a wisp of cotton. There should be a bilateral blink to corneal touch. Patients who wear contact lenses regularly may have diminished or absent reflex.

Decreased or unequal sensation is abnormal. Record the location of the involved areas of the face.

Decreased or unequal sensation is abnormal. Trigeminal neuralgia is characterized by stabbing pain radiating along the trigeminal nerve, caused by degeneration of or pressure on the nerve.[11]
The absence of a blink may require further evaluation.

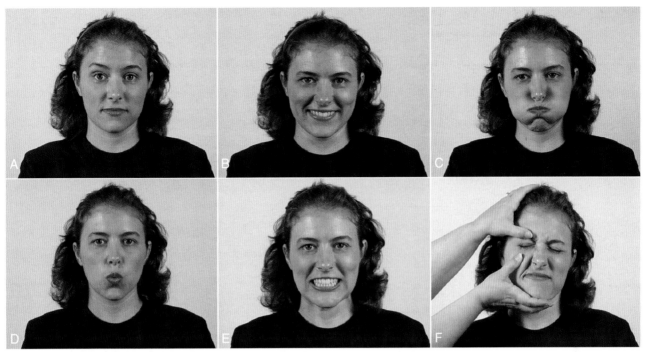

FIG. 15.11 Examination of the facial nerve (CN VII). Ask the patient to make the following movements: (A) Raise eyebrows and wrinkle forehead. (B) Smile. (C) Puff out cheeks. (D) Purse lips and blow out. (E) Show teeth. (F) Squeeze eyes shut while you try to open them. (From Chipps, Clanin, and Campbell, 1992.)

PROCEDURES WITH EXPECTED FINDINGS

- Assess the facial cranial nerves (CN VII) for movement. Inspect the face at rest and during conversation. Have the patient raise the eyebrows, purse the lips, close the eyes tightly, show the teeth, smile, and puff out the cheeks. The patient should be able to correctly perform each request, and the movements should be smooth and symmetric (Fig. 15.11A–F).

ASSESS ears for hearing.

Assessment of sensorineural hearing loss using the Rinne and Weber tests is described in Chapter 10. The tone should be heard equally in the Weber test. Air conduction is longer than bone conduction.

ASSESS tongue for taste.

Taste, the sensory component of CN VII and CN IX, usually is not assessed unless the patient reports a problem. Assess taste over the anterior and posterior tongue.

- For the anterior two thirds of the tongue (CN VII), instruct the patient to stick out the tongue and leave it out during the assessment process. Use a cotton applicator to place on the patient's anterior tongue small quantities of salt, sugar, and lemon, one at a time. Repeat the procedure on the other side of the tongue. The patient should be able to correctly identify salty, sweet, and sour tastes (Fig. 15.12).[9]

- For the posterior one third of the tongue (CN IX), repeat the procedure used for the anterior tongue. The patient should be able to taste salt, sweet, and sour tastes.

ABNORMAL FINDINGS

Asymmetry, facial weakness, drooping of one side of the face or mouth, or inability to maintain position until instructed to relax may require further evaluation.

Sensorineural hearing loss may be indicated using the Weber test by lateralization of sound to the unaffected ear or the Rinne test when air conduction is longer than bone conduction in the affected ear but by a less than 2:1 ratio.

An inability to identify tastes or consistently identifying a substance incorrectly may require further evaluation. Loss of smell and taste may occur together. Patients who are chronic smokers may have decreased taste.

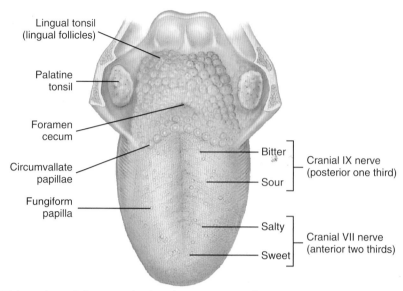

FIG. 15.12 Location of the taste bud regions assessed for sensory function of the facial and glossopharyngeal cranial nerves.

PROCEDURES WITH EXPECTED FINDINGS

INSPECT oropharynx for gag reflex and movement of soft palate.

Assess the glossopharyngeal nerves (CN IX) and the vagus nerves (CN X) together for movement of the soft palate and gag reflex. Instruct the patient to say "ah" to assess CN X. There should be equal upward movement of the soft palate and uvula bilaterally. If necessary, assess the gag reflex by touching the posterior pharynx with the end of a tongue blade; the patient should gag momentarily. Movement of the posterior pharynx and presence of a gag reflex indicates the CN IX are intact. See Chapter 10 for more detail.

ASSESS the tongue for symmetry, movement, and strength.

Ask the patient to protrude his or her tongue. Notice the symmetry. Then ask him or her to move the tongue toward the nose, the chin, and side to side (Fig. 15.13).

Assess the muscle strength of the tongue by asking the patient to press the tip of the tongue inside the check while you resist the pressure from outside of the patient's cheek with your fingers. Repeat the procedure on the other side. The tongue should be moist, pink, and symmetric without lumps, nodules, or ulcers. Tongue strength should be evident by resistance to outside pressure.

ABNORMAL FINDINGS

Asymmetry of the soft palate or tonsillar pillar movement, any lateral deviation of the uvula, or absence of the gag reflex may indicate disorders of the medulla oblongata. For example, tumors in the medulla oblongata may cause pressure on CN IX or CN X.

Asymmetric movement or weakness of the tongue may indicate impairment of the hypoglossal cranial nerve (CN XII). The tongue deviates toward the impaired side.

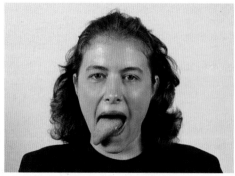

FIG. 15.13 Examination of the hypoglossal nerve (CN XII). (From Chipps, Clanin, and Campbell, 1992.)

PROCEDURES WITH EXPECTED FINDINGS

ASSESS shoulders and neck muscles for strength, movement, and symmetry.

Have the patient turn his or her head to the side against your hand; repeat with the other side (see Fig. 14.15A). Observe the contraction of the opposite sternocleidomastoid muscle and notice the force of movement against your hand. Movement should be smooth, and muscle strength should be strong and symmetric.

Evaluate the spinal accessory nerves (CN XI) for movement. Ask the patient to shrug his or her shoulders upward against your hands (see Fig. 14.20). Contraction of the trapezius muscles should be strong and symmetric.

ASSESS cerebellar function.

Assess the cerebellum when the patient reports or the nurse observes impaired balance or incoordination.

Use at least two techniques for each area assessed (e.g., balance and coordination of upper and lower extremities). Choose these techniques based on the patient's age and overall physical ability. For example, not every patient should have to perform deep knee bends.

ASSESS for balance.

- Perform the Romberg test. Have the patient stand with feet together, arms resting at sides with eyes open, and then eyes closed. Stand close to the patient with arms ready to "catch" the patient if he or she begins to fall off balance. There will be slight swaying, but the upright posture and foot position should be maintained.

- Have the patient close his or her eyes and stand on one foot and then the other. He or she should be able to maintain position for at least 5 seconds.

- Have the patient walk in tandem, placing the heel of one foot directly against the toes of the other foot. The patient should be able to maintain this heel-toe walking pattern along a straight line (Fig. 15.14).

- Have the patient hop first on one foot and then on the other. He or she should be able to follow directions successfully and have enough muscle strength to accomplish the task (Fig. 15.15).

ABNORMAL FINDINGS

Weakness or pain when pushing against your hand or asymmetry may require further evaluation.

Unilateral or bilateral muscle weakness or any pain or discomfort may require further evaluation.

If the patient moves a foot to maintain balance with eyes closed but not open, the problem is probably proprioceptive. If the patient moves a foot to maintain balance with eyes open and closed, the problem is probably a cerebellar or vestibular disorder and is documented as a positive Romberg sign.[12]

Inability to maintain single-foot balance for 5 seconds may require further evaluation.

Inability to walk heel-to-toe or using a wide-based gait to maintain the upright posture may require further evaluation.

Inability to hop or maintain single-leg balance may require further evaluation.

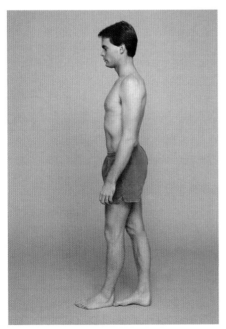

FIG. 15.14 Evaluation of balance with heel-toe walking on a straight line. (From Seidel et al., 2006.)

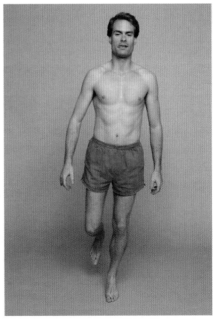

FIG. 15.15 Evaluation of balance with the patient hopping in place on one foot. (From Seidel et al., 2006.)

PROCEDURES WITH EXPECTED FINDINGS

- Have the patient hold one hand outward and perform several shallow or deep knee bends. He or she should be able to follow directions successfully, with muscle strength adequate to accomplish the task.
- Have the patient walk on toes, then heels. He or she should be able to follow directions, walking several steps on the toes and then on the heels. The patient may need to use the hands to maintain balance but should be able to walk several steps.

ASSESS for upper extremity coordination.

- Have the patient alternately tap thighs with hands using rapid pronation and supination movements. Timing should be equal bilaterally, and movement purposeful; the patient should be able to maintain a rapid pace (Fig. 15.16).

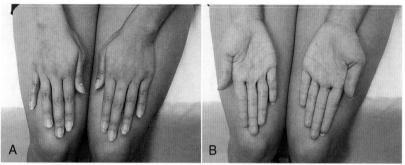

FIG. 15.16 Examination of coordination with rapid alternating movements. Ask patient to tap top of thighs with both hands, alternately with palms down (A) and palms up (B).

- Have the patient close eyes and stretch arms outward. Use index fingers to alternately touch the nose rapidly. The patient should be able to touch the nose repeatedly in a rhythmic pattern.
- Assess the patient's ability to perform rapid, rhythmic, alternating movement of fingers by having him or her touch each finger to the thumb in rapid sequence. Assess each hand separately. The patient should be able to perform movement rapidly and purposefully, touching each finger to the thumb (Fig. 15.17).
- Have the patient rapidly move his or her index finger back and forth between his or her nose and your finger 46 cm (18 inches) apart. Assess one hand at a time. The patient should be able to maintain the activity with a conscious, coordinated effort (Fig. 15.18).

ABNORMAL FINDINGS

Inability to perform activity because of difficulty with balance or lack of muscle strength may require further evaluation.

Inability to retain balance, poor muscle strength, or inability to complete the activity may require further evaluation.

Notice an inability to maintain a rapid pace. An intention tremor (i.e., an involuntary muscle contraction during a purposeful movement of an extremity that disappears when the extremity is not moving) may indicate cerebellar dysfunction.

Cerebellar dysfunction may cause the patient to miss touching his or her nose several times or cause the arms to drift downward.

Notice an inability to coordinate fine, discrete, rapid movement. An intention tremor may be observed during the movement, indicating a cerebellar dysfunction.

Inability to maintain continuous touch both with the patient's own nose and your finger, inability to maintain the rapid movement, or obvious difficulty coordinating may require further evaluation.

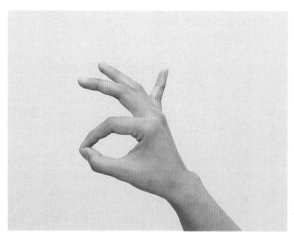

FIG. 15.17 Examination of finger coordination. Ask patient to touch each finger to thumb in rapid sequence.

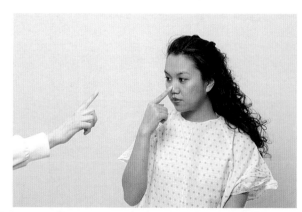

FIG. 15.18 Examination of fine-motor function. Ask patient to alternately touch own nose and the nurse's index finger with the index finger of one hand.

PROCEDURES WITH EXPECTED FINDINGS

ASSESS for lower extremity coordination.

With the patient in the supine position, ask him or her to place the heel of one foot to the knee of the other leg, sliding it all the way down the shin (Fig. 15.19). Repeat on the other leg. The patient should be able to run the heel down the opposite shin purposefully.

Patients with cerebellar disease may overshoot the knee and oscillate back and forth. When experiencing a loss of position sense, the patient may lift the heel too high and have to look to ensure that it is moving down the shin.

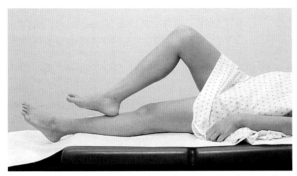

FIG. 15.19 Examination of lower-extremity coordination. Ask patient to run heel of one foot down shin of other leg. Repeat with opposite leg.

ASSESS for sensory function.

Perform these assessments when the patient reports abnormal or absent sensation or for patients with diabetes.

Ask the patient to close his or her eyes during these assessments of sensory function. Areas routinely assessed are the hands, lower arms, abdomen, lower legs, and feet. If sensation is intact, no further evaluation is needed; if impaired, assess sensation systemically from digits up or from shoulder or hip down to identify the area that is without sensation. Compare bilateral responses in each sensory assessment area. Try to map out the area involved using the dermatome map (see Fig. 15.8) to identify the spinal nerve providing sensation to that area of the body.

- To assess sensation to light touch (superficial touch), use a cotton ball and the lightest touch possible to assess each designated area (with the patient's eyes closed; Fig. 15.20A). The patient should perceive light sensation and be able to correctly point to or name the spot touched.

Absence of sensation may be caused by compression of the nerve, whereas inflammation of the nerve may cause abnormal sensation. Pressure in the parietal lobe (e.g., a tumor) can alter sensation. Diabetes mellitus may cause absent or abnormal sensation.

Patient reports of not feeling the light touch, incorrectly identifying the area touched, or reporting an asymmetric response may require further evaluation.

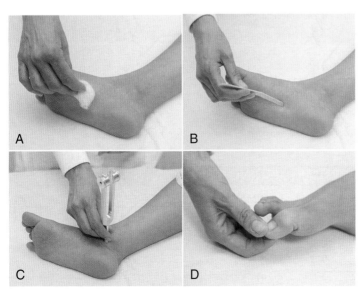

FIG. 15.20 Evaluation of peripheral nerve sensory function. (A) Superficial tactile sensation. (B) Superficial pain sensation. (C) Vibratory sensation. (D) Position sense of joints.

PROCEDURES WITH EXPECTED FINDINGS

- Assess sharp (pain) and dull sensations by using the pointed tip of a paper clip (or broken tongue blade) to lightly prick each designated area (with the patient's eyes closed Fig. 15.20B). Alternate sharp and dull sensations to more accurately evaluate the patient's response. The patient should be able to distinguish sharp from dull sensations and identify the area touched.
- Vibratory sense. Place a vibrating tuning fork on a bony area such as the styloid process of the radius (wrist), medial or lateral malleolus (ankle), and sternum (chest), and ask the patient to describe the sensation (Fig. 15.20C). He or she should feel a sense of vibration. Also ask the patient to report when he or she no longer feels vibration; then stop vibration of the tuning fork by touching it with your fingers without moving it from its location on the bony prominence.

- Joint position or assessment of proprioception. Assess the great toe on each foot and one finger on each hand. Grasp the lateral aspect of the patient's joint to avoid giving a clue about the direction of movement. Move the joint 1 cm up or down (Fig. 15.20D). The patient should be able to describe how the position has changed for all joints assessed.[9]
- Stereognosis. Place a small, familiar object in the patient's hand, e.g., a key, paper clip, or coin, and ask him or her to identify it (Fig. 15.21A). The object should be properly identified.
- Assess two-point discrimination. Touch selected parts of the body simultaneously (Fig. 15.21B). Use the points of two cotton-tipped applicators or reshape a paper clip so that two prongs can be pressed lightly against the patient's skin simultaneously. Ask the patient how many points he or she detects. The expected values for two-point discrimination are listed in Box 15.2.

ABNORMAL FINDINGS

Patient reports of not feeling the sharp or dull touch, being unable to distinguish between sharp and dull, or reporting an asymmetric response may require further evaluation.

Patient reports of an unequal or a decreased vibratory sensation require further evaluation. The patient may not be able to distinguish the change in sensation from vibration to nonvibration or may not feel the vibration in one or more locations. Referring to the dermatome drawing (see Fig. 15.8) helps identify the spinal nerve supplying this area. This may be found in patients with diabetes mellitus and those who have had a CVA or spinal cord injury.
If the patient reports an inability to distinguish the change in position, this may indicate impairment of the sensory (afferent nerves) or parietal lobe.
Altered stereognosis may indicate a parietal lobe or posterior sensory nerve tract dysfunction.[9]
An inability to distinguish two-point discrimination may indicate a parietal lobe or sensory nerve tract dysfunction.[12] Report the anatomic location of the sensory alteration.

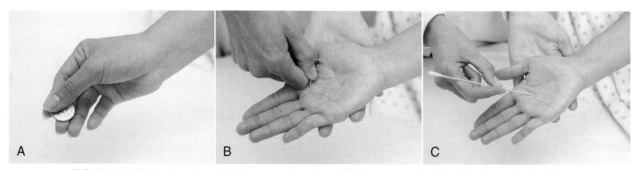

FIG. 15.21 Evaluation of cortical sensory function. (A) Stereognosis: identification of a familiar object by touch. (B) Two-point discrimination. (C) Graphesthesia: draw letter or number on palm and ask patient to identify by touch.

BOX 15.2 MINIMAL DISTANCES FOR DISTINGUISHING TWO POINTS

LOCATION	MINIMAL DISTANCE
Tongue	1 mm or 1/32 inch*
Fingertips	2–8 mm or 1/15* to 5/15 inch
Toes	3–8 mm or 3/32* to 5/15 inch
Palm of hand	8–12 mm or 5/15 to ½ inch
Chest and forearms	40 mm or 1½ inches
Back	40–70 mm or 1½–2¾ inches
Upper arms and thighs	75 mm or 3 inches

*Too small to measure with conventional ruler.

PROCEDURES WITH EXPECTED FINDINGS

- Extinction. Using a pointed tip of a cotton-tip applicator or paper clip, simultaneously touch the same place on each side of the body (e.g., both hands). Ask the patient how many sensations are felt and their locations. He or she should be able to identify both of the sensations and their locations.
- Graphesthesia. Use a blunt instrument to draw a number or letter on the patient's palm, back, or another area (Fig. 15.21C). He or she should be able to recognize the number or letter drawn.
- Point location. Touch an area of the patient's skin and immediately withdraw the stimulus. Ask the patient to point to the area touched. He or she should be able to point to the area touched.
- Peripheral sensation can be assessed using a monofilament on the plantar surface of the foot. The procedure is found in Chapter 3, with an accompanying photograph (see Fig. 3.25).

ASSESS extremities for deep tendon reflexes.

Assess reflexes when the patient reports or nurse notices a change in expected reflex response.

Assess deep tendon reflexes for muscle contraction in response to direct or indirect percussion of a tendon. Assess both right and left extremities. Box 15.3 outlines the scoring system. See Table 15.2 for the spinal level of each reflex. Hold the reflex hammer between your thumb and index finger, and briskly tap the tendon with a flick of the wrist. The patient must be relaxed and sitting or lying down.

- To elicit the *triceps reflex*, ask the patient to let his or her relaxed arm fall onto your arm. Hold the arm, with the elbow flexed at a 90-degree angle, in one hand. Palpate and then strike the triceps tendon just above the elbow with either end of the reflex hammer (Fig. 15.22A). (Some nurses prefer the flat end because of the wider striking surface.) An alternative arm position is to grasp the upper arm and allow the lower arm to bend at the elbow and hang freely; then strike the triceps tendon. The expected response is the contraction of the triceps muscle that causes visible or palpable extension of the elbow.
- The biceps reflex is elicited by asking the patient to let his or her relaxed arm fall onto your arm. Hold the arm with elbow flexed at a 90-degree angle and place your thumb over the bicep tendon in the antecubital fossa and your fingers over the biceps muscle. Using the pointed end of the reflex hammer, strike your thumb instead of striking the tendon directly (Fig. 15.22B). The expected response is the contraction of the biceps muscle that causes visible or palpable flexion of the elbow.
- The *brachioradialis reflex* is elicited by asking the patient to let his or her relaxed arm fall into your hand. Hold the arm with the hand slightly pronated. Using either end of the reflex hammer, strike the brachioradialis tendon directly about 1 to 2 inches (2.5 to 5 cm) above the wrist (Fig. 15.22C). The expected response is pronation of the forearm and flexion of the elbow.
- The *patellar reflex* is assessed with the patient sitting with legs hanging free. Flex his or her knee at a 90-degree angle, and strike the patellar tendon just below the patella (Fig. 15.22D). The expected response is the contraction of the quadriceps muscle, causing extension of the lower leg. When no response is found, divert the patient's attention to another muscular activity by asking him or her to pull the fingers of each hand against the other. While the patient is pulling, strike the patellar tendon.

BOX 15.3 SCORING DEEP TENDON REFLEXES

Assess the five deep tendon reflexes (triceps, biceps, brachioradial, patellar, and Achilles) using a reflex hammer. Compare the reflexes bilaterally. Reflexes are graded on a scale of 0–4, with 2 being the expected findings. Findings are recorded as follows:

0 = No response
1+ = Sluggish or diminished
2+ = Active or expected response
3+ = Slightly hyperactive, more brisk than normal; not necessarily pathologic
4+ = Brisk, hyperactive with intermittent clonus associated with disease

ABNORMAL FINDINGS

Identifying only one sensation may indicate a lesion of the parietal lobe, which causes the extinction of sensation on the side opposite the lesion.

If the patient cannot distinguish the number or letter, he or she may have a parietal lobe lesion.

Difficulty or an inability to identify the area touched may require further evaluation.

An inability to feel a monofilament indicates reduced peripheral sensation. This finding may occur in patients with diabetes mellitus who have peripheral neuropathy.[9]

Notice responses that may range from a hyperactive to a diminished response. Observe whether the abnormal reflex response is unilateral or bilateral.
Hyperactive reflexes are found in spinal cord injuries, calcium and magnesium deficits, and hyperthyroidism.[9] Diminished reflexes are found in calcium or magnesium excesses, hypothyroidism, spina bifida, or Guillain-Barré syndrome.

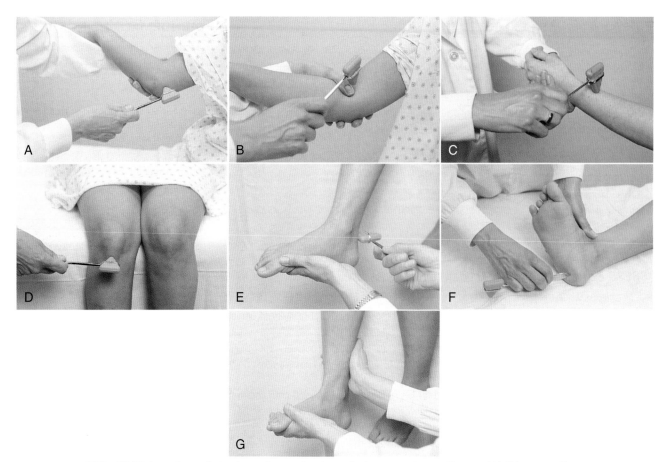

FIG. 15.22 Location of tendons for evaluation of deep tendon reflexes. (A) Triceps reflex. (B) Biceps reflex. (C) Brachioradialis reflex. (D) Patellar reflex. (E) Achilles reflex. (F) Babinski reflex. (G) Ankle clonus.

PROCEDURES WITH EXPECTED FINDINGS

- The *Achilles tendon* is assessed by flexing the patient's knee and dorsiflexing the ankle 90 degrees. Hold the bottom of the patient's foot in one hand while you use the flat end of the reflex hammer to strike the Achilles tendon at the level of the ankle malleolus (Fig. 15.22E). The expected response is the contraction of the gastrocnemius muscle, causing plantar flexion of the foot.
- Check for the plantar reflex (Babinski reflex). Using the end of the handle on the reflex hammer, stroke the lateral aspect of the sole of the foot from heel to ball, curving medially across the ball of the foot (Fig. 15.22F). The expected findings should be plantar flexion of all toes.
- Assess ankle clonus if reflexes are hyperactive. With the patient's knee in a partly flexed position, support the lower leg with one hand. With the other hand, sharply dorsiflex the foot and maintain it in flexion (Fig. 15.22G). There should be no movement of the foot.

ASSESS the level of consciousness.

Assessment of consciousness is needed when the patient is not alert and oriented.

When interacting with an unconscious patient, *always* assume that he or she can hear *everything* you say; thus tell the patient which actions you are going to perform before you do them. A change in the level of consciousness (LOC) is the earliest and most sensitive indicator of alterations in cerebral function. Consciousness is determined by awareness, arousal, and cognition.

ABNORMAL FINDINGS

Dorsiflexion of the great toe with fanning of the other toes is termed a *positive Babinski sign* and may indicate pyramidal (motor) tract disease.

Notice rhythmic muscle movements between dorsiflexion and plantar flexion.

When the cerebral cortex is impaired, the patient has altered cognition. When the reticular activating system in the brainstem is impaired, the patient becomes unaware of time, place, or person and becomes difficult to arouse. This impairment may occur from a head injury, tumor, or encephalitis.

PROCEDURES WITH EXPECTED FINDINGS

An indication of awareness is the patient's mental status determined by orientation, memory, attention, calculation, recall, and language, as well as judgment, insight, and abstraction. Chapter 7 describes the assessment of mental status.

A determination of arousal is assessed by how much stimulation is needed to elicit a response from the patient. The Glasgow Coma Scale (GCS) is a standardized scale for assessing LOC by determining the patient's ability to (1) open the eyes when verbal or painful stimuli are applied; (2) speak when spoken to; and (3) obey requests for movement (Fig. 15.23).[13] Box 15.4 provides guidelines for applying painful stimuli.

ABNORMAL FINDINGS

As LOC begins to decline, disorientation to time occurs first, followed by disorientation to place and, finally, disorientation to person.

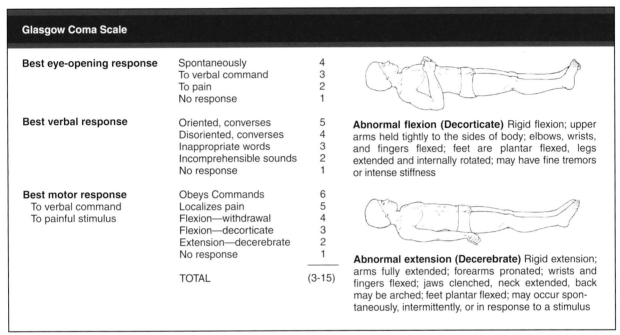

Glasgow Coma Scale

Best eye-opening response	Spontaneously	4
	To verbal command	3
	To pain	2
	No response	1
Best verbal response	Oriented, converses	5
	Disoriented, converses	4
	Inappropriate words	3
	Incomprehensible sounds	2
	No response	1
Best motor response	Obeys Commands	6
To verbal command	Localizes pain	5
To painful stimulus	Flexion—withdrawal	4
	Flexion—decorticate	3
	Extension—decerebrate	2
	No response	1
	TOTAL	(3-15)

Abnormal flexion (Decorticate) Rigid flexion; upper arms held tightly to the sides of body; elbows, wrists, and fingers flexed; feet are plantar flexed, legs extended and internally rotated; may have fine tremors or intense stiffness

Abnormal extension (Decerebrate) Rigid extension; arms fully extended; forearms pronated; wrists and fingers flexed; jaws clenched, neck extended, back may be arched; feet plantar flexed; may occur spontaneously, intermittently, or in response to a stimulus

FIG. 15.23 Glasgow coma scale. The patient's best response in each category is matched to the criteria for scoring. (Modified from Chipps, Clanin, and Campbell, 1992).

BOX 15.4 APPLYING PAINFUL STIMULI TO ASSESS A PATIENT

The Glasgow Coma Scale may require the application of painful stimuli to determine how much stimulation is required to elicit a response. These stimuli are used to assess arousal and awareness, which are components of consciousness regulated by the brain and brainstem. For example, the application of painful stimuli is needed when the patient does not open the eyes spontaneously as you approach him or her or after you speak. Spontaneous eye opening indicates the arousal mechanisms in the brainstem are functioning.[13] Similarly, application of pain is needed to elicit the best motor response to evaluate the integrity of the motor strip in the frontal lobe (see Fig 15.3A) when the patient does not respond to a request for movement, such as "squeeze my hand."

- Before applying pain, however, attempt to create a response by shaking the patient on the shoulder or leg and shouting at him or her.
- If this does not produce a response, resort to painful stimuli. When painful stimuli are used, they should be applied until the patient responds in some way or for at least 15 seconds. They should be used for no more than 30 seconds if there is no response.[13]

- Begin peripherally by using a pen or pencil to apply pressure to a finger, either to the nail bed, side of the nail bed, or fingertip.[13]
- If this does not elicit a response, move centrally using any of the following stimuli to observe for movement:
  - Squeeze and twist the trapezius muscle using the thumb and index finger (see Fig. 14.3); the desired movement is flexion of the arm.[13]
  - Apply pressure to the ear lobe using the thumb and index finger.
  - Push upward on the supraorbital notch above the eye. Do not push inward on the eyeball but on the bony orbit above the eyeball.
  - Apply pressure to the mid sternum by turning your knuckles to the right and left.
  - If no movement is noticed, no response is documented.

DOCUMENTING EXPECTED FINDINGS

Oriented to person, place, and time. Speech understandable and of sufficient volume. Cranial nerves II to XII intact. Balanced gait with upright posture. Muscle strength 5/5 and movement coordinated bilaterally. Sensation intact. Deep tendon reflexes 2+ bilaterally. No clonus present.

CLINICAL JUDGMENT

Neurologic System

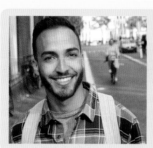

Case Presentation

Josh Stillmen, a 19-year-old male college student, presents to the student health services with a headache. He is accompanied by his roommate, who explains that the patient was playing a game of pickup football with friend and was struck in the left side of the head during a collision with another player. The incident occurred about 4 hours ago, and the headache has been getting worse. His vital signs are within normal limits.

Reflecting

The nurse reflects on Josh's clinical presentation and this clinical encounter; he was subsequently diagnosed with a temporal hematoma and closed head injury. He was admitted to the hospital overnight for observation. Fortunately, no additional intervention was necessary. This experience contributes to the nurse's expertise when encountering a similar situation.

Noticing / Recognizing Cues

Based on the presenting information, the experienced nurse recognizes the potentially emergent nature of Josh's condition. The nurse knows that a head collision can potentially result in significant injury – particularly if it is a high-velocity incident. The nurse observes Josh sitting upright unassisted and alert and oriented to time, place, and person. The nurse palpates a lump over the left temporal region of the scalp and observes a hematoma; the skin is intact.

Responding / Taking Action

The nurse initiates appropriate initial interventions by immediately notifying the attending physician and ensures that Josh receives prompt medical care.

Interpreting / Analyzing Cues & Forming Hypotheses

The nurse follows the cognitive cues, recalling several possible causes for Josh's headache: scalp trauma (hematoma, laceration), closed head injury (CHI), or both. The nurse also knows that CHI can present in many ways, depending on the type of injury. To determine if he potentially has a CHI, the nurse gathers additional data:

- Was there a loss of consciousness at the time of injury?
  Josh says, "I am not sure", but his roommate says, "Josh was knocked out for a few minutes".
- Is there evidence of neurologic changes?
  Josh does not recall playing football or sustaining the injury. The roommate reports that Josh keeps asking the same questions over and over again and adds "He is not acting like himself – he seems kind of agitated". The nurse notes that his pupils are equal, round, and react to light and accommodation.

The experienced nurse not only recognizes the abnormal clinical findings (loss of consciousness, headache, memory impairment, and agitation) but also interprets this information in the context of a young man who had a recent high-velocity blow to the head.

AGE-RELATED VARIATIONS

This chapter discusses assessment techniques with adult patients. These data are important to assess for individuals of all ages, but the approach and techniques used to collect the information may vary, depending on the patient's age.

older child and adolescent follows the same procedures as for adults and reveals similar expected findings. Chapter 19 presents further information regarding the neurologic assessment of infants, children, and adolescents.

INFANTS AND CHILDREN

There are several differences in the assessment of the systems of infants and young children. Neonates and infants have age-dependent reflexes that are assessed. Children's motor development is compared with standardized tables of normal age and sequences of motor development. Assessment of the

OLDER ADULTS

Assessing the neurologic system of an older adult usually follows the same procedures as for the younger adult. Assessing for balance and gait of older adults is often performed to identify those at risk for falls. Chapter 21 presents further information regarding the neurologic assessment of older adults.

COMMON PROBLEMS AND CONDITIONS

DISORDERS OF THE CENTRAL NERVOUS SYSTEM

Multiple Sclerosis

Progressive demyelination of nerve fibers of the brain and spinal cord results in MS. The estimated prevalence of MS in the United States is 700,000.[14] The onset is typically between ages 20 and 50, with symptoms first appearing at an average age of 30 to 35 years, affecting women three times more often than men.[15] **Clinical Findings:** Manifestations vary, depending on the areas of the central nervous system that are affected by the demyelination. Common symptoms are fatigue, depression, and paresthesias. Other manifestations are focal muscle weakness; ocular changes (diplopia, nystagmus); bowel, bladder, and sexual dysfunction[15]; gait instability; and spasticity.

Meningitis

Bacteria or viruses can cause meningitis, an acute inflammation of the meninges. Rates of meningococcal disease have been declining in the United States since the late 1990s. In 2015, 375 cases of meningeal disease were reported.[16] **Clinical Findings:** Meningitis produces severe headache, fever, nausea, and vomiting. A sign of meningeal irritation is nuchal rigidity or a stiff neck, which is an involuntary resistance by the patient when the nurse attempts to flex the neck. Photophobia and a decreased level of consciousness may also be present, which may progress to coma in 5% to 10% of patients with bacterial meningitis. Seizures occur in about one-third of all cases.[7]

Encephalitis

An acute inflammation of the brain is termed encephalitis. In the United States, encephalitis is responsible for about 20,000 cases and 1400 deaths annually. **Clinical Findings:** Manifestations of encephalitis vary, depending on the virus implicated and the part of the brain involved. Initial manifestations are nonspecific, such as fever, headache, nausea, and vomiting. The onset of encephalitis appears on day 2 or 3, and may vary

from minimal changes in mental status to coma. Manifestations may include hemiparesis, tremors, seizures, cranial nerve palsies, personality changes, memory impairment, and dysphasia.[7]

Spinal Cord Injury

Any traumatic disruption of the spinal cord can result in a spinal cord injury (SCI). Injury to the cervical spinal cord may result in quadriplegia or tetraplegia, whereas injury to the thoracic and lumbar spinal cord may result in paraplegia. The number of people with SCI living in the United States is estimated to be 288,000 persons.[17] **Clinical Findings:** Manifestations of complete spinal cord transection include paresthesia or anesthesia, and signs are spastic paralysis below the level of injury with loss of bowel and bladder control. When the injury to the spinal cord is incomplete, it results in variable manifestations that correlate to the location and extent of injury to the spinal cord.

Head Injury

Head injury includes any injury or trauma to the scalp, skull, or brain. A serious form of head injury is *traumatic brain injury* (TBI).[7] Open head injuries result from fractures or penetrating wounds; closed head injuries result from blunt head injury–producing cerebral concussion or contusion. The incidence of TBI (as measured by combined emergency department [ED] visits, hospitalizations, and deaths) in 2014 was 2.87 million.[18] **Clinical Findings:** Manifestations of head injury vary, depending on the severity of the trauma and the areas of the brain involved. Residual deficits in memory, cognition, emotional functioning, and motor and sensory abilities depend on the extent of injury to the brain.

Parkinson Disease

PD is a chronic and progressive movement disorder resulting from the degeneration of the dopamine-producing neurons in the substantia nigra of the basal ganglia. The Parkinson's Foundation Prevalence Project estimates that 930,000 people

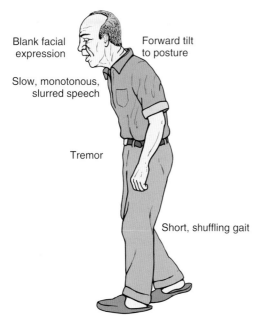

Blank facial expression

Forward tilt to posture

Slow, monotonous, slurred speech

Tremor

Short, shuffling gait

FIG. 15.24 Posture and shuffling gait associated with parkinson disease. (From Christensen and Kockrow, 2011.)

in the United States will be living with PD by the year 2020.[19] **Clinical Findings:** Symptoms develop slowly over years and include tremors, mainly at rest, described as pill-rolling tremors in hands; bradykinesia; limb rigidity; and gait and balance problems. Symptoms unrelated to movement include apathy, depression, constipation, sleep disorders, loss of smell, and cognitive impairment (Fig. 15.24).[20]

Cerebrovascular Accident (Stroke)

A CVA occurs when brain cells die from ischemia as a result of a thrombus or embolus in part of the brain or from hemorrhage into the brain. Other terms for a CVA are brain attack and stroke.[21] Stroke is the fifth leading cause of death in the United States. About 795,000 people in this country have a stroke each year.[1] **Clinical Findings:** The cerebral ischemia results in impairment of motor activity, bowel and bladder elimination, intellectual function, spatial-perceptual alterations, personality, affect, sensations, swallowing, and communication.[21] Manifestations are directly related to the area of the brain involved and the extent of ischemic area. For example, ischemia to the left frontal lobe may result in

paralysis of the right arm or leg. There may be sudden unilateral numbness or weakness of the face, arm, or leg. The patient may complain of trouble walking, dizziness, or loss of balance or coordination. There may be sudden confusion, difficulty swallowing (dysphagia), difficulty speaking or understanding speech (aphasia), or partial loss of vision.

DISORDERS OF PERIPHERAL NERVES

Myasthenia Gravis

Myasthenia gravis is a chronic autoimmune neuromuscular disease characterized by muscle weakness that improves with rest and administration of anticholinesterase drugs.[22] There are three types of myasthenia: (1) ocular, which affects only the eyes; (2) bulbar, which involves the nerves that innervate the muscles needed for swallowing (CN IX, CN X, CN XI, and CN XII); and (3) generalized, which affects skeletal muscles of the arms, legs, and trunk. It affects about 20 per 100,000 people worldwide.[23] **Clinical Findings:** Manifestations vary with the type of myasthenia. Ocular myasthenia produces muscle weakness confined to the muscles of the eye, causing ptosis and diplopia. Patients with bulbar myasthenia have dysphagia and dysarthria. Generalized myasthenia produces weakness of the face, arms, hands, legs, neck, trunk, and thorax, including the muscles of breathing.[22]

Guillain-Barré Syndrome

This acute syndrome is characterized by widespread demyelinization of motor nerves of the peripheral nervous system. The incidence in the United States is 1.2 to 3/100,000.[24] Patients usually have a respiratory or gastrointestinal viral infection weeks before the onset. Between 80% and 90% of patients recover from this syndrome, with few or no residual deficits; however, patients may die when respiratory depression develops rapidly. **Clinical Findings:** The usual manifestation is an ascending paralysis that begins with weakness and paresthesia in the lower extremities and ascends to the upper extremities and face. If ascending paralysis reaches the thorax, respiratory depression may result. There is a descending variation of Guillain-Barré syndrome that begins with the facial, glossopharyngeal, vagus, and hypoglossal cranial nerves and moves downward more commonly to the hand, but it can reach the feet. Deep tendon reflexes are absent.[9]

CLINICAL APPLICATION AND CLINICAL JUDGMENT

See Appendix B for answers to exercises in this section.

CASE STUDY

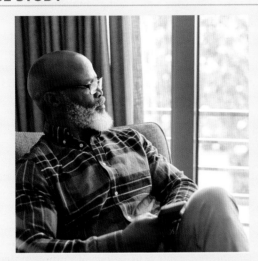

Leo Thompson is a 54-year-old African American man admitted to the hospital with a diagnosis of acute CVA. The following data are collected by the nurse during an interview and examination.

Interview Data

Mr. Thompson's wife tells the nurse that he was fine until this morning, when he suddenly had a headache, fell to the floor, and could not get up. Mrs. Thompson adds that her husband made only mumbling noises and she could not understand him. He has type 2 diabetes mellitus and hypertension. He stopped smoking last year.

Examination Data

- *Neurologic examination:* Awake, alert man. Unable to talk but able to follow requests. Cries and avoids eye contact with his wife and nurse. Cranial nerves III, IV, V, VI, and VIII are intact bilaterally. Patient has asymmetry and unequal movements of his face, with a drooping of the left side of his face. He has asymmetric shoulder shrug, with weakness noticed on his left side. He has supination and pronation of his right hand but is unable to perform with his left hand. Light touch with sharp and dull sensation is present on his right arm and leg; there is no sensation on his left arm or leg. Right arm and leg muscle strength is 5, left arm muscle tone 0, and left leg 1. He is unable to move around in bed unassisted at this time. Assessment of balance is deferred.

Clinical Judgment

1. What cues do you recognize that suggest deviations from expected findings, suggesting a need for further investigation?
2. For which additional information should the nurse ask or assess?
3. Based on the data, which risk factors for CVA does Mr. Thompson have?
4. With which team member would the nurse collaborate to meet this patient's needs?

REVIEW QUESTIONS

1. During a health history, a patient reports having difficulty swallowing. Based on this report, which assessment technique does the nurse use to collect more data about the patient's ability to swallow?
   1. Ask the patient to puff out her cheeks, purse her lips, and blow out.
   2. Observe the soft palate when the patient says "ahh."
   3. Observe the patient while she swallows water from a paper cup.
   4. Wearing gloves, grasp the patient's tongue and palpate all sides.

2. As a patient is walking into the exam room, the nurse notices his unsteady gait. What findings does the nurse anticipate during the neurologic exam?
   1. When the patient stands with his feet together and eyes closed, his upright posture is maintained.

2. The nurse notices no patient response after striking the right patellar tendon with a reflex hammer.
3. The patient is able to move the heel of one foot down the shin of the other leg while lying supine.
4. A tremor is observed in his hands while he touches his finger to his thumb on the same hand.

3. During a symptom analysis, the patient reports a pain that radiates from the right lateral thigh, over the knee, and around to the right medial ankle. The nurse refers to the dermatome map (see Fig. 15.8) to determine that the patient's description of pain is consistent with dysfunction of which spinal nerve?
   1. Second lumbar (L2)
   2. Third lumbar (L3)
   3. Fourth lumbar (L4)
   4. Fifth lumbar (L5)

4. Which question gives the nurse additional information about a patient's report of his hands shaking for the last 2 months?
   1. "Does the shaking occur when your hands are at rest or when you are picking up an item?"
   2. "Do you experience any abnormal sensations, such as tingling or coldness, at the same time?"
   3. "What actions do you take to relieve the shaking when it occurs?"
   4. "Have you ever experienced this shaking before?"

5. Which technique does the nurse use to assess the triceps reflex?
   1. Holds the patient's relaxed arm with the elbow extended while striking the appropriate tendon with a reflex hammer
   2. Holds the patient's relaxed forearm with the hand slightly pronated while striking the appropriate tendon with a reflex hammer
   3. Holds the patient's relaxed arm with elbow flexed at a 90-degree angle, places a thumb over the appropriate tendon, and strikes the thumb with the reflex hammer
   4. Holds the patient's relaxed arm with elbow flexed at a 90-degree angle in one hand and strikes the appropriate tendon just above the elbow with a reflex hammer

6. Which patient behavior indicates to the nurse that the patient's facial cranial nerve (CN VII) is intact?
   1. The patient's eyes move to the left, right, up, down, and obliquely.
   2. The patient moistens the lips with the tongue.
   3. The sides of the mouth are symmetric when the patient smiles.
   4. The patient's eyelids blink periodically.

7. The nurse asks a patient to stand with her feet together, her arms placed at her sides, and her eyes closed. The nurse then observes the patient moving her foot to maintain balance and opening her eyes. Based on this finding, which additional assessment does the nurse perform to confirm an abnormality with balance?
   1. Ask the patient to walk in tandem, putting the heel of one foot directly against the toes of the other foot.
   2. Ask the patient to sit down and alternatively tap the thighs with your hands using rapid supination and pronation movements.
   3. Place a vibrating tuning fork in the patient's ankle and ask when she no longer detects the vibration.
   4. With the patient in a seated position, support one lower leg while sharply dorsiflexing the foot and maintain it in flexion.

8. What is the earliest and most sensitive indication of altered cerebral function?
   1. Memory impairment
   2. Loss of deep tendon reflexes
   3. Inability to communicate
   4. Change in level of consciousness

9. What is the expected patient response when assessing the function of CN XI (spinal accessory)?
   1. Demonstrates full, active range of motion of the neck
   2. Moves shoulders against resistance equally
   3. Follows an object with eyes without nystagmus
   4. Sticks out tongue without tremor or deviation

10. You had to yell his name to get him to open his eyes; he could not tell you his name or location, and he could raise his hands when asked. Using the Glasgow Coma Scale (see Fig. 15.23), what score would you give to this patient?
    1. 12
    2. 13
    3. 14
    4. 15

Breasts and Axillae

evolve

http://evolve.elsevier.com/Wilson/assessment

ANATOMY AND PHYSIOLOGY

The breasts are paired mammary glands located within the superficial fascia of the anterior chest wall. Breasts are a feature of all mammals, evolving as milk-producing organs to provide nourishment for offspring. During embryologic development, these glands develop along paired "milk lines," an embryonic ridge that extends between the limb buds of what will become the axillae and the inguinal regions. Normally, only one gland develops on each side in the pectoral region. After birth, the glands undergo little additional development in the male. However, in the female, the breasts undergo considerable development during adolescence under the influence of estrogen and progesterone.

FEMALE BREAST

The breast of the mature female has a distinctive shape; however, the "normal" breast size varies greatly. The breasts extend vertically from the second to the sixth ribs and laterally from the sternal margin to the midaxillary line. To facilitate description (or location of lesions), breasts are divided into quadrants by imaginary vertical and horizontal lines intersecting at the nipple (Fig. 16.1).

The female breast is composed of three types of tissue: glandular, fibrous, and subcutaneous and retromammary fat. The glandular tissue is arranged into 15 to 20 lobes per breast, radiating around the nipple in a spoke-like pattern. Each lobe is composed of 20 to 40 lobules, or alveoli, containing the milk-producing acini cells (Fig. 16.2). The largest amount of glandular tissue lies in the upper outer quadrant of each breast. From this quadrant, the breast tissue extends into the axilla, forming the axillary tail of Spence.

The breast is supported by a layer of subcutaneous fibrous tissue and by multiple fibrous bands termed Cooper ligaments. These suspensory ligaments extend from the connective tissue layer and run through the breast, attaching to the underlying muscle fascia. Subcutaneous and retromammary fat surrounds the glandular tissue and composes most of the breast.

Centrally located on the breast, the nipple is surrounded by the pigmented areola. The nipples are composed of epithelium intertwined with circular and longitudinal smooth muscle fibers. These muscles contract in response to sensory, tactile, or autonomic stimuli, producing erection of the nipple and causing the lactiferous ducts to empty. A number of sebaceous glands, termed *Montgomery glands,* are located within the areolar surface, aiding in lubrication of the nipple during lactation.

Throughout the reproductive years, the breasts undergo a cyclic pattern of size change, nodularity, and tenderness during the menstrual cycle. The breasts are smallest during days 4 through 7 of the menstrual cycle. Three to four days before the onset of menses, many women experience breast fullness, tenderness, and pain because of hormonal changes and fluid retention.

The breasts undergo a dramatic change during pregnancy and lactation in response to luteal and placental hormones. These changes include an increase in the number of lactiferous ducts and the size and number of alveoli. During lactation, milk produced by acini cells empties into the lactiferous ducts. These ducts drain milk from the lobes to the surface of the nipple.

MALE BREAST

The male breast undergoes very little additional development after birth, and the gland remains rudimentary. It consists of a thin layer of undeveloped tissue beneath the nipple. The areola of the nipple is small when compared with that of the female. During puberty, the male breast may become slightly enlarged, producing a temporary condition termed *gynecomastia.* Although gynecomastia is usually unilateral, it may occur bilaterally. The older male may also have gynecomastia secondary to a decrease in testosterone.

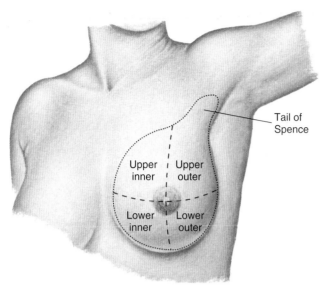

FIG. 16.1 Quadrants of the left breast and axillary tail of spence.

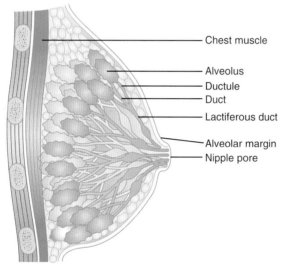

FIG. 16.2 Anatomy of the breast, showing position and major structures. (From Mahan and Escott-Stump, 2008.)

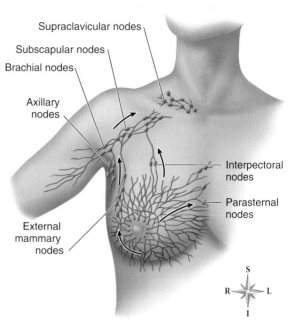

FIG. 16.3 Lymphatic drainage of the breast. (From Thibodeau and Patton, 2012.)

LYMPHATIC NETWORK

Each breast contains an extensive lymphatic network, which drains into lymph nodes in several areas. As blood flows through the capillary bed, fluid is forced out into the interstitial space and into the cells. Most of the fluid is immediately resorbed into the capillaries; however, fluid left in the interstitial spaces is eventually absorbed by the lymph system and carried through the lymph nodes. More than 75% of lymph drainage from the breast flows outward toward the axillary lymph node groups and then upward to the subclavicular and supraclavicular nodes. Other routes for lymph drainage include flow through the anterior axillae (pectoral) nodes (above the breast), internal mammary nodes (in the thorax), and subdiaphragmatic nodes (toward the abdomen), and through cross-mammary pathways to the opposite breast (Fig. 16.3).[1]

HEALTH HISTORY

Nurses interview patients to collect subjective data about their present health status, past health history, family history, and personal and psychosocial history because they relate to the assessment of breasts and axilla.

GENERAL HEALTH HISTORY

Present Health Status

Do you take any medications (prescription and over-the-counter) or herbal supplements? If yes, what do you take and how often? Why do you take them?

Some medications are associated with noncyclic breast discomfort or nipple discharge (Box 16.1); taking vitamin E supplement may reduce symptoms. Hormone therapy for menopausal symptoms (combined estrogen and progestin) increases risk for breast cancer.[2] Transgender people may be on gender-confirming hormone therapy specifically to increase or decrease breast size. Transgender women on hormone replacement have a higher breast cancer risk than the general male population.[3]

Have you noticed recent changes to the way your breasts look or feel? Has the appearance of your nipples changed?

Reported changes in the appearance of the breast provide clues to potential problems such as lesions or inflammation.

BOX 16.1 MEDICATIONS THAT CAUSE BREAST PAIN OR NIPPLE DISCHARGE

Medications Known to Contribute to Breast Pain
- Oral contraceptives
- Postmenopausal estrogen and progesterone hormone therapy
- Spironolactone
- Methyldopa
- Digoxin
- Haloperidol
- Selective serotonin reuptake inhibitors

Medications Contributing to Nipple Discharge

Analgesics
- Morphine
- Methadone
- Codeine

Cardiovascular Agents
- Methyldopa
- Methadone
- Codeine

Hormones
- Oral contraceptives
- Estrogen

Psychotropics
- Haloperidol
- Monoamine oxidase inhibitors
- Selective serotonin reuptake inhibitors

RISK FACTORS

Breast Cancer

- *Gender:* Females account for 99% of breast cancer cases.
- *Age:* Risk increases with age; the large majority of women with a new diagnosis of breast cancer are more than age 45 with a peak incidence in women ages 65–84.
- *Race:* White women have the highest incidence of breast cancer.
- *Genetic:* Inherited mutations of *BRCA1* or *BRCA2* genes account for 5%–10% of breast cancer cases in women and 5%–20% in men.
- *Family history:* Breast cancer in a first-degree family relative (on either maternal or paternal side) especially before age 50 increases risk; risk is highest if relative is mother or sister.
- *Personal medical history:*
  - A history of breast cancer increases risk of subsequent episodes.
  - A history of proliferative breast disease with a biopsy-confirmed atypical hyperplasia increases risk.
  - Exposure to ionizing radiation to the chest area as child or young adult (for treatment of other cancer such as Hodgkin disease) increases risk.
- *Reproductive history:*
  - Long menstrual history (menarche before age 12 and/or menopause after age 55) increases risk.
  - Nulliparity increases risk.
  - First full-term pregnancy after age 30 increases risk.
- *Breast density:* Increased breast density is associated with a higher risk of breast cancer.
- *Estrogen replacement:* Hormone replacement therapy for more than 5 years after menopause increases risk. (M)
- *Physical inactivity* (M)
- *Alcohol intake:* Increased alcohol intake (two to five drinks a day) is associated with increased risk. (M)
- *Obesity:* Obesity, especially after age 50, or increased weight gain as an adult increases breast cancer risk. (M)

M, Modifiable risk factor.
From American Cancer Society: *Cancer facts and figures,* 2020, Atlanta, 2020; Centers for Disease Control and National Cancer Institute: *U.S. Cancer Statistics Working Group. U.S. Cancer Statistics Data Visualizations Tool, based on November 2018 submission data (1999–2016),* 2019. Retrieved from: www.cdc.gov/cancer/dataviz; Centers for Disease Control: *What are the risk factors for breast cancer?* 2018. Retrieved from: https://www.cdc.gov/cancer/breast/basic_info/risk_factors.htm.

Past Health History

How old were you when you began menstruating? How old were you when you reached menopause (if appropriate)?
Menarche before age 12 or menopause after age 55 increases the risk for breast cancer.[2,4] Longer lifetime exposure to estrogen and progesterone hormones (associated with menstrual cycles) is thought to be associated with this risk.

Have you ever been pregnant? If yes, at what age did you have your children?
Nulliparous or first child born after age 30 is a risk factor for breast cancer.[2,4]

Have you ever had a mammogram? If yes, when was your last one? What were the findings from the mammogram? How frequently do you have a mammogram?
Mammography is considered an effective method for breast cancer screening in women of average risk for breast cancer between ages 50 and 74 years of age.[5]

Have you ever had a breast problem such as fibrocystic changes to the breast, fibroadenoma, benign breast disease, or breast cancer? If yes, describe. When did it occur? How was it treated?
A history of breast cancer, including ductal carcinoma in situ or lobular carcinoma in situ, increases the risk of recurrence. Some benign breast conditions such as atypical hyperplasia may also be associated with increased risk for breast cancer.[4] Fibrocystic changes to the breast and fibroadenoma complicate the evaluation of the breasts because the presence of cysts makes it difficult to detect new masses or lumps. Determining the time frame and previous treatment provides baseline information.

Have you ever had surgery on a breast (e.g., biopsy, mastectomy, lumpectomy, or breast reduction or augmentation)? If yes, when was it and why did you have it?
This background information may affect findings noted with examination.

Have you ever had radiation treatment to your chest?
High-dose radiation treatment to the chest at a young age (for treatment of lymphoma) is a risk factor for breast cancer.[4]

Family History

Is there a history of breast cancer, breast disease, or ovarian cancer in your family? If yes, in whom? At what age did this relative have breast cancer or disease?
A family history of breast or ovarian cancer is a risk factor for breast cancer, particularly if it involves first-degree relatives (mother, sister, or daughter). Having one first-degree relative with breast cancer approximately doubles a woman's risk; two first-degree relatives with breast cancer triples the risk.[2]

🌐 ETHNIC, CULTURAL, AND SPIRITUAL VARIATIONS

Breast Cancer Incidence, Screening, and Mortality

- White women have the highest rate of new breast cancer, closely followed by black women. American Indian/Alaska Native have the lowest rate of new breast cancer.
- Black women have the highest rates of mammography screening. Asian women have the lowest rate of mammography cancer screening of any ethnic group, closely followed by American Indian and Hispanic.
- Median age at diagnosis for black women is 60 compared to age 64 for white women.
- Black women have the lowest 5-year survival rate for breast cancer, compared to women of any other racial or ethnic group. Access to care and delays in follow-up may partly explain the survival gap between black and white women.

From Komen SG: *Comparing breast cancer screening rates among different groups*, 2019. Retrieved from: https://ww5.komen.org/BreastCancer/DisparitiesInBreastCancerScreening.html.

Personal and Psychosocial History

Do you drink alcohol? If yes, how many drinks do you have each day?
Regular alcohol consumption over 1 drink a day is associated with increased risk for breast cancer; the risk is directly related to the amount regularly consumed.[2,4]

FREQUENTLY ASKED QUESTIONS

A patient asked me about breast self-examination. What is that?
In the past, women were taught to do monthly *breast self-examination* (BSE) on themselves as a screening for breast cancer. Although BSE is no longer recommended for cancer screening in women, they are advised to maintain *breast awareness*. Women should know how their breasts normally look and report changes to their health care provider.

PROBLEM-BASED HISTORY

Commonly reported problems related to the breasts in women are pain or tenderness, breast lump, nipple discharge, and pain or lumps in the axillae, and in men it is breast swelling or enlargement. As with symptoms in all areas of health assessment, a symptom analysis is completed using the mnemonic OLD CARTS, which includes the *Onset*, *Location*, *Duration*, *Characteristics*, *Aggravating factors*, *Related symptoms*, *Treatments*, and *Severity* (see Box 2.6).

Breast Pain or Tenderness

Where does it hurt? Is the pain in one breast or both? Is there a specific location, or is the pain generalized? When did the pain in your breast(s) first begin? Have you had any recent trauma or injury to your breast?
Along with breast mass, breast pain (mastalgia) is one of the most common breast-related symptoms.[6,7] Breast pain is classified as cyclic (related to menstrual cycle and typically bilateral) or noncyclic (not related to menstrual cycle and is usually unilateral and focal). Thus determining the onset and location of breast pain is important.

Describe the pain. Rate the severity of the pain on a scale from 0 to 10.
Determine the characteristics and severity of the pain. Some women with breast cancer report a burning or pulling sensation in addition to a vague pain. Rapidly growing cysts or infection may be very painful.

Have you noted any recent changes in your breasts such as changes in size, shape, lumps, rash, or discharge since the pain began?
Question the patient for potential causes and related symptoms with the breast pain.

Have you noticed any specific activities that initiate the pain or make it worse? For example, when you exercise or when wearing a certain bra or when not wearing a bra? Does the pain prevent you from carrying out routine activities?
Strenuous activity can bring on pain, as can the other specific causes noted. Determine any aggravating factors for the pain.

How much caffeine do you consume each day or each week?
A diet high in methylxanthines (found in foods containing caffeine such as coffee, tea, energy drinks, chocolate, some types of soda pop) may cause benign breast disease such as fibrocystic changes.[6]

Is the breast tenderness associated with a swollen feeling to the breasts? If yes, when do you notice the swelling? Is it related to your menstrual cycle?
Cyclic bilateral breast edema or fullness is a normal occurrence caused by hormonal fluctuations associated with the menstrual cycle. Significant edema should be further evaluated, especially if it is unilateral, has other associated findings, or influences the woman's ability to participate in usual activities.

Breast Lump

Where is the breast lump? When did you first notice it?
Establish the onset and location of all breast lumps. Some lumps may be present over a period of several years. If they do not undergo change, they may be insignificant but still should be examined. Any new lumps or changes in a

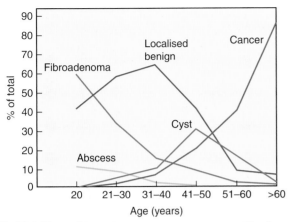

FIG. 16.4 Type of breast mass among women with discrete breast lump by age groups. (From Dixon, 2018.)

previously identified and documented lump should be of particular concern (Fig. 16.4).

Is the lump always present or does it seem to come and go? Is there a relationship between the lumps and your menstrual cycle?
Lumps that change in size in relation to the menstrual cycle may be influenced by hormonal fluctuations.

Is the lump tender to the touch? If yes, does the severity of the tenderness change related to menstruation?
Determine the characteristics of the lump. Some lumps are tender, whereas others are painless. The degree of pain or tenderness may be affected by hormonal fluctuations.

Have you recently experienced injury to the breasts? If yes, did the lump develop after the injury?
Lumps resulting from an injury may be associated with a hematoma. Typically, these resolve in a short period of time.

Have you noticed other symptoms associated with this lump?
Determine associated changes to the breast (i.e., redness, edema, localized heat, rash, and dimpling), which are all symptoms requiring further evaluation.

Nipple Discharge
When did you first notice the discharge from your nipple? Have you ever noticed it before? Does it affect one or both nipples?
Determine onset, location, and duration. Nipple discharge is the third most commonly reported breast symptom, accounting for 2% to 5% of medical visits by women, and represents a symptom in 5% to 12% of breast cancers.[7,8] Unilateral nipple discharge is concerning because it is more commonly associated with a pathologic condition than bilateral nipple discharge.[8]

Describe the color of the discharge. Is it thick or thin? Is there an odor associated with the discharge? Does
the discharge occur at specific times, such as always before your menstrual period or with breast manipulation?
Nipple discharge may indicate a pathologic condition. A bloody or blood-tinged discharge is alarming and must be investigated.

Does the discharge occur spontaneously or only when expressed? If spontaneous, does it happen continuously or does it come and go?
Spontaneous discharge is considered an abnormal finding, and whether it occurs intermittently or constantly is important. Discharge that is expressed may result from medications or endocrine disorders.

Have you noticed other symptoms?
Determine if there are any other associated breast symptoms or onset of other symptoms.

Axillary Lumps or Tenderness
When did you first notice the lumps or tenderness under your arms?
Because the tail of Spence extends up into the axilla and most lymphatic drainage flows toward the axillary nodes, a symptom analysis for lumps and tenderness is needed.

Where is the lump or tenderness located? Under one arm or both arms? Do the symptoms come and go or are they always present? Has the tenderness or lump become worse?
Determine the location and characteristics of the lump or tenderness.

Do you shave your underarms? If yes, how often? Do you notice a relationship to shaving and the tenderness? Do you use deodorant or antiperspirant?
Shaving and the use of deodorants or antiperspirants can cause discomfort and a mild inflammation to the axilla.

What have you done to treat this tenderness, if anything?
Explore self-care practices; this may be helpful to guide future treatment strategies.

Breast Swelling or Enlargement (Men)
Describe the change you have been experiencing to your breast. When did you first notice it? Have the changes occurred on one or both sides? Have they been associated with weight gain?
Gynecomastia is the enlargement of one or both breasts in the male. Although it may occur at any time, it is most prevalent during puberty, among older adult men, or among men who are overweight. Although breast cancer in men is rare, the most common initial symptom is a breast mass.

Have you experienced any other symptoms such as pain or discharge?
Although a painless palpable mass is the most common initial finding with male breast cancer, nipple discharge may be the only symptom. Nipple discharge of any kind in a man requires further evaluation.[9]

HEALTH PROMOTION FOR EVIDENCE-BASED PRACTICE

Breast Cancer

An estimated 279,100 women were diagnosed with breast cancer in 2020 in the United States, making it the most frequently diagnosed nonskin cancer in women. In addition, breast cancer is the second leading cancer-related cause of death in women; an estimated 42,690 women were expected to die from breast cancer in 2020.

Screening Recommendations US Preventive Services Task Force

BRCA-Related Cancer Risk Assessment

- Women who have family members with breast, ovarian, tubal, or peritoneal cancer should be screened for a family history associated with increased risk for genetic mutations (*BRCA1* or *BRCA2*).
- Women with positive screening for family history associated with increased risk for *BRCA1* or *BRAC2* should receive genetic counseling and, if indicated, *BRCA* testing.

Mammography Screening Recommendations

The following are recommendations for mammography screening for asymptomatic women age 40 and over who do not have preexisting breast cancer or a breast condition (such as ductal carcinoma or lobular carcinoma in situ), and who are not at high risk for breast cancer (underlying genetic mutation or a history of chest radiation at an early age):

- Women aged 40–49: decision to begin mammography screening is individualized based on personal value on the potential benefit as opposed to potential harm from false-positive tests.
- Women at average risk have the greatest benefit during ages 50–74.
- Women at greater-than-average risk (those with a parent, sibling, or child who has had breast cancer) may benefit more than women at average risk by beginning screening between the ages of 40 and 49 years.
- Women aged 50–74: screening mammography every 2 years.
- Women aged 75 years and older: insufficient evidence to recommend or not recommend screening mammography.

From American Cancer Society: *Cancer facts and figures, 2020,* Atlanta, 2020; U.S. Preventative Services Task Force: *BRCA-related cancer: Risk assessment, genetic counseling, and genetic testing,* 2013. Available at: www.uspreventiveservicestaskforce.org/Page/Topic/recommendation-summary/brca-related-cancer-risk-assessment-genetic-counseling-and-genetic-testing?ds=1&s=breast%20cancer%20screening; U.S. Preventive Services Task Force: *Final Recommendation Statement: Breast Cancer Screening,* 2016. Available at: www.uspreventiveservicestaskforce.org/Page/Document/RecommendationStatementFinal/breast-cancer-screening.

EXAMINATION

FEMALE BREAST EXAMINATION

Routine techniques

- INSPECT both breasts.
- INSPECT the skin of the breasts.
- INSPECT the areolae.
- INSPECT the nipples.
- INSPECT the breasts in various postures.
- PALPATE the breasts and axillae.
- PALPATE the nipples.

Equipment needed

Gloves in the presence of nipple drainage or open lesions

PROCEDURES WITH EXPECTED FINDINGS

ROUTINE TECHNIQUES: FEMALE BREAST

Always explain the procedure to the patient before you begin. Let her know that you will be touching her breasts and be sure to obtain her permission before you begin the examination. Initially position the patient so she is sitting on the examination table facing you. She should be sitting erect with her gown dropped to the waist.

PERFORM hand hygiene.

INSPECT the breasts for size, symmetry, and shape.

Start by inspecting the breasts with the patient sitting with her arms at her sides. Breasts may be slightly unequal in size. Breast size may vary significantly, but symmetry or only slight asymmetry should be considered normal. The breast shape should be smooth, convex, and even (Fig. 16.5). Some women (including transgender women) have breast implants. Gently lift each breast with your fingers and inspect the lower and outer aspects for dimpling, retraction, or bulging.

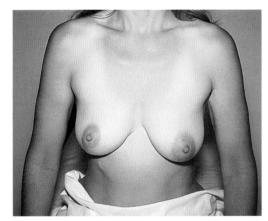

FIG. 16.5 Breasts should appear bilaterally symmetric.

ABNORMAL FINDINGS

Note evidence of marked asymmetry of breast size or shape. Significant and rapid changes in the size of one breast could indicate an inflammatory process or a growth. Dimpling, retraction, or bulging could indicate a malignancy (Fig. 16.6).

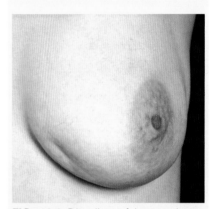

FIG. 16.6 Dimpling of breast, lower inner quadrant. (From Dixon, 2018.)

FREQUENTLY ASKED QUESTIONS

I am embarrassed to think about performing a breast examination on a patient. What can be done to overcome this?

This is a common feeling for a beginner to have. Probably the most important thing to consider first is your own feelings about breast examination in general. Are you uncomfortable about the thought of touching someone else's breasts? Is the discomfort associated with your own perceived inability or lack of experience?

Another key point is to consider the therapeutic purpose for the examination; remember that this is simply a process of data collection and an opportunity for patient teaching. Like most other skills, you will become less nervous with experience. As you gain experience, you will also gain confidence. You will also feel more confident about performing a breast examination if you have established a rapport with your patient. Typically, you will perform less-invasive examination procedures first; thus, by the time you get to the breast examination, you and the patient will feel more at ease with one another.

PROCEDURES WITH EXPECTED FINDINGS

INSPECT the skin of the breasts for surface characteristics, color, and venous patterns.

The skin of the breast should appear smooth, with an even color. The skin color should be similar to skin on the rest of the body, although it may be lighter in color compared with sun-exposed skin surfaces. The venous patterns (visible veins under the skin) should be bilaterally similar. The venous pattern may be pronounced in obese or pregnant females.

ABNORMAL FINDINGS

Note any localized or generalized areas of discoloration. Inflammation (e.g., cellulitis or breast abscess) in the breast tissue may cause surface erythema and heat (Fig. 16.7).

A rash on both breasts is likely caused by dermatitis; unilateral breast rash, especially surrounding the areola, could be associated with Paget's disease of the breast (a rare type of breast cancer).

Unilateral hyperpigmentation is also considered an abnormal finding. Obese women or women with large breasts may have a red rash with demarcated borders from candidiasis resulting from excessive moisture.

Unilateral venous patterns on the breast may occur secondary to dilated superficial veins from an increased blood flow to a malignancy. Roughened, tough, or thickened skin is considered abnormal. Edema may give the skin an orange-like texture and appearance termed *peau d'orange* (Fig. 16.8).

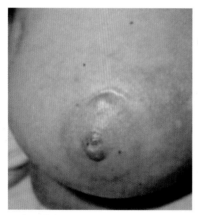

FIG. 16.7 Erythema of the breast. (From Swartz, 2010.)

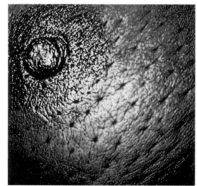

FIG. 16.8 Peau d'orange appearance caused by edema. (From Gallager et al., 1978.)

PROCEDURES WITH EXPECTED FINDINGS

| | ABNORMAL FINDINGS |

INSPECT the areolae for color, shape, and surface characteristics.

The color of the areola may vary, depending on the patient's skin color. Fig. 16.9A to C shows the variations of areola color, ranging from pink to black. The areola should be round or oval and appear bilaterally similar. Montgomery glands (Fig. 16.9B) may appear as slightly raised bumps on the areola tissue. Hairs on the nipple may also be seen.

Abnormal findings include areolae that are unequal bilaterally, have an irregular shape, or have lesions or changes in color.

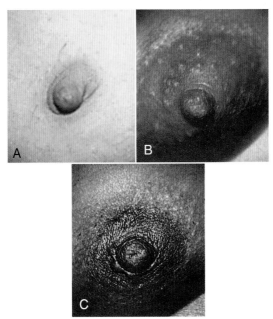

FIG. 16.9 Variations in color of areola. (A) Pink. (B) Brown. (C) Black. Note presence of Montgomery glands in B. (B and C, From Ball et al., 2015.)

INSPECT the nipples for position, symmetry, surface characteristics, lesions, bleeding, and discharge.

Most women's nipples protrude, although some may appear to be flat or actually inverted. All should be considered normal if they have remained unchanged throughout adult life and the nipples are symmetric bilaterally. Nipple inversion (a nipple that is recessed as opposed to protruding) can be a normal or an abnormal finding (Fig. 16.10). Consider it normal if it is not a new finding and if it can be everted with manipulation.

Nipples that point in different directions or those that are not symmetric should be considered abnormal. Recent nipple inversion or nipple *retraction* (a nipple that is pointing or pulled in a different direction) suggests malignancy, and the patient should be referred for further evaluation (Fig. 16.11).

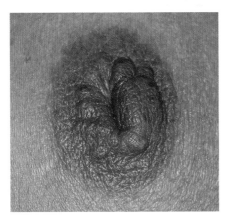

FIG. 16.10 Nipple inversion. (Courtesy Lemmi and Lemmi, 2013.)

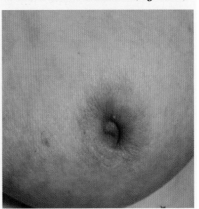

FIG. 16.11 Nipple retraction. (From Barber and Sharma, 2019.)

PROCEDURES WITH EXPECTED FINDINGS

Nipples are normally smooth and intact without evidence of crusting, lesions, bleeding, or discharge. Notice presence of supernumerary nipples, which are considered a normal variation although uncommon. These nipples look similar to pink or brown moles and generally appear along the embryonic "milk line" (Fig. 16.12).

ABNORMAL FINDINGS

Deviations include nipple edema, redness, pigment changes, ulceration or crusting, erosion or scaling, and wrinkling or cracking. A red, scaly nipple with discharge and crusting that lasts more than a few weeks could indicate Paget's disease (Fig. 16.13). Nipple discharge is usually considered an abnormal finding. Table 16.1 presents various types of discharge and possible causes.

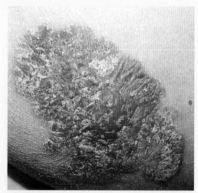

FIG. 16.13 Paget's disease. (From Habif, 1996.)

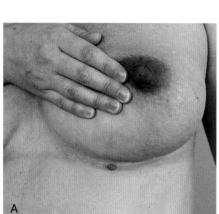

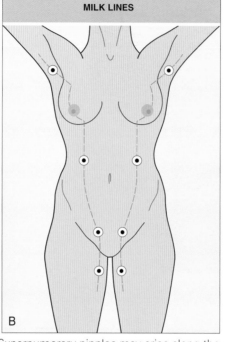

FIG. 16.12 (A) Supernumerary nipple. (B) Supernumerary nipples may arise along the "milk line." (A, From Mansel and Bundred, 1995. B, From Bolognia et al., 2012.)

TABLE 16.1 **NIPPLE DISCHARGE**			
COLOR OF DISCHARGE	**POSSIBLE CAUSE**	**COLOR OF DISCHARGE**	**POSSIBLE CAUSE**
Serous (yellow)	Usually normal	Milky	Pituitary adenoma
Serosanguineous	Carcinoma		Pharmacologic causes
(straw colored)	Ductal ectasia		Galactorrhea
Sanguineous (bloody)	Carcinoma	Purulent	Infectious process
	Intraductal papilloma		Ductal ectasia
	Ductal ectasia	Multicolored	Fibrocystic changes
	Vascular engorgement	(green, gray, brown)	Carcinoma
Clear (watery)	Pharmacologic causes		Infectious process
	Carcinoma		Ductal ectasia

PROCEDURES WITH EXPECTED FINDINGS

The following techniques are usually performed as part of a *clinical breast examination* (CBE) and involve inspection and palpation of the breasts and axillae. This may also be done to evaluate breast symptoms.[10]

INSPECT the breasts in various positions for bilateral pull, symmetry, and contour.

This procedure is done to detect abnormalities, particularly when breasts are observed from multiple views and in various positions.

Procedure and Findings: Ask the patient to remain seated and raise her arms over her head (Fig. 16.14A). This position adds tension to the suspensory ligaments and accentuates dimpling or retractions. Observe and compare the breasts, areolae, and nipples. The breasts should appear equal on both sides (bilaterally symmetric).

With her arms still raised, have the patient lean forward (Fig. 16.14B). The nurse may hold onto the patient's hands to provide balance.

Inspect the breasts for symmetry as previously described. The breasts should hang equally with a smooth contour, and pull should be symmetric. Having the patient lean forward is an especially useful technique if she has large and pendulous breasts because the breasts fall away from the chest wall and hang freely.

Next, inspect the breasts while the seated patient pushes her hands onto her hips or pushes her palms together, therefore contracting the pectoral muscles (Fig. 16.14C). There should be no deviations in contour and symmetry of the breasts.

ABNORMAL FINDINGS

Asymmetry or appearance of attachment (fixation), bulging, or retraction of either breast is abnormal.

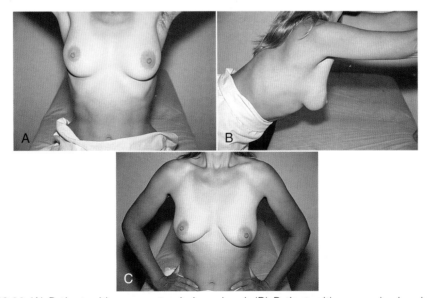

FIG. 16.14 (A) Patient with arms extended overhead. (B) Patient with arms raised and leaning forward. (C) Patient sitting and pressing her hands on hips.

PROCEDURES WITH EXPECTED FINDINGS	ABNORMAL FINDINGS

PALPATE the axillae for evidence of enlarged lymph nodes, lesions, or masses.

Palpation of axillary lymph nodes is included with clinical breast examination because lymph nodes are accessible and may provide clues regarding the presence of inflammation or lesions. Small masses and/or tumors may be evident first by detection of a slight abnormality within the axilla.

Procedure: (If the patient has a rash or an open lesion in the axilla, wear examination gloves.) You must have short fingernails to prevent injury to the patient.

Instruct the patient to relax both arms at her sides. Using your left hand, lift the patient's left arm and support it so her muscles are loose and relaxed (Fig. 16.15). While in this position, use your right hand to palpate the axilla.

Reach your fingers deep into the axilla and slowly and firmly slide your fingers along the patient's chest wall, first down the middle of the axilla, then along the anterior border of the axilla, and finally along the posterior border. Then, turn your hand over and examine the inner aspect of the patient's upper arm. Repeat the same palpation in the right axilla using your left hand. During all maneuvers, position the patient's arm with your other hand to maximize the examining area. In all positions, palpate for areas of enlargement, masses, or lymph nodes or isolated areas of tenderness.

Findings: Lymph nodes or masses are not typically palpable in the axillae. If they are noticed, they should be small, soft, mobile, and nontender.

Infections in the breast, arm, and even the hand may cause lymphatic drainage into the axillary area. Enlargement and tenderness of lymph nodes in the axilla may indicate such an infection. Hard, fixed nodules or masses may suggest metastatic carcinoma or lymphoma.

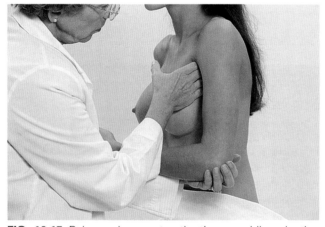

FIG. 16.15 Raise and support patient's arm while palpating axilla.

PALPATE the breasts for tissue characteristics.

Position: The preferred position for breast palpation is supine with a small pillow or towel placed under the shoulder on the same side as the breast to be examined. Instruct the patient to place her arm over her head. The combination of the slight shoulder elevation and the arm positioning flattens the breast tissue evenly over the chest wall. A sitting position may be used if the patient has difficulty lying down, if she is young and has very small breasts, or if she has very large breasts, making palpation difficult in a supine position.

PROCEDURES WITH EXPECTED FINDINGS

Procedure: Using the finger pads of the first two or three fingers of your examining hand, gently, firmly, and systematically palpate all quadrants of the breast and the tail of Spence (Fig. 16.16). Use a systematic approach to breast palpation that begins and ends at a designated point. This ensures that all areas of the breast are palpated.

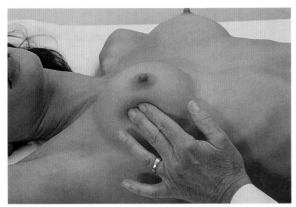

FIG. 16.16 Palpate the breasts using your finger pads.

Several motions may be used for breast palpation (Table 16.2), although one study suggests the vertical strip approach as the preferred method.[11] Press firmly enough to feel the underlying tissue but not so firmly that the tissue is compressed against the rib cage. Do not lift your fingers from the chest wall during the palpation because this breaks the continuity of the palpation. Instead, gently slide your fingers over the breast tissue, moving along the designated pattern of palpation.

If the sitting position is used for a woman with very large breasts, ask the patient to lean forward slightly and position your hands between the breasts as shown in Fig. 16.17. While supporting the inferior side of the breast with one hand, palpate the breast with the other hand, starting at the top of the breast, and slowly slide the finger pads down the breast. Repeat the technique until all breast tissues of both breasts are examined. If a mass is identified, palpate the mass for characteristics, including its location, estimated size, shape, consistency, tenderness, mobility, delineation of borders, and retraction (Fig. 16.18). Characteristics that should be included when assessing a mass are presented in Box 16.2.

Findings: The breast should feel firm, smooth, and elastic, without the presence of masses, lumps, or nodules. Typically, the breast should be nontender on palpation. After pregnancy or menopause, the breast tissue may feel softer and looser. During the premenstrual period the patient's breasts may be engorged, be slightly tender, and have generalized nodularity. Most women have a firm transverse ridge along the lower edge of the breast termed the *inframammary ridge*. This firm ridge is normal and should not be mistaken for a breast mass.

ABNORMAL FINDINGS

Abnormal findings include masses or isolated areas of tenderness or pain. Conditions that may cause lumps or masses include breast cancer, fibroadenoma, and fibrocystic changes to the breast. These are discussed in greater detail in the Common Problems and Conditions section later in this chapter. Breast engorgement (in patients who are not pregnant or premenstrual) is also an abnormal finding.

TABLE 16.2 METHODS FOR BREAST PALPATION

Circular Method

Place the finger pads of your middle three fingers against the outer edge of the breast. Press gently in small circles around the breast until you reach the nipple. Try not to lift your fingers off the breast as you move from one point to another.

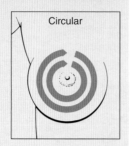

Wedge Method

Place the finger pads of your middle three fingers on the areola and palpate from the center of the breast outward. Return your fingers to the areola and again palpate from the center outward, covering another section of the breast (in a spoke-like fashion). Repeat this until the entire breast has been covered.

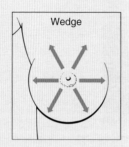

Vertical Strip Method

Place the finger pads of your middle three fingers against the top outer edge of the breast. Palpate downward and then upward, working your way across the entire breast.

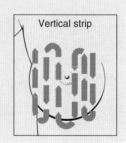

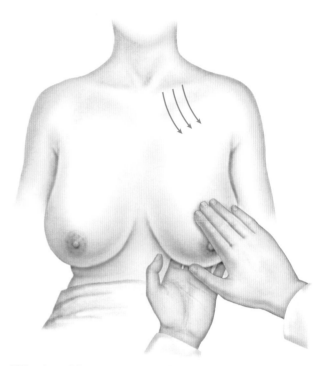

FIG. 16.17 Manual palpation of large breasts. (From Seidel et al., 2003.)

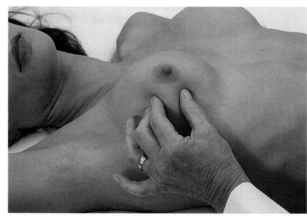

FIG. 16.18 Palpate the borders and mobility of a breast mass.

BOX 16.2 BREAST MASS CHARACTERISTICS

Note and record the following:

- *Location:* Which breast is being examined; which quadrant (may describe as position on the clock or draw on chart to show location)?
- *Size:* Estimate the width, length, and thickness in centimeters.
- *Shape:* Is the mass oval, round, lobed, irregularly shaped, or indistinct?
- *Consistency:* Is the mass hard, soft, firm, or rubbery?

- *Tenderness:* Is the mass tender during palpation?
- *Mobility:* Does the lump move during palpation or is it fixed to the overlying skin or the underlying chest wall?
- *Borders:* Are the edges of the mass discrete or poorly defined?
- *Retractions:* Is there any dimpling of the tissue around the mass?

Modified from Ball J, Dains J, Flynn J, et al: *Seidel's guide to physical examination,* ed 8, St. Louis, 2015, Elsevier/Mosby.

PROCEDURES WITH EXPECTED FINDINGS

PALPATE the nipples for surface characteristics and discharge.

Procedure and Findings: Wear examination gloves if there is a history of nipple discharge or if discharge is observed. With the patient in the supine position, palpate the nipples. They should be soft and pliable with no masses or discharge. If a discharge is present, notice the color, consistency, quantity, and odor. Try to determine the origin of the discharge by gently palpating the areola completely around the nipple with your index finger (Fig. 16.19). Observe for the appearance of discharge through one of the duct openings.

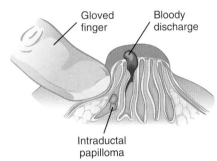

Gloved finger — Bloody discharge — Intraductal papilloma

FIG. 16.19 Express nipple discharge by palpating on the areola.

ABNORMAL FINDINGS

Thickening of the nipple tissue, a mass, and loss of elasticity are signs consistent with malignancy. Nipple discharge is considered an abnormal finding, except during pregnancy or lactation or as a side effect of some medications. Table 16.1 presents types of discharge and possible causes. Discharge may occur secondary to fluid retention of the ducts, infection, hormonal flux, or carcinoma.

MALE BREAST EXAMINATION

Routine techniques

- INSPECT the breasts, nipples, and areolae.
- PALPATE the breasts and nipples.
- PALPATE the axillae.

Equipment needed

Gloves in presence of nipple drainage or open lesions

PROCEDURES WITH EXPECTED FINDINGS

ROUTINE TECHNIQUES: MALE BREAST

PERFORM hand hygiene

INSPECT the breasts and nipples for symmetry, color, size, shape, rash, and lesions.

Procedure and Findings: With the patient in a seated position with his arms at his sides, inspect both breasts. The breasts should be flat, symmetric, and without rash or lesions. Men who are overweight often have a thicker fatty layer of tissue on the chest, giving the appearance of breast enlargement. If this is noticed, determine if he has a history of weight gain. If the patient reports that his breasts became full as he gained weight, the condition is most likely within expected limits. If the transgender man wears a chest binder (to create a masculine appearance), inspect for skin breakdown or skin lesions that may result from prolonged or excessive binding.

The nipples and areolar areas should be intact; smooth; and of equal color, size, and shape bilaterally.

ABNORMAL FINDINGS

Note any asymmetry or distinct differences between the two sides. Note any ulcerations, masses, or swelling. If the patient reports a sudden bilateral or unilateral breast enlargement with associated tenderness, the nurse should consider the situation abnormal and refer the patient for further evaluation.

PROCEDURES WITH EXPECTED FINDINGS

PALPATE the breasts, nipples, and areolae for surface characteristics, tenderness, size, and masses.

With the patient in the same position, palpate the breasts and areolar areas. The tissue should feel smooth, intact, and nontender. Notice evidence of tenderness, unilateral enlargement, or masses.

PALPATE the axillae for lymph nodes.

The procedure for palpation of axillary lymph nodes in men is the same as previously described for women. Lymph nodes are typically not palpable in the axilla. If they are noticed, they should be small, soft, mobile, and nontender.

ABNORMAL FINDINGS

Unilateral or bilateral breast enlargement in men is termed *gynecomastia*. Breast cancer can occur in men, usually manifesting as a hard, painless, irregular nodule often fixed to the area under the nipple. These are discussed in greater detail in Common Problems and Conditions later in this chapter.

The presence of a lump is considered abnormal. See abnormal findings of axillae previously described in the female examination.

DOCUMENTING EXPECTED FINDINGS

Female Breast Examination
Breasts moderate size, even color, bilaterally symmetric, and hang equally with smooth contour. Venous patterns bilaterally similar. Breasts firm, smooth, elastic, without tenderness, lumps, or nodules. Areolae round, nipples protruding, symmetric, soft, pliable, smooth, and intact without discharge. Axillary lymph nodes not palpated.

Male Breast Examination
Nipples and areolae intact; smooth; evenly pigmented; and of equal color, size, and shape bilaterally. Tissue smooth, intact, and nontender. Axillary lymph nodes not palpated.

AGE-RELATED VARIATIONS

This chapter discusses conducting an examination of the breasts with adult patients. These data are important to assess for individuals of all ages, but the approach and techniques used to collect the information may vary depending on the patient's age.

INFANTS AND CHILDREN

The breast assessment among infants and children requires only inspection. Neonates of both genders may have slightly enlarged breasts secondary to the mother's estrogen. Maternal hormones are also responsible for a small, watery, whitish discharge referred to as "witch's milk" seen in a small percentage of newborns during the first few weeks of life. Chapter 19 presents further information regarding the assessment of the breasts in these age groups.

ADOLESCENTS

Breast development (known as *thelarche*) initially begins in preadolescence and continues through adolescence. Girls are often sensitive about having their breasts exposed for examination; thus the nurse must take the time to reassure them and ensure privacy. Males may experience an unexpected enlargement of the breasts (known as gynecomastia) as a result of obesity or body change transition during early puberty. Chapter 19 presents further information regarding breast assessment among adolescent patients.

OLDER ADULTS

Atrophic changes to the female breast begin by age 40 and continue through menopause. As the glandular tissue atrophies, the breast tissue is gradually replaced with fat and connective tissue. Postmenopausal women should continue to have regular breast examinations because of the increased risk of breast cancer with age. Chapter 21 presents further information regarding breast assessment among older adults.

SITUATIONAL VARIATIONS

PATIENTS WITH A MASTECTOMY

Women who have had a mastectomy require the same breast assessment as all other women. Many women experience anxiety or fear because they worry about the recurrence of cancer or metastasis. Some women may also have personal issues regarding body image and feel self-conscious about exposing the chest. The nurse should be sensitive to this but also reassure the patient that performing a comprehensive examination is necessary. In addition to examining the remaining breast in the usual manner, the nurse should assess the mastectomy site and the scar because malignancy recurrence is possible at the scar site (Fig. 16.20A). The mastectomy site and axilla should be examined for color changes; redness; rash; irritation; and visible signs of edema, thickening, or lumps. Note areas that may have had muscle resection. Also note any signs of lymphedema in the affected upper extremity. Lymphedema is a localized accumulation of lymph fluid in the interstitial spaces caused by removal of the lymph nodes.

Using the finger pads of your examining hand, palpate the side with the mastectomy, especially around the area of the scar. Use a small circular motion, assessing for thickening, lumps, edema, or tenderness, and then use a sweeping motion to palpate the entire chest area on the affected side to ensure that no abnormalities have been missed. Finally, palpate the axillary and supraclavicular areas for lymph nodes. If the patient has had breast reconstruction or augmentation, perform the breast examination in the usual manner, paying particular attention to scars (Fig. 16.20B).

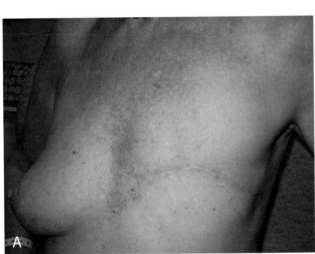
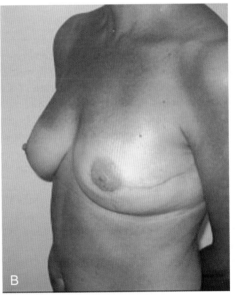

FIG. 16.20 (A) Appearance of chest following left total mastectomy. (B) Appearance of breast following nipple-areola sparing mastectomy of left breast. (From Rivolin, et al, 2012.)

COMMON PROBLEMS AND CONDITIONS

BENIGN BREAST DISEASE

Noncancerous breast conditions account for 90% of clinical breast problems. *Benign breast disease* is a term that represents a number of breast-related symptoms and problems, including breast pain or tenderness, swelling, lumps, discharge, and inflammation. Benign breast disease in women is a very common finding and results in a diagnosis in approximately 1 million women annually in the United States.[12]

Fibrocystic Changes to the Breast

The phrase *fibrocystic changes to the breast* refers to a variety of conditions associated with multiple benign masses within the breast caused by ductal enlargement and the formation of fluid-filled cysts. These are commonly seen among middle-age women. **Clinical Findings:** Typically, cysts manifest as one or more palpable masses that are round, well-delineated, mobile, and tender (Fig. 16.21). The degree of discomfort experienced can range from slightly tender to very painful, with the cysts often fluctuating in size and tenderness with the menstrual cycle.[13] Symptoms tend to subside after menopause. Table 16.3 presents typical findings compared to other causes of a breast mass.

Fibroadenoma

The most common type of benign breast disease is a fibroadenoma – a mass consisting of glandular and fibrous tissue (Fig. 16.22). Although this condition can occur at any age, it

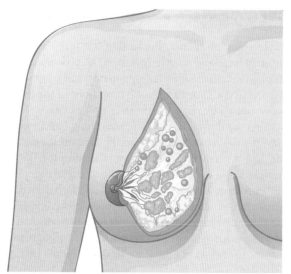

FIG. 16.21 Fibrocystic changes to the breast. The cysts are depicted as green masses.

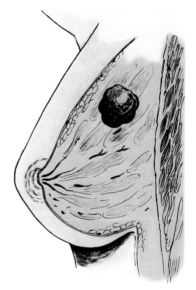

FIG. 16.22 Fibroadenoma.

is frequently a condition afflicting young women between the ages of 15 and 35. An estimated 10% of all women will develop a fibroadenoma during their lifetime.[14] **Clinical Findings:** Fibroadenoma usually manifests unilaterally as a small, solitary, firm, rubbery, nontender lump. It is generally mobile and well-delineated. This tumor does not change premenstrually (see Table 16.3).[15]

Ductal Ectasia

This benign breast disease is characterized by inflammation and dilation involving one or multiple subareolar ducts. It affects perimenopausal and postmenopausal women. **Clinical Findings:** The initial symptom is a sticky nipple discharge that is commonly dark green or black.[16] The woman may experience burning or itching of the nipple and edema in the areolar area. The discharge may become purulent or sanguineous. A complication that can occur is a breast abscess.

Intraductal Papilloma

This small, benign tumor growth in the major ducts usually forms within 1 to 2 cm of the areolar edge. One or more ducts may be affected. Affecting an estimated 2% to 3% of women, intraductal papilloma occurs most often between 40 and 60 years of age.[17] **Clinical Findings:** The clinical presentation usually associated with intraductal papilloma is a spontaneous, bloody discharge from the nipple; occasionally, a painful mass is palpated.[13]

BREAST CANCER

A major health problem for women is breast cancer. It is the most common nonskin-related malignancy and the second leading cause of cancer deaths in American women.[2]

Invasive Breast Cancer

The most common type of breast cancer is an invasive malignancy arising from the ducts or lobules. Breast cancer is most prevalent in women ages 40 to 60 years (see Table 16.3), accounting for an estimated 279,100 new cases in the United States in 2020.[2] **Clinical Findings:** A breast malignancy usually manifests as a solitary, unilateral, nontender lump, thickening, or mass (Fig. 16.23). As the mass grows, there may be breast asymmetry, discoloration (erythema or ecchymosis),

TABLE 16.3 DIFFERENTIATION OF BREAST MASSES			
	FIBROCYSTIC CHANGES TO BREAST	FIBROADENOMA	CANCER
Age range	20–49	15–55	30–80
Occurrence	Usually bilateral	Usually bilateral	Usually unilateral
Number	Multiple or single	Single; may be multiple	Single
Shape	Rounded	Rounded or discoid	Irregular or stellate
Consistency	Soft to firm; tense	Firm, rubbery	Hard, stone like
Mobility	Mobile	Mobile	Fixed
Skin or nipple retraction	Absent	Absent	Often present
Tenderness	Usually tender	Usually nontender	Usually nontender
Borders	Well delineated	Well delineated	Poorly delineated; irregular
Variations with menses	Yes	No	No

Ball et al: Seidel's guide to physical examination, ed 8, St. Louis, 2015, Elsevier/Mosby.

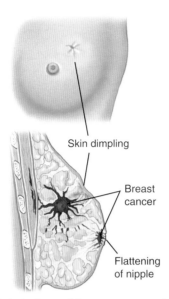

FIG. 16.23 Clinical signs of breast cancer: nipple retraction and dimpling of skin. (From LaFleur Brooks and LaFleur Brooks, 2012.)

Skin dimpling

Breast cancer

Flattening of nipple

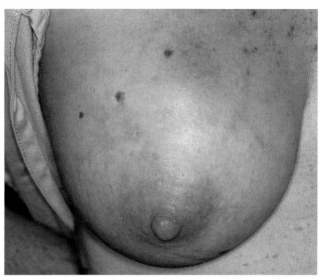

FIG. 16.24 Mastitis 4 weeks after delivery. (Courtesy Lemmi and Lemmi, 2013.)

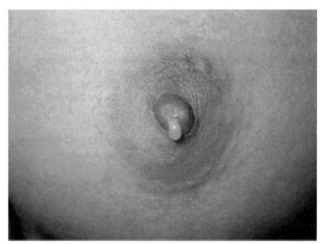

FIG. 16.25 Galactorrhea. (From Bouloux, 1993.)

unilateral vein prominence, peau d'orange, ulceration, dimpling, puckering, or retraction of the skin. The lesion is sometimes fixed to underlying tissue. Its borders are irregular and poorly delineated. The nipple may be inverted or diverted to one side. A serosanguineous or clear nipple discharge may be present. There may be crusting around the nipple or erosion of the nipple or areola. Lymph nodes may be palpable in the axilla.

Noninvasive Breast Cancer

There are two types of breast cancers categorized as noninvasive: ductal carcinoma in situ (DCIS) and lobular carcinoma in situ (LCIS). The term *in situ* is used to describe an early, noninvasive stage of cancer.[18] DCIS is a true precursor of invasive ductal carcinoma and is considered the more important of the two. LCIS is a risk factor for subsequent development of breast cancer. An estimated 48,530 new cases of DCIS were diagnosed in the United States in 2020.[2] **Clinical Findings:** The most common manifestation of DCIS or LCIS is an abnormal mammogram. Occasionally, DCIS is clinically detected as a lump with well-defined margins or nipple discharge.

OTHER BREAST CONDITIONS

Mastitis

Mastitis is an inflammatory condition of the breast usually caused by a bacterial infection. The condition occurs frequently in lactating women, secondary to milk stasis or a plugged duct. The incidence is highest in the first few weeks after delivery and decreases thereafter.[19] In nonlactating women, mastitis may also result from foreign bodies such as nipple rings and breast implants or from trauma. **Clinical Findings:** The infection generally occurs in one area of the breast, which appears as red, edematous, tender, warm to the touch, and hard. Axillary lymph nodes are often enlarged and tender. The patient usually has associated fever and chills and often experiences general malaise (Fig. 16.24).

Galactorrhea

The term *galactorrhea* means inappropriate lactation. Causes include endocrine-related disorders such as a pituitary tumor; systemic diseases such as renal failure; and adverse effects of many medications, especially those that interfere with or suppress dopamine (e.g., codeine, morphine, metoclopramide, phenothiazines, and reserpine). Although the incidence is unknown, it is estimated that as many as 20% of women experience galactorrhea at some point during their lifetime, but it is rare among men.[20] **Clinical Findings:** The manifestation is milky-appearing nipple discharge (Fig. 16.25).[21] There are no other specific symptoms because any additional signs or symptoms are likely based on the underlying cause (e.g., headache or change in vision if caused by a pituitary tumor).

Gynecomastia

Gynecomastia is a noninflammatory enlargement of one or both male breasts and represents the most common breast problem in men. It can occur at any age. In neonates, the cause is typically associated with maternal hormones. At puberty, the condition is idiopathic and transient.[22] **Clinical Findings:** Gynecomastia may be unilateral or bilateral and manifests as enlargement of the male breast (Fig. 16.26).

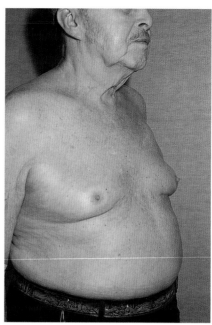

FIG. 16.26 Gynecomastia in an adult male. (From Swartz, 2010.)

CLINICAL APPLICATION AND CLINICAL JUDGMENT

See Appendix B for answers to exercises in this section.

CASE STUDY

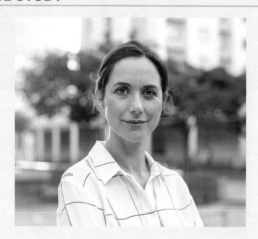

Julie Fisher is a 46-year-old woman who came to the clinic because she had discovered a lump in her left breast. The following data were collected during an interview and examination.

Interview Data

Ms. Fisher tells the nurse that she first noticed the lump approximately 9 months ago. Because it seemed small and didn't hurt, she didn't worry about it that much. Recently, she noticed that the lump felt bigger and decided that she should have someone to look at it. Ms. Fisher tells the nurse, "I am pretty sure it's not cancer because I'm much too young and healthy." The nurse asks her if she has noticed any redness or dimpling of the breast. Ms. Fisher tells the nurse, "No, not really." She tells the nurse that she started having regular menstrual cycles at age 11 and has not reached menopause. She has never been married and has no children.

Examination Data

- *General survey:* Alert, well-nourished female; hesitant to expose her breast for examination.
- *Breast examination:* Inspection reveals breasts of typical size with right and left breast symmetry. The skin of both breasts is smooth with even pigmentation. The nipples protrude slightly with no drainage noted. The left nipple is slightly retracted. Slight dimpling is noted on the left breast in the upper outer quadrant when arms are raised over her head. Right breast is firm, smooth, elastic, without lumps or tenderness. Palpation of the left breast reveals a small, firm lump in the upper outer quadrant. The left nipple produces a serosanguineous discharge when squeezed; the right nipple is unremarkable.

Clinical Judgment

1. What cues do you recognize that suggest deviation from normal findings, suggesting a need for further investigation?
2. What additional information should the nurse ask or assess for?
3. Which risk factors for breast cancer does Ms. Fisher have?
4. With which additional health care professionals should the nurse consider collaborating to meet the patient's health care needs?

REVIEW QUESTIONS

1. Which finding is considered abnormal when conducting a breast examination on a 68-year-old woman?
   1. Dark pink areola
   2. Pendulous breasts
   3. Serous nipple drainage
   4. Granular texture

2. A 51-year-old woman has found a small lump in her breast. Which data from her history are risk factors for breast cancer?
   1. Her husband's mother died from breast cancer at age 43.
   2. She drinks a glass of wine each night with dinner.
   3. Menarche occurred at age 14; menopause occurred at age 46.
   4. She underwent radiation treatment for Hodgkin disease at age 17.

3. What is the reason for palpating axillary lymph nodes during a clinical breast examination?
   1. Axillary nodes fluctuate during the month in response to the menstrual cycle.
   2. Axillary node tenderness is the most common initial symptom of breast cancer.
   3. The lymph network in the breast primarily drains toward the axillary lymph nodes.
   4. This is a matter of convenience because of the close proximity of the axillae to the breasts.

4. A 19-year-old college student comes to the student health center because she discovered a small, nontender, firm, rubbery lump in her right breast. What is the most common cause of breast lumps in women her age?
   1. Breast cancer
   2. Fibroadenoma
   3. Ductal ectasia
   4. Breast abscess

5. A man seeks treatment for "recent breast enlargement." On examination the nurse notes bilateral enlargement of the breasts. Which question asked by the nurse is most appropriate based on this finding?
   1. "What medications are you currently taking?"
   2. "Have you recently been lifting weights?"
   3. "Did your mother have large breasts?"
   4. "Have you ever had cancer?"

Reproductive System and the Perineum

This chapter begins with an overview of the anatomy and physiology of the female reproductive system, followed by that of the male reproductive system, rectum, and anus. The history questions are applicable to both genders, except when noted (e.g., obstetric history). Examination of the female is followed by examination of the male. Common problems and conditions begin with infections that affect either gender, followed by disorders specific to women and then those specific to men. Conditions of the anus and rectum are described, followed by prolapse or hernia, which affect either gender.

CONCEPT OVERVIEW

The concepts featured in this chapter are reproduction and sexuality. *Reproduction* refers to the process of creating a pregnancy through birth, whereas *sexuality* refers to human expression as sexual beings, through gender identity, sexual orientation, and sexual behaviors. Like most concepts, reproduction and sexuality are broad in scope, ranging from positive functioning and sexual well-being to infertility and/or sexual dysfunction. Reproduction and sexuality are separate concepts, yet they are closely interrelated and have clear connections to several other concepts. Hormonal regulation underlies the physical features associated with gender and gender expression, sexual desire, sexual expression, and reproductive function; these are reflected by the concept of development. Optimal gas exchange and perfusion are not only required for sexual responses, but also undergo significant changes during pregnancy. Sexual dysfunction or reproductive problems are often associated with concepts such a mood and affect, anxiety, and stress. These interrelationships are depicted in the concept illustration. Understanding the interrelationships of these concepts helps the nurse recognize risk factors when conducting a health assessment and is an important step associated with clinical judgment. The following case provides a clinical example featuring several of the interrelated concepts shown in the illustration.

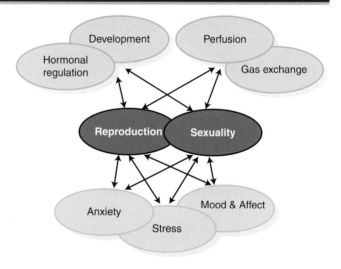

Rebecca Porter and her partner Javier Martin have been trying to get pregnant for 10 months without success. As time has passed, Rebecca has become obsessed with tracking her menstrual cycles and having sex to coincide with ovulation. She worries that either she or Javier has a hormonal problem, preventing them from getting pregnant. Their carefree, enjoyable sexual experience with each other has been replaced with stress associated with having sex on certain days. Javier has become insecure about his masculinity, and Rebecca's mood shifts from anxiety about ovulation to depression when dealing with disappointment when menstruation begins.

ANATOMY AND PHYSIOLOGY

FEMALE REPRODUCTIVE SYSTEM

The anatomy of the female reproductive system consists of the external genitalia (mons pubis, labia, and vestibule) and internal structures (vagina, uterus, fallopian tubes, and ovaries). Physiologically, major glands of the endocrine system affect the development and function of the female reproductive system, including the hypothalamus, pituitary gland, and adrenal glands. The breasts are also often considered part of the female reproductive system and are described in Chapter 16. Physiologic functions discussed in this chapter are limited to the menstrual cycle and menopause. The process of pregnancy is discussed in Chapter 20.

External Genitalia

The term *vulva* is used to describe the external genital. While no two vulvas look exactly the same, vulvas do have the same structures, including the mons pubis, labia majora, labia minora, vestibule, and perineum (Fig. 17.1). The external genital organs function primarily to protect the internal genital organs, facilitate the transport of sperm, and provide sexual pleasure.

Mons Pubis

The mons pubis is a layer of tissue that lies over the pubic bone (symphysis pubis). Prior to puberty, the mons pubis contains very little fat and is flatter in appearance. During puberty, under the influence of estrogen and progesterone, pubic hair begins to grow and the transformation to a fatty pad of tissue occurs, resulting in the mounded appearance and serving as a cushion. The mons pubis contains sebaceous and sweat glands involved in the release of pheromones, the scent of which is known to stimulate sexual arousal. During menopause, the pubic hair becomes sparse, coarser, and grayer while the mons pubis loses some of its fatty tissue and becomes flatter in appearance, once again.

Labia

The labia majora and the labia minora are two sets of longitudinal skin folds. They could just as aptly be referred to as "outer" and "inner" labia, as *majora* and *minora* are reflective of size, which is not always the case. The labia majora (outer lips) are a pair of relatively large fatty folds of tissue that enclose and further protect other external genital organs. The labia majora extend from the mons pubis toward the anus; they merge beneath the vaginal introitus in an area known as the perineum. Prior to puberty, the labia majora are thin and hairless. During puberty, the labia majora thicken with fatty tissue, and the exterior folds will grow hair while the interior folds remain hairless and will begin to release lubricating secretions. During menopause, the hair becomes sparse and the tissue becomes drier and thinner. The labia minora are located just inside the labia majora and are typically thin, smooth folds of skin that vary widely in size, pigmentation, and shape; labia minora may protrude beyond the labia majora in some females but not in others. The length of the labia minora emerges just anterior to the clitoris and extends on either side of the vestibule, merging just posterior to the vaginal introitus. The labia minora connect in three places: anteriorly to form the clitoral prepuce, medially to form the clitoral frenulum, and posteriorly to form the posterior fourchette. Devoid of fatty tissue, the labia minora have a rich supply of blood vessels, resulting in a deeper, pinker color, swelling, and increased sensitivity during sexual arousal.

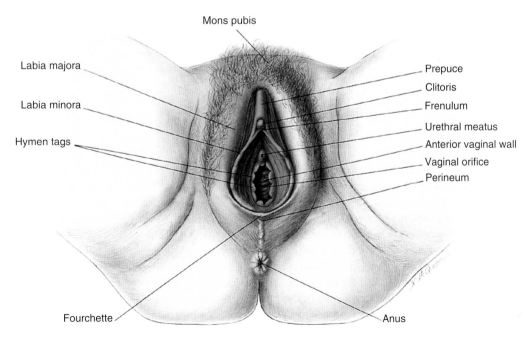

FIG. 17.1 Female external genitalia. (From Stenchever et al., 2001.)

Vestibule

The vaginal vestibule is the area that lies between the labia minora and contains the clitoris, the urethral (urinary) meatus, the introitus (vaginal opening), the hymen, and the Bartholin and Skene glands. The *urethral meatus* is located just below the clitoris and appears as an irregularly shaped slit. The *vaginal introitus* lies immediately below the urethral meatus and varies in size and shape. The *hymen* (also referred to as hymenal tissue or hymenal tags) is a collar or semi-collar of tissue that surrounds the vaginal introitus. Although it does not cover the vaginal opening, it does separate the external genitalia from the vagina. At puberty, the estrogenized hymen becomes thickened, elastic, and distensible. The hymen's appearance changes with age and life experiences (i.e., intercourse, vaginal childbirth).

The ducts of the Skene glands and the Bartholin glands open within the vestibule. The tiny *Skene glands* are numerous and are located in the paraurethral area. During sexual intercourse, they secrete a lubricating fluid. The ducts usually are not visible. *Bartholin glands* are small and round, located on either side of the introitus, at approximately the 5 and 7 o' clock positions. The ducts of the Bartholin glands open onto the sides of the vestibule in the space between the hymen and the labia minora. The ductal openings are usually not visible. During sexual excitement, the Bartholin glands secrete a mucoid material into the vaginal orifice for lubrication.

Perineum

The perineal surface is the triangular-shaped area between the vulva (beginning at the posterior fourchette) and the anus. The pelvic floor consists of a group of muscles that form a suspended sling supporting the pelvic contents. These muscles attach to various points on the bony pelvis and form functional sphincters for the vagina, rectum, and urethra.

Internal Structures

The internal structures include the vagina, uterus, fallopian tubes, and ovaries (Fig. 17.2). They are supported by four pairs of ligaments: cardinal, uterosacral, round, and broad ligaments (Fig. 17.3).

Vagina

The vagina is a canal composed of smooth muscle and is lined with a mucous membrane that extends posteriorly from the vestibule to the uterus. It inclines posteriorly at an angle of approximately 45 degrees to the vertical plane of the body. Transverse ridges of mucous membranes line the vaginal canal in the reproductive years. The uterine cervix enters superiorly and anteriorly into the vaginal canal to form a recess, or fornix, around the cervix. The fornix is divided into anterior, posterior, and lateral fornices. The vagina carries menstrual flow from the uterus and is the receptive organ for the penis during sexual intercourse. During birth, the vagina becomes the terminal portion of the birth canal.

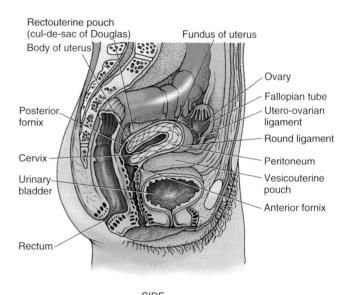

SIDE

FIG. 17.2 Midsagittal view of female pelvic organs. (From Ignatavicius and Workman, 2016.)

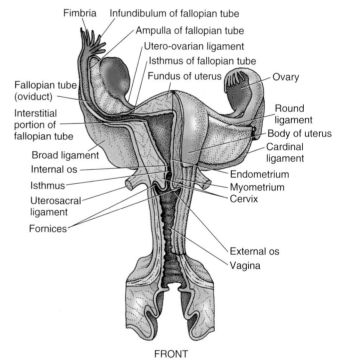

FRONT

FIG. 17.3 Cross-sectional view of internal female genitalia and pelvic contents. (From Ignatavicius and Workman, 2016.)

Uterus

The uterus is a hollow, thick, pear-shaped, muscular organ. It is suspended and stabilized in the pelvic cavity by the four pairs of ligaments (listed previously). It is fairly mobile, usually loosely suspended between the bladder and rectum. The cervix is a mucus-producing gland that is the lowest portion of the uterus. The cervical opening, or the os, is visible on the surface of the cervix. It appears as a small, round opening in a nulliparous woman (never having borne a child) or as an irregular slit in parous women.

The portion of the uterus above the cervix is known as the corpus. It is composed of three sections: the isthmus (the narrow neck from which the cervix extends into the vagina); the main body of the uterus; and the fundus, which is the bulbous top portion of the uterus (see Fig. 17.3). The fundus maintains its position by the attached round ligaments.

Fallopian Tube

The fallopian tubes extend from the fundus laterally 3 to 5 inches (7.5 to 12.5 cm) to the ovaries. The fimbriated ends of the fallopian tubes (uterine tube) partially project around the ovary to capture and draw ova into the tube for fertilization (see Fig. 17.3). The ova are transported to the uterus by rhythmic contractions of the tubal musculature and the cilia that line the fallopian tubes.

Ovaries

The almond-shaped ovaries are connected to the uterine body by the ovarian ligaments. The primary functions of the ovaries include protection and storage of the ova (eggs) a female is born with, ovulation, and secretion of reproductive hormones. Ovulation is the release of an ovum (egg), which usually occurs monthly as part of the menstrual cycle. The two dominant female sex hormones produced by the ovaries are estrogen and progesterone. These hormones have several functions, including triggering sexual maturation at puberty, development of secondary sex characteristics, and regulation of the menstrual cycle.

Menstrual Cycle

The menstrual cycle refers to the physiologic process of the female reproductive system regulated by the hypothalamus, the anterior pituitary, and the ovaries. The hypothalamus secretes releasing hormones that stimulate the anterior pituitary to release follicle-stimulating hormone (FSH) and luteinizing hormone (LH). FSH synthesizes and secretes estrogen from the ovaries, while LH stimulates progesterone secretion. Menstrual cycles can vary in length, the duration of bleeding (menses or period), and the amount of menstrual bleeding (flow) with each menses. Cycle length is determined from the first day of one menstrual period to the first day of the next menstrual period and can vary from 21 to 35 days. The duration of bleeding is usually 4 to 6 days, though this can also vary. The amount of flow is approximately 25 to 60 mL per period; clinically, the amount of flow may be reported in terms of the number of tampons or pads used. The five stages of a typical 28-day menstrual cycle are described in detail in Box 17.1 and illustrated in Fig. 17.4.

Menarche denotes the first menstrual cycle or first menstrual bleeding; this is commonly referred to as a "first period." The average age at menarche is 12.4 years, with a range of between 9 and 15 years of age. Genetics, nutrition, weight, general health, and personal life stressors are factors that directly impact the menstrual cycle throughout the lifespan.

Menopause

A period of decreased hormonal function starts between ages 35 and 40. This period is termed the *climacteric*, a long transition phase extending many years. It includes endocrine, somatic, and psychological changes, involving a complex relationship between the ovarian and hypothalamic-pituitary factors. During this period, a series of changes associated with aging and estrogen depletion occur. *Menopause* is defined as the permanent cessation of menses and is considered complete after the woman has experienced an entire year with no menses. Ovulation usually ceases 1 to 2 years before menopause. The age at which women reach menopause varies greatly, with the average age being 52 years.[1]

MALE REPRODUCTIVE SYSTEM

The anatomy of the male reproductive system can be categorized into external genitalia (penis, scrotum) and internal structures (testes, ducts, and glands).

BOX 17.1 STAGES OF THE MENSTRUAL CYCLE

Stage 1: Menstrual Phase (Days 1–4).
  The menstrual cycle begins with the menstrual phase. During this phase estrogen and progesterone levels have decreased, triggering a shedding of the upper layers of the endometrium and menstrual bleeding. See Fig. 17.4.
Stage 2: Postmenstrual or Preovulatory Phase (Days 5–12).
  The follicle-stimulating hormone (FSH) stimulates follicular growth during this stage. The ovary and maturing follicle produce estrogen, which supports egg development within the follicle.
Stage 3: Ovulation (Day 13 or 14).
  Ovulation is characterized by a steep rise in estrogen and luteinizing hormone (LH). The egg is expelled from the follicle and drawn into the fallopian tube by the fimbriae

and cilia. A subsequent rise in progesterone causes the thickening of the uterine wall.
Stage 4: Secretory Phase (Days 15–20).
  After ovulation, the FSH and LH hormones decline. The egg moves into the uterus, and the follicle becomes a corpus luteum. Secretion of progesterone rises and predominates while estrogen declines. The uterine wall continues to thicken in anticipation of receiving a fertilized egg.
Stage 5: Premenstrual Phase (Days 21–28).
  If fertilization of the egg and subsequent implantation do not occur, the corpus luteum degenerates, and progesterone production decreases. Estrogen levels begin to rise again as a new follicle develops. When the thickened uterine wall begins to shed, menstruation starts, which marks the beginning of another menstrual cycle.

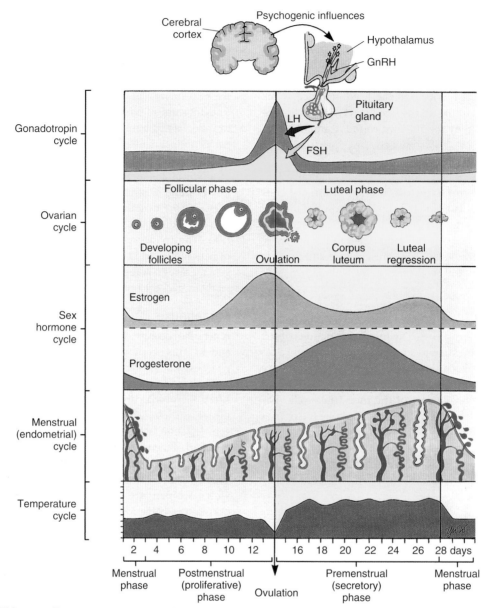

FIG. 17.4 Female menstrual cycle. Diagram shows the interrelationship of the cerebral, hypothalamic, pituitary, and uterine functions throughout a standard 28-day menstrual cycle. The variations in basal body temperature are also shown. *FSH*, Follicle-stimulating hormone; *LH*, luteinizing hormone. (From Thibodeau and Patton, 2007.)

External Genitalia

Scrotum

The scrotum is a pouch covered with thin, darkly pigmented, rugous (wrinkled) skin (Fig. 17.5). A septum divides the scrotum into two pendulous compartments, or sacs. Each sac contains a testis, which contains seminiferous tubules arranged within lobules, and an epididymis, which is suspended by the *spermatic cord* (i.e., a network of nerves, blood vessels, and the vas deferens; Fig. 17.6). Because sperm production requires a temperature slightly below body temperature, the testes are suspended outside the body cavity; the temperature of the scrotum is controlled by a layer of muscle under the scrotal skin that contracts or relaxes in response to

the outside temperature. When the temperature is cold, the scrotal sac and its contents move close to the body; conversely, when the temperature rises, the scrotal sac relaxes and the testes drop downward.

Penis

The penis serves two functions: it is the final excretory organ in urination, and during intercourse, it introduces sperm into the vagina. The body of the penis contains two layers of tissue—the corpus cavernosa and the corpus spongiosum—which encase the urethra (see Fig. 17.5). The corpus cavernosa are smooth, spongy tissues that become firm when engorged with blood, forming an erection. The corpus spongiosum expands at its distal end to form the glans penis,

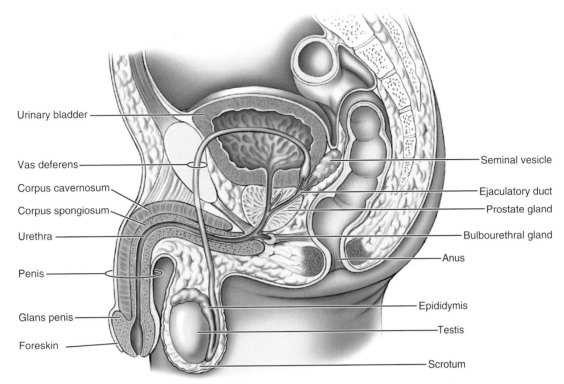

Urinary bladder

Vas deferens

Corpus cavernosum

Corpus spongiosum

Urethra

Penis

Glans penis

Foreskin

Seminal vesicle

Ejaculatory duct

Prostate gland

Bulbourethral gland

Anus

Epididymis

Testis

Scrotum

FIG. 17.5 Male reproductive organs. (From Herlihy et al., 2011.)

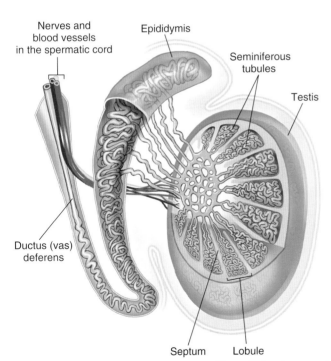

Nerves and blood vessels in the spermatic cord

Epididymis

Seminiferous tubules

Testis

Ductus (vas) deferens

Septum   Lobule

FIG. 17.6 Scrotum and its contents. (From Thibodeau and Patton, 2007.)

which is lighter pink in color than the rest of the penis. It is exposed when the prepuce (the foreskin) is either pulled back or surgically removed (circumcision). The corona is the ridge that separates the glans from the shaft of the penis. The skin covering the penis is thin, hairless, and a little darker than the

rest of the body; it adheres loosely to the shaft to allow for expansion with erection.

Erection is a neurovascular reflex that occurs when increased arterial dilation and decreased venous outflow cause the two corpora cavernosa to become engorged with blood. This reflex can be induced by psychogenic and local reflex mechanisms, both under the control of the autonomic nervous system. The psychogenic erection can be initiated by any type of sensory input (auditory, visual, tactile, or imaginative), whereas local reflex mechanisms are initiated by tactile stimuli. Ejaculation (i.e., the emission of semen from the vas deferens, epididymides, prostate, and seminal vesicles) is followed by constriction of the vessels supplying blood to the corpora cavernosa and gradual return of the penis to its relaxed, flaccid state.

Internal Structures

Testes

The testes are paired sex organs located within the scrotum. They are oval shaped, with a smooth surface and rubbery texture. The primary function of the testes is the production of sperm (spermatogenesis). Each testicle contains a series of coiled ducts (seminiferous tubules) where spermatogenesis occurs. As sperm are produced, they move toward the center of the testis, traveling into the efferent tubules adjacent to the epididymis (see Fig. 17.6).

Ducts

There are a series of ducts that are collectively responsible for the transportation of sperm. Once formed in the testes, sperm move into the comma-shaped *epididymis*—a long and elaborately coiled duct that lies on the posterolateral surface of each testis (see Fig. 17.6). As sperm move through the epididymis, they receive nutrients and mature. Eventually, they exit the epididymis through the vas deferens.

The *vas deferens* (also known as the *ductus deferens*) transport sperm from the epididymis to the ejaculatory duct. It is enclosed within the spermatic cord (a connective tissue sheath) along with arteries, veins, and nerves as it ascends through the inguinal canal. The cord enters the inguinal canal through the external inguinal ring; this ring is vulnerable to hernias, or protrusion of the abdominal contents. In the abdominal cavity, the vas deferens travels up and around to the posterior aspect of the bladder, where it unites with the seminal vesicle (see Fig. 17.5). The union of the seminal vesicles with the vas deferens forms the *ejaculatory duct* just before the entrance into the prostate gland. Within the ejaculatory duct, sperm are transported downward through the prostate gland and into the prostatic portion of the urethra.

The innermost tube of the penis, the *urethra,* is usually about 18 to 20 cm from bladder to meatus. It extends out of the base of the bladder, traveling through the prostate gland into the pelvic floor and through the penile shaft (see Fig. 17.5). The urethral orifice is a small slit at the tip of the glans. The urethra is the terminal passageway for both urine and sperm. During ejaculation, sperm travel from the ejaculatory duct through the urethra and out of the body.

Glands

Three glands (seminal vesicles, prostate gland, and bulbourethral glands) produce and secrete fluid that makes up most of the fluid in the ejaculate (semen). These secretions serve as a medium for the transport of sperm and also provide an alkaline environment that promotes sperm motility and survival.

The *seminal vesicles* (small pouches lying between the rectum and the posterior bladder wall) join the ejaculatory duct at the base of the prostate (see Fig. 17.5). The *prostate gland* lies beneath the urinary bladder and surrounds the upper portion of the urethra. The posterior surface of the prostate lies adjacent to the anterior rectal wall. Two of the three prostate lobes are palpable through the rectum (right and left lateral lobes). These lobes are divided by a slight groove known as the median sulcus. The third lobe (median lobe) is anterior to the urethra and cannot be palpated. *Bulbourethral glands,* located on either side of the urethra just below the prostate, also secrete fluid that contributes to the semen, providing a medium for transport of the sperm.

RECTUM AND ANUS

The rectum and anus are the terminal structures of the gastrointestinal (GI) tract. They are presented in this chapter because they make up the posterior portion of the perineum in the male and female and because they are usually examined in conjunction with examination of the reproductive system.

Rectum

The proximal end of the rectum lies at the distal end of the sigmoid colon and extends down for approximately 12 cm to the anorectal junction (Fig. 17.7). Three semilunar folds of tissue called *rectal valves* (superior, middle, and inferior rectal valves) lie within the rectal wall and extend across half the circumference of the rectal lumen. The function of these valves is not well understood but is thought to support feces while allowing flatus to pass. The most distal of these valves (the inferior rectal valve) can be palpated with digital examination.

Anal Canal and Anus

The anal canal extends from the anorectal junction to the anus (see Fig. 17.7). It is lined with mucous membranes arranged in longitudinal folds called *rectal columns* that contain a network of arteries and veins (frequently referred to as the *internal hemorrhoidal plexus*). Between each of the columns is a recessed area called the *anal crypt,* into which the perianal glands empty. Surrounding the anal canal are two concentric rings of muscle: the internal and external sphincters. The internal sphincter consists of smooth muscle and is under involuntary control. The external sphincter, consisting of skeletal muscle, is under voluntary control, allowing for control of defecation. The lower portion of the anal canal is sensitive to painful stimuli, whereas the upper portion is relatively insensitive.

The anus is the terminal portion of the rectum, located just posterior to the perineum. It is hairless, moist mucosal tissue surrounded by hyperpigmented perianal skin. Normally the anus is closed, except during defecation.

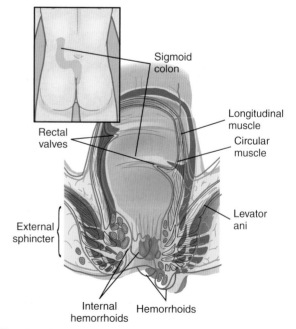

Sigmoid colon

Longitudinal muscle

Circular muscle

Rectal valves

Levator ani

External sphincter

Internal hemorrhoids

Hemorrhoids

FIG. 17.7 Anatomy of the anus and rectum. (From Lewis et al., 2014.)

HEALTH HISTORY

Nurses interview patients to collect subjective data about their present health status, past health history, family history, personal and psychosocial history, and sexual and obstetric history, which may affect the health condition of their reproductive systems.

GENERAL HEALTH HISTORY

Present Health Status

Do you have any chronic illnesses? If yes, describe.
Many chronic illnesses may affect reproductive functioning in women and men. For example, endocrine disorders may impact a woman's menstrual cycle, while diabetes mellitus, vascular insufficiency, cardiac disease, and respiratory disease can contribute to erectile dysfunction (ED).

Do you take any medications? If yes, what do you take and how often?
Both prescription and over-the-counter medications should be noted. Ask if the medications are taken as prescribed. Many medications can affect reproductive system functioning or libido. For example, medications such as oral contraceptives and broad-spectrum antibiotics can alter the balance of the normal vaginal flora in women. In men, some medications such as diuretics and antihypertensive agents can cause impotence.

Do you take any herbal supplements? If yes, what do you take and how often? What are they for?
Herbal supplements may be taken to increase testosterone levels. Other supplements may be taken to reduce symptoms of menstrual pain or menopause.

Past Health History

Have you had any reproductive problems in the past? If yes, describe.
Identify previous problems with the reproductive system because this information may be helpful when documenting current problems or risk factors for other medical problems. For example, women with endometriosis have been shown to have an increased risk of ovarian cancer.[2]

Have you ever had a sexually transmitted infection? If yes, what type of infection did you have? How was it treated?
Some sexually transmitted infections (STIs) (also known as sexually transmitted disease [STD]) are chronic and place sexual partners at risk. A history of some STIs, such as human papillomavirus (HPV), increases the risk for certain cancers (cervical cancer and rectal cancer).[3] STI can also increase the risk for pelvic inflammatory disease (PID).

Have you ever had surgery on your reproductive organs or rectum? If yes, when? How has it affected you?
If a woman reports that she has had a hysterectomy, ask if it was an abdominal or a vaginal approach and if she had a total

RISK FACTORS

Cervical Cancer

- Persistent infection with human papillomavirus virus
- Sexual intercourse at an early age and a lifetime history of multiple sex partners or partners with multiple sexual partners
- Suppressed immune system
- Cigarette smoking (M)
- Multiple childbirths
- Long-term use of oral contraceptives
- Obesity (M)
- Family history of cervical cancer

M, Modifiable risk factor.
From American Cancer Society: *Cancer facts and figures 2020*, Atlanta, GA, American Cancer Society. Retrieved from: https://www.cancer.org/cancer/cervical-cancer/causes-risks-prevention/risk-factors.html; Center for Disease Control: *What are risk factors for Cervical Cancer?* 2018. Retrieved from: https://www.cdc.gov/cancer/cervical/index.htm; PDQ® Adult Treatment Editorial Board: *PDQ cervical cancer treatment*, Bethesda, MD, 2019, National Cancer Institute. Retrieved from: https://www.cancer.gov/types/cervical/hp/cervical-treatment-pdq.

(uterus, fallopian tubes, and ovaries removed) or a partial (only uterus removed) hysterectomy. In addition, ask the patient why she had the hysterectomy, when it was performed, if she had any accompanying bowel or bladder repairs, and what problems or concerns she has had since the surgery. Men may have had surgery to treat an enlarged prostate, prostate cancer, hydrocele, varicocele, or testicular cancer. Both men and women may have had surgical procedures to prevent pregnancy (vasectomy or a tubal ligation) or involving the anus or rectum (such as hemorrhoidectomy).

Do you have a history of cancer? If yes, which type of cancer? How was it treated?
In women, a history of breast cancer or nonpolyposis colon cancer is a risk factor for some types of female reproductive cancers. In men, a history of testicular cancer increases the risk of recurrence in the other testicle.[4]

RISK FACTORS

Testicular Cancer

- Age (highest incidence in young men ages 20–34)
- Cryptorchidism (undescended testicle)
- Family history (increased risk if father or brother had testicular cancer)
- History of testicular cancer in other testicle
- Race (highest incidence among white men)

From: American Cancer Society: *Risk factors for testicular cancer*, 2020. Retrieved from: https://www.cancer.org/cancer/testicular-cancer/causes-risks-prevention.html; Cancer treatment Centers of America: *Testicular Cancer Risk Factors*, 2019. Retrieved from: https://www.cancercenter.com/cancer-types/testicular-cancer/risk-factors; PDQ® Adult Treatment Editorial Board: *PDQ Testicular Cancer Treatment*, Bethesda, MD, 2019, National Cancer Institute. Retrieved from: https://www.cancer.gov/types/testicular/patient/testicular-treatment-pdq.

Have you received the hepatitis A or B vaccine? Have you received the HPV vaccine?

Preexposure vaccination is one of the most effective methods for preventing some sexually transmitted diseases (STDs). The hepatitis B virus (HBV) vaccination series, the hepatitis A virus (HAV) vaccination series, and the HPV vaccination series are recommended for males and females during adolescence and young adulthood.

Family History

Women: Has any woman in your family ever had cancer of the cervix, ovary, uterus, breast, or colon? If yes, who? When?

A family history of these cancers (particularly in a first-degree relative) increases risk for certain female reproductive cancers.[4]

RISK FACTORS

Ovarian Cancer

- Strong family history of ovarian cancer
- Personal history of breast cancer
- *BRCA1* and *BRCA2* gene mutations
- Pelvic inflammatory disease and Lynch syndrome
- Nulliparity
- Obesity (M)
- Estrogen use for postmenopausal hormone replacement therapy (M)
- Age (increased risk with aging)

M, Modifiable risk factor.
From American Cancer Society: *Cancer facts and figures* 2020 Atlanta, 2020, American Cancer Society. Retrieved from: https://www.cancer.org/cancer/ovarian-cancer/causes-risks-prevention/risk-factors.html; Center for Disease Control: *What are the Risk Factors for Ovarian Cancer?* 2017. Retrieved from: http://www.cdc.gov/cancer/ovarian/basic_info/risk_factors/htm; PDQ® Screening and Prevention Editorial Board: *PDQ Ovarian, Fallopian Tube, and Primary Peritoneal Cancer Prevention*, Bethesda, MD, 2019, National Cancer Institute. Retrieved from: https://www.cancer.gov/types/ovarian/patient/ovarian-prevention-pdq.

Men: Has any man in your family ever had cancer of the prostate or testicle? If yes, who? When?

A family history of these cancers (particularly in a first-degree relative) increases risk for certain prostate and testicular cancers.

Personal and Psychosocial History

How often do you have an examination of your genitalia by a health care professional? What were the results?

Assess health care behaviors. Ideally, a well-woman visit should include screening, evaluation, and counseling based on age, history, and identified risk factors; "routine" screening is individualized and patient-centered.[5] The same can be said for men. Men should have an examination of their genitalia and prostate on a regular basis, depending on their age, history, risk factors, and preexisting health conditions. For instance, ED is a significant predictor of underlying cardiovascular disease and can be a result of diabetes mellitus.[6,7]

RISK FACTORS

Prostate Cancer

- *Age:* 56% of new cases occur in men over age 65.
- Race: African American men have the highest incidence of prostate cancer—two times higher than white men.
- *Family history:* First-degree relative with prostate cancer increases risk.
- Dietary: High dietary fat intake, high dairy, and calcium intake. (M)
- Genetic: Lynch syndrome (a form of colorectal cancer), *BRCA1*, *BRCA2*.

M, Modifiable risk factor.
From American Cancer Society: *Cancer facts and figures 2020*, Atlanta, 2020, American Cancer Society. Retrieved from: https://www.cancer.org/content/dam/cancer-org/research/cancer-facts-and-statistics/annual-cancer-facts-and-figures/2019/cancer-facts-and-figures-2019.pdf; Centers for Disease Control: *Prostate cancer, who is at risk? 2018*. Retrieved from: http://www.cdc.gov/cancer/prostate/basic_info/risk_factors.htm; PDQ® Screening and Prevention Editorial Board: *PDQ Prostate Cancer Prevention*, Bethesda, MD, 2019, National Cancer Institute. Retrieved from: https://www.cancer.gov/types/prostate/hp/prostate-prevention-pdq.

Sexual History

Are you currently in a sexual relationship? If yes, do you prefer relationships with men, women, or both? In which type of sex do you engage (penile-vaginal, penile-anal, recipient anal, oral)?

The type of sex in which one participates may provide useful information for risk assessment of STIs. Cross-infections from mouth, anus, and genitals can occur. Men and women need to feel accepted when discussing their health concerns. If the nurse seems genuinely interested and concerned, the patient may appreciate the opportunity to discuss sexuality issues or problems.

How frequently do you engage in sexual activities? Are you and your partner(s) satisfied with the sexual relationship? Do you communicate comfortably about sexual activity?

Determining the frequency of sexual activity and the patient's satisfaction are important. Questions related to sexual activities and satisfaction are often found on health history forms; however, health care providers have been found to focus on physiologic function and/or offer little discussion related to sexuality unless an issue is raised by the patient.[6,7]

Do you or your partner(s) have multiple partners? How many sexual partners have you had in the past 3 months?

This information may be used to determine the patient's risk for STI.

How do you protect yourself from STI? Do you use a protective barrier such as a condom every time you have intercourse?

Determine the patient's level of understanding and practice regarding safe sex and STI prevention. Individuals may not have accurate information. When used correctly and consistently, condoms are highly effective in preventing sexual transmission of human immunodeficiency virus (HIV), chlamydia, gonorrhea, and trichomoniasis. While condoms do not fully protect one from herpes simplex virus (HSV) or HPV, they do help in the prevention of both viral infections.[3]

Are you currently using any birth control measures? If yes, which type(s)? How effective do you think it (they) has (have) been? Do you have any difficulty with the birth control measures? Do you use birth control measures every time you have intercourse?
All women who have the potential to become pregnant or men who have the potential to create a pregnancy should be questioned about contraceptive practices. Information should be gathered about the appropriate use of contraception, length of use, and satisfaction with the product.

How old were you when you first had intercourse? Was it by choice? Have you ever been forced into sexual acts as a child or an adult? If so, how has this impacted you and your partner?
Inquire about current or past sexual abuse. Although most cases of sexual assault are committed by men who know their victims, men and women can be victims of sexual assault and abuse.[8] Research has shown that victims of sexual assault or abuse may wait years before reporting or disclosing; delay in disclosure is even more likely when the perpetrator is a family member.[9] Sexual abuse or assault often cause ongoing sexual difficulties for the victims and their partners; male partners of women who are sexually assaulted often feel angry, guilty, and helpless. Sexual assault crosses all socioeconomic, racial, and cultural boundaries—no one is immune—thus, screening of all patients is essential.

Do you or your partner(s) frequently use drugs or alcohol before you engage in sexual activity? Have you ever traded sex for drugs, alcohol, or food?
Drug and alcohol use is associated with high-risk sexual behavior. Some individuals addicted to drugs or alcohol rely on sexual activity as a means to gain access to the substances to which they are addicted.

OBSTETRIC HISTORY

Menstruation

What was the date of the first day of your last menstrual period (LMP)? How often do you have periods? How long do they usually last?
A menstrual history consists of the LMP, usual menstrual interval, and the duration of menses. Women who are menopausal should be asked at what age menopause occurred.

How would you describe your usual amount of flow—light, moderate, heavy? How many pads or tampons do you use over the course of a day? An hour?

Normal flow is difficult to determine, but any change from the "normal" for the patient should be noted.

Have you noticed any change in your periods recently?
Early identification of changes in or abnormal menstrual patterns may improve the identification of other potential health concerns. Abnormal bleeding could be caused by pregnancy, hormonal imbalance, weight changes, thyroid condition, coagulopathy, medication, uterine lesions, or malignancy.[10]

How old were you when you started having periods?
Menarche typically occurs between ages 12 and 14 years, although the range spans ages 9 to 15. By age 15 years, 98% of females will have begun menstruating; if menses have not begun by this age, an evaluation for primary amenorrhea may be indicated. Early onset of menarche (before age 11) is a risk factor for endometrial and ovarian cancer.[4]

Pregnancy

Have you ever been pregnant? If so, how many times? How many babies have you had? Have you had any miscarriages, abortions, or infants who died before they were born? If yes, how many?
Gravida refers to the number of pregnancies; *para* refers to the number of pregnancies that reached 20 weeks or longer. See Chapter 20 for more information regarding documentation of obstetric history.

Do you think you may be pregnant now? If yes, what symptoms have you noticed?
Symptoms may include missed or abnormal periods, nausea or vomiting, breast changes or tenderness, and fatigue.

Have you ever had difficulty becoming pregnant? If yes, have you seen a health care provider? What have you tried to do to become pregnant? How do you feel about not being able to become pregnant?
Inquiring about difficulty becoming pregnant is as important as asking about actual pregnancy. If couples trying unsuccessfully to become pregnant are highly distressed, they may need a nurse to provide a referral for counseling or to encourage them to discuss their feelings.

PROBLEM-BASED HISTORY

Commonly reported problems related to the reproductive system and perineum for men and women include pain, genital lesions, vaginal or penile discharge, problems with urination, and rectal bleeding. Common problems unique to women include problems or changes with the menstrual cycle and menopausal symptoms. Common problems unique to men include difficulty with erection. As with symptoms in all areas of health assessment, a symptom analysis is completed using the mnemonic OLD CARTS, which includes the *O*nset, *L*ocation, *D*uration, *C*haracteristics, *A*ggravating factors, *R*elated symptoms, *T*reatment, and *S*everity (see Box 2.6).

Pain

When did the pain begin? Where is it located? Describe its characteristics. On a scale of 0 to 10, how would you rate the severity of the pain?

Men and women may experience lower abdominal, pelvic, or rectal pain from a number of problems involving the reproductive system, urinary tract (urethra, bladder, ureters), rectum, anus, or pelvic floor dysfunction.[11] Women with unexplained pelvic pain should be screened for infection including chlamydia. Pain is also a common symptom of endometriosis. Rectal discomfort may be associated with a number of factors, including poor hygiene, infection, hemorrhoids, and abscess. Symptoms such as burning with urination suggest urinary tract infection (UTI).

Among men, pain in the groin or scrotum may occur from inguinal hernia or problems in the spermatic cord, testicles, or prostate gland. Testicular pain can occur secondary to almost any problem of the testis or epididymis, including epididymitis, orchitis, hydrocele, testicular torsion, and testicular cancer.

What factors aggravate the pain?

A number of factors can affect pain in the reproductive system, such as menstrual cycles, sexual activity, mobility, or even diet. Identifying factors that aggravate the pain may help identify the underlying cause.

Do you have related symptoms such as discharge or bleeding, abdominal distention or tenderness, or pelvic fullness?

Determine if there are any related symptoms that occur with the pain to help identify the cause. Vaginal and penile discharges are described later in the chapter.

What alleviates the symptoms or what have you done to treat the pain? How effective was the treatment?

Alleviating factors include rest or positioning. Knowledge of previous self-treatment measures may be helpful in identifying appropriate treatment strategies.

Genital Lesion

When did you first become aware of the lesion? Where exactly is it located? What does it look like? Is it tender?

A lesion or sore on the genitalia is often caused by STD or cancer but may also be associated with other problems. Establish when the lesion was first noticed because this may be important in identifying the cause.

Do you have any related symptoms (e.g., pain, bleeding, discharge, burning pain with urination, or pelvic fullness)?

These are symptoms commonly associated with STD.

Have you had a sexual relationship with someone who has an STD? If so, when? Have you ever been treated for any of these infections? If so, was the treatment successful?

Sexual contact with a partner with untreated STI increases a person's risk for STI.

RISK FACTORS

Sexually Transmitted Diseases

Sexually transmitted diseases (STDs) can occur with oral, vaginal, or anal sex, regardless of gender or orientation

- Unprotected sex (not using a protective barrier consistently and correctly) (M)
- Multiple partners (having sex with multiple partners and/or having sex with an individual who has multiple partners)
- Age (younger people, particularly women are at greater risk)
- Substance use (alcohol or illicit drug use is associated with high-risk sexual behavior) (M)
- Trading sex for money or drugs, having sex with a sex worker or IV drug user (M)
- History of having an STD
- Having sex with a partner with untreated STD (M)
- Not vaccinated against human papillomavirus or hepatitis B (M)

M, Modifiable risk factor.
From American College of Obstetricians and Gynecologists. FAQ009: *How to prevent sexually transmitted infections,* 2017. Retrieved from: https://www.acog.org/Patients/FAQs/How-to-Prevent-Sexually-Transmitted-Infections-STIs?IsMobileSet=false; Centers for Disease Control and Prevention: *How you can prevent sexually transmitted diseases,* 2016. Retrieved from: https://www.cdc.gov/std/prevention/default.htm.

Vaginal or Penile Discharge

When did the discharge begin? What color is it? Describe its odor and consistency.

Identify the onset of the symptom. Penile discharge suggests infection. Among women, normal discharge is clear or cloudy with minimal odor. A change may suggest a vaginal infection. Specific appearance or odor of the discharge may help identify the causative organism. For example, bacterial vaginosis produces an unpleasant fishy odor with vaginal discharge in some women.

Do you have other symptoms such as pain or itching?

Pain and itching are related symptoms. Irritation from the discharge can cause itching, rash, or pain with intercourse. Pelvic, abdominal, or urinary pain associated with discharge suggests infection.

If sexually active, does your partner have a discharge? Have you or your partner had a recent change or addition in sex partners?

A common cause of penile and vaginal discharge is a STI.

Problems With Menstruation

What kinds of problems with menstruation are you experiencing?

Ask the patient to describe the specific problems she has been experiencing as a starting point.

Have you noticed clotted blood during your periods? If yes, when did it begin? Is it becoming worse over time?

Menorrhagia is a term for heavy menses. Clotting of blood indicates a heavy flow or vaginal pooling. *Metrorrhagia* is a term for bleeding at irregular intervals.

Do you have cramps or other pains associated with your period? Do they occur each month? What relieves the discomfort? Do the cramps or pains interfere with your normal activities?

Dysmenorrhea is a term for painful or difficult menses and often causes significant cramping. It is often associated with hormone imbalance or endometriosis.

Do you ever have spotting between periods?

Spotting (very light bleeding) between periods or midcycle bleeding may indicate hormone imbalance, ovulation, or a need for dose adjustment if the patient is taking hormonal contraceptives or hormone replacement.[10]

Do you have unexplained vaginal bleeding?

Vaginal bleeding not associated with menstrual cycles could indicate endometrial cancer.

Do you have any other problems or symptoms before menses, such as headaches, bloated feeling, weight gain, breast tenderness, irritability, or moodiness? Do they seem to be associated with your periods, or do they occur at other times? Do they interfere with your routine activities?

Hormone fluctuation associated with the menstrual cycle may cause the patient to have symptoms that are frequently referred to as premenstrual syndrome (PMS). Asking how routine activities are affected by symptoms helps the nurse gain a better understanding of the significance of the symptoms.

Menopausal Symptoms

When did your menstrual periods slow or stop? Describe the menopausal symptoms you are experiencing.

Amenorrhea means absent menses. The perimenopausal period for most women occurs between ages 42 and 58. Common symptoms experienced during menopause include hot flashes, excessive sweating, back pain, palpitations, headaches, vaginal dryness, painful intercourse, changes in sexual desire, or mood swings.[10]

Are you being treated for any symptoms associated with menopause? Are you taking hormone replacement? If yes, what are you taking and how much? Have you noticed any adverse effects?

Hormone replacement therapy (HRT) includes taking estrogen for women without a uterus or taking estrogen and progesterone for women with a uterus. Adverse effects of estrogen include headache, nausea, fluid retention, breast pain or enlargement, and vaginal bleeding. A link between cardiovascular disease and estrogen replacement therapy has also been found. Adverse effects of progesterone include weight gain and increased appetite, fluctuations in mood (irritability and depression), breast tenderness, and spotting.

 ETHNIC, CULTURAL, AND SPIRITUAL VARIATIONS

Menopausal Symptoms

Cultural and societal influences can impact a woman's experience of menopause, including her emotional and physical relationships. In one study that examined the prevalence of postmenopausal symptoms in North America and Europe, the top five symptoms of vaginal dryness, hot flashes, night sweats, disrupted sleep, and weight gain were determined to be the most prevalent in women from the United States, the United Kingdom, and Canada and less prevalent in women from Sweden and Italy, compared with other countries. The lead author of the study concluded that in cultures and societies where aging is embraced and associated with wisdom, such as Sweden and Italy, menopausal symptoms are significantly less bothersome.

From Minkin MJ, Reiter S, Maamari R: Prevalence of postmenopausal symptoms in North America and Europe, *Menopause* 22(11):1231–1238, 2015.

Difficulty With Erection

When did you first notice problems with attaining or maintaining an erection? Did this problem develop suddenly or over a period of time? Do you have this problem consistently, or does the problem come and go?

ED is a common problem, yet a very delicate topic. In one study, more than half of men with ED had not discussed their condition with a health care provider.[12] ED is highly age dependent; 4% of men in their 50s and 17% of men in their 60s are unable to achieve an erection. By age 75, the incidence jumps to 47%.[13]

Do you have an idea about what might be contributing to the problem?

ED may be associated with medications, chronic illness (e.g., hypertension or treatment for prostate cancer), sexual dissatisfaction, or emotional problems. It may also be an indicator for underlying complications among men with diabetes. When a patient has difficulty with erection, he can be referred to a urologist who specializes in this area.

Problems With Urination

What kind of problem or change with urination are you experiencing? Is it hard to urinate? Do you have to urinate more frequently than normal?

Infection is the most common urinary problem among men and women. Many older men experience urinary obstruction caused by an enlarged prostate. (Problems with urination is also discussed in Chapter 13.)

Have you experienced any pain or burning with urination? Is the urine clear or cloudy? Discolored? Bloody? Foul smelling? If yes, do you have other symptoms such as frequent urination in small amounts? Feeling that you cannot wait to urinate? Incontinence?

These symptoms may accompany problems such as UTI or acute cystitis among men and women and prostatitis among men. Urethritis in the young, sexually active male may indicate an STD such as chlamydia or gonorrhea.[3]

Do you think you are urinating more frequently than you consider normal? Do you awaken at night because you have to urinate?
Medications, especially diuretics and antihistamines, may cause increased urination. Increased nocturia (awakening at night to urinate), urinary frequency, and urgency may increase when the patient has a urinary disorder or prostate enlargement.

Men: Do you have any trouble initiating or maintaining a urine stream? Is the stream narrower or weaker than usual? Afterward, do you feel that you still have to urinate?
Prostate enlargement, common among older men, gradually obstructs the urethra, impeding urine flow. Common symptoms may include hesitancy, straining, loss of force, or decreased caliber of the stream, terminal dribbling, sensation of residual urine, and recurrent episodes of acute cystitis.

Rectal Bleeding
When did the rectal bleeding start? Is the problem constant or does it come and go? Describe the color and amount of blood.
Determine the onset and duration of the problem. Determine the characteristics of the bleeding. Bleeding from high in the intestinal tract produces black, tarry stools (melena), whereas bleeding near the rectum is associated with bright red bleeding (hematochezia). Black or dark, non-tarry stools may occur when taking certain medications such as iron supplements.

Have you had accompanying abdominal cramping or pain? Have you been constipated? Have you felt fatigued?
Identify related symptoms. Some conditions such as ulcerative colitis can cause rectal bleeding accompanied by abdominal cramping. The passage of hard, dry stools can contribute to rectal bleeding. Fatigue is a significant finding in patients who develop anemia secondary to rectal bleeding.

HEALTH PROMOTION FOR EVIDENCE-BASED PRACTICE
Sexually Transmitted Disease

Background
STDs have a major impact on sexual, reproductive, and neonatal health. There are an estimated 20 million new cases of sexually transmitted disease (STD) cases each year in the United States. While adolescents and young adults (15–24 years) are at a higher risk for acquiring an STD, the incidence in the older population (age > 50 years) is growing too. The nation experienced steep and sustained STD increases between 2013 and 2017, with a 22% increase in cases of chlamydia, a 67% increase in cases of gonorrhea, and a 76% increase in cases of syphilis. Women tend to suffer more serious consequences of STDs compared with men; disparities persist in rates of infection among racial and ethnic minority groups—in this case, black and Hispanic—when compared with rates among whites. Access to and routine use of affordable, quality health care, including STD prevention and treatment, are essential to reducing STD disparities in the United States.

Recommendations to Reduce Risk (Primary Prevention)
- Abstinence or reduction of the number of sex partners
- Use of barrier protection (male or female condoms) during sex
- Preexposure vaccinations with the hepatitis B virus (HBV) vaccination, the hepatitis A virus (HAV) vaccination, and the human papillomavirus (HPV) vaccine

Screening Recommendations (Secondary Prevention)
- *HIV:* Screening should be offered to all adolescents and all other individuals based on level of risk (such as MSM). All pregnant women should be screened at the first prenatal visit.
- *Chlamydia:* Annual screening is recommended for all sexually active women under age 25 and other individuals at increased risk. Pregnant women under age 25 and all other pregnant women with high-risk behaviors should be screened at the first prenatal visit and again during the third trimester.
- *Gonorrhea:* Annual screening is recommended for all sexually active women under age 25 and other individuals who are at increased risk. All pregnant women under age 25 and pregnant women with high-risk behaviors should be screened at the first prenatal visit.
- *Syphilis:* Routine screening is not recommended for those of average risk; all high-risk individuals should be screened. Screen all pregnant women at the first prenatal visit and again during the third trimester or at delivery if they have high-risk behaviors.
- *Hepatitis B Surface Antigen.* All pregnant women should be tested for the presence of antigens.

MSM, Men who have sex with men.
From Centers for Disease Control and Prevention: Sexually transmitted disease treatment guidelines 2015, *MMWR* 64(3) 1–137, 2015.

HEALTH PROMOTION FOR EVIDENCE-BASED PRACTICE

Reproductive Cancers

Background

Reproductive cancers will account for an estimated 317,260 new cases and 67,830 estimated deaths in 2020. Uterine cancer in females and prostate cancer in males are the most prevalent; the incidence of anal cancer is on the rise, and the number of people has tripled since the 1970s, correlated with infection with the human papillomavirus (HPV). In theory, both cervical and anal cancer could be prevented before it develops, provided there is adequate screening for precancerous lesions. Screening for these cancers will also be an issue in transmen and transwomen—which should not be overlooked.

Recommendations to Reduce Risk (Primary Prevention)

- Practice healthy behaviors (e.g., smoking cessation, safe sex practices, and maintaining healthy body weight) because these may reduce the incidence of certain cancers.

Screening Recommendations (Secondary Prevention)

Routine screening for individuals at average risk for endometrial cancer, ovarian cancer, prostate cancer, and testicular cancer is not recommended. Screening is recommended for:

Cervical Cancer

- Women ages 21–30 should be screened with the Pap test every 3 years.
- Women ages 30–65 can be tested with Pap test every 3 years, or Pap/HPV co-testing every 5 years.

Ovarian Cancer

- Women with increased risk (strong family history of two or more first- or second-degree relatives with ovarian or breast cancer) should be referred for genetic counseling.

From American Cancer Society: *Cancer facts and figures 2020*, Atlanta, 2019, American Cancer Society; U.S. Preventive Services Task Force: *Guide to clinical preventive services, 2014.* AHRQ Pub. No. 14-05158.

EXAMINATION

FEMALE EXAMINATION

Routine techniques	Techniques for special circumstances
• INSPECT the pubic hair and skin over the mons pubis and inguinal area. • INSPECT and PALPATE the labia majora, labia minora, and clitoris. • INSPECT the urethral meatus, hymen, vaginal introitus, and perineum. • INSPECT and PALPATE the sacrococcygeal area. • INSPECT the perianal areas and anus.	• PALPATE the Skene and Bartholin glands. • PALPATE the vaginal wall. • PALPATE the rectal wall. • PALPATE the anal sphincter. • EXAMINE the stool. **Techniques Performed by an APRN** • INSPECT the cervix and vaginal walls. • OBTAIN specimens for laboratory testing. • PALPATE the uterus and ovaries.

Equipment needed
• Examination gloves • Light source • Speculum • Swabs • Lubricating gel

APRN, Advanced practice registered nurse.

PREPARING FOR THE FEMALE EXAMINATION

Before you begin this procedure, prepare the room. Assemble the equipment; obtain a sheet, pillow, and gown; and be sure that the room temperature is warm. Consider also having a hand mirror available, allowing the women to see the exam, as applicable. Women may feel apprehensive about having their genitalia examined, especially if the nurse is male. If necessary, arrange for a female assistant. Before bringing the woman to the examination room, ask her to empty her bladder. Provide for privacy as the woman prepares for the examination. She should be instructed to undress and put on a gown. Some women may be more comfortable wearing their socks.

Assist the woman into the lithotomy position, with body supine and knees apart. Provide adequate draping with a sheet. Position her with her buttocks at the edge of the examination table. Ask her to place her arms at her sides or across her chest but not over her head (this tightens the abdominal muscles). Position the sheet completely over the patient's lower abdomen and upper legs, exposing only the vulva for your examination. Push the sheet down so you can see the woman's face as you proceed. The lithotomy position may make her feel embarrassed and vulnerable. If she seems uncomfortable or embarrassed, you may ask her if she would like her head elevated so she can see you better.

As you start the examination, reassure her that you will tell her everything that you are going to do before you actually do it. Touch the inner aspect of her thigh before you touch the external genitalia. (Don't be tentative with your touch; once you make physical contact, maintain it throughout the procedure.)

Be sure to talk to the woman throughout the examination to tell her what you are doing, what you are seeing or feeling, and how long it will be until you are finished. As a final consideration for preparation, keep in mind that if the patient has had gender-affirming surgery, examination findings may vary.

PROCEDURES WITH EXPECTED FINDINGS

ROUTINE TECHNIQUES: FEMALE GENITALIA AND RECTAL EXAMINATION

PERFORM hand hygiene and don examination gloves.

INSPECT the pubic hair and skin over the mons pubis and inguinal area for distribution and surface characteristics.

Hair distribution varies but usually covers an inverse triangle with the base over the mons pubis; some hair may extend up midline toward the umbilicus. Some women shave their pubic hair as a matter of preference. When this is the case, it is considered a normal variation. The skin should be smooth and clear (Fig. 17.8).

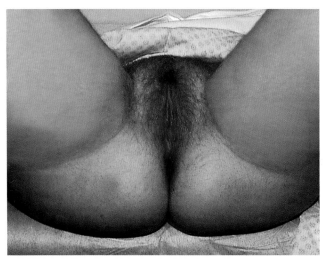

FIG. 17.8 Inspection of the external genitalia. (From Original Wilson/Giddens.)

INSPECT the labia majora, labia minora, and clitoris for pigmentation and PALPATE for surface characteristics.

Procedure: Gently touch the patient on the inner thigh and tell her that you are going to spread the labia apart. Spread the labia majora to view the inner surface of the labia majora, labia minora, and the surface of the vestibule (Fig. 17.9) with one hand. Palpate the labia minora between your thumb and the second fingers of your other hand. The clitoris is located midline between the labia minora.

Findings: The skin pigmentation of the labia majora should be darker than the patient's general skin tone; and the tissues may appear shriveled or full, gaping or closed, with a smooth skin surface and a dry or moist texture. The tissue should appear symmetric and without drainage, lesions, or sores. The tissue should feel smooth and soft without nodules or masses, and the palpation should elicit no statements of discomfort from the patient. The labia minora may appear symmetric or asymmetric, and the inner surface should be moist and dark pink. The tissue should feel smooth and soft. The clitoris is normally a smooth, pink, and moist cylindric structure about the size of an eraser head.

ABNORMAL FINDINGS

Notice any male hair distribution (diamond-shaped pattern), patchy loss of hair, or absence of hair in any patient over 16 years of age. Observe for presence of skin lesions or infestations (nits or lice) of skin or pubic hair. *Candida infections* are red, eroded patches with scaling and pustules and are associated with immobility, systemic antibiotics, and immunologic deficits.

Inflammation, irritation, excoriation, ulceration, lesions, nodules, drainage, asymmetry, and pain are abnormal findings. Discoloration and tenderness may be the result of traumatic bruising.

PROCEDURES WITH EXPECTED FINDINGS

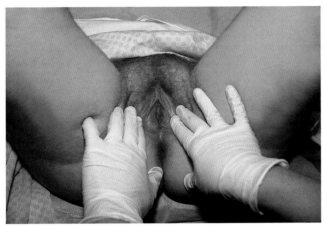

FIG. 17.9 Inspection of the labia. (From Original Wilson/Giddens.)

INSPECT the urethral meatus, hymen, vaginal introitus, and perineum for positioning and surface characteristics.

The urethral meatus should appear as a midline irregular opening or slit just superior to the vaginal introitus. The vaginal introitus may appear as a thin vertical slit or a large orifice, notice the characteristics of the hymen; the tissues should appear moist. The posterior skin surface of the perineum between the vaginal introitus and the anus should appear smooth and without lesions or discoloration. If the patient has had an episiotomy, a scar (midline or mediolateral) may be visible.

INSPECT the sacrococcygeal area for surface characteristics and PALPATE for tenderness.

The sacrococcygeal area is located between the sacrum and the coccyx. The skin surface should be smooth, without lesions. There should be no tenderness with palpation.

INSPECT the perianal area and anus for color and surface characteristics.

The anus should exhibit increased pigmentation and coarse skin, and the skin should be intact. The anus should be closed tightly. If a lesion is seen, identify the location of the abnormality in terms of the position of a clock, with the 12 o'clock position being toward the symphysis pubis and the 6 o'clock position toward the sacrococcygeal area. Ask the patient to bear down. While the patient is straining, observe for the presence of internal hemorrhoids, polyps, tumors, and rectal prolapse. None should be seen.

BOX 17.2 CLINICAL NOTE

Sexually transmitted diseases (STDs) can occur on the genitalia, on the anus, and in the oral cavity. Furthermore, STDs can be present concurrently in more than one location. Therefore, if an STD is suspected, an examination of other areas is warranted.

ABNORMAL FINDINGS

Notice any discharge from the surrounding (Skene) glands or the urethral opening, polyps, inflammation, or a lateral position of the meatus. Surrounding inflammation, discolored or foul-smelling vaginal discharge, bleeding or blood clots, edema, skin discoloration indicative of tissue bruising, or lesions are abnormal. Notice scars, skin tags, fissures, lumps, or excoriation.

A dimple with an inflamed tuft of hair or a tender palpable cyst in the sacrococcygeal area suggests a pilonidal cyst or sinus.

Note lesions or fissures around the anus. Lesions associated with STD frequently appear on or around the anus (Box 17-2). Lesions that may be seen include external hemorrhoids, ulcerations, warty growths (condylomata acuminata), skin tags, inflammation, fissures, and fistulas. Internal hemorrhoids, polyps, tumors, and rectal prolapse are also abnormal findings.

PROCEDURES WITH EXPECTED FINDINGS

| **ABNORMAL FINDINGS** |

SPECIAL CIRCUMSTANCES: FEMALE GENITALIA AND RECTUM

The examination procedures discussed in this section are done as a continuation of the female examination; thus patient positioning is the lithotomy position, as previously described.

PALPATE the Skene and Bartholin glands for surface characteristics, discharge, and tenderness.

This is performed if the patient has pain or vaginal discharge.

Procedure: With the labia spread apart, insert the index finger of your dominant hand (palm surface up) into the vagina as far as possible. Exert upward pressure on the anterior vaginal wall surface and milk the Skene glands by moving your finger outward toward the vaginal opening (Fig. 17.10). The glands are located in the paraurethral area and usually are not visible or palpable.

Next, palpate the lateral tissue of the vagina bilaterally. Use your thumb and index finger to palpate the entire area, paying attention to the posterolateral portion of the labia majora where the Bartholin glands are located (Fig. 17.11).

Findings: The glands usually are not visible or palpable. There should be no tenderness or discharge.

PALPATE the vaginal wall for tone.

This is indicated in the presence of a history of incontinence or vaginal discomfort.

Procedure: With the labia spread apart, insert the index finger of your dominant hand (palm surface up) into the vagina as far as possible and instruct the patient to squeeze the vaginal orifice around your finger. Remove your finger from the vagina. Holding the labia apart, ask the patient to bear down as you inspect for vaginal wall bulging and urinary incontinence. Ask the patient to cough and again inspect for bulging and incontinence.

Notice any tenderness or discharge; collect a sample of any discharge for culture. Discharge from the Skene and Bartholin glands usually indicates an infection. Edema in the area of the Bartholin glands that is painful and "hot to the touch" may indicate an abscess of that gland. The abscess is generally pus filled and is gonococcal or staphylococcal in origin. A nontender mass, which is the result of chronic inflammation of the gland, usually indicates a Bartholin cyst.

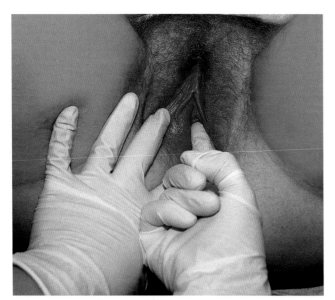

FIG. 17.10 Palpation of skene gland. (From Original Wilson/Giddens.)

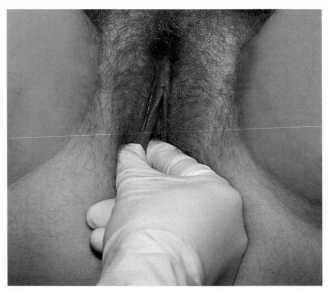

FIG. 17.11 Palpation of bartholin gland. (From Original Wilson/Giddens.)

PROCEDURES WITH EXPECTED FINDINGS

Findings: The nulliparous patient is usually able to squeeze tightly so you feel the vaginal wall tissue firmly around your examining finger (Fig. 17.12). If the woman has had children by vaginal delivery, she may not squeeze as tightly. No bulging or incontinence should be observed.

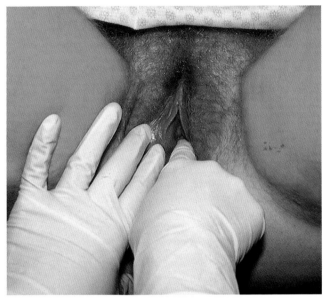

FIG. 17.12 Assessing vaginal tone. (From Original Wilson/Giddens.)

PALPATE the rectal wall for surface characteristics.

This is indicated when a patient presents with rectal pain, bleeding, or fullness.

Procedure: Lubricate the index finger of a gloved hand. Place the index finger, palm side up, over the anus. Ask the patient to bear down; while she is doing so, gently insert your index finger into the rectum.

With the index finger inserted as far as possible, instruct the patient to bear down. This brings more rectal wall into the range of palpation. Gently rotate the finger in the rectum to evaluate the characteristics of the rectal wall.

Findings: The rectal wall should feel smooth and be without any areas of masses, fistulas, fissures, or tenderness.

ASSESS the anal sphincter for muscle tone.

Perform this procedure when decreased tone or pain are reported.

Procedure: After palpating the rectal wall, ask the patient to tighten the external sphincter around your finger.

Findings: The anal sphincter should tighten evenly around the examination finger.

ABNORMAL FINDINGS

Inability of patient to constrict the vaginal orifice around your finger is abnormal. Bulging of the anterior wall may indicate a cystocele. Bulging of the posterior vaginal wall may indicate a rectocele. If the cervix is visible at the opening of the vagina, it may indicate signs of a uterine prolapse. The presence of urine during either bearing down or coughing may indicate stress incontinence.

Report any areas of masses, polyps, nodules, irregularities, and tenderness.

Notice the presence of rectal stricture. A hypotonic sphincter can occur with neurologic deficits, following rectal surgery, or with anal/rectal trauma (especially trauma associated with frequent anal sex). Hypertonic sphincter may be associated with lesions, inflammation, scarring, or anxiety related to the examination. Extreme pain with anal palpation almost always indicates a local inflammation such as a fissure, fistula, or cyst.

PROCEDURES WITH EXPECTED FINDINGS

EXAMINE stool for characteristics and presence of occult blood.

This examination is done as a screening measure for colorectal cancer.

After palpating the rectal wall, slowly remove the gloved finger from the patient's rectum. Inspect the gloved finger for color and consistency of stool. It should be brown and soft. Use a guaiac test to evaluate for occult blood. A negative response is expected. Occult blood test can also be done in the privacy of a patient's home by providing the fecal immunochemical test (FIT) or the guaiac- fecal occult blood test (FOBT) kit to the patient.

ABNORMAL FINDINGS

Report the presence of blood, pus, mucus, or abnormal color of stool (Table 17.1). A positive guaiac test indicates the presence of blood; ingestion of red meat and medications such as NSAIDs can result in false-positive results, while high doses of Vitamin C can result in false-negative results.

TABLE 17.1 STOOL COLORS AND SIGNIFICANCE

COLOR	SIGNIFICANCE
Bright red	Hemorrhoidal or lower rectal bleeding
Tarry black	Upper intestinal tract bleeding or excessive iron or bismuth ingestion
Light tan or gray	Obstruction of the biliary tract (obstructive jaundice)
Pale yellow	Malabsorption syndrome

TECHNIQUES PERFORMED BY AN ADVANCED PRACTICE NURSE

Specialty practice may require advanced techniques that are beyond the skill set of a nurse generalist. Knowing the purposes of these techniques may be helpful when caring for patients who require advanced assessment techniques. The female pelvic examination is done by an APRN as a routine annual examination or when a patient presents with pelvic pain or discharge.

- **Speculum Examination.** Using a speculum of appropriate size, the nurse carefully inserts it into the vagina (with the blades closed) by sliding the speculum over fingers that have been inserted in the vagina. After the speculum is inserted, the blades are opened (Fig. 17.13) and the nurse practitioner performs the following as part of the examination:
  - **INSPECT** the cervix for surface characteristics, color, position, size and shape, and discharge.
  - **INSPECT** the vaginal walls for color and surface characteristics.
  - **OBTAIN** specimens for laboratory testing such as Papanicolaou (Pap) test or cultures.

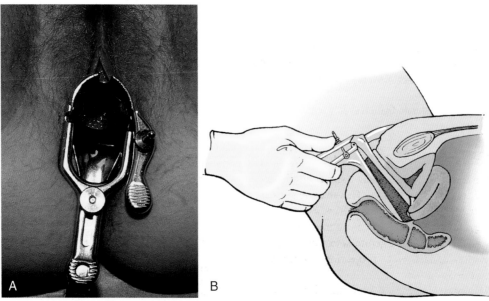

FIG. 17.13 (A) Speculum that has been properly placed. (B) Cross-sectional view. ([B] From Monahan, 2007).

- **Bimanual Examination.** After removing the vaginal speculum, the nurse practitioner palpates the internal reproductive structures (Fig. 17.14). This includes the following steps:
  - **PALPATE** the vagina for surface characteristics and discomfort.

- **PALPATE** the cervix and uterus for position, size, surface characteristics, mobility, and discomfort.
- **PALPATE** the uterus and ovaries for size, shape, and tenderness (using both a vaginal and a rectovaginal approach).

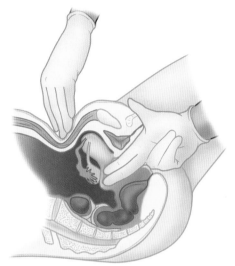

FIG. 17.14 Bimanual palpation of the uterus and ovaries.

DOCUMENTING EXPECTED FINDINGS

Female Exam

Pubic hair inverse triangle pattern with smooth, clear, and intact skin. Labia symmetric, smooth, soft, and moist with pigment darker than general skin tone. Clitoris midline between labia minora with smooth, pink, moist cylindric structure. Urinary meatus midline with an irregular opening. Vaginal introitus moist and appears as a thin vertical slit. No tenderness or discharge noted in the areas of Skene or Bartholin glands.

Skin of perineum intact and smooth. Anus more darkly pigmented; skin is coarse and tightly closed. Rectal wall smooth and intact. Septum between vagina and rectum thin, smooth, and intact. Anal sphincter tone tight, and stool soft and brown.

MALE EXAMINATION

Routine techniques	Techniques for special circumstances
• INSPECT the pubic hair. • INSPECT and PALPATE the penis. • INSPECT the scrotum. • INSPECT the inguinal region and the femoral area. • INSPECT and PALPATE the sacrococcygeal areas. • INSPECT the perianal area and anus.	• PALPATE the scrotum. • PALPATE the testes, epididymides, and vas deferens. • PALPATE the anus. • PALPATE the anal canal and rectum. • EXAMINE stool. **Techniques Performed by an APRN** • TRANSILLUMINATE the scrotum. • PALPATE the inguinal canal. • PALPATE the prostate.

Equipment needed
• Examination gloves • Lubricating gel • Light source

APRN, Advanced practice registered nurse.

PREPARING FOR THE MALE EXAMINATION

Men may feel apprehensive about having their genitalia examined, especially if the nurse is female. This may be seen as an invasion of privacy rather than accepted as a necessary component of the examination. As a nurse you must be aware of these concerns and approach the genitalia examination in a professional, matter-of-fact way, projecting confidence throughout the examination (Box 17.3).

Most of the examination can be conducted in either a standing or lying position; a specific position will be mentioned in the examination procedure as applicable. If the patient has had gender-affirming surgery, examination findings may vary.

BOX 17.3 CLINICAL NOTE

When examining male genitalia, use a firm, deliberate touch. If an erection occurs, reassure the patient that this is a normal physiologic response to touch and that he could not have prevented it. Do not stop the evaluation; stopping focuses further on the erection and reinforces the patient's embarrassment.

PROCEDURES WITH EXPECTED FINDINGS

ROUTINE TECHNIQUES: MALE GENITALIA

PERFORM hand hygiene and don examination gloves.

INSPECT pubic hair for distribution and skin for surface characteristics.

Hair distribution varies widely but is normally in a diamond-shaped pattern that may extend to the umbilicus. The hair should appear coarser than scalp hair. It should be free of parasites; and the skin should be intact, smooth, and clear.

INSPECT the penis for surface characteristics and color; PALPATE the penis for tenderness and discharge.

The dorsal vein should be apparent on the dorsal surface of the shaft of the penis. The skin is usually dark and hairless, with a wrinkled surface and frequently apparent vascularity. In uncircumcised men the prepuce is present and folded over the glans (Fig. 17.15A); in circumcised men the amount of prepuce varies (Fig. 17.15B). If the patient has not been circumcised, ask him to retract the foreskin. The foreskin should retract easily and completely over the glans.

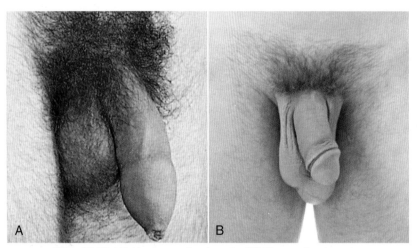

FIG. 17.15 (A) Uncircumcised penis. (B) Circumcised penis.

🌐 ETHNIC, CULTURAL, AND SPIRITUAL VARIATIONS

Circumcision

Historically, many cultures have practiced circumcision for a variety of reasons, including medical, religious, cultural, and ethnic traditions. The estimated overall circumcision rate in the United States is between 76% and 92%; this is the highest rate among developed nations. The frequency of circumcision varies depending on religious affiliation, geographic location, and socioeconomic status. Ritual circumcision is a common practice for Jews and Muslims around the world. The current evidence suggests that while health benefits may outweigh risks, an infant's well-being and thus the informed decision regarding circumcision is best left to the parents, in consultation with a medical provider.

From Angel CA: *Circumcision. Emedicine.medscape.com*, 2018. Retrieved from: https://emedicine.medscape.com/article/1015820-overview.

ABNORMAL FINDINGS

Note patchy growth, loss, or absence of hair; distribution of hair in a female pattern (triangular, with the base over the pubis); nits or pubic lice; scars; lower abdominal or inguinal lesions; or a rash. *Tinea cruris* ("jock itch") is a common fungal infection found in the groin that appears as large, clearly marginated, red patches that are pruritic. *Candida infections* are red eroded patches with scaling and pustules and are associated with immobility, systemic antibiotics, and immunologic deficits.

Inability to retract the foreskin, discomfort on retraction, or difficulty returning the foreskin to the original position should be considered abnormal. *Phimosis* is a very tight foreskin that cannot be retracted over the glans (Fig. 17.16). *Paraphimosis* is the inability to return the foreskin over the glans (Fig. 17.17).

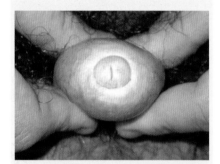

FIG. 17.16 Phimosis. (From Yura and Flury, 2017).

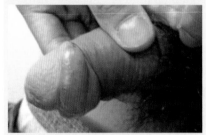

FIG. 17.17 Paraphimosis. (From Morteza and Yen, 2020.)

PROCEDURES WITH EXPECTED FINDINGS

Inspect the glans and under the fold of the prepuce. The glans should be smooth, pink, and bulbous. Note any erythema, lesions, edema, nodules, or presence of discharge. (If discharge or smegma is present, obtain a specimen on a slide for microscopic examination.) The prepuce fold is wrinkled and loosely attached to the underlying glans; it is darker than the glans. Note: Circumcised penises have varying lengths of foreskin remaining; some have multiple folds, and others have none.

Inspect the urethral meatus. It should be located centrally at the distal tip of the glans and should appear as a slit-like opening. No discharge should be present. Palpate the glans anteroposteriorly to open the distal end of the urethra (Fig. 17.20). The surface should be pink and smooth, and no discharge should be present.

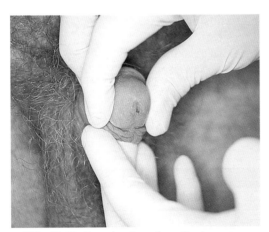

FIG. 17.20 Examination of urethral meatus.

Palpate the entire shaft of the penis between the thumb and first two fingers. The penis shaft should be nontender and smooth with a semifirm consistency.

INSPECT the scrotum for color, texture, surface characteristics, and position.

Move the penis out of the way with the back of your hand (or ask the patient to hold the penis out of the way) while you inspect the scrotum (Fig. 17.21). The scrotal sac is divided in half by the septum; the two sides often appear asymmetric; the left side tends to hang lower than the right because of a longer spermatic cord (see Fig. 17.15B). The scrotal surface is usually more deeply pigmented than the body skin; the color should be consistent throughout. The scrotal skin has a coarse-appearing surface and should be without lesions. Small bumps on the scrotal skin are known as *sebaceous cysts* or *sebaceous glands*; they are considered a normal finding. Be sure to lift the scrotum to examine the underside as well. This area is deeply pigmented, hairless, and has a rugous surface.

ABNORMAL FINDINGS

Erythema or edema may indicate *balanitis*, an inflammation of the glans that commonly occurs in patients with phimosis (Fig. 17.18).

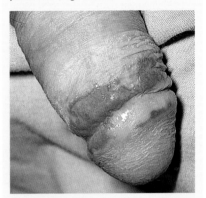

FIG. 17.18 Balanitis. (From Swartz, 2010.)

Note if the meatus is located either on the upper surface of the penis (epispadias) or on the bottom of the penis (hypospadias). Note if a discharge is present. The discharge may be yellow-green or milky white or have a foul odor (Fig. 17.19). Notice any erythema, edema, discharge, or crusting.

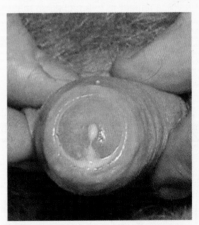

FIG. 17.19 Purulent penile discharge. (From Swartz, 2010.)

Note tenderness, edema, nodules, or induration.

Scrotal lesions or scrotal redness (either generalized or isolated) are considered abnormal and may indicate an infection. Excessive differences between the right and left sides are an abnormal finding.

PROCEDURES WITH EXPECTED FINDINGS

Temperature affects the appearance of the scrotum. When the environmental temperature is very cold, the testes retract slightly upward, causing the scrotum to become smaller and tighter in appearance. Conversely, when the temperature is hot, the testes extend downward and the scrotal sac hangs loosely.

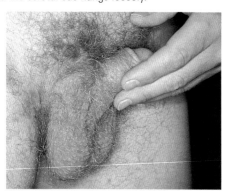

FIG. 17.21 Inspect the scrotum and ventral surface of the penis as the patient positions his penis.

INSPECT the inguinal region and the femoral area for bulges.

The patient should assume a standing position for this part of the examination. While standing in front of and facing the patient, ask him to bear down. While he is straining, inspect the inguinal canal and femoral area (just above where the femoral artery is palpated) for the presence of a bulge. There should be no bulges.

The presence of bulges of the external ring or femoral area suggests a hernia. See Table 17.2 and Fig. 17.25 (in the next section).

INSPECT the sacrococcygeal areas for surface characteristics and PALPATE for tenderness.

Ask the patient to turn around so that the nurse is facing his backside. The sacrococcygeal area is located between the sacrum and the coccyx. The skin surface should be smooth, without lesions. There should be no tenderness with palpation.

A dimple with an inflamed tuft of hair or a tender palpable cyst in the sacrococcygeal area suggests a pilonidal cyst or sinus.

TABLE 17.2 COMPARISONS OF HERNIAS

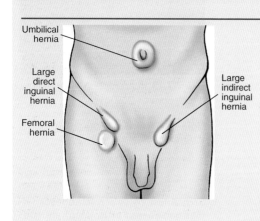

Umbilical hernia

Large direct inguinal hernia

Femoral hernia

Large indirect inguinal hernia

DESCRIPTION AND FINDINGS

Indirect Hernia
* Most frequent type of hernia; may occur in both sexes and in children (mostly males).
* Sac herniates through the internal inguinal ring; can remain in the inguinal canal, exit through the external canal, or pass into the scrotum.
* The patient usually complains of pain with straining. The hernia may decrease when the patient lies down.

Direct Hernia
* Less common; occurs frequently in males over age 40; uncommon in women.
* The sac herniates through the external inguinal ring. It rarely enters the scrotum.
* The patient has a bulge that is usually painless. The hernia pushes against the nurse's fingertips when the patient bears down. The hernia may decrease when the patient lies down.

Femoral Hernia
* Least common type of hernia; occurs frequently in women.
* The sac extends through the femoral ring, canal, and below the inguinal ligament.
* There is pain in the inguinal area. The right side is more frequently affected than the left side. Pain may be severe.

Illustration from Monahan and Drake, 1998.

PROCEDURES WITH EXPECTED FINDINGS

ABNORMAL FINDINGS

INSPECT the perianal area and anus for pigmentation and surface characteristics.

Ask the patient to bend over. Spread the buttocks with both hands to inspect this area. The anus should exhibit increased pigmentation and coarse, intact skin. The anus should be tightly closed. No lesions or inflammation should be present. If a lesion is present, identify the location of the abnormality in terms of the position of a clock, with the 12 o'clock position being toward the symphysis pubis and the 6 o'clock position toward the sacrococcygeal area. Ask the patient to bear down while you inspect the anal area. Again, no lesions should be observed.

Note the presence and location of inflammation and lesions. Lesions that may be seen include external hemorrhoids, ulcerations, warty growths (condylomata acuminata), skin tags, inflammation, fissures, and fistulas. While the patient is straining, note the presence of internal hemorrhoids, polyps, tumors, and rectal prolapse.

SPECIAL CIRCUMSTANCES: MALE GENITALIA AND RECTUM

PALPATE the scrotum for surface characteristics and tenderness.

This procedure is performed to screen for scrotal masses or when the patient reports pain or edema.

Palpate each half of the scrotum (Fig. 17.22). The surface should feel coarse, with the skin intact and loose over a muscle layer. The thickness of the skin of the scrotum changes with temperature and age. In cold or cool temperatures, the scrotal skin feels thickened. As the individual ages, the skin thins. The scrotum should be nontender.

Note any marked tenderness or edema.

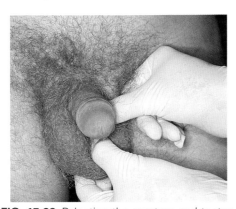

FIG. 17.22 Palpating the scrotum and testes.

PALPATE the testes, epididymides, and vas deferens for location, consistency, tenderness, and nodules.

This procedure is performed to screen for testicular cancer or when the patient reports pain or edema.

Palpate the testes simultaneously with both hands, using the thumb and the first two fingers. Notice that the testis is present in each sac; they should be equal in size, mildly sensitive but nontender to moderate compression, smooth and ovoid, and movable. Transgender women undergoing hormone therapy as part of the transition process may have decreased testicular size or they may be retracted.[14]

On the posterolateral surface of each testis, palpate the epididymis; it will feel like a tubular, comma-shaped structure that collapses when gently compressed between your fingers and thumb. This area should be smooth and nontender.

Notice if the testes have not descended into the sac or are enlarged (unilaterally or bilaterally), atrophied, markedly tender, nodular or irregular, or fixed. A painless mass with scrotal edema needs further evaluation for testicular cancer.
If a problem is noticed with the epididymis, determine its position in relation to the testis (i.e., proximal or distal); whether it can be moved with your fingers; and if it disappears when the patient lies down. Report any tenderness, irregular placement, enlargement, induration, or nodules.

The vas deferens lies within the spermatic cord. To palpate, grasp both spermatic cords between the thumb and forefinger and palpate, starting at the base of the epididymides, moving upward to the inguinal ring. Because the vas deferens lies within the spermatic cord along with arteries and veins, it is difficult to identify specifically with palpation. The vas deferens feels like a smooth, cordlike structure. It should be nontender and palpable from the epididymis to the external inguinal ring.

Report any tenderness, tortuosity (twisting), thickened or beaded area, or induration.

PROCEDURES WITH EXPECTED FINDINGS

ABNORMAL FINDINGS

RECTAL EXAMINATION

Preparing the patient: The male patient should assume the left lateral position with the hips and knees flexed, a knee-chest position, or the standing position with the hips flexed and the patient bending over the examination table with feet pointed together (Fig. 17.23A–C).

PALPATE the anus for sphincter tone.

Perform this procedure when pain or reduced rectal tone is suspected.

Ask the patient to bear down. Place the finger pad surface of a gloved and lubricated index finger at the anal opening; as the sphincter relaxes, slowly insert the finger, pointing toward the patient's umbilicus (Fig. 17.24A and B). Ask the patient to tighten the anus around your examining finger. The sphincter should tighten evenly around your finger with minimum discomfort to the patient.

A hypotonic sphincter can occur with neurologic deficits, following rectal surgery, or with anal/rectal trauma (especially trauma associated with frequent anal sex). Hypertonic sphincter may be associated with lesions, inflammation, scarring, or anxiety related to the examination. Extreme pain with anal palpation usually indicates a local inflammation such as a fissure, fistula, or cyst.

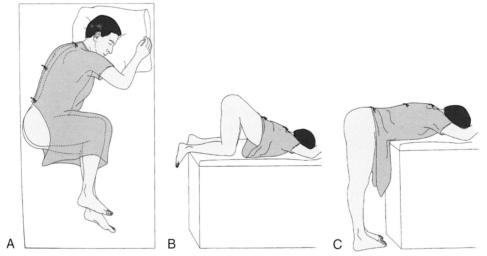

FIG. 17.23 Positions for rectal examination. (A) Left lateral or Sims position. (B) Knee-chest position. (C) Standing position. (From Barkauskus et al., 2002.)

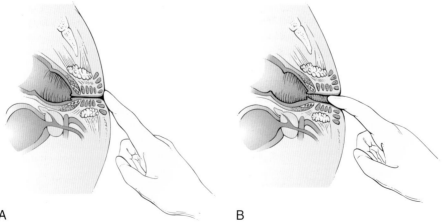

FIG. 17.24 Rectal examination. (A) Relax sphincter with gentle pressure with the palmar surface of the finger. (B) Insert the finger into the anal canal. (From Swartz, 2011.)

PROCEDURES WITH EXPECTED FINDINGS	ABNORMAL FINDINGS

PALPATE the anal canal and rectum for surface characteristics.

This procedure is performed to detect masses in the rectum.

Rotate the finger around the musculature of the anal ring to palpate the surface characteristics. The area should be smooth, with even pressure on your finger. Insert the finger as far as possible into the rectum to palpate the rectal walls. There should be a continuous smooth surface, and the patient should experience only minimal discomfort.

Nodules, irregularities, masses, presence of hard stool, or tenderness are abnormal findings.

EXAMINE stool for characteristics and presence of occult blood.

Perform this procedure to detect blood in the stool.

Slowly remove the gloved finger from the patient's rectum. Inspect the gloved finger for the color and consistency of the stool. It should be brown and soft. Use a guaiac test to evaluate for occult blood. A negative response is the expected finding.

Alternatively, the occult blood test can be done in the privacy of the patient's home by providing the FIT or the guaiac fecal occult blood test (gFOBT) kit to the patient.

Report the presence of blood, pus, mucus, or abnormal color of stool (see Table 17.1). A positive guaiac test indicates the presence of blood; ingestion of red meat and medications such as NSAIDs can result in false-positive results, while high doses of Vitamin C can result in false-negative results.

TECHNIQUES PERFORMED BY AN ADVANCED PRACTICE REGISTERED NURSE

Specialty practice may require advanced techniques that are beyond the skill set of a nurse generalist. The following examination procedures are performed by an APRN as a routine annual examination or when a patient presents with scrotal mass, possible hernia, or symptoms associated with an enlarged prostate. Knowing the purposes of these techniques may be helpful when caring for patients who require advanced assessment techniques.

- **TRANSILLUMINATE the scrotum for evidence of fluid and masses.** This technique is performed when a scrotal mass, fluid, or irregularity are suspected. The APRN uses a bright penlight or transilluminator and presses the light source up against the scrotal sac.

- **PALPATE the inguinal canal for evidence of indirect hernia or direct hernia.** When a hernia is suspected, the APRN inserts a gloved index or middle finger into the lower aspect of the scrotum and follows the spermatic cord up through the inguinal ringer and into the inguinal canal (Fig. 17.25). The patient is asked to cough, and the APRN feels for a mass or a bulge.

- **PALPATE the prostate for size, contour, consistency, mobility, and tenderness.** This technique is performed to detect an enlarged prostate or to screen for prostate cancer. The APRN nurse dons gloves and palpates the posterior surface of the prostate gland by palpating the anterior surface of the rectum (Fig. 17.26).

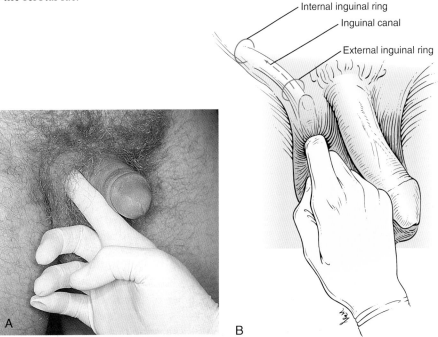

Internal inguinal ring
Inguinal canal
External inguinal ring

FIG. 17.25 (A) Palpating for inguinal hernia. (B) Position of gloved finger inserted through inguinal canal. ([B] From Swartz, 2011.)

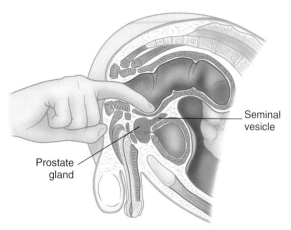

FIG. 17.26 Palpation of the anterior surface of the prostate gland. Feel for the lateral lobes and median sulcus.

Prostate gland

Seminal vesicle

DOCUMENTING EXPECTED FINDINGS

Male Exam

Pubic hair diamond pattern with smooth, clear, and intact skin. Penis uncircumcised, hairless, wrinkled surface and dorsal vein noted. Shaft smooth and nontender. Glans smooth, pink, and bulbous. Urinary meatus slitlike opening in center of glans, with pink, smooth urethra without discharge. Sacrococcygeal area smooth, clear, and nontender. Scrotum deeply pigmented, hairless, coarse with rugous surface and intact skin. Testicles smooth, ovoid, and movable bilaterally; epididymis smooth and nontender bilaterally. No bulges detected in inguinal area.

Skin of perineum intact and smooth. Anus more darkly pigmented with coarse skin; tightly closed. Anal sphincter tone tight, and stool soft and brown.

AGE-RELATED VARIATIONS

This chapter discusses conducting an examination of the reproductive system with adult patients. These data are important to assess for individuals of all ages, but the approach and techniques used to collect the information may vary depending on the patient's age.

INFANTS AND CHILDREN

Infants and children have functionally immature reproductive systems. For this reason, examination is usually limited to the inspection of external genitalia. Further examination may be warranted if the parents, caregivers, or nurse notice a problem. The nurse should always maintain an awareness of the potential for sexual abuse among infants and children. Chapter 19 presents further information regarding reproductive assessment for this age group.

ADOLESCENTS

The onset of puberty (pubescence) marks the beginning of sexual development for boys and girls. A focus for this age group is assessing sexual maturity and the patient's response. Adolescents are often self-conscious about the changes; for this reason, the nurse must provide privacy, ensure confidentiality, and be reassuring. Chapter 19 presents further information regarding the assessment of the reproductive system among adolescents.

OLDER ADULTS

The history and examination of older adults are similar to that which has been previously described for the younger adult. Sexual response and physical changes to the genitalia occur as a result of the aging process. Chapter 21 presents further information related to the assessment of the older adult.

COMMON PROBLEMS AND CONDITIONS

INFECTIONS

Bacterial Vaginosis

Bacterial Vaginosis (BV) is caused by an alteration of the normal vaginal flora with other bacteria; a number of bacteria can cause BV, including *Gardnerella vaginalis, Mobiluncus,* and *Mycoplasma hominis.* The prevalence in the United States is estimated to be 21.2 million (29.2%) among women ages 14 to 49.[15] **Clinical Findings:** The typical signs and symptoms of BV include malodorous (often described as fishy) vaginal discharge and vulvar itching and irritation.

Candida Vaginitis

Candidiasis is a fungal (yeast) infection usually caused by *Candida albicans.* The Centers for Disease Control and Prevention (CDC) estimates that 75% of all women have had at least one

fungal infection; 40% to 45% will have two or more infections at some point during their lifetime.[3] *Candida* infections are more prevalent in women who have diabetes mellitus or who are pregnant. **Clinical Findings:** Some women have asymptomatic infections. Those who have symptoms frequently experience vulvar pruritus associated with a thick, cheesy, white vaginal discharge. Vaginal soreness and external dysuria (caused by the splashing of urine on inflamed tissue) may occur. Erythema and edema to the labia and vulvar skin may be visible.

Sexually Transmitted Disease

STD, also commonly referred to as *STI,* represents a large number of infections that are transmitted through sexual activity. There are well over 50 different STDs. Listed here are those that the nurse may observe in conjunction with the examination of the genitalia.

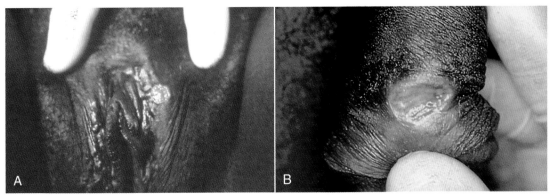

FIG. 17.27 (A) Syphilis chancre on vulva. (B) Syphilis chancre on the penis. ([A] Courtesy CDC Public Health Image Library. [B] From Goldstein and Goldstein, 1997.)

Chlamydia

The most common STD in the United States is chlamydia, occurring most frequently among sexually active adolescents and young adults under the age of 25.[3] It is transmitted from genital-genital, oral-genital, and anal-genital contact. Neonatal exposure during vaginal delivery can cause ophthalmia neonatorum—a purulent conjunctivitis and keratitis. **Clinical Findings, Women:** Chlamydia infection is asymptomatic in up to 75% of women because it often does not cause enough inflammation to produce symptoms.[3] When symptoms occur, the most common are urinary (e.g., dysuria, frequency, or urgency) and vaginal (e.g., spotting or bleeding after sexual intercourse or purulent cervical discharge). The most important examination findings in a chlamydia infection include purulent or mucopurulent cervical discharge, cervical motion tenderness, or cervical bleeding on the introduction of a cotton swab (friability). **Clinical Findings, Men:** This infection usually occurs in the urethra, but it can also affect the rectum. The most common symptoms associated with urethral infection include dysuria, discharge, and urethral itch. If untreated, urethral infection can spread to the epididymis causing epididymitis.

Gonorrhea

Caused by the aerobic, gram-negative diplococcus *Neisseria gonorrhoeae*, this is currently the second most frequently reported STD in the United States.[3] It is transmitted from genital-genital, oral-genital, and anal-genital contact. Neonatal exposure during vaginal delivery can cause corneal ulceration. **Clinical Findings, Women:** In most women, gonorrhea causes a yellow or green vaginal discharge, dysuria, pelvic or abdominal pain, and abnormal menses. Vaginal itching and burning may be severe. **Clinical Findings, Men:** The most common clinical manifestation of gonorrhea is urethritis. Specific clinical findings include mucopurulent or purulent discharge and dysuria.[3] If untreated, gonorrhea can lead to epididymitis.

Syphilis

Syphilis, a systemic disease, is caused by a spirochete, *Treponema pallidum*, which is transmitted congenitally or by sexual contact. Syphilis infection begins as a local infection in the primary phase and can become systemic. It progresses through four stages if left untreated: primary, secondary, latent, and tertiary. Primary and secondary phases occur within months of exposure; latent and tertiary syphilis occur over a number of years.[10] Fetal exposure (from an infected mother) results in congenital syphilis. **Clinical Findings, Adults:** The clinical manifestations of syphilis vary, depending on the phase of infection. Primary syphilis produces a single, firm, painless open sore or chancre with indurated borders at the site of entry on the genitals or mouth (Fig. 17.27A). In men, the most common location is on the shaft of the penis (see Fig. 17.27B). This ulcer typically appears about 21 days after infection and usually heals within 3 to 6 weeks. Secondary syphilis occurs 6 to 12 weeks after the initial lesion. Individuals develop a rash characterized by red macules and papules over the palms of the hands and soles of the feet. Round or oval flat, grayish lesions known as *condyloma latum* develop in the anogenital area. Latent syphilis follows the secondary stage and can last from 2 to 20 years; during this period, the patients are asymptomatic. Tertiary infection has destructive effects on the neurologic, cardiovascular, ophthalmic, and musculoskeletal systems. **Clinical Findings, Neonates:** Infected neonates are often premature with intrauterine growth retardation. Manifestations include retinal inflammation, glaucoma, destructive bone and skin lesions, and central nervous system involvement.

Trichomoniasis

Trichomoniasis is a highly contagious STD caused by the protozoan *Trichomonas vaginalis*, which inhabits the vagina and lower urinary tract, particularly the Skene ducts. **Clinical Findings:** Although some women are asymptomatic, the primary symptom is a malodorous greenish-yellow vaginal discharge often accompanied by vulvar irritation.[3] The walls of the vagina and the cervix may have petechial "strawberry patches" (Fig. 17.28). Men are usually asymptomatic, but when symptoms occur, they include irritation inside the penis, burning after urination or ejaculation, or penile discharge.

Herpes Genitalis

Herpes is a sexually transmitted viral infection caused by the Herpes simplex virus (HSV). HSV type 1 (HSV1) and HSV

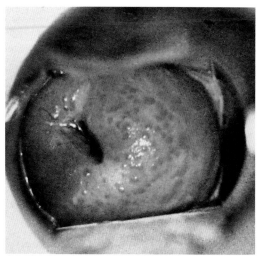

FIG. 17.28 Trichomoniasis. The vaginal mucosa and cervix are inflamed and speckled with petechial lesions. (From Zitelli and Davis, 2007.)

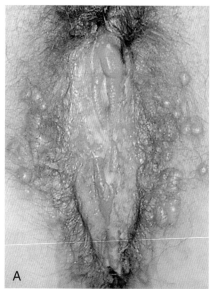

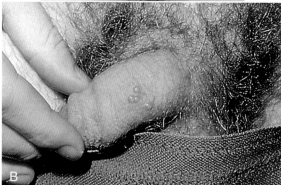

FIG. 17.29 Herpes lesions. (A) Female. (B) Male. ([A] From Swartz, 2010. [B] From Goldstein and Goldstein, 1997.)

type 2 (HSV2) are two different antigen subtypes of the HSV. HSV1 is more commonly associated with gingivostomatitis and oral ulcers (fever blisters), whereas HSV2 is usually associated with genital lesions. However, both types can be transmitted to both sites through genital-oral contact.

Clinical Findings, Women: Herpes genitalis is far more common among women than in men, and women usually have a more severe clinical course. Typical early symptoms include burning or pain with urination, pain in the genital area, and fever. Examination findings reveal single or multiple vesicles that can be found on the genital area or the inner thigh. After vesicles rupture, small, painful ulcers are observed (Fig. 17.29A). **Clinical Findings, Men:** The typical clinical manifestations for men include lesions that appear anywhere along the shaft of the penis or near the glans (Fig. 17.29B). The lesion is identified because of the red superficial vesicles, which are frequently quite painful. Many men with HSV2 are unaware that they have an infection because the symptoms may be mild.

Human Papillomavirus (Genital Warts, Condylomata Acuminatum)

One of the most common STDs is human papillomavirus (HPV) because it is highly contagious and because these infections are often asymptomatic or unrecognized.[3] HPV infection is associated with early onset of sexual activity, multiple sex partners, and infrequent use of barrier protection. Although it previously was considered benign, HPV has been linked to malignancies of the cervix and penis. **Clinical Findings:** HPV can cause wartlike growths that are termed *condylomata acuminata* (Fig. 17.30A and B). The warts typically appear as soft, papillary, pink-to-brown, elongated lesions that may occur singularly or in clusters on the internal genitalia, the external genitalia, and the anal-rectal region. When in clusters, they take on a cauliflower-like appearance.

Pediculosis Pubis (Crabs, Pubic Lice)

Pediculosis pubis is a parasitic infection usually transmitted by sexual contact. **Clinical Findings:** The primary symptom of pubic lice infestation is severe pruritus in the perineal area. Patients may also notice the lice or nits (eggs) in the pubic hair. Examination findings include excoriation and an area of erythema; on close inspection, the lice and nits can be seen. Nits are tiny, yellow-white eggs that are attached to the hair shaft. The adult lice are larger, are tan to grayish-white in color, and have a crablike appearance when viewed under a magnifying glass. Lice feces appear as tiny dark spots (resembling pepper) and may be seen adjacent to the hair shafts.

Pelvic Inflammatory Disease

PID is a polymicrobial infection of the upper reproductive tract affecting any or all of the following structures: the endometrium, fallopian tubes, ovaries, uterine wall, or broad ligaments. It usually is caused by untreated gonococcal and chlamydia infections. PID is a leading cause of infertility in the United States.[10] **Clinical Findings:** PID can occur as an acute or chronic disease; thus symptoms may vary. Acute PID is associated with very tender

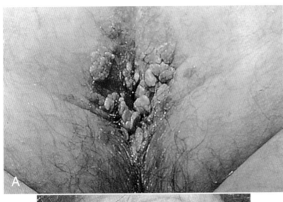

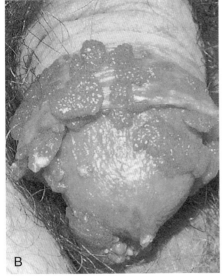

FIG. 17.30 Condyloma acuminatum. (A) Female. (B) Male. (Courtesy Lemmi and Lemmi, 2013.)

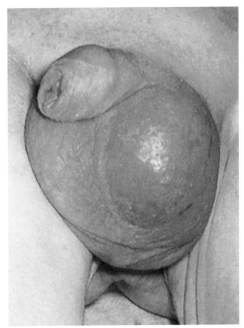

FIG. 17.31 Epididymitis. (From Lloyd-Davies et al., 1994.)

adnexal areas (ovaries and fallopian tubes). Typically the pain is so severe that the patient is unable to tolerate bimanual pelvic examination. Other symptoms include fever, chills, dyspareunia, and abnormal vaginal discharge. Chronic PID is associated with tender, irregular, and fixed adnexal tissues.

Epididymitis

An inflammation of the epididymis and vas deferens is referred to as *epididymitis*. It is usually caused by the spread of infection from the urethra or bladder. Among sexually active men under the age of 35, it is often associated with STDs involving chlamydia and gonorrhea.[3] **Clinical Findings:** Classic symptoms include dull, unilateral scrotal pain that develops over a period of hours to days. The scrotum becomes erythematous and edematous (Fig. 17.31). Related symptoms may include fever and dysuria. A hydrocele may be seen with transillumination.

BENIGN REPRODUCTIVE CONDITIONS AFFECTING WOMEN

Premenstrual Syndrome

PMS is a group or cluster of recurrent symptoms experienced by women associated with their menstrual cycle. It is thought to be associated with fluctuations in hormone levels and changes in altered sensitivity of the neurotransmitter serotonin.[16] A history of emotional and sexual abuse in childhood or as an adolescent is associated with PMS in adulthood.[16] **Clinical Findings:** A combination of emotional, cognitive, and physical symptoms begins during the last half of the menstrual cycle and diminishes after menstruation begins. Common emotional symptoms include mood swings, depression or sadness, irritability, tension, anxiety, restlessness, and anger. Common cognitive symptoms include difficulty concentrating, confusion, forgetfulness, and being accident prone. Physical symptoms may include excessive energy or fatigue, nausea or changes in appetite, insomnia, back pain, headaches, general muscular pain, breast tenderness, and fluid retention.

Endometriosis

This is a benign, progressive disease process characterized by the presence and growth of uterine tissue outside the uterus (Fig. 17.32). It affects an estimated 10% of women of reproductive age in all ethnic and social groups.[10] **Clinical Findings:** Common symptoms include pelvic pain, dysmenorrhea, and heavy or prolonged menstrual flow. In some women, clinical examination findings include small, firm, nodular-like masses palpable along the uterosacral ligaments. The uterus may be tender. However, in many women with endometriosis, a clinical examination does not detect any abnormality.

Uterine Leiomyomas

Leiomyomas (also called fibroids) are very common benign uterine tumors that commonly affect women over age 35, affecting as many as 60% of women over their lifetime. The tumors can occur singly or in multiples and can range in size from microscopic lesions to large tumors that fill the entire

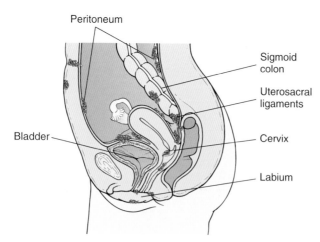

FIG. 17.32 Common sites of endometriosis. (From Lewis et al., 2011.)

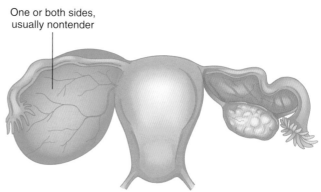

FIG. 17.34 Ovarian cyst. (From McCance et al., 2010.)

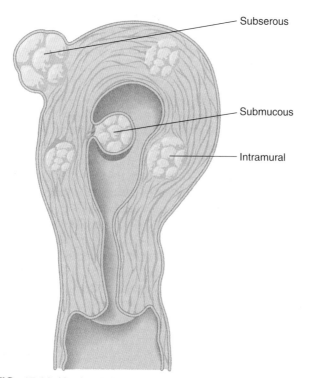

FIG. 17.33 Uterine leiomyomas (Fibroids). (From McCance et al., 2010.)

abdominal cavity. Leiomyomas are most prominent during reproductive years and tend to shrink after menopause. **Clinical Findings:** Most women with leiomyomas are asymptomatic. Those who have symptoms often report pelvic pressure and heaviness, urinary frequency, dysmenorrhea, pelvic or back pain, and abdominal enlargement. If large enough, the leiomyomas can be detected by palpation during a pelvic examination. The tumors typically feel firm, smooth, and irregular in shape (Fig. 17.33).

Ovarian Cysts

Benign cystic growths within the ovary (ovarian cysts) may be solitary or multiple occurring unilaterally or bilaterally.

Ovarian cysts usually occur in young menstruating women.[10] **Clinical Findings:** Most ovarian cysts are asymptomatic. When symptoms occur, they often include tenderness and a dull sensation or feeling of heaviness in the pelvis. If a cyst ruptures, a sudden onset of abdominal pain occurs. Examination findings for an ovarian cyst include a nontender, fluctuant, mobile, and smooth mass on the ovary (Fig. 17.34).

MALIGNANT REPRODUCTIVE CONDITIONS AFFECTING WOMEN

Cervical Cancer

Cancer of the cervix is usually caused by HPV infection; an estimated 13,800 new cases were diagnosed in the United States in 2020.[4] **Clinical Findings:** The most common symptom is abnormal vaginal bleeding, such as bleeding between normal menstrual periods, bleeding after intercourse, or menstrual bleeding that is heavier or lasts longer than normal. On examination a lesion may be visible; the lesion usually has a hard, granular surface that bleeds easily and has irregular borders (Fig. 17.35).

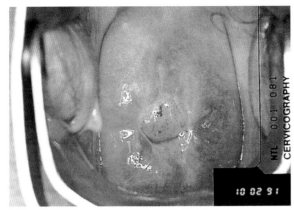

FIG. 17.35 Cervical cancer. The lesion is seen on the cervical os. (From Symonds and Macpherson, 1994.)

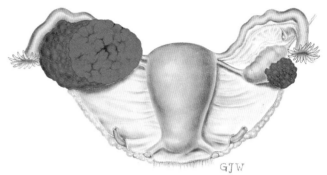

FIG. 17.37 Cancer of the ovaries. (From Belcher, 1992.)

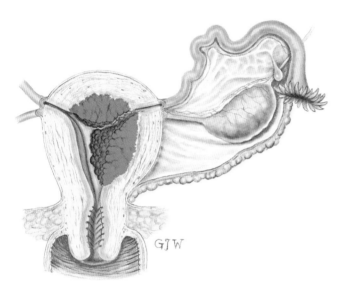

FIG. 17.36 Endometrial cancer. (From Belcher, 1992.)

Endometrial Cancer

The most common gynecologic malignancy is endometrial cancer with an estimated 65,600 new cases diagnosed each year in the United States.[4] It occurs most often in postmenopausal women, especially women taking estrogen. **Clinical Findings:** The cardinal symptom is abnormal uterine bleeding or spotting, although a watery vaginal discharge is frequently noted several weeks to months before the bleeding (Fig. 17.36).

Ovarian Cancer

Ovarian cancer has the highest mortality rate of the gynecologic cancers because it is typically undetected; thus it is known as the "whispering disease." An estimated 13,900 die each year from ovarian cancer in the United States.[4] It commonly occurs among white women over age 50 who live in western industrialized nations. **Clinical Findings:** There are usually no symptoms until advanced stages of the disease. The most common symptom of ovarian cancer is abdominal distention or fullness. By the time ovarian malignancies are palpable, the disease is usually advanced (Fig. 17.37).

REPRODUCTIVE CONDITIONS AFFECTING MEN

Testicular Torsion

This condition is caused by the twisting of the testicle and spermatic cord and cutting off the blood supply. It is considered a surgical emergency. Testicular torsion may occur at any age, but the prevalence is highest during adolescence. **Clinical Findings:** The hallmark finding of testicular torsion is a history of sudden onset of severe testicular pain and scrotal swelling. The testicle often becomes slightly discolored. It is not associated with physical activity or trauma.

Hydrocele

An accumulation of fluid within the scrotum creates a hydrocele. In adults, the cause of hydrocele is often unknown but may result from infection or a malignancy. **Clinical Findings:** Gradual scrotal enlargement is the most common symptom. The scrotum appears enlarged; edema appears on the anterior surface of the testis but may also extend up into the spermatic cord area. Transillumination of the scrotum is indicated when a hydrocele is suspected. A light red glow indicates the presence of fluid; failure to glow suggests a mass.

Spermatocele

A spermatocele is a cystic mass that occurs within the epididymis or spermatic cord. It is filled with sperm and seminal fluid. **Clinical Findings:** This condition is usually painless but is characterized by significant edema in the involved testicle. A separate mass is palpated within the testis, adjacent to the epididymis or spermatic cord (Fig. 17.38).

Varicocele

This condition is caused by an abnormal dilation and tortuosity of the veins along the spermatic cord (Fig. 17.39A and B). The cause is often multifactorial; the dilation is thought to be caused by differences in venous drainage between the right and left sides of the spermatic cord. Varicocele is a condition primarily affecting boys and young men. **Clinical Findings:** The patient may describe a pulling sensation or a dull ache or have scrotal pain. The veins above the testis tend to feel thickened; a palpable mass is usually detected in the scrotum. Ninety percent of varicoceles occur on the left side.

Testicular Cancer

The most common malignancy in men ages 20 to 34 is testicular cancer, with 9600 new cases diagnosed each year in the United States.[4] **Clinical Findings:** The classic manifestation is a painless testicular mass that is usually discovered by the patient or his sexual partner. On examination, a hard and irregular mass is felt within the testis. If the mass is large enough, deformity of the scrotum may be observable.

Benign Prostatic Hyperplasia

Benign prostatic hyperplasia (BPH) is an enlargement of the prostate gland that usually affects older men (Fig. 17.40). At least some degree of BPH will eventually develop in all men with advanced age, causing minor-to-moderate symptoms. **Clinical Findings:** Common symptoms include the sensation of not completely emptying the bladder after urinating, frequent urination, difficulty starting the urinary stream and/or

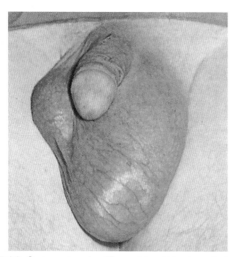

FIG. 17.38 Spermatocele. (From Lloyd-Davies et al., 1994.)

a weak urinary stream, and urgency. The classic rectal examination finding is an enlarged prostate that is smooth and projects into the rectum.

Prostatitis

An inflammation of the prostate gland is termed *prostatitis*. It is the most common urologic diagnosis in men under age 50 and the third most common in men over age 50.[17] There are four recognized categories of prostatitis: acute bacterial prostatitis (ABP); chronic bacterial prostatitis (CBP); chronic pelvic pain syndrome (CPPS); and asymptomatic inflammatory prostatitis. **Clinical Findings:** The clinical manifestations of prostatitis vary. The patient with ABP classically has fever, chills, pain in the back and rectal or perineal area, and urinary obstructive symptoms (difficulty urinating, bladder fullness); examination reveals an enlarged prostate that is usually tender with induration. CBP commonly causes recurrent UTI, pain, dysuria, and scrotal or penile pain; examination findings may be nonspecific or reveal an enlarged, tender, and boggy prostate. CPPS is characterized by urinary urgency, frequency, nocturia, dysuria, and pain or discomfort; examination findings may be normal or may include a soft and boggy prostate. Asymptomatic prostatitis is often detected based on abnormal urinalysis (increased white cells) or a digital examination finding, such as a boggy prostate.

Prostate Cancer

The prostate is the leading site of cancer in men with an estimated 191,900 new cases diagnosed in 2020.[4] Approximately 80% of men who reach age 80 have evidence of prostate cancer at autopsy.[17] **Clinical Findings:** The patient is usually asymptomatic until the cancer begins causing urinary obstruction, resulting in difficulty urinating. On palpation, the prostate feels hard and irregular. The median sulcus is obliterated as the prostate tumor grows (Fig. 17.41).

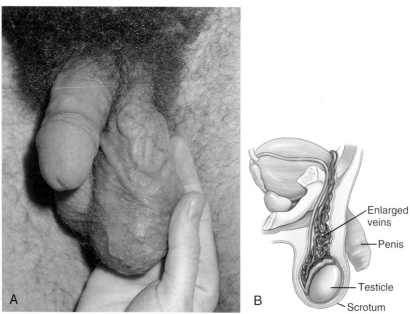

- Enlarged veins
- Penis
- Testicle
- Scrotum

FIG. 17.39 Varicocele. (A) Examination finding. (B) Anatomic finding. ([A] From Swartz, 2010. [B] From LaFleur Brooks and LaFleur Brooks, 2012.)

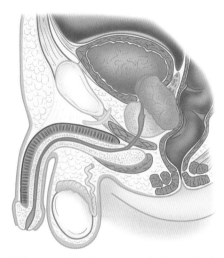

FIG. 17.40 Benign prostatic hyperplasia.

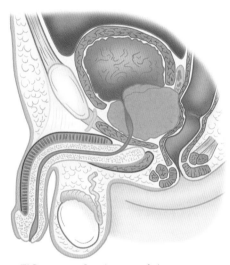

FIG. 17.41 Carcinoma of the prostate.

CONDITIONS OF THE ANUS AND RECTUM

Hemorrhoids

Hemorrhoids are dilated veins of the hemorrhoidal plexus resulting from increased portal venous pressure. This is an extremely common condition with estimates that more than 50% of the population older than 50 have experienced hemorrhoids; both genders are equally affected.[18] **Clinical Findings:** External hemorrhoids originate outside the external rectal sphincter and appear as flaps of tissue. If they become irritated or thrombosed, symptoms include localized itching and perhaps bleeding, and they may appear as blue or purple shiny masses at the anus. Internal hemorrhoids originate above the interior sphincter. Although they may be present in the rectum, they may not be seen unless they become thrombosed, prolapsed, or infected (See Figs. 17.7 and 17.42A and B).

Anorectal Fissure

An anorectal fissure is a tear of the anal mucosa causing intense pain. It occurs in all age groups but is seen most often in young healthy adults; the incidence is similar between genders. **Clinical Findings:** The fissure appears as a crack within the anus, usually located midline in the posterior wall of the rectum (Fig. 17.43).[18] The patient experiences severe rectal pain, itching, and rectal bleeding.

Anorectal Abscess and Fistula

A pus-filled cavity in the anal or rectal area is referred to as an *anorectal abscess.* A fistula is an inflamed tract that forms an abnormal passage from within the anus or the rectum to the outside skin surface, usually in the perianal area. A fistula is often caused by the drainage of an abscess.[18] **Clinical Findings:** The principal symptom of an abscess is rectal pain; frequently the patient also has a fever. An area of inflammation adjacent to or within the anus is observed with edema, erythema, and induration. Often the pain is so severe that the

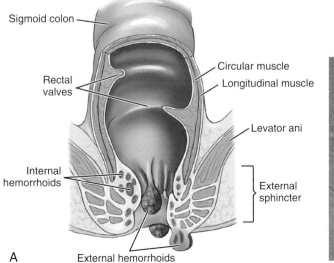

Sigmoid colon

Rectal valves

Circular muscle

Longitudinal muscle

Levator ani

Internal hemorrhoids

External sphincter

A

External hemorrhoids

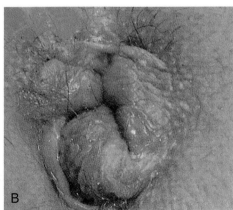

B

FIG. 17.42 (A) Internal and external hemorrhoids. (B) External hemorrhoid. ([A] From LaFleur Brooks, 2009. [B] From Ball et al., 2015. Courtesy Gershon Efron, MD, Sinai Hospital of Baltimore.)

patient cannot tolerate palpation of the area. If a fistula is present, the opening on the skin usually appears as red, raised granulation tissue; the drainage is serosanguineous or purulent (Fig. 17.44).

Rectal Polyp

A rectal polyp is a protruding growth from the rectal mucosa. It may grow outward, as on a stalk (pedunculated), or adhering to the mucosa (sessile) (Fig. 17.45A and B). Most colorectal cancers arise from mutated adenomatous polyps. **Clinical Findings:** A common symptom is rectal bleeding, although

often the patient is unaware that a polyp exists. Occasionally a polyp may protrude from the anus and appear as small, soft nodules. Polyps may be difficult to palpate and are often identified during a colonoscopy examination.

Carcinoma of the Rectum and Anus

Rectal and anal cancer occur when a malignant tumor grows within the rectal mucosa, anal canal, or anus (Fig. 17.46). Anal cancer, as a result of HPV infection, is being diagnosed at an increasing rate in both males and females.[3] An estimated 52,000 new cases of anal or rectal cancers were

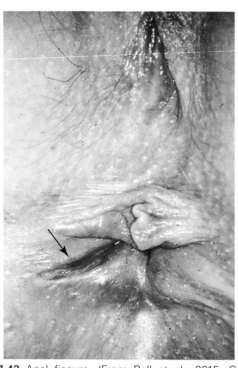

FIG. 17.43 Anal fissure. (From Ball et al., 2015. Courtesy Gershon Efron, MD, Sinai Hospital of Baltimore.)

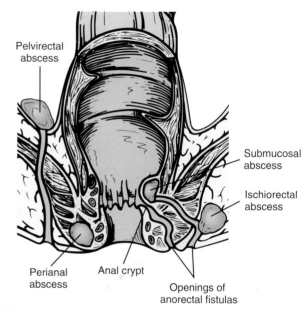

Pelvirectal abscess

Submucosal abscess

Ischiorectal abscess

Perianal abscess

Anal crypt

Openings of anorectal fistulas

FIG. 17.44 Common sites of anorectal fistula and abscess formation. (From Lewis et al., 2011.)

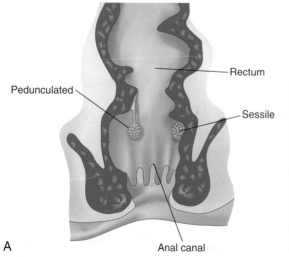

Pedunculated

Rectum

Sessile

Anal canal

A

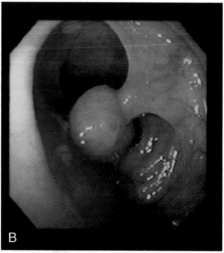

B

FIG. 17.45 (A) Types of rectal polyps. (B) Endoscopic image of a pedunculated polyp. ([B] From McCance and Huether, 2010. Courtesy David Bjorkman, MD, University of Utah School of Medicine, Department of Gastroenterology.)

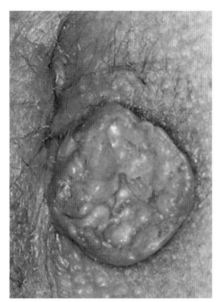

FIG. 17.46 Squamous cell carcinoma on anus. (From Meyerhardt, et al., 2010.)

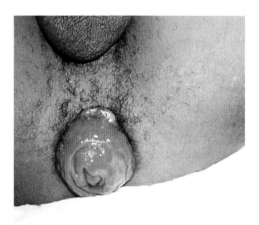

FIG. 17.47 Prolapse of the rectum. (From Seidel et al., 2006. Courtesy Gershon Efron, MD, Sinai Hospital of Baltimore.)

diagnosed in the United States in 2020.[4] **Clinical Findings:** Patients may remain asymptomatic for a long period of time. The most common symptom is rectal bleeding. If palpable, a malignant rectal tumor manifests as an irregular mass on the rectal wall with nodular, raised edges.

PROLAPSE OR HERNIATION

Hernia

A hernia is a protrusion of part of the peritoneal-lined sac through the abdominal wall. The three most common types of hernias seen when examining the inguinal area are indirect inguinal, direct inguinal, and femoral. **Clinical Findings:** Signs and symptoms of the various types of hernias are presented in Table 17.2.

Rectal Prolapse

Rectal prolapse is a full-thickness protrusion of the rectal wall through the anus (turning inside out). The incidence is hard to determine because many people have mild forms of this condition and never seek treatment. It can occur at any age, but most cases involve women over age 60. **Clinical Findings:** Symptoms of rectal prolapse include rectal bleeding, a mass, and change in bowel habits (e.g., fecal incontinence or soiling with mucous discharge). The patient may report that an intestine or a hemorrhoid is hanging out of the anus. The prolapsed rectum appears as a pink mucosal bulge that is described as a "doughnut" or "rosette" (Fig. 17.47).

Uterine Prolapse

Uterine prolapse is associated with a retroverted uterus that descends into the vagina. In first-degree prolapse, the cervix remains within the vagina (Fig. 17.48A). In second-degree prolapse, the cervix is in the introitus (Fig. 17.48B). In third-degree prolapse, the cervix and vagina drop outside the

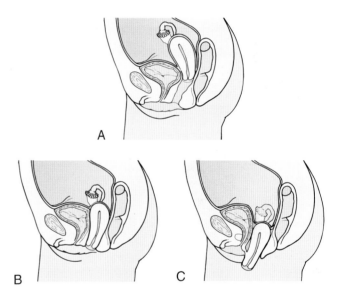

FIG. 17.48 Uterine prolapse. (A) First-degree prolapse of the uterus. (B) Second-degree prolapse of the uterus. (C) Third-degree prolapse of the uterus. (From Lewis et al., 2011.)

introitus (Fig. 17.48C). **Clinical Findings:** The primary symptoms include a feeling of heaviness, fullness, or the sensation of "falling out" in the perineal area. The cervix is visualized low within the vagina, at the vaginal opening, or protruding from the vaginal opening.

Cystocele

Cystocele is a protrusion of the urinary bladder against the anterior wall of the vagina. **Clinical Findings:** The woman may experience a sensation of fullness or pressure, stress incontinence, occasional urgency, and a feeling of incomplete emptying after voiding. A soft bulging mass of the anterior vaginal wall is usually seen and felt as the woman bears down (Fig. 17.49A and B).

Rectocele

Rectocele is a hernia-type protrusion of the rectum against the posterior wall of the vagina. **Clinical Findings:** The woman often complains of a heavy feeling within the vagina. Other commonly reported symptoms include constipation, a feeling of incomplete emptying of the rectum after a bowel movement, and a feeling of something "falling out" in the vagina. Bulging of the posterior vagina is observed as the woman bears down (Fig. 17.49C).

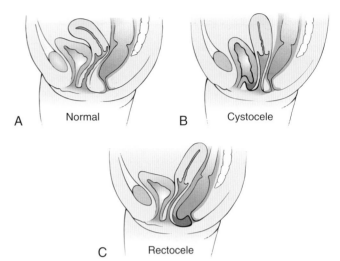

FIG. 17.49 (A) Normal anatomic position. (B) Cystocele (protrusion of the urinary bladder wall through the vagina). (C) Rectocele (protrusion of the rectal wall through the vagina). (From Swartz, 2010.)

CLINICAL APPLICATION AND CLINICAL JUDGMENT

See Appendix B for answers to exercises in this section.

CASE STUDY

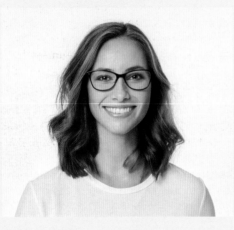

Mia Richards is a 33-year-old woman who comes to the urgent care center. The nurse collects the following data:

Interview Data

Ms. Richards tells the nurse, "I have a really bad pain in front of my butt. It hurts so much that I can't even wipe with a tissue after I go to the bathroom. There is no way I could have a bowel movement right now." Ms. Richards states that the pain started 2 days ago and is "much worse now." When asked about her sexual activity, she says, "I'm with a guy, but it's not exclusive or anything. We see other people and try not to be real serious."

Examination Data

- *External examination:* Typical hair distribution, urethral meatus intact, no redness or discharge. The perineum is intact. Extreme pain response to palpation of vaginal opening; edema, redness, and mass detected on the right side. Spontaneous, foul-smelling, dark-yellow discharge noted with palpation over Bartholin glands.
- *Internal examination:* Deferred because of extreme pain associated with inflammation.

Clinical Judgment

1. What cues do you recognize that suggest deviation from normal findings, suggesting a need for further investigation?
2. For which additional information should the nurse ask or assess?
3. Based on the data, which risk factors for STD does Ms. Richards have?
4. With which additional health care professionals should you consider collaborating to meet her health care needs?

REVIEW QUESTIONS

1. Which finding does the nurse recognize as abnormal when examining a male patient?
   1. Testes are palpable and firm within the scrotal sac bilaterally
   2. Discharge observed from the penis when the glans is compressed
   3. Foreskin lies loosely over the penis
   4. Glans a lighter skin tone than the rest of the penis

2. A 22-year-old white male comes to the emergency department with a concern about a mass in his testicle. In addition to his age and race, which fact is a known risk factor for testicular cancer?
   1. He had an undescended testicle at birth.
   2. His mother had breast cancer.
   3. He was treated for gonorrhea 18 months ago.
   4. He had a hydrocele during infancy.

3. Which data collected from the history of a 32-year-old female patient should be followed with a symptom analysis?
   1. Has never had a mammogram.
   2. Experiences light to moderate bleeding during the menstrual cycle.
   3. Periods began at age 12; has never been pregnant.
   4. Has pelvic pain and vaginal discharge.

4. While taking the health history of a 23-year-old female patient, the nurse considers risk factors for STD. Which data from the patient suggest a need for patient education?
   1. She has been in a monogamous sexual relationship for 2 years; she uses a condom to prevent pregnancy.
   2. She has been sexually involved with one man for the last 2 weeks; she uses spermicidal gel to prevent pregnancy.
   3. She has a Pap test each year, and the results have been negative.
   4. She uses oral contraceptives to prevent pregnancy.

5. A patient has a herpes lesion on her vulva. While examining her, the nurse should take which measures?
   1. Wear examination gloves while in contact with the genitalia.
   2. Place the patient in an isolation room.
   3. Wash the genitalia with alcohol or povidone-iodine (Betadine) before the examination.
   4. Inspect the genitalia only; reschedule the patient for a full examination after the lesion has healed.

6. To inspect the glans penis of the uncircumcised male, the nurse retracts the foreskin. After inspection, she is unable to replace the foreskin over the glans. The nurse recognizes that this situation could potentially lead to which complication?
   1. Decreased sperm production
   2. Urinary tract infection
   3. Tissue necrosis of the penis
   4. Testicular cancer

7. Which finding is expected during a rectal exam?
   1. The rectal wall is smooth.
   2. Severe pain is reported when the finger is introduced through the anus.
   3. Hard stool is present in the rectum.
   4. The anus is surrounded by white flat lesions.

8. The nurse recognizes which symptom as commonly associated with prostate enlargement?
   1. Constipation
   2. Rectal bleeding
   3. Weak urinary stream
   4. Penile discharge

9. During an examination, the nurse palpates the Skene glands. Which technique best describes this process?
   1. Exerting pressure over the clitoris, slide the finger downward (posteriorly) toward the vaginal opening.
   2. Palpate the fourchette and slide the finger forward (anteriorly) toward the vaginal opening.
   3. Exert pressure on the anterior vaginal wall and slide the finger outward toward the vaginal opening.
   4. Grasp the labia majora between the index finger and thumb and milk the labia outward.

10. A patient tells the nurse that her stools have bright red blood in them. The nurse suspects which problem?
    1. Gallbladder disease
    2. Hemorrhoids
    3. Rectal polyps
    4. Upper intestinal bleeding

Developmental Assessment Throughout the Life Span

evolve

http://evolve.elsevier.com/Wilson/assessment

Physical, behavioral, and cognitive development is a vital part of assessment. Nurses compare and contrast a patient's physical characteristics with those described in standardized norms. For example, the growth of infants is assessed to determine if their bones and muscles are developing as expected for a specific age. Deviations from these expectations or the norm may indicate a health problem that nurses can address with the parents, caregivers, and/or providers. Nurses also collect data related to behavioral and cognitive development from patients and compare these data with the developmental tasks that have been identified for those age groups. When deviations from the norm are found, nurses discuss the findings with patients, parents, caregivers, and/or providers.

This chapter is organized by chronologic age divisions, which correlate with developmental periods. Each division discusses physical, behavioral, and cognitive development and developmental tasks for that age group. However, during the first 6 years, physical growth and development are so dramatic that additional data are used to describe motor development, social-adaptive behaviors, and language development.

- *Motor development* has two components: gross- and fine-motor behavior. Gross-motor behavior refers to postural reactions such as head balance, sitting, creeping, standing, and walking. Fine-motor behavior refers to the use of hands and fingers in the prehensile approach to grasping and manipulating an object.
- *Social adaptive behavior* refers to the interactions of the infant or child with other people, and the ability to organize stimuli, perceive relationships between objects, dissect a whole into its component parts, reintegrate these parts in a meaningful fashion, and solve practical problems. Examples are smiling at other people and learning to feed self.
- *Language behavior* is used broadly to include visible and audible forms of communication, whether facial expression, gesture, postural movements, or vocalizations (words,

phrases, or sentences). Language also includes the comprehension of communication by others.

THEORIES OF DEVELOPMENT

By using theories of development, nurses can describe and predict the growth and development of patients throughout the life span. Two widely used theories of behavioral and cognitive development are described briefly; these theories were developed by Erik Erikson and Jean Piaget.

Personality Development: Erikson's Theory

Erik Erikson (1902–1994) believed that the ego was the primary seat of personality functioning.[1] In addition to the ego, he believed that society and culture influenced behavior. Erikson believed that people developed through a predetermined unfolding of their personalities in eight stages. An analogy of a rosebud unfolding may be useful in thinking about development. Each petal opens at a certain time in a certain order, which is predetermined. If the natural order is disturbed, by pulling off a petal prematurely or out of order, the development of the mature rose is affected.[2] Each stage involves certain developmental tasks that are psychosocial in nature and described as polar opposites or conflicts (Table 18.1). For example, in the first stage, during infancy the conflict is trust versus mistrust. Infants learn that they can depend on their caregivers to meet their needs for food, protection, comfort, and affection. When the infant develops trusting relationships with others, usually the mother, the lasting outcome tends to be ambition, enthusiasm, and motivation. By contrast, when trust is not developed, the person tends to develop apathy and indifference; however, Erikson believed that a balance was needed at each stage. For example, infants need to learn to trust, but they also need to learn a little mistrust so they do not grow up to become gullible.[2]

TABLE 18.1 ERIKSON'S EIGHT STAGES OF HUMAN DEVELOPMENT

STAGE (APPROXIMATE)	PSYCHOSOCIAL STAGE	LASTING OUTCOMES	SIGNIFICANT RELATIONSHIPS
Infancy Birth to 1 year	Basic trust versus basic mistrust	Drive and hope	Mother
Toddler 2–3 years	Autonomy versus shame and doubt	Self-control and will power	Parents
Preschool 3–6 years	Initiative versus guilt	Direction and purpose	Family
Middle childhood (school age) 7–12 years	Industry versus inferiority	Method and competence	Neighborhood, school
Adolescence 12–19 years	Identity versus role confusion	Devotion and fidelity	Peer groups, role models
Young adulthood 20s	Intimacy versus isolation	Affiliation and love	Partners, friends
Middle adulthood Late 20s–50s	Generativity versus stagnation	Production and care	Household, work mates
Older adulthood 50s and beyond	Ego integrity versus despair	Renunciation and wisdom	Mankind or "my kind"

"Figure of Erickson's Stages of Personality Development" from Childhood and Society by Erik H. Erikson. © 1950, © 1963 by W.W. Norton & Company, Inc., renewed © 1978, 1991 by Erikson. Used by permission of W.W. Norton & Company, Inc. Significant relationships from webspace.ship.edu/cgboer/erikson.html.

Accomplishing each successive task provides the foundation for a healthy self-identity. Each stage builds on the previous stages and must be accomplished for the person to successfully complete the next stage. People with whom a person interacts and environmental factors influence the accomplishment of these tasks; however, the motivation to achieve a healthy identity arises from within each person. Although each conflict is described at a particular developmental stage, all of the conflicts exist in each person to some extent throughout life. Even though the conflict may be resolved at one time in a person's life, it may recur in similar circumstances.[1]

Cognitive Development: Piaget's Theory

Jean Piaget (1896–1980) described stages of cognitive development from birth to approximately 15 years of age. *Cognition* is defined as how a person perceives and processes information. He believed the child's main goal was to establish equilibrium between self and environment.

Piaget believed that the child's view of the world developed from simple reflex behavior to complex logical and abstract thought. To fully develop cognition, the child needs a functioning neurologic system and sufficient environmental stimuli. Piaget described four distinct, sequential levels of cognitive development (Table 18.2). Each stage represents a change in how children understand and organize their environments, and each stage is characterized by more sophisticated types of reasoning. All children move through the stages in sequential order but not necessarily at the same age.[3]

DEVELOPMENTAL TASKS

As individuals grow, they are able to perform more complex tasks. For example, as infants' bones, muscles, and nervous systems mature, they progress from sitting to standing to walking. This progression increases the tasks that they are able

TABLE 18.2 PIAGET'S LEVELS OF COGNITIVE DEVELOPMENT

STAGE	AGE	CHARACTERISTICS
Sensorimotor	0–2 years	Thought is dominated by physical manipulation of objects and events.
Preoperational	2–7 years	Function is symbolic, using language as major tool.
Concrete operations	7–11 years	Mental reasoning processes assume logical approaches to solving concrete problems.
Formal operations	11–15 years	True logical thought and manipulation of abstract concepts emerge.

Modified from Schuster C, Ashburn S: The process of human development: a holistic life-span approach, Boston, 1992, Lippincott.

to accomplish. Likewise, as their nervous system matures, they are able to interact with family members to develop communication skills. Infants who live in an environment with many family members may have more opportunities to develop communication skills earlier because of the increased number of people with whom they interact. Families, peers, and associates expect individuals in their spheres of influence to conform in certain ways. These expectations are culturally appropriate and influence individuals' functioning in various roles and statuses for their age and gender.[4]

Each culture has its own developmental tasks and expectations. These tasks also vary from region to region in the United States and even from one socioeconomic class to another within one geographic area, which may account for differences among people of various ethnic and cultural backgrounds. A developmental task is a drive from within the individual to develop in such a way as to attain a goal. The thrust to change usually comes from within the person, but it may be motivated by the demands and expectations of others.[4] A conflict may arise in families who move to the United States from foreign countries. Their children are expected to follow the culture of the parent's country of origin, but they also are influenced by the American culture. The developmental tasks presented in this chapter are intended as a guide because there are many normal variations based on ethnic and cultural influences. The boxes in this chapter describe developmental tasks throughout the life span:

- Infants (birth to 1 year)
- Toddlers (1 to 3 years)
- Preschoolers (3 to 5 years)
- School-age children (6 to 12 years)
- Adolescents (13 to 18 years)
- Young adults (19 to 35 years)
- Middle adults (36 to 65 years)
- Older adults
  - Young-old (66 to 74 years)
  - Middle-old (75 to 84 years)
  - Old-old (85 to 100 years)
  - Centenarians (100 to 104 years)
  - Semisupercentenarians (105 to 109 years)
  - Supercentenarians (110 years and older)

EXPECTED GROWTH AND DEVELOPMENT BY AGE GROUP

Infants

Infancy refers to the first year of life. The rapid growth and development that occur during these first 12 months are evident from the data given in Table 18.3, which lists changes in the infant by month, whereas subsequent tables document changes by intervals of 6 months to 1 year. During this time, extensive physical development occurs in addition to the acquisition of psychosocial skills.

Physical Growth

Weight, height, and head circumference are measured to assess infant growth. Growth proceeds from head to toe (cephalocaudal), as evidenced by the infant's development of head control before sitting and mastery of sitting before standing. Healthy newborns weigh between 5 lb 8 oz and 8 lb 13 oz (2500 and 4000 g). The newborn period is the first 28 days of life. Commonly, newborns lose 10% of their birth weight in the first week but regain it in 10 to 14 days. In general, they double their birth weight by 4 to 6 months of age and triple it by 12 months of age. The infant grows 1 inch (2.5 cm) each month for the first 6 months, followed by 0.5 inch (1.3 cm) a month from ages 6 to 12 months. Expected head circumference for term newborns averages from 13 to 14 inches (33 to 36 cm). The average head size is 17 inches (43 cm) at 6 months and 18 inches (46 cm) at 12 months.[5] By 6 months, teeth begin to erupt, with a total of six to eight teeth by the end of the first year.

Behavioral and Cognitive Development

A summary of the expected developmental milestones of infants is found in Table 18.3. Erikson's developmental task of infancy, or the oral-sensory stage, is to develop trust without completely eliminating the capacity for mistrust.[2] Infants develop trust relationships with the mother or primary caregiver. The quality and consistency of the mother-infant relationship are important. Infants who receive consistent, loving care learn that they can depend on people around them to meet their needs. By contrast, care that is inconsistent, abusive, or undependable may result in the mistrust of people.

Piaget identified sensorimotor development as the primary task at this age. Infants use their sensorimotor abilities to master motor milestones and launch relationships with others.[3] Not only can infants advance from crawling to walking and eating some foods, but they also have the ability to win the hearts and attention of others with an intentional smile and showing preference for familiar caregivers. Bonding takes place with caregivers at approximately 1 month. Different cries can be identified as being related to different needs, expressive language progresses with the first word, and receptive language is developed enough to understand and briefly respond to simple commands. Learning at the sensorimotor level of cognitive development occurs through the five senses

TABLE 18.3 EXPECTED DEVELOPMENT OF INFANTS

AGE	FINE-MOTOR	GROSS-MOTOR	SOCIAL-ADAPTIVE	LANGUAGE
1 mo	Follows with eyes to midline Hands predominantly closed	Turns head to side Keeps knees tucked under abdomen When pulled to sitting position, has gross head lag and rounded, swayed back	Regards face	Responds to bell Cries in response to displeasure Makes sounds during feeding
2 mo	Follows objects well; may not follow past midline Limited finger motion	Holds head in same plane as rest of body Can raise head and maintain position; looks downward	Smiles responsively	Vocalizes (not crying) Cries become differentiated Coos
3 mo	Follows past midline When in supine puts hands together; holds hands in front of face Pulls at blanket and clothes	Raises head to 45-degree angle Maintains posture Looks around with head May turn from prone to side position When pulled into sitting position, shows only slight head lag	Shows interest in surroundings	Laughs Coos, babbles, chuckles

TABLE 18.3 EXPECTED DEVELOPMENT OF INFANTS—cont'd

AGE	FINE-MOTOR	GROSS-MOTOR	SOCIAL-ADAPTIVE	LANGUAGE
4 mo	Grasps rattle Plays with hands together Inspects hands Carries objects to mouth	Actively lifts head up and looks around (Fig. 18.1) Rolls from prone to supine No head lag when pulled to sitting position When held in standing position, attempts some weight support	Becomes bored when left alone Begins to show memory	Squeals Vocalizations change with mood
5 mo	Can reach and pick up object May play with toes	Able to push up from prone position and maintain weight on forearms Rolls from prone to supine Maintains straight back when in sitting position	Smiles spontaneously Playful, with rapid mood changes Distinguishes family	Uses vowel-like cooing sounds with consonantal sounds (e.g., *ah-goo*)
6 mo	Holds spoon or rattle Drops object and reaches for second offered object Holds bottle	Begins to raise abdomen off table Sits, but posture still shaky May sit with legs apart; holds arms straight as prop between legs Supports almost full weight when pulled to standing	Recognizes parents Holds out arms to be picked up	Begins to imitate sounds Uses one-syllable sounds (e.g., *ma, mu, da, di*)
7 mo	Can transfer object from one hand to other Grasps objects in each hand Bangs cube on table	Sits alone; still uses hands for support When held in standing position, bounces Puts feet to mouth	Fearful of strangers Plays peekaboo Keeps lips closed when dislikes food	Says four distinct vowel sounds "Talks" when others are talking
8 mo	Beginning thumb-finger grasping Releases object at will Grasps for toys out of reach	Sits securely without support Bears weight on legs when supported May stand holding on	Responds to word *no* Dislikes diaper changes	Makes consonant sounds *t, d, w* Uses two syllables such as *da-da* but does not ascribe meaning to them
9 mo	Continued development of thumb-finger grasp May bang objects together Use of dominant hand evident	Steady sitting; can lean forward and still maintain position Begins creeping (abdomen off floor) Can stand holding onto object when placed in that position	Seems interested in pleasing parent Shows fears of going to bed and being left alone	Responds to simple commands Comprehends *no-no*
10 mo	Practices picking up small objects Points with one finger Offers toys to people but unable to let go of objects	Can pull self into sitting position; unable to let self down again Stands while holding on to furniture	Stops behavior in response to *no-no* Repeats actions that attract attention Plays interactive games such as pat-a-cake Cries when scolded	Says *da-da, ma-ma* with meaning Comprehends *bye-bye*
11 mo	Holds crayon to mark on paper Drops object deliberately for it to be picked up	Moves about room holding onto objects Prepares to walk independently; wide-base stance Stands securely, holding on with one hand	Experiences satisfaction when task is accomplished Reacts to restrictions with frustration Rolls a ball to another on request	Imitates speech sounds
12 mo (1 yr)	May hold cup and spoon and feed self fairly well with practice Can offer toys and release them Releases cube in cup	Able to twist and turn and maintain posture Able to sit from standing position May stand alone, at least momentarily	Shows emotions of jealousy, affection, anger, fear May develop habit of "security blanket" or favorite toy	Recognizes objects by name Imitates animal sounds Understands simple verbal commands (e.g., "Give it to me")

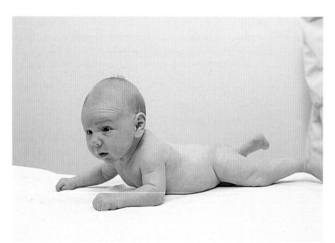

FIG. 18.1 At 4 months infant actively lifts head and looks about.

as infants interact with the environment. Infants learn object permanence, which means that objects and people still exist when they are out of sight. The developmental tasks of infancy are listed in Box 18.1. Preventive services recommended for infants are in Table 18.6 in the column labeled "Birth to 6 years."

Toddlers

Toddlerhood is the period of growth and development from 12 to 36 months. During this period, the child moves about more independently. Toddlers have a strong need to explore and master their environments. Parents who want to encourage their children's exploratory and inquiring spirit, along with the mastery of motor skills, often feel overwhelmed and exhausted at the end of the day. This exhaustion may occur when parents try to keep up with the toddlers to encourage their explorations while keeping them safe.

Physical Growth

A slower but steady growth in height and weight occurs during toddlerhood. By 24 months, chest circumference exceeds head circumference. The usual increase in height is 3 inches (7.5 cm) a year. Children are half their adult height by age 2. The average weight gain is 4 to 6 lb (1.8 to 2.7 kg) per year. By 30 months, the birth weight is quadrupled. The usual appearance of a toddler includes a potbelly, swayback, and short legs.[6] The toddler may be ready for daytime control of bowel and bladder function by age 24 months. Teeth continue to erupt, with 20 teeth expected by 30 months.

Behavioral and Cognitive Development

The developmental task for toddlers is to achieve a degree of autonomy while minimizing shame and doubt. The terms *holding on* and *letting go* are used to describe this stage. Now that toddlers are walking and talking, they yearn for independence; however, they lack judgment to maintain their safety. They learn when it is safe to hold on to furniture and when to let go. The parents or caregivers try to balance their control between allowing independent exploration of the environment and keeping the toddlers safe from injury. Holding on and letting go also apply to bowel control established at this time. In their attempts to be independent, toddlers may fail to achieve their goals. Repeated failures may lead to feelings of shame and doubt in their abilities, particularly when parents try to help them do what the children should learn to do independently. When parents do not have enough patience to allow children to accomplish tasks, such as tying shoes alone, the children may doubt their ability to accomplish tasks.[2]

Cognitive development of toddlers remains in the sensorimotor level. Piaget's preoperational stage begins at approximately 2 years of age, when toddlers learn by trial and error and exploration (Fig. 18.2). Using their motor skills, they

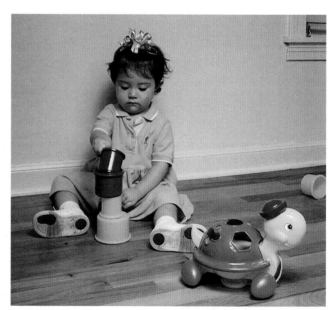

FIG. 18.2 The toddler takes great pleasure in building a tower of four blocks.

move around the environment and pick up objects; using their senses; they see, feel, smell, taste, and hear what they find.[3]

Developmental tasks of toddlers are listed in Box 18.2. A summary of the expected development milestones, including fine- and gross-motor, social-adaptive, and language behaviors, is found in Table 18.4. Preventive services recommended for toddlers are in Table 18.6 in the column labeled "Birth to 6 years."

Preschoolers

The age ranges for preschooler are from 3 to 5 years. As children's locomotion and language mature, they move away from the protective yet confining care of parental figures. They begin to understand concepts and meanings in a more "real" sense and begin increased forms of independent play and decision-making.

Physical Growth

Typical preschoolers grow 2.5 to 3.5 inches (6.5 to 9 cm) a year. By age 4, birth length has doubled, and weight increases by 4.5 to 6 lb (2 to 3 kg) a year. Appearance changes as the long bones grow more than the trunk and preschoolers lose their baby fat and potbellies.[7] By age 5, children begin to lose deciduous teeth, and the first permanent teeth erupt.

Behavioral and Cognitive Development

During the preschool years, children become more autonomous, can communicate easily, achieve bowel and bladder continence, have an active imagination, can demonstrate basic social skills, can delay gratification, use more acceptable outlets to express frustration, and can expand their environment beyond home. The task of this age group is to learn initiative without an overabundance of guilt. Preschoolers continue to explore their environments with greater skills and a new enthusiasm and motivation. When children are

---

BOX 18.2 DEVELOPMENTAL TASKS OF TODDLERS

- Achieving physiologic equilibrium following birth
  - Learning the know-how and where-when of elimination
  - Learning to manage one's body effectively
- Learning to adjust to other people
  - Responding to others' expectations
  - Recognizing parental authority and controls
  - Learning the dos and don'ts of the immediate world
- Learning to love and be loved
  - Meeting emotional needs through widening spheres and variety of contacts
- Developing system of communication
  - Acquiring basic concepts such as yes/no
  - Mastering basic language fundamentals
- Learning to express and control feelings
  - Healthy management of feelings of fear and anxiety
  - Handling feelings of frustration, disappointment, and anger appropriately for age
  - Moderating demanding attitudes
- Laying a foundation for self-awareness
  - Exploring the rights and privileges of being an individual

From Duvall EM, Miller BC: *Marriage and family development,* ed 6, New York, 1985, Harper & Row.

TABLE 18.4 EXPECTED DEVELOPMENT OF TODDLERS

AGE	FINE-MOTOR	GROSS-MOTOR	SOCIAL-ADAPTIVE	LANGUAGE
15 mo	Can put raisins into bottle Takes off shoes and pulls toys Builds tower of two cubes Scribbles spontaneously Uses cup well but rotates spoon	Walks alone well Able to seat self in chair Creeps up stairs Cannot throw ball without falling	Tolerates some separation from parents Begins to imitate parents' activities (e.g., sweeping, mowing lawn)	Says 10 or more words "Asks" for objects by pointing Uses *no* even when agreeing with request
18 mo	Builds tower of three to four cubes (see Fig. 18.2) Turns pages in book two or three at a time Manages spoon without rotating	May walk up and down stairs holding hand May show running ability	Imitates housework Temper tantrums may be more evident Has beginning awareness of ownership (e.g., *my toy*)	Says 50 or more words Points to two or three body parts
24 mo (2 yr)	Able to turn doorknob Able to take off shoes and socks Able to build seven- to eight-block tower Dumps raisins from bottle following demonstration	May walk up stairs by self, two feet on each step Able to walk backward Able to kick ball	Demonstrates parallel play Pulls people to show them something Increased independence from mother	Has vocabulary of 50–400 words Uses two- or three-word phrases Uses pronouns *I, you* Uses first name Refers to self by name
30 mo (2½ yr)	Able to build eight-block tower Scribbling techniques continue Feeds self with increased neatness Dumps raisins from bottle spontaneously	Able to jump from object Walking becomes more stable; wide-base gait decreases Throws ball overhanded	Separates easily from mother In play, helps put things away In toileting, only needs help to wipe Begins to notice gender differences	Gives first and last name Uses plurals Refers to self by appropriate pronoun Names one color

praised for their activities, they learn that they are meeting others' expectations and become independent and self-sufficient. At this stage, their conscience (i.e., that inner voice that provides a sense of right and wrong) develops.

Cognitive development continues at the preoperational level. Children begin the symbolic function, in which they develop concepts and classifications to associate one event, object, or person with a similar one. Children demonstrate this when they act out an event they have seen or experienced but emphasize only one aspect of the event. At this level, children become egocentric (i.e., they are self-centered and unable to understand others' viewpoints).[3]

The developmental tasks of preschoolers are listed in Box 18.3. A summary of the expected development of preschoolers, including fine- and gross-motor, social-adaptive, and language behaviors, is found in Table 18.5. Preventive services recommended for preschoolers are in Table 18.6 in the column labeled "Birth to 6 years."

School-Age Children

The beginning of school is a developmental landmark for children. Entering school brings a new influential environment into their lives. Information about concepts, life, and interpersonal relationships expands beyond the confines of the home. Teacher and peer influences may be noticed in school-age children's reactions and behavior. The school-age period lasts from approximately 6 to 12 years of age.

Physical Growth

The growth continues at a slow pace, with weight gain between 4.4 to 6.6 lb (2 to 3 kg) and height increase of 2 inches (5 cm) per year.[8] Growth rates for boys and girls are similar until the growth spurt starts between 10 and 12 years of age. By age 8 or 9, there is increased smoothness and speed in motor control, making the child more agile and graceful. Bone replaces cartilage and continues to harden. Bones of the face and jaw grow at a faster rate than they have in previous years. The school-age child is slimmer, with less body fat and a lower center of gravity. Eyes and hands are well coordinated, and muscles are stronger and more developed. These changes in growth improve fine-motor activities such as drawing, needlework, and playing musical instruments, and gross-motor activities such as jumping, biking, and swimming. By age 12, the rest of the teeth (except the wisdom teeth) erupt.

Behavioral and Cognitive Development

The task for this age group is to develop a capacity for industry while avoiding an undue sense of inferiority. Interactions with children and teachers at school broaden children's social contacts. Industry influences a desire to achieve. Children learn how to compete and cooperate with others. School relationships provide social support outside the home environment, and peer approval becomes important. A sense of inferiority develops when the child is allowed little success because of interactions with rejecting teachers, peers, or parents. Experience of racism, sexism, and other forms of discrimination contribute to feelings of inferiority. A

> ### BOX 18.3 DEVELOPMENTAL TASKS OF PRESCHOOLERS
>
> - Settling into healthy daily routines
>   - Enjoying a variety of active play
>   - Being more flexible and capable of accepting change
>   - Mastering good eating habits
>   - Mastering the basics of toilet training
>   - Developing physical skills
> - Becoming a participating member of the family
>   - Assuming responsibility within the family
>   - Giving and receiving affection and gifts freely
>   - Identifying with the parent of the same gender
>   - Developing an ability to share parents with others
>   - Recognizing the family's unique ways
> - Beginning to master impulses and conform to expectations of others
>   - Outgrowing impulsivity
>   - Learning to share, take turns, enjoy companionship
>   - Developing sympathy and cooperation
>   - Adopting situationally appropriate behavior
> - Developing healthy emotional expressions
>   - Acting out feelings during play
>   - Delaying gratification
>   - Expressing hostility/making up
>   - Discriminating between a variety of emotions and feelings
> - Learning to communicate effectively with others
>   - Developing a vocabulary and speech ability
>   - Learning to listen, follow directions, increase attention span
>   - Acquiring social skills that allow more comfortable interactions with others
> - Developing ability to handle potentially dangerous situations
>   - Respecting potential hazards
>   - Effectively using caution and safety practices
>   - Being able to accept assistance when needed
> - Learning to be autonomous with initiative and a conscience of his or her own
>   - Becoming increasingly responsible
>   - Taking initiative to be involved in situations
>   - Internalizing expectations and demands of family and culture
>   - Being self-sufficient for stage of development
> - Laying foundation for understanding the meaning of life
>   - Developing gender awareness
>   - Trying to understand the nature of the physical world
>   - Accepting religious faith of parents, learning about spirituality
>
> From Duvall EM, Miller BC: *Marriage and family development*, ed 6, New York, 1985, Harper & Row.

maladaptation that may occur is inertia, in which the child feels so inferior that he or she stops making the effort to achieve goals or accomplish tasks.[2]

The cognitive development for this age is concrete operations, when children learn inductive reasoning and logical operations. In school they learn to use numbers, read, and classify.[3] By the time children enter school, their development of fine- and gross-motor, social-adaptive, and language skills

TABLE 18.5 EXPECTED DEVELOPMENT OF PRESCHOOLERS

AGE	FINE-MOTOR	GROSS-MOTOR	SOCIAL-ADAPTIVE	LANGUAGE
36 mo (3 yr)	Can unbutton front buttons Copies vertical lines within 30 degrees Copies zero Begins to use fork	Walks up stairs, alternating feet on steps Walks down stairs, two feet on each step Pedals tricycle Jumps in place Able to perform broad jump	Dresses self with help with back buttons Pulls on shoes Parallel play Able to share toys	Vocabulary of 900 words Uses complete sentences Constantly asks questions
48 mo (4 yr)	Able to copy plus sign (+) Picks longer line three out of three times Uses scissors Can lace shoes	Walks down stairs, alternating feet on steps Able to button large front buttons Able to balance on one foot for approximately 5 seconds Catches ball	Associative play Imaginary friend common Boasts and tattles Selfish, impatient, rebellious	Gives first and last name Has 1500-word vocabulary Uses words without knowing meaning Questioning is at a peak
60 mo (5 yr)	Able to dress self with minimal assistance (Fig. 18.3) Able to draw three-part human figure Draws square (■) following demonstration Colors within lines	Hops on one foot Catches ball bounced to him or her two out of three times Able to demonstrate heel-toe walking Jumps rope	Eager to follow rules Less rebellious Relies on outside authority to control the world	Has 2100-word vocabulary Recognizes three colors Asks meanings of words Uses sentences of six to eight words

TABLE 18.6 PREVENTIVE SERVICES THROUGHOUT THE LIFE SPAN[a]

	BIRTH TO 6 YEARS	7–18 YEARS	19–64 YEARS	OVER 65 YEARS
Screening	Height and weight Obesity (age 6) Phenylalanine level at birth Vision screen (ages 3–5)	Height and weight Obesity (ages 7–18) Blood pressure (18) Unhealthy alcohol use (18) Human immunodeficiency virus (HIV) (ages 15-18)	Height and weight Obesity Blood pressure Unhealthy alcohol use Human immunodeficiency virus (HIV) (age 19-64) Fecal occult blood test, sigmoidoscopy, or colonoscopy (age 50–64) Pap test (women age 21–64) Mammogram (women age 50–64)	Height and weight Obesity Blood pressure Unhealthy alcohol use Human immunodeficiency virus (HIV) (age 65) Fecal occult blood test, sigmoidoscopy, or colonoscopy (age 65–75) Pap test (women age 65) Mammogram (ages 65–74) Bone measurement testing to screen for osteoporosis in women

Continued

TABLE 18.6 PREVENTIVE SERVICES THROUGHOUT THE LIFE SPAN—cont'd

	BIRTH TO 6 YEARS	7–18 YEARS	19–64 YEARS	OVER 65 YEARS
Counseling	**Injury prevention:** Infant/child safety seats for children <5 years Lap-shoulder belt for children >5 years Smoke detector in home Bicycle helmet; bicycle safety Hot water heater temperature <120°F (49°C) Window and stair guards; pool fences Safe storage of drugs, toxic substances, firearms, and matches Poison control number 1-800-222-1222 **Substance abuse:** Effects of passive smoke Antitobacco message **Diet and exercise:** Breast-feeding, iron-enriched formula and foods (infants and toddlers) Limit fat and cholesterol, maintain caloric balance; emphasize grain, fruits, vegetables (ages 2–10) Regular physical activity Regular dental care Brush with fluoride toothpaste and floss daily Advice about baby bottle tooth decay	**Injury prevention:** Lap-shoulder seat belts Helmet use Smoke detector in home Safe storage of firearms **Substance abuse:** Avoid tobacco use Avoid underage drinking Avoid alcohol and drug misuse **Sexual behavior:** Sexually transmitted infection prevention: abstinence, avoid high-risk behavior; use condoms or female barrier with spermicide Contraception **Diet and exercise:** Limit fat and cholesterol, maintain caloric balance; emphasize grain, fruits, vegetables; regular calcium intake Regular physical activity Regular dental care Brush with fluoride toothpaste and floss daily	**Injury prevention:** Lap-shoulder seat belts Helmet use Smoke detector in home Safe storage of firearms **Substance abuse:** Tobacco cessation Avoid alcohol and drug misuse **Sexual behavior:** Sexually transmitted infection prevention: abstinence, avoid high-risk behavior; use condoms or female barrier with spermicide Contraception **Diet and exercise:** Limit fat and cholesterol, maintain caloric balance; emphasize grain, fruits, vegetables; regular calcium intake (women) Regular physical activity Regular dental care Brush with fluoride toothpaste and floss daily	**Injury prevention:** Lap-shoulder seat belts Helmet use Fall prevention Smoke detector in home Safe storage of firearms Hot water heater temperature <120°F (49°C) **Substance abuse:** Tobacco cessation Avoid alcohol and drug misuse **Sexual behavior:** Sexually transmitted infection prevention: abstinence, avoid high-risk behavior; use condoms or female barrier with spermicide **Diet and exercise:** Limit fat and cholesterol, maintain caloric balance; emphasize grain, fruits, vegetables; regular calcium intake (women) Regular physical activity Regular dental care Brush with fluoride toothpaste and floss daily
Immunizations[b]	DTaP, Hep A, Hep B, Hib, IPV, IIV yearly, MMR, PCV13, PPSV23, RV, varicella See www.cdc.gov for schedule	HPV, IIV yearly, MenACWY, MenB, Tdap See www.cdc.gov for schedule	HPV, IIV or LAIV yearly, MMR, Td booster every 10 years, RZV or ZVL, VAR; See www.cdc.gov for schedule	IIV or LAIV yearly, PCV13, PPSV23, RZV or ZVL, See www.cdc.gov for schedule

[a]US Preventive Services Task Force recommended interventions (i.e., screening tests, and chemoprophylactic regimens) for the prevention of target conditions. Counseling interventions, dental health, and immunizations recommended by the Center for Disease Control. The patients who receive these services are asymptomatic individuals of all age groups and risk categories. The recommendations are based on a standardized review of current scientific evidence.

[b]Vaccine abbreviations: *DTaP*, diphtheria, tetanus, and acellular pertussis; *Hep A*, hepatitis A; *Hep B*, hepatitis B; *Hib*, Haemophilus influenzae type b conjugate; *HPV*, human papilloma virus; *IIV*, influenza; *IPV*, inactivated poliovirus; *LAIV*, influenza live attenuate; *MenACWY*, meningococcal serogroups A,C,W,Y; *MenB*, Meningococcal serogroup B; *MMR*, measles, mumps, and rubella virus; *PCV13*, pneumococcal conjugate vaccine; *PPSV23*, pneumococcal polysaccharide vaccine; *RZV*, Zoster recombinant; *RV*, rotavirus; *Td*, tetanus toxoid; *Tdap*, tetanus, diphtheria, acellular pertussis; *VAR*, varicella; *ZVL*, zoster live.

USPSTF A and B Recommendations. U.S. Preventive Services Task Force. June, 2019. Available at: https://www.uspreventiveservicestaskforce.org/Page/Name/uspstf-a-and-b-recommendations; www.cdc.gov/vaccines/schedules, 2018.

"Chemoprophylaxis for newborn" from Wheeler, B: Health promotion of the newborn and family. In Hockenberry MJ, Wilson D, editors: *Wong's nursing care of infants and children*, ed 11, St Louis, 2018, Elsevier/Mosby, pp 243.

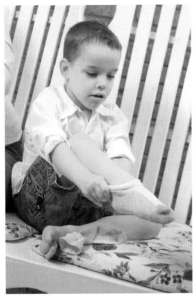

FIG. 18.3 Preschooler develops the ability to help dress self. (©Andy Dean Photography/Shutterstock.com.)

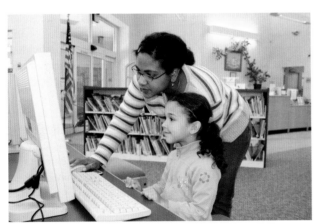

FIG. 18.4 School-age children learn the basic skills required for school. (©Rob Marmion/Shutterstock.com.)

changes more gradually (Fig. 18.4). Tasks for the school-age child are listed in Box 18.4. Assessment tools for school-age children focus on mental abilities and social and emotional behaviors. Preventive services recommended for school-age children are in Table 18.6 in the columns labeled "Birth to 6 years" and "7 to 18 years."

Adolescents

The hallmark of adolescence is puberty, which marks the end of childhood and the onset of adulthood. Adolescence occurs from approximately 13 to 18 years of age.

Physical Growth

The growth spurt that occurs during puberty varies greatly and accounts for 20% to 25% of the final adult height. Growth frequently occurs during spring and summer months. The peak height velocity (PHV) occurs at approximately 12 years of age in girls, 6 to 12 months before menarche.

BOX 18.4 DEVELOPMENTAL TASKS OF SCHOOL-AGE CHILDREN

- Learning the basic skills required for school (see Fig. 18.4)
  - Mastering reading and writing
  - Developing reflective thinking
  - Mastering physical skills
- Mastering money management
  - Obtaining money through socially acceptable ways
  - Buying wisely
  - Saving
  - Delaying gratification
  - Understanding the role of money and place in life
- Becoming an active and cooperative member of the family
  - Participating in family discussions
  - Joining in family decision-making
  - Being responsible for household chores
  - Participating in reciprocal gift giving
- Extending abilities to relate to others
  - Asserting rights
  - Developing leadership skills
  - Following social mores and customs
  - Cooperating in group situations
  - Maintaining close friendships
- Managing feelings and impulses
  - Coping with frustrations
  - Managing anger appropriately
  - Expressing feelings in the right time, place, and manner, and to the right person
- Identifying the gender role
  - Differentiating expectations based on gender
  - Understanding reproduction and gender-specific physical development
  - Managing physical growth spurts
  - Conceptualizing life as a mature man or woman
- Identifying self as a worthy individual
  - Gaining status and respect
  - Growing in self-esteem and self-confidence
  - Establishing unique identity
- Developing conscience and morality
  - Determining right from wrong
  - Developing moral-guided control over behavior
  - Learning to live according to identified values

From Duvall EM, Miller BC: *Marriage and family development,* ed 6, New York, 1985, Harper & Row.

The PHV is used as a predictor of menarche. On average, girls grow 2 to 8 inches (5 to 20 cm) in height and gain 15.5 to 55 lb (7 to 25 kg) in weight during adolescence. By contrast, boys usually reach PHV at approximately 14 years of age, after the growth of testicles and penis and the appearance of axillary and mature pubic hair. On average, boys gain 4 to 12 inches (10 to 30 cm) in height and 15 to 66 lb (7 to 30 kg) in weight during adolescence.[9]

Behavioral and Cognitive Development

The task during adolescence is to achieve ego identity and avoid role confusion. The adolescent reviews the learning, experiences, and values that he or she accepted in earlier stages and modifies them into a unique and personalized

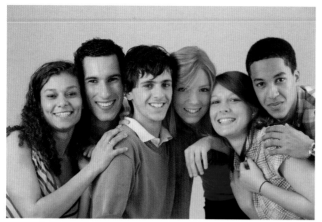

FIG. 18.5 The peer group is a major influence in adolescent development. (©auremar/Shutterstock.com.)

identity. During this identity clarification process, adolescents may decide that previously accepted ideas and beliefs need to be changed. They may behave in new and different ways, much to the chagrin of their parents, as they "try on" differing roles and values. Adolescents begin testing and evaluating previously accepted notions about life, living, spirituality, relating, gender identity, and being. Some influences to change may come from peers (Fig. 18.5). Gender identity development is described in the adjacent box. The early values of the child are often the accepted values from the parental authority in the family. Role confusion develops for adolescents who are unsuccessful in developing their own identity. They may develop low self-esteem, have poor-to-no direction in their lives, and have difficulty making career choices.

Formal operations is the term Piaget gave to the adolescent years. Adolescents are able to perform abstract reasoning and form logical conclusions, and can form hypotheses and devise ways to test them. They use analytic skills in making judgments about their actions and future lives. Advanced intellectual skills allow them to reexamine accepted ideas, which can be a strain within the family but leads to a stronger sense of self and independence.[3] Developmental tasks for the teen years include those listed in Box 18.5.

Assessment tools for this age group focus on social and emotional behaviors, in addition to identifying and reducing stress. Preventive services recommended for adolescents are in Table 18.6 in the column labeled "7 to 18 years."

Young Adults

Young adults (approximately 19 to 35 years of age) move away from the dependent role in the family of origin to establishing their own lifestyle.

Physical Growth

Height and weight are generally complete by young adulthood. Health, motor coordination, and physiologic performance usually peak between ages 20 and 30. The epiphyses of the long bones fuse by the early twenties and muscular development is at its peak.[10]

Behavioral and Cognitive Development

The task of young adults is to achieve some degree of intimacy as opposed to remaining isolated. These individuals begin to express their identity through work, recreation, and interpersonal relationships. Productivity, self-sufficiency, and intimacy in love relationships are driving tasks for young adults, even though they may shift back and forth in career choices, commitment, and goals as they continually redefine themselves. The young adult is ready to enter the adult world and assume a position as a responsible citizen. Achievements are the result of self-direction, with goals that may change as an outcome of reevaluation. Mature relationships with others are important in both the work and home environments. Many young adults choose to marry and start a family. Role confusion may develop when young adults have difficulty

GENDER IDENTITY DEVELOPMENT

At birth, babies are assigned a sex, male or female, based on assessment of external genitalia. This refers to the "sex" or "assigned gender." The term "gender identity" refers to the internal sense that individuals have about who they are, which develops from an interaction of biologic traits, developmental influences, and environmental conditions. This identity may be male, female, somewhere in between, a combination of both, or neither.

Gender identity develops in stages:

- At approximately the age of two, children become conscious of the physical differences between boys and girls;
- Before age three, most children can easily label themselves as either a boy or a girl; and
- By age four, most children have a stable sense of their gender identity.

Research suggests that gender is present from birth and cannot be changed. For most children, however, their gender identity is consistent with the identify assigned at birth.[1,2] For some, however, gender identity can be fluid, shifting depending on varying circumstances.

"Gender expression" refers to a wide range of ways people display their gender through clothing, hair styles, mannerisms, or social roles. Exploring different ways of expressing gender is common in children and may challenge expectations of others. Children who later identified as being transgender or gender diverse (TGD) reported first having recognized their gender as "different" at an average age of 8.5 years; however, they did not disclose their feelings until an average of 18 years.[2]

1. Rafferty J: Gender identity development in children. Retrieved from https://www.healthychildren.org/English/ages-stages/gradeschool/Pages/Gender-Identity-and-Gender-Confusion-In-Children.aspx. Last updated September 18, 2018.
2. Rafferty J: Ensuring comprehensive care and support for transgender and gender-diverse children and adolescents, *Pediatrics* 142 (4), October, 2018. Retrieved from https://pediatrics.aappublications.org/content/142/4/e20182162. American Academy of Pediatrics Policy Statement.

- Accepting physical changes
  - Coming to terms with physical maturation
  - Accepting one's own body
- Achieving a satisfying and socially accepted role
  - Learning masculine/feminine role
  - Realistically understanding gender role
  - Adopting acceptable practices
- Developing more mature peer relationships
  - Being accepted by peer group (see Fig. 18.5)
  - Making and keeping friends of both genders
  - Dating
  - Loving and being loved
  - Adapting to a variety of peer associations
  - Developing skills in managing and evaluating peer relationships
- Achieving emotional independence
  - Outgrowing childish parental dependence
  - Developing a mature affection for parents
  - Being autonomous
  - Developing mature interdependence
- Getting an education
  - Acquiring basic knowledge and skills
  - Clarifying sex-role attitudes toward work and family roles
- Preparing for marriage and family life
  - Formulating gender-role attitudes
  - Enjoying responsibilities
  - Developing responsible attitudes
  - Distinguishing between infatuation and mature love
  - Developing mutually satisfying personal relationships
- Developing knowledge and skills for civic competence
  - Communicating as a citizen
  - Becoming involved in causes outside oneself
  - Acquiring problem-solving skills
  - Developing social concepts
- Establishing one's identity as a socially responsible person
  - Developing philosophy of life
  - Implementing worthy ideals and standards
  - Assuming social obligations
  - Adopting a mature sense of values and ethics
  - Dealing effectively with emotional responses

From Duvall EM, Miller BC: *Marriage and family development,* ed 6, New York, 1985, Harper & Row.

- Establishing one's autonomy as an individual
- Planning a direction for one's life
- Getting an appropriate education
- Working toward a vocation
- Appraising love and sexual feelings
- Becoming involved in love relationships
- Selecting a mate
- Getting engaged
- Being married

From Duvall EM, Miller BC: *Marriage and family development,* ed 6, New York, 1985, Harper & Row.

important to the predictive power of these inventories. If an individual has many, varied interests, his or her inventory scores may be less reliable and less valid.

Along with career choices, mate selection is a primary interest area for many individuals in early adulthood. The field of premarital and couple counseling has rapidly expanded since the 1940s, along with the increasing divorce rate in the United States. Various tools and internet services are used to match couples based on compatibilities.

Adult intelligence develops through interactions of biologic and environmental factors. Intellectual abilities of adults can be sustained or improved until late adulthood. Two types of adult intelligence have been described: fluid (mechanical) and crystallized (practical). Fluid intelligence provides for cognitive abilities, such as information processing and problem solving, including attention, reasoning, spatial orientation, or perceptual speed. This type of intelligence develops through central nervous system function and declines with age and physiologic change. Crystallized intelligence is associated with skills and knowledge learned as part of growing up in a given culture, such as verbal comprehension, vocabulary, and the ability to evaluate life experiences. This type of intelligence dominates throughout adulthood. Although fluid intelligence begins to decline at approximately ages 35 to 40, crystallized intelligence is maintained longer.[11, 12]

Middle Adults

Entry into the middle years, approximately between ages 36 and 65, may be met with the feeling that one's best years have passed, especially in light of today's emphasis on youth.

Physical Growth

There are obvious physical signs of aging, such as wrinkling of the skin, graying or loss of hair, and changes in muscle tone and mass. Changes in vision and hearing may affect social relationships and learning unless corrective actions are taken.

Behavioral and Cognitive Development

During this time, many decisions are made concerning career, partner, children, lifestyle, and living arrangements. The task is to reach a balance between generativity and stagnation.

moving from adolescence and their dependence on parents or family to developing their own identity and adult role responsibilities. Developmental tasks listed in Box 18.6 are usually accomplished during this stage. Preventive services recommended for young adults are in Table 18.6 in the column labeled "19 to 64 years."

The focus of assessment for young adults is on career choice and mate selection. Many assessment tool inventories have been developed for young adults who are contemplating career choices. In these inventories, basic interest areas are compared with occupational themes. The inventory responses cluster similar interest areas and relate them to an occupation or vocational choice. Stability in interest areas is

Generativity involves showing concern for the generations to follow. This may be accomplished by raising children and grandchildren or may be in the form of writing, teaching, inventing, or performing community service projects to contribute to the welfare of those who follow. Stagnation develops when the person is so self-absorbed that he or she ceases to be a productive member of society. Persons who have successfully met the developmental tasks of earlier stages may find this a period of stability, self-understanding, and self-actualization. For others, this is the time of the midlife crisis, when they feel that life is stagnant or incomplete. Frustration drives them to search for new directions and goals in life. During middle age, one reaps the benefits of career success, support of family and friends, and experiences of earlier years. Fluid intelligence continues a slow decline, while crystal intelligence is maintained.

Nearly half of adults in their 40s and 50s have a parent age 65 or older and are either raising a young child or supporting a grown child. These adults are often referred to as the *sandwich generation*. Hispanics are more likely than whites or blacks to be in this group. Approximately 30% of Hispanic adults have a parent age 65 or old older and a dependent child. This compares with 24% of whites and 21% of blacks. Assistance given to parents and children include financial and emotional support. While some aging parents need financial support, others also need help with day-to-day living. Middle-aged adults who make up the core of the sandwich generation are dealing with these challenges and, perhaps, creating new family dynamics.[13]

Developmental tasks for this stage are listed in Box 18.7. Preventive services recommended for middle adults are in Table 18.6 in the column labeled "19 to 64 years."

Older Adults

For many adults, the later years, beginning with age 65, are productive years met with a sense of pleasure and enjoyment. Older adults represent the fastest-growing population in the United States[14] (Fig. 18.6) and probably the least understood.

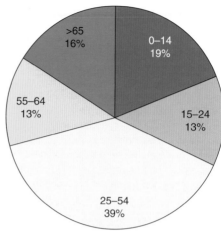

FIG. 18.6 Graph of percentages of population by age ranges. Data from: Data from United States Central Intelligence Agency. World Fact Book. Retrieved from: https://www.cia.gov/library/publications/resources/the-world-factbook/geos/us.html

Physical Growth

Although many physical changes accompany aging, many older adults are active members of society and have independent lifestyles. Box 21.1 in Chapter 21, Assessment of the Older Adult, lists selected anatomic and physiologic changes associated with this age group.

Behavioral and Cognitive Development

The task of development is to achieve ego integrity with a minimal amount of despair. Ego integrity is achieved when older adults can look back at their lives and accept the course of events and the choices they made as being necessary. Despair may develop with the death of one's spouse and friends, or the adjustment related to retirement. Society is becoming more aware of the presence of ageism and stereotyping of a person because of age. Older adults are encouraging positive attitudes about aging and making society aware of the developmental tasks they experience and the barriers to leading a healthy, happy life in a society that values youth. Ego integrity develops as older adults give back to society and interact with grandchildren (Fig. 18.7).

BOX 18.7 DEVELOPMENTAL TASKS OF MIDDLE ADULTS

- Providing a comfortable and healthful home
- Allocating resources to provide security in later years
- Dividing household responsibilities
- Encouraging both husband and wife roles within and beyond the family
- Maintaining emotional and sexual intimacy
- Incorporating all family members into the family circle as the family enlarges and cares for the extended family
- Participating in activities outside the home
- Developing competencies that maintain family functioning during crises and encourage achievement

From Duvall EM, Miller BC: *Marriage and family development*, ed 6, New York, 1985, Harper & Row.

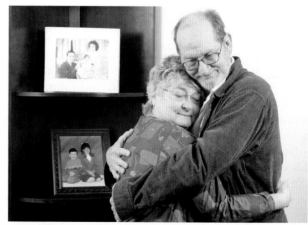

FIG. 18.7 Love and affection are important to older persons. (From Sorrentino and Gorek, 2007.)

Fluid intelligence continues to decline, while crystal intelligence is maintained. Cognitive development in the older adult was reported in a longitudinal study of subjects ranging from 73 to 99 years of age. Researchers found that although many subjects reported some decline in abilities, more than half displayed no decline. A study of 18 people ages 100 to 106 found that these centenarians reported rich late-life learning experiences, the majority of which occurred through social interaction.[4]

Because of the variation between a 65-year old and an 85-year old, old age has been categorized into young-old from ages 65 to 74, middle-old from ages 75 to 84, and old-old as 85 years and older.[14] Developmental tasks with different age groups are identified in Box 18.8. Preventive services recommended for older adults are in Table 18.6 in the column labeled "Over 65 years."

FAMILY DEVELOPMENT

Most individuals in the United States grow up within the social unit of a family. However, the definition and composition of family structures have changed over the years. Families are no longer only the traditional two married heterosexual parents with children who live under one roof. Blended families are composed of stepchildren and children from the current unit. Homosexual couples join as family units, some of which include children. There are single-parent families: some from divorce, some never married, and some formed because of adoption or artificial fertilization. There are also intergenerational families in which multiple generations live together under one roof or in which grandparents or even great-grandparents raise and care for their grandchildren. An Ethnic, Cultural, and Spiritual Variations box describes some cultures in which extended families may be maintained. A *family* is defined as two or more individuals who share bonds of commitment, loyalty, and affection. The family unit typically shares some degree of time, financial, and physical resources and responsibilities for the unit's maintenance (Fig. 18.8). Developmental tasks for the family are summarized in Table 18.7.

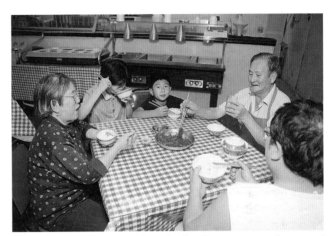

FIG. 18.8 The family unit typically shares some degree of time, financial, and physical resources and responsibilities for the unit's maintenance.

BOX 18.8 DEVELOPMENTAL TASKS OF YOUNG-OLD AND OLD-OLD ADULTS

Young-Old (Approximately 65–85 years)
- Preparing for and adjusting to retirement
- Adjusting to lower and fixed income of retirement
- Establishing physical living arrangements
- Adjusting to new relationships with adult children and their offspring
- Managing leisure time
- Adjusting to slower physical and intellectual responses
- Dealing with the death of parents, spouse, and friends

Old-Old (over 85 years)
- Learning to combine new dependency needs with continued need for independence
- Adapting to living alone
- Accepting and adjusting to possible institutional living
- Establishing affiliation with age group
- Adjusting to increased vulnerability to physical and emotional stress
- Adjusting to loss of physical strength, illness, and approach of one's own death
- Adjusting to losses of spouse, home, and friends

From Touhy T, Jett K: Ebersole and Hess' *Toward healthy aging: human needs & nursing response*, ed 8, St Louis, 2012, Elsevier.

TABLE 18.7 DEVELOPMENTAL TASKS OF THE FAMILY

STAGES	THEMES
Married couple	Without children; establishing satisfying marriage; adjusting to pregnancy; fitting into kin network
Childbearing	Oldest child birth to 30 months; nurturing infants; establishing home
Family with preschoolers	Oldest child 2½–6; adapting to needs of children; decreased energy and privacy as parents
Family with school-age children	Oldest child 6–13; being part of community of school-age families; encouraging educational achievement of children
Family with teenagers	Oldest child 13–20; balancing freedom and responsibility; establishing postparental interests
Family launching young adults	First child gone until last child leaves home; maintaining supportive home base
Middle-age parents	Empty nest to retirement; refocusing on marriage; maintaining kin ties
Aging family members	Retirement to death of both spouses; coping with bereavement; adapting home for aging; adjusting to retirement; living alone

From Duvall EM, Miller BC: *Marriage and family development*, ed 6, New York, 1985, Harper & Row.

In stepfamilies, a biologic parent lives elsewhere, and the children may move between the homes of two biologic families. Virtually all members of a stepfamily sustain primary relationship loss. The parent and stepparents must repeatedly deal with a part-time relationship with the stepchild, if the stepchild is involved with the other biologic parent. The relationship between the adult parents outside of the stepfamily predates the new marriage and the relationship with the stepparent. This can create conflicts and loyalty divisions in parenting strategies, and with the child. Children within a stepfamily struggle with being members of more than one household, whereas stepparents cope with parenting a child to whom they are not related.

In single-parent families, the child lives with one biologic or adoptive parent. In some cases, the child and the single parent sustain a loss from the absent biologic parent of the child. There is great variation in the involvement of the absent parent in the life of the child; some are actively involved, whereas others have minimal to no involvement. Other children may be added to the single-parent family from the same or different biologic parentage. Financial difficulties are a common stressor for single-parent families because only one adult is present to care for the children, maintain the home, and provide for the family.

🌐 ETHNIC, CULTURAL, AND SPIRITUAL VARIATIONS

Cultural Differences Within Families

In many cultures, the extended family is important in the care of children. In African American families, when mothers are unable to provide emotional and physical support for their children, grandmothers, aunts, and extended family members readily provide assistance or take responsibility for the children.

Chinese family members emphasize loyalty to the family and tradition. Personal independence is not valued. Often, children live with grandparents or aunts and uncles so that individual family members can obtain a better education or to reduce financial burden.

Mexican-American families are patriarchal, with some evidence of a slow change to a more egalitarian pattern in recent years. Children are highly valued because they ensure the continuation of the family and cultural values.

Navajo families have separate dwellings but are grouped together by family relationships. The Navajo family unit consists of the nuclear family and relatives such as sisters, aunts, and their female descendants. The elderly play an important role in keeping rituals and instructing children and grandchildren.

From Purnell L: *Transcultural health care: A culturally competent approach*, ed 4, Philadelphia, 2012, F.A. Davis.

GENERATIONAL DIFFERENCES

A generation is approximately 30 years, representing the difference in age between parents and their children. As children grow, they have different experiences from their parents due to multiple factors such as world events, technology, economic, and social shifts. These different experiences give a generation a unique history.[12] Five generations have been identified based on the approximate years of birth (which vary among resources).

- Silent or Traditionalists (born 1925–1945; in 2020 their ages are 75 to 95)
  - Influences: World War II, New Deal, and Korean War. Raised by parents who survived the Great Depression
  - View of money: Save money, pay cash
  - Respect authority. Hard working, Value family/community
- Baby boomers (born 1946–1964; in 2020 their ages are 56 to 74)
  - Post war babies who grew up to be radicals in the 1970s and yuppies in the 1980s.
  - Influences: Civil Rights movement, Vietnam war, sexual revolution, and cold war with Russia
  - View of money: Buy now, pay later
  - Team oriented, strong work ethic, most educated compared with other generations. Highest divorce rate and second marriages in history, value success
- Generation X (born 1965–1981; in 2020 their ages are 39 to 55)
  - Influences: Watergate, energy crisis, dual-income families
  - Latchkey kids, first day care generation, increased divorce rate
  - Self-starters, results driven, strong sense of entitlement, want work/life balance, value time
  - Think globally
- Generation Y or Millennials (born 1982–1996; in 2020 their ages are 24 to 38)
  - Influencers: 9/11 terrorists attack, school shootings
  - Parents protected them from evils of the world, grew up as children of divorce
  - Change using technology (have not lived without computers), value individuality and diversity
  - Open to new ideas, optimistic[15]
- Generation Z or Centennials (born 1997 to today; in 2020 their ages are birth to 23)
  - Influencers: social media, constant connectivity, on-demand entertainment and communication.[16]

CLINICAL APPLICATION AND CLINICAL JUDGMENT

See Appendix B for answers to exercises in this section.

CASE STUDY

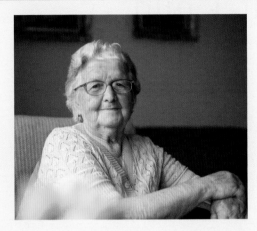

Mrs. Caberra is a 78-year-old woman who is brought to the geriatric clinic by her son and daughter-in-law. Mrs. Caberra's son tells the nurse that his father died 5 months ago and ever since then his mother has "gone downhill." Mr. Caberra indicates that his mother is no longer keeping her house clean or cooking appropriate meals. Her personal hygiene habits have also dramatically changed. She has lost interest in getting her hair done, and she no longer likes to dress for the day. Mr. Caberra tells the nurse, "When I suggest a retirement

home, she becomes very angry and tells me to mind my own business. I'm just worried about Mom, and I want to make sure that someone is taking care of her." During this conversation Mrs. Caberra sits quietly. She interjects only to say, "I've taken care of you, your brother, and your father. Now all of a sudden you think I'm helpless and want to lock me away." Mrs. Caberra appears clean, although her hair is matted and her clothes are badly wrinkled and don't match. Her speech is clear, but her overall affect is very dull. She doesn't make eye contact with her son or the nurse. A physical examination demonstrates expected bodily functioning consistent with her age.

Clinical Judgment

1. List the subjective data described in the case study.
2. List the objective data described in the case study.
3. Which of Erikson's developmental stages is Mrs. Caberra experiencing?
4. Based on what is known from the interview, which developmental tasks of older adults may Mrs. Caberra be struggling with?
5. Which additional assessment data are needed?

REVIEW QUESTIONS

1. Which immunizations does the nurse ask about when interviewing a 75-year-old patient?
   1. Measles, mumps, and rubella
   2. Tetanus and influenza
   3. Hepatitis A and B
   4. Inactivated polio vaccine

2. Which statement reflects an expected developmental task of a 40-year-old man?
   1. "I'll be completing my degree this year, and then I plan to marry my fiancé."
   2. "I'm staying active with plenty of volunteer activities every day of the week."
   3. "My wife and I have divided the chores with the children since we're both working."
   4. "My life is going to be different now that I have more leisure time to enjoy my hobbies."

3. Which finding is expected when assessing an 11-year-old child?
   1. Five-pound (2.3 kg) weight gain and beginning of a growth spurt
   2. Loss of deciduous teeth and eruption of permanent teeth
   3. Development of mature relationships and beginning of dating
   4. Acting out feelings during play and sports

4. A nurse is assessing an infant who is able to pull up to a sitting position, turn from prone to side position, laugh and babble, and show interest in her surroundings. These behaviors are consistent with an infant of which age?
   1. 7 months old
   2. 5 months old
   3. 3 months old
   4. 1 month old

5. A 15-year-old boy approaches the school nurse and describes how uncomfortable he is around the girls because most of them are taller than he is. What is the nurse's best response to this adolescent?
   1. "Let's discuss your diet to determine if you are eating enough nutrients."
   2. "Genetics play an important part in height; if your parents are short, you may be short as well."
   3. "Sleep is necessary for growth. Are you getting adequate sleep?"
   4. "The growth spurt during adolescence occurs in girls 18 to 24 months before it occurs in boys."

Assessment of the Infant, Child, and Adolescent

evolve

http://evolve.elsevier.com/Wilson/assessment

Pediatric nurses care for children from birth through adolescence, making health assessment a unique challenge. To adequately assess children, the nurse considers differences in anatomy and physiology that occur with growth; developmental milestones specific to age; and the psychosocial issues unique to infants, toddlers, preschoolers, school-age children, and adolescents. Pediatric patients are assessed in the context of their family, which adds to the complexity; thus nurses performing pediatric assessments must be skilled at interviewing and observing families, caregivers, and children. In performing the physical examination, the nurse adjusts the approach and techniques to meet the unique needs of each age group. Table 19.1 presents definitions for these age groups.

TABLE 19.1 PEDIATRIC AGE GROUPS

AGE GROUP TERM	AGE RANGE
Neonate/Newborn	Birth–28 days
Infant	1–12 months
Toddler	1–3 years
Preschool	3–5 years
School age	6–12 years
Adolescent	12–18 years

ANATOMY AND PHYSIOLOGY

Children differ anatomically and physiologically from adults in many important ways; generally, the younger the child, the greater these differences. The nurse considers the changing anatomy and physiology as a child grows and matures. Of particular importance are differences that exist at birth, including immaturities of the central nervous system (CNS), respiratory and cardiovascular function, and immune function. These immaturities are evident in such things as heart and respiratory rates, reflexes, infection risks, and pain responses. Differences in anatomy and physiology also place young children at unique risk for certain illnesses, such as otitis media, because of their short, straight eustachian tube. Even the adolescent, who may be adultlike in size and appearance, is still undergoing maturation of body systems, including the reproductive system, the central nervous system, and cognitive function. Box 19.1 summarizes basic variations in anatomy and physiology in infants, children, and adolescents.

HEALTH HISTORY

Nurses interview patients to collect subjective data about their present health and any past medical experiences. The pediatric health history is adapted to the age and developmental level of the child. The basic format of the history is similar to that of the adult, with additional age-specific data collected in the areas of perinatal history, growth and development, and behaviors. In addition, observing the interaction between parent and child throughout the history and examination is important. As in the adult, a complete history is obtained during well-child visits. A more limited, focused history is performed when the child presents with an illness.

BOX 19.1 SELECTED ANATOMIC AND PHYSIOLOGIC DIFFERENCES IN CHILDREN

Skin

- Newborns, especially preterm, have thinner, more permeable skin than older children and adults.
- Newborns and young infants have decreased subcutaneous fat and a large body surface area, which can lead to thermoregulation problems.
- Apocrine sweat glands and sebaceous gland activity increase in adolescents, resulting in oilier skin and acne.

Head

- The cranial bones are soft and not fused at birth. The posterior fontanelle closes by 2 months, and the anterior fontanelle closes by 18 months. This allows for continuing head growth.
- Infants' and small children's heads are larger in proportion to their body.
- The brain and CNS are immature at birth; major development occurs during the first year of life and continues throughout childhood. The immature brain is particularly vulnerable to injury.

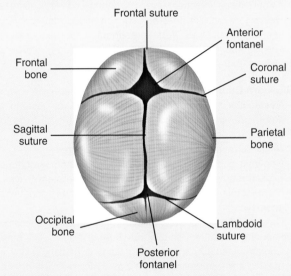

Ears, Nose, Throat, Mouth

- The eustachian tubes are shorter and straighter in infants and young children, increasing their susceptibility to ear infections.
- Newborns and young infants are obligate nose breathers.
- The airway is vulnerable to obstruction because the nasal passages are small, the trachea narrower and less rigid, and the tongue large.

- Twenty deciduous teeth appear between 6 and 24 months of age; permanent teeth begin to erupt at about age 6.

Lungs

- Young infants rely on the diaphragm and abdominal muscles for breathing; the chest wall is thinner and more flexible.
- The respiratory rate is faster in newborns, infants, and young children.

Heart

- Several anatomic shunts are present in the newborn heart, closing shortly after birth.
- The heart rate is faster in infants and young children; the rate frequently increases on inspiration (sinus arrhythmia).
- The heart lies more horizontally in the chest; the PMI is higher (fourth ICS) and more lateral in young infants and toddlers.
- Innocent murmurs are common throughout childhood.

Musculoskeletal

- Bones are softer in children, making them more vulnerable to fractures.
- Infants and young toddlers are usually bowlegged; preschoolers and young school-age children are often "knock-kneed."

Lymph System

- Lymph tissue increases during childhood, reaching a peak between 6 and 9 years. Children at this age often have large tonsils.

Neurologic

- Major growth of the nervous system occurs during the first year of life; motor control develops in a cephalocaudal direction, from head to trunk to extremities.
- Primitive reflexes are present at birth and disappear in a predictable pattern throughout early infancy.
- Infants, including preterm infants, perceive and react to pain. This pain response is manifested primarily by physiologic changes (heart rate, blood pressure, oxygen saturation).

Breasts

- Breasts remain undeveloped until the onset of puberty.

Reproductive System

- Genitalia of males and females do not undergo development until the onset of puberty.

CNS, Central nervous system; *ICS,* intercostal space; *PMI,* point of maximum impulse.
Image from Duderstadt K: *Pediatric physical examination: an illustrated handbook,* St. Louis, 2006, Mosby.

Much of the pediatric history is obtained from the parent (or other adult) accompanying the child, and including the child as much as appropriate for his or her age is important (Fig. 19.1). After the parent's concerns are explored, additional health history questions can be asked directly to school-age children and adolescents using language and concepts appropriate to their age. Giving adolescents an opportunity to talk with the nurse without a parent present

is important. In many states, adolescents have a legal right to confidential care for specific problems, including sexually transmitted infections, contraception, pregnancy, mental health issues, and substance abuse. For these reasons the adolescent should be given an opportunity to discuss these issues privately. The American Medical Association's *Guidelines for Adolescent Preventive Services* (GAPS)[1] includes health history questionnaires that can be completed by adolescents and

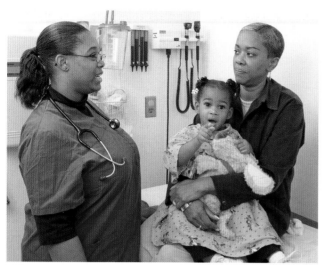

FIG. 19.1 Most data are obtained from the adult accompanying the child.

their parents. These forms provide a valuable first step in data collection for this age group.

COMPONENTS OF THE PEDIATRIC HEALTH HISTORY

Biographic Data

In addition to the information included in the adult history (name, gender, age, date of birth, race, and culture), biographic data also include the name of the person giving the history (the informant) and that person's relationship to the child. Also inquire if there is a nickname the child is accustomed to.

Reason for Seeking Health Care

Record the reason for the visit in the words of the parent or child/adolescent, documenting which person provided data. Many pediatric visits are for well-child care. If this is the case, record the reason for the visit (e.g., "6-month well-child care") and appropriateness of the visit based upon the American Academy of Pediatrics recommended child health visit schedule. If the child is seen for acute or chronic illnesses, the reason for the visit is often a symptom (e.g., "cough and runny nose × 10 days"). The reason for seeking care should be brief (i.e., no more than a sentence or two).

History of Present Illness

The history of present illness is recorded in the same way as for the adult. The nurse records a complete symptom analysis when an illness is present using the mnemonic OLD CARTS, which includes the *O*nset, *L*ocation, *D*uration, *C*haracteristics, *A*ggravating factors, *R*elated symptoms, *T*reatment, and *S*everity (see Box 2.6). In addition, important data to include are questions related to changes in sleeping, eating, and elimination patterns of the infant or child because these changes offer important clues regarding the severity of the illness. A history of present illness is not included in a well visit.

Present Health Status

As in the adult history, the nurse asks the parents or accompanying adult about the child's health conditions, including chronic illnesses such as asthma. In addition, the nurse asks about medications including over the counter and herbal medications the child is taking and allergies the child has experienced to medications, foods, and environmental triggers.

Past Health History

For newborns, infants, and children age 2 and under, the past health history includes the mother's health during the course of the pregnancy and information about the birth and neonatal period. Collectively these data are referred to as the perinatal history and are presented in Box 19.2. The perinatal history may also be important for older children with congenital problems or other problems that may be related to pregnancy or birth complications (e.g., fetal alcohol syndrome or cerebral palsy). Also included in the past health history is a developmental history, which details the age of achievement for major developmental milestones. Specific questions asked depend on the age and developmental level of the child. Chapter 18 presents further information regarding developmental assessment and milestones.

Other components of the past health history are similar to the adult history and include a summary of childhood illnesses; chronic illnesses and treatments; hospitalizations and surgeries; accidents or injuries; and the dates of the last medical, vision, and dental care. Particularly important in pediatric health care is the immunization history, which should be reviewed at every well-child visit and each visit for acute illness. The immunization schedule is presented in Table 18.6.

Family History

The health history of three generations are documented, including the child and any siblings, the parents, and both sets of grandparents. The ages and health status of all family members are recorded, with particular attention to congenital problems, infant and child deaths, and hereditary illnesses. As in the adult, a family history of chronic illness (including diabetes, cardiovascular disease, malignancy, or mental health disorders) is noted. Smoking among family members and problems with alcohol or substance abuse are particularly important to note.

Personal and Psychosocial History

An overview of the child's current level of function and data about social and family relationships, behaviors and health habits, and mental health is obtained. With young children these data are collected primarily from the parent. As children reach adolescence, sensitive parts of the history should be obtained without the parent present. This provides the adolescent with the opportunity to give a confidential history and discuss issues privately.

Personal Status

Ask the parent to describe the child's personality and temperament. Engage older children (over age 6) in a conversation about how they think their life is going, things they like about themselves, and things they do well or not so well. Determine if the school-age child is in an age-appropriate grade and if there are any issues related to school performance and attendance pattern. Ask about personal habits and behavior patterns such as nail biting, thumb sucking, rituals (e.g., "security blanket" or toy), and unusual behaviors (e.g., head banging, rocking, overt masturbation, walking on toes). Also ask for a description of the child's typical day.

Family and Social Relationships

A comprehensive pediatric history includes assessment of social relationships, including family and friends.

Family composition. Ask about individuals who live in the home and their relationship to the child, the primary caregiver(s) in the family, recent changes in family composition and health, family members or other important persons who interact frequently with the child but live outside the home (noncustodial parents, grandparents, other extended family, nannies, or day care providers). Inquiring about pets in the home is important, because pet dander (hair, skin cells, and feathers) can cause allergic symptoms in children and exacerbate allergic disorders.

Family life. Ask questions about family activities, impact of culture on family, parenting style and skills, discipline methods and their effectiveness, family rules, child care arrangements, parent and family support system, family conflict or chaos, family violence.

Family socioeconomic status. Parents should be asked about their occupation and employment; sources of income, including government assistance (Medicaid, food stamps, the Special Supplemental Nutrition Program for Women, Infants, and Children [WIC]); insurance coverage; history of homelessness or unstable living arrangements; ability of parents to meet child's basic physical needs (food, shelter, clothing, medical care, supervision).

Friends. The history also includes the child's relationships with friends, classmates, and siblings; ages of friends; ability to make friends easily; activities shared with friends; history of bullying or being bullied; fighting; violence among peers. Adolescents should be asked specifically about peers, gang activity and violence in their school and peer group, engagement with social media, dating, and sexual activity.

Diet and Nutrition

When taking a diet history, inquire about the typical daily diet, intolerances or allergies, supplements (particularly vitamin D for breast-fed infants), family mealtime routines, snacks, and any concerns of the parent or child about diet or weight. For newborns and infants, determine the type (breast or formula) and amount/frequency of feeding in 24 hours, age of introduction of solid foods (cereal, fruits, vegetables, meats, eggs) and other liquids (e.g., water, juice, cow's milk). Note excess intake of milk or juice, which may impact appetite and decrease the intake of more nutritious foods. Also inquire about the use of bottles for dietary intake (for infants and toddlers) and the transfer to the use of a cup and discontinuation of bottle use.

The diet history of children should include a description of the typical diet, including any diet restrictions that may place them at risk for nutritional deficiencies. Ask about habits that increase the risk for dental caries (e.g., constant sipping of milk or juice, consumption of soda and sweet and sticky foods). Assess where most meals are eaten (at home, school, or in restaurants) and identify children who frequently consume "fast food," "junk food," and sweet drinks. Adolescents should be asked specifically about their perception of their current weight and behaviors associated with eating disorders, including food restrictions, extreme diet/exercise routines, binging or purging, and the use of laxatives. Adequate calcium and iron intake should also be evaluated. Adequate calcium intake in childhood and adolescence supports healthy bone development. Menstruating teens are at risk for anemia, especially if their iron intake is deficient.

BOX 19.3 **CLINICAL NOTE**

Sudden infant death syndrome prevention strategies include sleeping in the supine position ("back to sleep") on a firm surface. Also recommended are using a pacifier at bedtime, avoiding pillows or other soft objects in the crib, and having infants sleep in their own bed in the parents' room.

From Moon RY: SIDS and other sleep-related infant deaths: expansion of recommendations for a safe infant sleeping environment, *Pediatrics* 128(5):e1341–e1367, 2011.

Sleep

The pediatric sleep history includes where and with whom the child sleeps; total amount of sleep, including naps; bedtime rituals; difficulty falling or staying asleep; and nightmares or night terrors. Parents should be asked about the sleep position of newborns and infants and the sleep environment (Box 19.3).

Mental Health

Many factors that can impact mental health will have been previously noted in either the past health history (maternal substance abuse in pregnancy, perinatal hypoxia, neurologic illness or injury) or the social history (e.g., developmental delays, family problems, body image disturbances, witnessed violence). The mental health history should explore the impact of these problems on the child, identify past psychiatric history, explore current stresses in the child's life, and identify signs and symptoms of mental health conditions. Questions should include frequent sense of boredom, suicidal thoughts or attempts, symptoms of depression or anxiety, and risk-taking behaviors (e.g., drug or alcohol use, fighting, risky sexual behaviors, school failure or truancy). Adolescents should be asked specifically about peers, bullying, gang activity and violence in their schools and peer groups, and alcohol and drug use. Determine the child's usual ability to cope with stress and any recent changes in coping, mood, or behavior. Asking children to identify to whom they can talk about problems in their lives is also important. Children who have poor coping skills, multiple stressors, do not have a trusted adult in their lives, and those who engage in multiple risk-taking behaviors are at particular risk for mental health issues. Note that the nurse's duty to maintain confidentiality ends when children or adolescents reveal that they are a danger to themselves or others.

The Pediatric Symptom Checklist (PSC)[2] can be used to identify parental concerns about behavioral and emotional issues in children ages 4 to 18. A second version of the form, the PSC Youth Report, is available for self-reporting of symptoms by older children and adolescents (Fig. 19.2). GAPS Questionnaires[1] (described previously) are also useful components of an adolescent mental health history.

Sexuality

Ask about pubertal changes, which occur earlier in girls than in boys. Girls should be asked about the age of menarche,

menstruation, including their last menstrual period and the frequency and duration of menses. Teenage males should be asked about testicular changes and self-examination. Teens should be asked privately about sexual activity. Questions about sexuality should be approached with great sensitivity, and the nurse must not make assumptions about sexual orientation. The sexually active adolescent should be evaluated for risk of pregnancy and/or sexually transmitted infections. Determining if sexual activity is consensual and whether coercion or force is involved is important and should be documented. See Chapter 17 for a complete discussion of the menstrual and sexual history.

A related contemporary topic for providers to consider when discussing sexuality in children and adolescents is one of commercial sexual exploitation of children (CSEC) or domestic minor sex trafficking (DMST). Assessment of children and adolescents should include elements of history taking that, when combined, lead to a heightened level of concern. For example, the Commercial Sexual Exploitation Identification Tool (CSE-IT) is a valid instrument designed for health care providers that outlines eight elements of a health history and physical exam that impact the level of concern about sexual exploitation of child/adolescent.[3] The index of suspicion of sexual exploitation is raised when vulnerable children experience instability in their housing or caregiving, report trauma or sexual abuse, have notable changes in their physical appearance or health, report activities or experiences in places where exploitation frequently occurs, or when vulnerable youth are with controlling partners or "caregivers."

Children are said to experience gender identification at a young age; many publications indicating that this occurs at 3 to 5 years of age. Children who experience gender dysphoria or incongruence between their experienced gender and their biologic sex are at increased risk of being the target of bullying and mental health problems. Therefore during a comprehensive physical examination parents should be asked questions related to gender identification, such as when playing make believe or "dress up" does your child prefer toys, games, or activities stereotypically used by the other gender? Asking questions such as these heightens parents' awareness of the process of gender identification and that this occurs at a young age.

Development

An accurate developmental history is based on the child's age as well as skills or tasks each performs. When a child is born prematurely, his or her "corrected age" must be determined, otherwise the infant may be identified as having developmental delays. For example, an infant born 8 weeks prematurely, the calculated age is determined by making an 8-week adjustment for the first 3 years. When the infant is 4 months of age, the corrected age would be 2 months and the child should be expected to perform activities appropriate for a 2-month-old infant. To assess the current developmental stage of infants and children, the nurse asks parents about new skills since the last well-child visit and achievement of

Pediatric Symptom Checklist (PSC)

Emotional and physical health go together in children. Because parents are often the first to notice a problem with their child's behavior, emotions, or learning, you may help your child get the best care possible by answering these questions. Please indicate which statement best describes your child.

Please mark under the heading that best describes your child:

	NEVER	SOMETIMES	OFTEN
1. Complains of aches and pains ... 1			
2. Spends more time alone ... 2			
3. Tires easily, has little energy ... 3			
4. Fidgety, unable to sit still ... 4			
5. Has trouble with teacher ... 5			
6. Less interested in school ... 6			
7. Acts as if driven by a motor ... 7			
8. Daydreams too much ... 8			
9. Distracted easily ... 9			
10. Is afraid of new situations ... 10			
11. Feels sad, unhappy ... 11			
12. Is irritable, angry ... 12			
13. Feels hopeless ... 13			
14. Has trouble concentrating ... 14			
15. Less interested in friends ... 15			
16. Fights with other children ... 16			
17. Absent from school ... 17			
18. School grades dropping ... 18			
19. Is down on himself or herself ... 19			
20. Visits the doctor with doctor finding nothing wrong ... 20			
21. Has trouble sleeping ... 21			
22. Worries a lot ... 22			
23. Wants to be with you more than before ... 23			
24. Feels he or she is bad ... 24			
25. Takes unnecessary risks ... 25			
26. Gets hurt frequently ... 26			
27. Seems to be having less fun ... 27			
28. Acts younger than children his or her age ... 28			
29. Does not listen to rules ... 29			
30. Does not show feelings ... 30			
31. Does not understand other people's feelings ... 31			
32. Teases others ... 32			
33. Blames others for his or her troubles ... 33			
34. Takes things that do not belong to him or her ... 34			
35. Refuses to share ... 35			

Total score _____

Does your child have any emotional or behavioral problems for which she/he needs help? ( ) N   ( ) Y
Are there any services that you would like your child to receive for these problems?   ( ) N   ( ) Y

If yes, what
services? _____

FIG. 19.2 Pediatric symptom checklist and pediatric symptom checklist youth report. (Jellinek et al., 1994.)

Continued

Pediatric Symptom Checklist - Youth Report (Y-PSC)

Please mark under the heading that best fits you:

	Never	Sometimes	Often
1. Complain of aches or pains	____	____	____
2. Spend more time alone	____	____	____
3. Tire easily, little energy	____	____	____
4. Fidgety, unable to sit still	____	____	____
5. Have trouble with teacher	____	____	____
6. Less interested in school	____	____	____
7. Act as if driven by motor	____	____	____
8. Daydream too much	____	____	____
9. Distract easily	____	____	____
10. Are afraid of new situations	____	____	____
11. Feel sad, unhappy	____	____	____
12. Are irritable, angry	____	____	____
13. Feel hopeless	____	____	____
14. Have trouble concentrating	____	____	____
15. Less interested in friends	____	____	____
16. Fight with other children	____	____	____
17. Absent from school	____	____	____
18. School grades dropping	____	____	____
19. Down on yourself	____	____	____
20. Visit doctor with doctor finding nothing wrong	____	____	____
21. Have trouble sleeping	____	____	____
22. Worry a lot	____	____	____
23. Want to be with parent more than before	____	____	____
24. Feel that you are bad	____	____	____
25. Take unnecessary risks	____	____	____
26. Get hurt frequently	____	____	____
27. Seem to be having less fun	____	____	____
28. Act younger than children your age	____	____	____
29. Do not listen to rules	____	____	____
30. Do not show feelings	____	____	____
31. Do not understand other people's feelings	____	____	____
32. Tease others	____	____	____
33. Blame others for your troubles	____	____	____
34. Take things that do not belong to you	____	____	____
35. Refuse to share	____	____	____

FIG. 19.2, cont'd

specific age-related milestones. For example, ask the parent of a 5-year-old if the child is able to dress self, jump rope, identify colors, and follow rules when playing games—all of which are expected developmental achievements in a 5-year-old. Asking about school performance is another key component of developmental assessment. Include current grade level, any special educational needs, school problems, and truancy. Adolescents should be asked about future school and career plans.

Health Promotion Activities

To assess health habits, ask about oral health; smoking; exercise; hobbies; and other activities, including the amount of "screen time" (e.g., television, computer, tablet, and cell phone) per day. Also evaluate the use of safety measures, including car seats, sunscreen, and bicycle helmets/sports equipment.

Home Environment

Inquire about characteristics of the home, including facilities (heat, running water, cooking facilities, adequate space, sleeping arrangements) and home safety (child-proofing; storage of firearms, medications, and chemicals; animals in the home; pool safety); characteristics of the community (available resources, crime, pollution, overcrowding, safety hazards). Teens should be questioned about employment during non-academic time.

Review of Systems

The review of systems for the infant, child, and adolescent is similar to that for an adult. The goal is to elicit symptoms and problems from the parent or caregiver that may not have been identified earlier in the history. Critical components of the review of systems in pediatrics include:

General Symptoms

- *Constitutional symptoms:* Fever, chills, night sweats, fatigue, tiring with feeding (infants), change in energy level or activity tolerance
- *Growth:* Unusual weight gain or loss; concerns about height, weight, or head size
- *Pain:* Symptoms or signs of pain in infants and toddlers or older children using age-appropriate pictorial pain scales (Figs. 19.3 and 19.4) or numeric pain scales, such as the Numeric Rating Scale—11 (Fig. 19.5)[4]

Skin, Hair, Nails

- *Skin:* Jaundice (newborn); rashes, birthmarks, or lesions; easy bruising; petechiae; itching; dry skin; acne (adolescents); piercings and tattoos (older children and adolescents)
- *Hair:* Infestations (such as lice), hair loss, seborrhea (infants)
- *Nails:* Nail changes; nail biting; ingrown or painful nails

Head, Eyes, Ears, Nose, and Throat

- *Head:* Concerns about head size or shape (newborns, infants); headaches; recent trauma

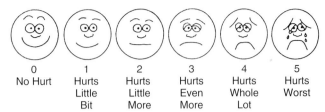

FIG. 19.3 Wong-baker FACES pain rating scale. Recommended for children 3 years of age and older. Ask the child to choose the face that best describes how he or she is feeling. (Copyright 1983, Wong-Baker FACES ® Foundation, www.WongBakerFACES.org. Used with permission. Originally published in Whaley & Wong's Nursing Care of Infants and Children. ©Elsevier Inc.)

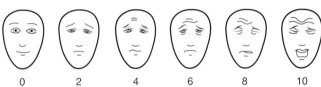

FIG. 19.4 Faces pain scale-revised (FPS-R). Recommended for children 6 years and older. **Directions for use:** These faces show how much something can hurt. This face (point to left-most face) shows no pain. The faces show more and more pain (point to each from left to right) up to this one (point to right-most face), which shows very much pain. Point to the face that shows how much you hurt (right now). (From Spagrud LJ, Piira T, von Baeyer CL: Children's self-report of pain intensity: The Faces Pain Scale—Revised, *Am J Nurs* 03[12]:62–64, 2003.)

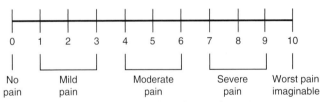

FIG. 19.5 Numeric rating scale—11.

- *Eyes:* Visual concerns, including not fixing on objects or following with both eyes (newborns, infants), reading difficulty, sitting too close to television or computer screen, bumping into things; redness, drainage, or crusting; itching or pain; abnormal eye movement or alignment
- *Ears:* Hearing concerns, including not responding to sound (newborns, infants), unusual vocalizations (infants), loud speech or loud television, child's complaint of decreased hearing, ear pain, discharge
- *Nose:* Congestion, drainage, frequent nosebleeds, snoring
- *Mouth/throat:* Teeth (tooth pain, tooth loss, caries); mouth pain or lesions; unusual coatings of tongue or mouth; throat pain; difficulty swallowing; voice changes
- *Neck:* Lymph node enlargement, swelling or masses in neck, stiff neck, unusual head/neck position

RISK FACTORS
Congenital or Perinatal Hearing Loss

Neonatal Risk Factors (Birth to 1 Month)
- Family history of congenital sensorineural hearing loss (SNHL)
- In utero infections associated with SNHL (herpes, syphilis, rubella, cytomegalovirus, or toxoplasmosis)
- Low Apgar scores at birth (0–3 at 5 min; 0–6 at 10 min)
- Birth weight less than 1500 g
- Respiratory distress at birth or need for mechanical ventilation for more than 10 days
- Presence of ear or other craniofacial malformations
- Severe hyperbilirubinemia
- Bacterial meningitis
- Administration of ototoxic medications for more than 5 days (or used in combination with loop diuretics)

Infant Risk Factors (1–24 Months)
- Any of the neonatal risk factors listed previously
- Recurrent otitis media with effusion for at least 3 months
- Infections associated with SNHL (meningitis, mumps, measles)
- Head trauma involving fracture of the temporal bone

From Wroblewska-Seniuk KE, Dabrowski P, Szyfter W, Mazela J: University newborn hearing screening: methods and results, obstacles, and benefits, *Pediatr Res Mar* 81(3):415–422, 2017; From The Joint Committee on Infant Hearing: Year 2007 position statement: principles and guidelines for early hearing detection and intervention programs, *Pediatrics* 120(4):898–921, 2007.

RISK FACTORS
Otitis Media

- Age: peak incidence 6–12 months
- Group child care (M)
- Bottle-fed infant (M)
- Use of a pacifier (M)
- Poor air quality: exposure to tobacco smoke, air pollution
- Cold weather
- History of allergies

M, Modifiable risk factor.

Breasts
- Breast engorgement (newborns of both sexes); breast changes (school age and adolescents); pain; unilateral breast changes; and any unexpected sequential development (see Fig. 19.42 later in chapter).

Respiratory System
- Cough; wheezing or noisy breathing; shortness of breath at rest or with activity; nighttime snoring; increased respiratory rate or effort

Cardiovascular
- Cyanosis or pallor; edema; known murmur or cardiovascular disease; syncope

Gastrointestinal System
- Usual pattern of bowel movements; changes in bowel function, including constipation and diarrhea; abdominal pain; nausea; vomiting; change in appetite

Urinary System
- Number of wet diapers per day (newborns, infants, toddlers); toilet training progress; bedwetting or daytime accidents in a previously toilet-trained child; signs of urinary tract infection (dysuria, urgency, frequency, foul odor); hematuria

Reproductive System
Questions need to be at an appropriate level based on the child's/teen's developmental and cognitive maturity.
- Boys: Healing of circumcision (newborns), rash or irritation, penile discharge, pain, itching, development of secondary sexual characteristics, testicular masses, trauma
- Girls: Rash, discharge, menstrual concerns (dysmenorrhea, irregular menses, heavy bleeding, amenorrhea)

Musculoskeletal System
- Asymmetric movement; poor muscle tone (newborns/infants); pain in joints or muscles; deformity or asymmetry; range-of-motion limitations; muscle or joint trauma; curvature of the spine; concerns about legs or feet (e.g., bow-legged, intoeing, limp)

Neurologic System
- Unusual and/or high-pitched cry; irritability; speech problems (stuttering, articulation, language delay or loss of previously attained language skills); fainting or dizziness; seizures; difficulty with coordination or gait, repeated and/or jerky movements.

EXAMINATION

Because the process and findings associated with infant, child, and adolescent examinations vary, the presentation of the examination is organized by age group (with the exception of vital signs and baseline measurements, which are presented across age groups). For each age group a separate discussion of examination issues and techniques is provided for each body system. Perform hand hygiene before beginning the examination.

Equipment needed: Thermometer, watch with second hand, pediatric stethoscope, pediatric blood pressure cuff, device to measure height, scale, tape measure, ophthalmoscope, otoscope with pneumatic attachment, penlight, tongue blade, examination gloves, pulse oximeter, and reflex hammer. For vision screening of toddlers use LEA symbols or HOTV letters; for children 3 to 6 years use Snellen E, for children 7 to 8 years use standard Snellen chart. Use Ishihara color blind test as needed. Use opaque card for cover-uncover test.

VITAL SIGNS AND BASELINE MEASUREMENTS

Vital signs are measured at every visit using appropriately sized instruments (i.e., blood pressure cuff) and processes.

Temperature

Procedure. The recommended approaches for temperature measurement in newborns, infants, and children up to age 5 are axillary, tympanic membrane (TM), and temporal artery sites. Oral measurement using an electronic thermometer is permissible with older children, but the nurse must be sure that the probe is held correctly in the mouth (thermometer under the tongue with the mouth closed). To take a tympanic measurement in a child younger than 3 years of age, pull down on the earlobe to straighten the ear canal. For children older than 3, pull up on the ear to straighten the canal. Research has shown that tympanic measurements in children may be unreliable, possibly due to errors in technique in which the sensor beam is directed at the sides of the ear canal rather than at the TM.[5,6] To take a temporal artery measurement, the nurse places a disposable cover on the probe and then places the probe on the center of the child's forehead. After depressing the scan button, the nurse slides the probe across the forehead into the hairline and behind the ear while keeping the probe in contact with the skin. When the scan button is released, the temperature illuminates on the screen.

Rectal temperatures should be taken as a last resort for routine assessments because children tend to fear intrusive procedures and because of the risk for rectal perforation. However, this is the preferred method of assessment in febrile children. A convenient position for taking a rectal temperature is with the child in a side-lying position with knees flexed toward the abdomen. This position is maintained with one of the nurse's hands while the lubricated thermometer is held in the rectum a maximum of 2.5 cm (less in newborns and young infants). See Chapter 4 for additional discussion of techniques.

Expected and abnormal findings. The temperature of infants, children, and adolescents should be similar to that of the adult (98.6°F or 37°C). However, temperature variations may be found in newborns because they have less effective heat-control mechanisms. Elevated temperatures among infants, children, and adolescents are often related to viral or bacterial infections, dehydration, and environmental exposure to heat. Low body temperature is commonly associated with environmental exposure or inability to self-regulate temperature, and requires additional clothing.

Heart and Respiratory Rates

Procedure. Heart and respiratory rates are assessed for the same qualities as in the adult (heart and respiratory rhythm; depth of respiration). This assessment should take place when the infant or child is quiet, using a pediatric stethoscope. The nurse listens to the apical pulse for a full minute and counts the respirations before proceeding to other parts of the assessment.

Respiratory rates are counted using inspection in the same way as for adults; however, infants and young children usually breathe diaphragmatically, which requires observation of abdominal movement. Respirations are counted for a full minute because an infant's respiratory rate may be irregular as a normal variation.

Expected and abnormal findings. Expected heart and respiratory rates for infants and children are listed in Table 19.2. Elevations in heart and respiratory rates are commonly seen with crying, fever, respiratory distress, and dehydration. A decreased heart rate is also abnormal and is often an ominous sign indicating a serious condition.

Blood Pressure

Blood pressure measurement should occur with every health visit for all children over the age of 3.[7] For an accurate blood pressure reading, the nurse must use the appropriate cuff size. The cuff size is determined by arm circumference measured at the middle of the arm (Table 19.3). Childhood obesity is common and may require the use of a larger cuff size. Measurements may be taken in the arm or leg of infants and younger children. Blood pressure standards for children ages 1 through 17 are based on gender, age, and height (see Table 19.2). Blood pressure tables that include both systolic and diastolic blood pressures according to blood pressure percentiles are available from the National Heart Lung and Blood Institute.[7] Although not common, hypertension can develop in childhood and adolescence; thus the differentiation of two terms, prehypertension and hypertension, is worth noting. *Hypertension* in children is defined as average

TABLE 19.2 **AVERAGE PEDIATRIC VITAL SIGNS**				
VITAL SIGN	NEWBORN	TODDLER	SCHOOL-AGE CHILD	ADOLESCENT
Heart Rate (beats/min)				
• Range	120–160	90–140	75–100	60–90
• Average	140	110	85	70
Respiratory Rate (breaths/min)	30–60	24–40	18–30	12–16
Blood Pressure (mm Hg)				
• Systolic range	60–90	80–112	84–120	94–139
• Diastolic range	20–60	50–80	54–80	62–88

TABLE 19.3 CUFF SIZES FOR PEDIATRIC BLOOD PRESSURE	
ARM CIRCUMFERENCE (cm)[a]	**NAME/SIZE OF CUFF**
5–7.5	Newborn (4 × 8 cm)
7.5–13	Infant (6 × 12 cm)
13–20	Child (9 × 18 cm)
22–26	Small adult (12 × 22 cm)

[a]Measured at middle of arm.

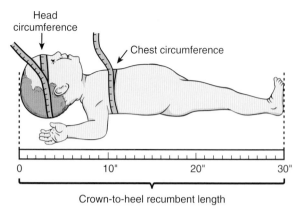

FIG. 19.6 Measurement of head and chest circumference and recumbent length. (Redrawn from Hockenberry et al., 2003.)

systolic blood pressure (SBP) and/or diastolic blood pressure (DBP) that is greater than or equal to the 95th percentile for gender, age, and height on three or more occasions. Any child whose SBP or DBP is 5 mm above the 99th percentile and is symptomatic (chest pain, shortness of breath, palpitations) needs immediate referral. *Prehypertension* in children is defined as average SBP or DBP levels that are greater than or equal to the 90th percentile but less than the 95th percentile on three or more occasions. As with adults, adolescents with blood pressure levels between 120/80 and 130/90 should be considered prehypertensive.[7]

Height and Weight

Routine height and weight measurements are taken during all visits until the end of the growth spurt between the ages of 18 and 20 and are plotted on a growth chart to allow tracking of the child's growth in comparison with the population standard. Different growth charts are used as infants begin to stand for this assessment. Growth charts for infants through adolescence are available on the Centers for Disease Control and Prevention website (www.cdc.gov). Body mass index (BMI) should be calculated on all children beginning at age 2 and recorded as the BMI percentile for age to allow for early recognition of weight-related issues. Obesity is a significant issue in childhood and is associated with the later development of chronic diseases such as Type 2 diabetes mellitus, hypertension, and heart disease.[8]

Height

Procedure. Recumbent length of newborns, infants, and young children is measured from the top of the head to the heel with the infant in a supine position (Fig. 19.6). The length is recorded in inches or centimeters.

Devices such as measuring mats or boards can be used to measure recumbent length. An infant measuring mat consists of a soft rubber graduated mat attached to a plastic head and footboard. The infant lies on the mat with the head against the headboard. The infant's knees are held together and pressed gently against the mat with one hand while the footboard is moved against the heels. A measuring board has a rigid headboard and a movable footboard. It is placed on a table, and the infant lies on the board so the head touches the headboard. The footboard is then moved until it touches the bottom of the infant's feet.

To measure the height of a child who can stand but is too short for the adult scale, the nurse uses a platform with a

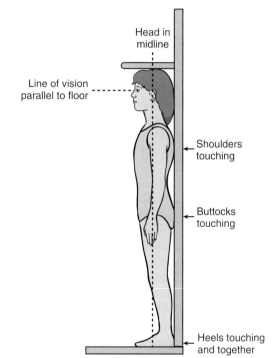

FIG. 19.7 Measurement of height using a platform with movable headboard.

movable headboard. The child stands erect on the platform, and the headboard is lowered until it touches the child's head (Fig. 19.7). A tape measure also can be attached to a wall so the child's height can be measured by having the child stand against the wall; however, this is a gross method of measurement and not considered accurate.

Expected and abnormal findings. Growth is plotted on the Centers for Disease Control growth charts and used to evaluate changes in growth since last visit and also to make comparisons with the general population of children of the same age. Growth during childhood is continuous, but uneven. Growth spurts typically occur during infancy and adolescence. Measures that fall outside the 5th or 95th percentile for age, or wide differences in percentiles between height and weight (e.g., 90th percentile for height and 10th percentile for

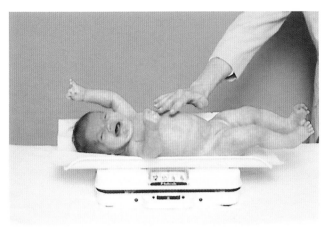

FIG. 19.8 Weighing an infant on an infant scale. (From Hockenberry and Wilson, 2011.)

weight), are considered abnormal findings. Steady growth that suddenly stops is also an abnormal finding.

Weight

Procedure. The platform scale is used for weighing newborns, infants, and small children (Fig. 19.8). The scale has curved sides to prevent the infant from rolling off. A paper is placed on the scale, and the unclothed and undiapered newborn is laid on the paper. The weight is recorded in kilograms or pounds and ounces to the nearest 0.5 oz. A standard scale is used for children who can stand independently on a standard scale.

Expected and abnormal findings. Healthy newborns typically weigh between 5 lb 8 oz and 8 lb 13 oz (2500 and 4000 g). Newborns may lose up to 10% of their birth weight in the first few days of life but should regain it in 10 to 14 days. A greater than expected weight loss or a slower than expected weight gain requires further evaluation. In general, infants double their birth weight by 4 to 6 months of age and triple it by 12 months of age.

EXAMINATION OF NEWBORNS AND INFANTS

In general, the nurse should conduct the physical examination of young infants (<6 months) on an examination table. For the older infant (>6 months) the nurse may find that having the caregiver hold the baby decreases fear and distress, thus making it easier for the nurse to conduct the examination.

The nurse should undress the infant completely for examination, keeping the diaper in place until the buttocks and genitalia are examined. Care must be taken to ensure that the infant remains warm during the examination period. The nurse prevents excessive chilling by keeping the room warm and covering areas of the infant not being examined. If the infant becomes chilled, the skin, hands, and feet may take on a transient mottling (blotching or marbling) appearance.

Unlike the physical examination in adults, which for the most part proceeds in a head-to-toe sequence, the physical examination of an infant requires that the nurse conduct the least invasive portions of the examination before proceeding to the more invasive components. The nurse should observe the infant for any signs of distress and while the baby is quiet, auscultate heart and lungs, palpate fontanels, pulses, and abdomen saving the musculoskeletal, ear, and oral examination (more invasive procedures) for last.

Skin, Hair, and Nails

No special procedures are necessary when inspecting or palpating the skin, hair, and nails other than keeping the young infant warm during the examination.

Skin

Expected findings. The skin color of the neonate (a newborn immediately after birth) depends partially on the amount of fat present. Preterm infants generally appear redder because they have less subcutaneous fat than full-term infants. In addition, the neonate may appear to have a red skin tone for a short period because of vasomotor instability. This color tends to fade within the first few days. In addition, immediately following birth the neonate's lips, nail beds, and feet may be dusky or appear cyanotic. Once the newborn is adequately warmed, the dusky color should fade, and a well-oxygenated pink tone should appear. Dark-skinned newborns should also have a dark pink tone, which is most evident on the palms of the hands and the soles of the feet. Physiologic jaundice may be present in the newborn between the second and fifth day of life. The skin, mucous membranes, and sclerae may appear to have a yellow tone. This normal phenomenon occurs in almost half of all newborns and is secondary to the increased number of red blood cells that hemolyze following birth[9] and may be accentuated with the mild dehydration that often occurs initially with breastfeeding.

Common primary skin lesions among newborns that are normal variations include the following:
- *Milia:* Small, whitish papules that may be found on the cheeks, nose, chin, and forehead of newborns (Fig. 19.9). These are benign and generally disappear by the third week of life.
- *Erythema toxicum:* A self-limited, benign rash of unknown etiology consisting of erythematous macules, papules, and pustules (Fig. 19.10). The rash may appear anywhere on the body except the palms of the hands and the soles of the feet. Although it may be present at birth, it usually appears by the third or fourth day of life.

Birthmarks in newborns may be pigmentation or vascular variations. Common birthmarks that are considered normal variations include:
- *Congenital dermal melanocytosis (Mongolian spot):* An irregularly shaped, darkened flat area commonly found over the sacrum and buttocks (Fig. 19.11). They are most prevalent in African American, Hispanic, Native American, and Asian children and often disappear by the time the child is 1 or 2 years of age.
- *Café-au-lait spot:* A large round or oval patch of light brown pigmentation that is generally present at birth (Fig. 19.12). Occasionally these spots may be associated with neurofibromatosis (a genetic disorder associated with tumor growth within the nervous system).

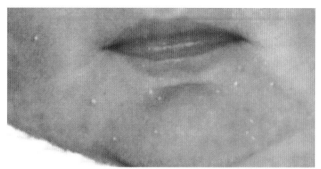

FIG. **19.9** Milia on the face of infant. (From Gleason and Juul, 2018.)

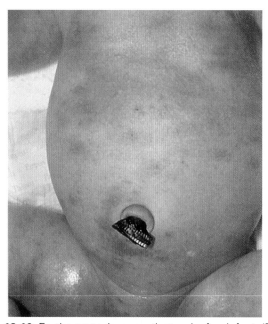

FIG. **19.10** Erythema toxicum on the trunk of an infant. (From Zitelli and Davis, 2018.)

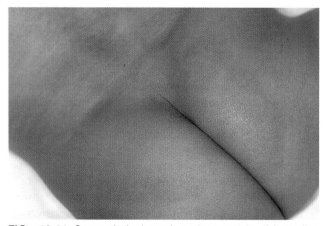

FIG. **19.11** Congenital dermal melanocytosis (Mongolian spot). (From Lemmi, 2000.)

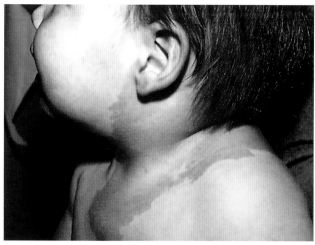

FIG. **19.12** Café-au-lait spot. (From Weston, Lane, and Morelli, 2002.)

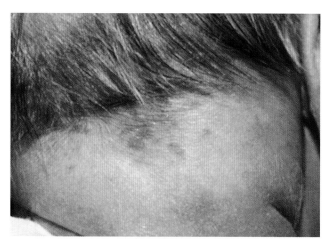

FIG. **19.13** Stork bite. (From Weston, Lane, and Morelli, 1996.)

- *Telangiectasis or flat capillary hemangioma (Stork bite):* A vascular birthmark appearing as a small red or pink spot often seen on the back of the neck or eyelids (Fig. 19.13). Stork bites usually disappear by 5 years of age.

  Abnormal findings. Some birthmarks considered abnormal include the following:
- *Nevus flammeus (Port wine stains):* Large, flat, bluish-purple capillary areas (Fig. 19.14 A). They are frequently found on the face and may have a triangular pattern along distribution of the fifth cranial nerve (CN). They do not disappear spontaneously.
- *Infantile hemangioma (also called Strawberry hemangioma):* Slightly raised, reddened areas with a sharp demarcation line (Fig. 19.14B). They initially increase in size and may become quite large (2 to 3 cm). These usually disappear by 5 years of age, but some require other treatments (such as laser) to resolve.
- *Cavernous hemangioma:* Reddish-blue round mass of blood vessels (Fig. 19.15). They may continue to actively grow in size and depth during the first year, and thus should be assessed frequently.

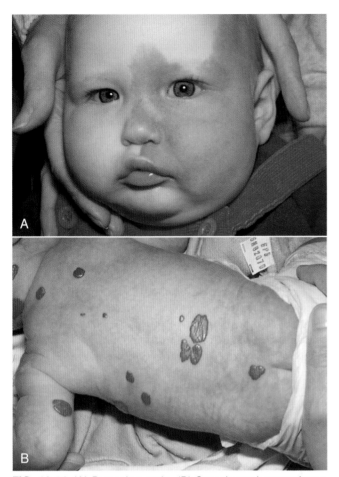

FIG. 19.14 (A) Port-wine stain. (B) Strawberry hemangioma. (From Zitelli, McIntire, and Nowalk, 2012.)

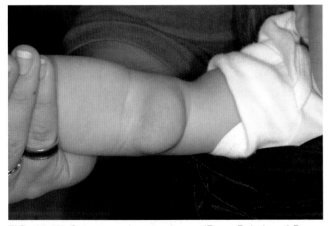

FIG. 19.15 Cavernous hemangioma. (From Rakel and Bope, 2004. Courtesy Richard P. Usatine.)

Hair and Nails

Expected findings. Scalp hair on the newborn is generally fine and soft. Seborrheic dermatitis (cradle cap) is a scaly crust that may appear on the scalp of infants (Fig. 19.16). The newborn's skin may be covered with fine, soft, immature hair called *lanugo hair* (Fig. 19.17). It may be found anywhere on the body but is common on the scalp, ears, shoulders, and back. Postterm infants may have long fingernails at birth.

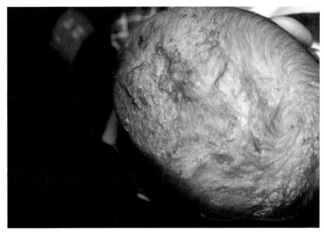

FIG. 19.16 Seborrheic dermatitis (Cradle cap). (From Kliegman et al., 2011.)

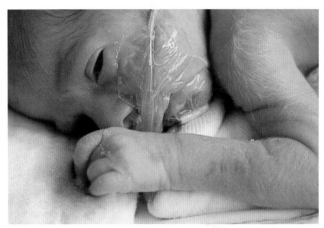

FIG. 19.17 Lanugo (Silky body hair) in premature infant. (Courtesy Lemmi and Lemmi, 2013.)

Head, Eyes, Ears, Nose, and Throat
Head

Procedure. Inspect and palpate the infant's head. Palpate the anterior and posterior fontanelles for fullness and mobility of the suture lines while the infant is in an upright position and calm (if the infant is lying down or crying, a false fullness may be felt). Head circumference should be measured at every well-baby visit through age 2 (or until the anterior fontanel is closed) and plotted on a growth chart as previously described for height and weight. To measure head circumference, a paper or plastic measuring tape is wrapped snugly around the infant's head at the largest circumference, usually just above the eyebrows, the pinna of the ears, and the occipital prominence at the back of the skull (Fig. 19.18). The tape measure is read to the nearest 0.5 cm. Head circumference is measured at least twice to check for accuracy; if the measurements differ, measure a third time.

Expected findings. The neonate's head may be asymmetric as a result of *molding*, in which the cranial bones override each other. Molding may result when the head passes through the birth canal; this generally lasts less than a week. Another

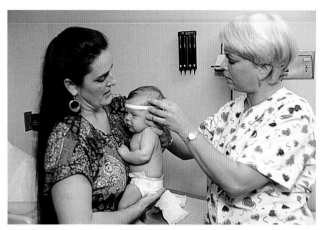

FIG. 19.18 Measuring head circumference in an infant.

BOX 19.4 HEAD CIRCUMFERENCE GROWTH RATES

- Full-term newborn to 3 months: 2 cm/month
- 3–6 months: 1 cm/month
- 6 months to 1 year: 0.5 cm/month

common finding in newborns is a cephalohematoma. This is a subperiosteal hematoma under the scalp that occurs secondary to birth trauma. The area, which appears as a soft, well-defined swelling over the cranial bone, generally is resorbed within the first month of life. The hematoma does not cross suture lines. The fontanelles should have a slight depression, should feel soft, and may have a slight pulsation. The anterior fontanelle in infants less than 6 months of age should not exceed 4 to 5 cm. It should get progressively smaller as the infant gets older and should be completely closed by 18 months of age. The infant's posterior fontanelle may or may not be palpable at birth. If it is palpable, it should measure no more than 1 cm, and it should close by 2 months of age. The infant should be able to turn his or her head from side to side by 2 weeks of age. Expected head circumference for term newborns averages from 33 to 36 cm and should be about 2 to 3 cm larger than chest circumference. By 4 months most infants demonstrate head control by holding the head erect and midline when in an upright position. By 2 years of age the child's head circumference is two thirds its adult size, and the chest circumference should exceed the head circumference (Box 19.4).

Abnormal findings. Marked asymmetry of the head is usually abnormal and may indicate craniosynostosis, a premature ossification of one or more of the cranial sutures. This condition occurs in 3 to 6 infants in 10,000 live births; most cases involve male infants.[10] A deeply depressed fontanelle may indicate dehydration; a bulging fontanelle may indicate increased intracranial pressure. A head circumference that is increasing rapidly suggests increased intracranial pressure. A head circumference below the fifth percentile suggests microcephaly. "Head bobbing" in infants is subtle sign of respiratory distress.

⊕ ETHNIC, CULTURAL, AND SPIRITUAL VARIATIONS

Infant Care

Native American and Alaskan Native infants may be secured to traditional cradle boards from birth, which may cause a flattening of the posterior skull.

Eyes

Procedure. Newborns may have edema of the eyelids, either from the trauma of birth or in response to prophylactic eyedrops or ointments. The edema may delay the examination for a few days. To begin the assessment, hold or rock the infant into an upright position to elicit eye opening. An alternative strategy is to hold the infant supine with the head gently lowered.

Observe if the eyes are small or of different sizes. Inspect the eyelids for edema and the epicanthal folds for position. Note the alignment and slant of the palpebral fissures and assess for wide or narrow eye positioning. Draw an imaginary line through the corners of the eyes (from the medial to the outer canthi) to assess the slant of the eyes. Observe the space between the eyes for wide-spaced eyes. Inspect the sclera for color. Also test for pupillary reaction at this time. Using the ophthalmoscope, assess light reflex; also attempt to visualize the red reflex in each eye.

Expected findings. Normal findings of the eye examination of an infant reveal eyes that are usually closed; often no eyebrows are present. The eyes are symmetric, and eyelashes may be long. Eyelids may have edema. The medial and lateral canthus are usually horizontal, in Asians an upward slant is expected. Infant sclerae may have a blue tinge caused by thinness; otherwise they are white. Tiny black dots (pigmentation) or a slight yellow cast may appear near the limbus of dark-skinned infants. Palpebral conjunctivae are pink and intact without discharge. There are no tears until about 2 to 3 months of age.

Infants should fix on and follow an object no later than 2 months age. The blink reflex also is present in newborns and infants. Pupils should constrict in response to bright light and are round, about 2 to 4 mm in diameter, and equal in size. A bilateral red reflex should be noted, which is a bright, round, red-orange glow seen through the pupil. It may be pale in dark-skinned newborns. The presence of the red reflex typically rules out most serious defects of the cornea, aqueous chamber, lens, and vitreous chamber.[9]

Specific age-related responses may be observed that indicate the infant's attention to visual stimuli.

- Birth to 2 weeks: Eyes do not reopen after exposure to bright light; there is increasing alertness to objects; the infant is capable of fixating on objects.
- Age 1 month: The newborn is nearsighted and cannot see objects unless they are close, but can fixate on and follow a bright toy or light.
- Ages 3 to 4 months: The infant can fixate on, follow, and reach for a toy because binocular vision is normally achieved at this age.

- Ages 6 to 12 months: The infant is capable of fixating on and following a toy in all directions.

Corneal light reflex should be symmetric. Transient strabismus is common during the first few months of life because of lack of binocular vision. However, if it continues beyond 6 months of age, a referral to an ophthalmologist is needed because early recognition and treatment can restore binocular vision.

Abnormal findings. A pronounced lateral upward slant of the eyes with an inner epicanthal fold is a common finding with Down syndrome. Other abnormalities include asymmetry of eyes, wide-set eyes (hypertelorism), or eyes that are close together (hypotelorism). Notice any discoloration of the sclerae such as dark blue sclerae or any dilated blood vessels. Hyperbilirubinemia may cause jaundiced (yellow) sclerae in newborns. Asymmetric corneal light reflex may indicate abnormality of eye muscles.

Excessive tearing before the third month or no tearing by the second month is a deviation from normal. A purulent discharge from the eyes shortly after birth is abnormal. It may indicate ophthalmia neonatorum and should be reported. Redness, lesions, nodules, discharge, or crusting of the conjunctiva is abnormal. Birth trauma may cause conjunctival hemorrhage. If the pupillary response is not present after 3 weeks, the infant may be blind. A dilated, fixed, or constricted pupil may indicate anoxia or neurologic damage. Absence of the red reflex (leukocoria) or asymmetric red reflex may indicate the presence of retinal hemorrhage; congenital cataracts; or retinoblastoma, a relatively rare congenital malignant tumor arising from the retina.[9]

Ears

Procedure. Examine the infant's external ears as previously described for the adult. A second individual (the "holder") is needed to restrain the infant, because the nurse must have both hands free to hold the ear and maneuver the otoscope to examine the auditory canal. The infant can be placed in either a prone or supine position. Instruct the holder to secure the infant's arms down at the sides with one hand and turn and hold the infant's head to one side with the other hand (Fig. 19.19A and B). To optimize visualization of the ear canal and tympanic membrane (TM), the nurse must alter the method of holding the auricle of the ear. Grasp the lower portion of the pinna and apply gentle traction down and slightly backward (as opposed to pulling the pinna up and back for the adult). This maneuver straightens the ear canal.

Hearing screening is recommended for all newborns.[11] Two common hearing screening tools used in many newborn nurseries are the Auditory Brainstem Response (ABR) test and the Otoacoustic Emissions (OAE) test. The ABR and OAE tests do not actually test hearing but rather assess the structural integrity of the auditory pathway. For this reason, hearing cannot be definitively considered normal until the child is old enough to perform an audiogram. When special tools for screening are unavailable, a simple hearing screening can be performed and should be included with an infant

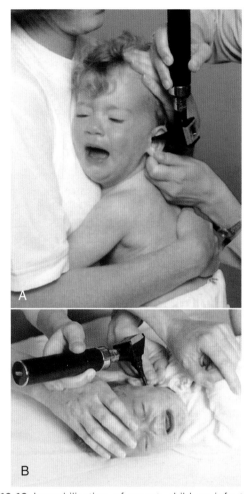

FIG. 19.19 Immobilization of young child or infant during otoscopic examination. Note that lower portion of pinna of ear is pulled down and slightly backward. (A) Prone position. (B) Supine position. (From Hockenberry and Wilson, 2011.)

examination. This is easily done by eliciting a loud noise (e.g., clapping hands or ringing bell) and observing for a response from the infant such as sudden body movement, startle response, or crying.

Expected findings. The ears should be symmetrically shaped and positioned. The top of the pinna of the ear should align directly with the outer canthus of the eye and be angled no more than 10 degrees from a vertical position (Fig. 19.20).

The TM of the infant may be difficult to visualize because it is more horizontal than in older children and adults. It may appear slightly reddened secondary to crying. In addition, because the TM does not become conical for several months, the light reflex may appear diffuse. By age 6 months the infant's TM takes on an adult type of appearance and is easier to visualize and examine.

Hearing behaviors should be readily observed. By ages 4 to 6 months the infant should turn the head toward the source of a sound and respond to the parent's voice or other sounds. By 6 to 10 months the child should respond to his or her name and follow sounds.

Abnormal findings. Low-set ears or ears with angulation greater than 10 degrees is often associated with a congenital condition such as Down syndrome. An unusually small or absent auricle is referred to as *microtia,* a congenital anomaly of the external ear (Fig. 19.21A–C). Microtia is classified from less severe (grade I) to the absence of an ear—termed *anotia* (grade IV). Preauricular skin tags are often associated with renal malformations.

Nose and Mouth

Procedure. When possible, examine the mouth when the infant is crying. Observe mucous membranes, posterior pharynx, tongue, gums, and any teeth. Palpate the buccal mucosa and gums for surface characteristics using a gloved hand and light source. While a gloved finger is in the infant's mouth, check the strength of his or her suck and palpate for an intact palate.

Infants who are uncooperative or unable to hold still may need to be carefully restrained. Ideally, a parent or other

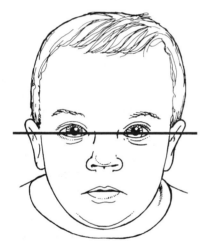

FIG. 19.20 Alignment of the outer canthus with the pinna of the ear is a normal finding. (From Seidel et al, 2011.)

adult holds the infant during the examination to ensure the infant's safety and permit the full viewing of the nose and mouth. Alternatively, the infant is restrained in a supine position, with the arms extended securely above his or her head (Fig. 19.22). The holder is then able to secure both the infant's arms and head. A second holder or the nurse may need to immobilize the infant's lower extremities.

The infant's nose is small and difficult to examine. Do not attempt to insert a speculum into the nares. Inspect the inside of the nose by tilting the infant's head back and shining a light into the nares. If an infant has nasal congestion, suction the nares with a bulb syringe or small-lumen catheter.

Expected findings. The nose should be appropriate to the size of the face. Infants are obligate nose breathers until about age 3 months. Should their nasal passages become occluded, they may have difficulty breathing. Sneezing is a common finding for an infant and is therapeutic because it helps to clear the nose. Milia may be present on the infant's nose. The infant's nares have only minimal movement with breathing. The buccal mucosa should appear pink, moist, and smooth. The infant's gums should appear smooth and full. Other expected findings may include the presence of small, white epithelial cells on the palate or gums. These are called *Bohn nodules* or *Epstein's pearls* (Fig. 19.23). The infant's tongue should be appropriate to the size of the mouth and fit well into the floor of the mouth. The palate should be intact. The infant should have a strong suck with the tongue pushing upward against the nurse's finger.

Abnormal findings. Nasal flaring is a hallmark of respiratory distress.[9] Because infants are obligatory nose breathers, any obstruction of the nares secondary to a congenital abnormality such as choanal atresia (occlusion between pharynx and nose), foreign body, or nasal secretions causes the infant to be irritable or distressed. If whitish patches are seen along the oral mucosa, scrape the area with a tongue blade to differentiate between milk deposits and a lesion. Milk deposits can be scraped off easily; candidiasis lesions also scrape off

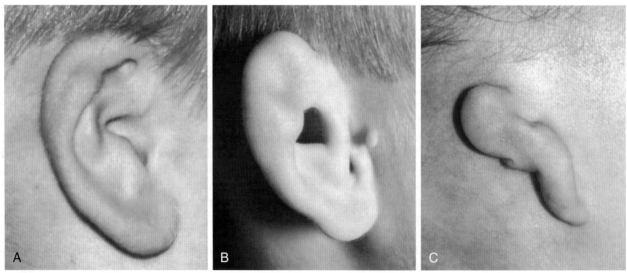

FIG. 19.21 Microtia. (A) Grade I. (B) Grade II. (C) Grade III. (From Sie et al., 2015.)

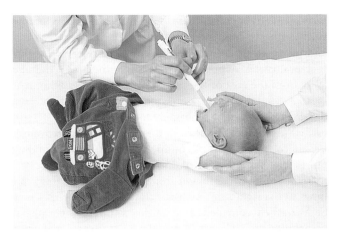

FIG. 19.22 Positioning of infant for examination of nose and mouth.

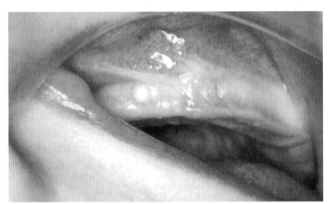

FIG. 19.23 Epstein pearls (Gingival cysts) in an infant. (From Scully and Welbury, 1994.)

but leave a red area that may bleed. Occasionally a natal loose tooth may be found. These teeth should be removed to prevent possible aspiration.

Neck

Procedure. To examine the neck, start with the infant in the supine position, grasp the infant's hand, and pull to sitting to lift the shoulders off the exam table. Observe the infant's muscle tone by watching the head position when bringing up to a sitting position. Inspect the neck for a midline trachea, abnormal skinfolds, and generalized neck enlargement. Return the infant to the supine position and palpate the neck for tone, presence of masses, and enlarged lymph nodes. The thyroid is not typically examined in the newborn.

Expected and abnormal findings. Up until about 20 weeks, newborns have head lag, which is characterized by a head that does not remain in line with the torso when the infant is pulled from a lying to sitting potion. Head lag after 20 weeks is an abnormal finding and has been shown to be one possible indicator of autism. Normally the newborn's lymph nodes are not palpable.[9] If the infant's neck is proportionately short or has webbing (loose, fanlike skinfolds), he or she should be evaluated for congenital abnormalities such as Down syndrome or Turner syndrome. If an enlargement of

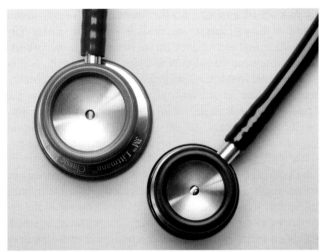

FIG. 19.24 The pediatric stethoscope has a smaller head compared with the adult stethoscope.

the infant's anterior neck is palpated, the infant should be referred to a primary care provider for further evaluation.

Lungs and Respiratory System

Procedure. Assessing the respiratory status of a newborn or infant follows the same sequence as for an adult. If possible, conduct the examination while the infant is calm because examination of a crying infant is difficult. Inspect the infant's chest to observe symmetry and respiratory effort. Auscultate the infant's breath sounds in the same manner as for the older child and adult; however, use a pediatric stethoscope with a small diaphragm (Fig. 19.24). Percussion and palpation are not routinely performed. Pulse oximetry is another way to assess oxygenation status of the infant.

Measure chest circumference when an abnormality of the thorax is observed or if the head and chest seem disproportionate in size. The chest circumference is measured at the nipple line pulling the tape measure firmly without causing an indentation in the skin. The measurement is noted between inspiration and expiration and recorded to the nearest 1/8 inch (0.5 cm) (see Fig. 19.6). Chest circumference should be plotted at birth and thereafter may be plotted on a growth chart as previously described for height and weight but is not a routine measurement.

Expected findings. Inspection of the infant's thorax should show a smooth, rounded, and symmetric appearance and easy respirations. Unlike the adult, the infant has a round thorax with equal anteroposterior and lateral measurements. The average chest circumference in an infant ranges from 30 to 36 cm. This measurement should be equal to or up to 2 to 3 cm smaller than the child's head circumference.

The respiratory pattern in the newborn may be irregular, with brief pauses of no more than 10 to 15 seconds. The respiratory rate in the newborn ranges from 30 to 60 breaths/min (see Table 19.2). Infants are obligate nose breathers until about age 3 months. The infant has a thin chest wall, which makes breath sounds difficult to localize with auscultation. They are commonly transmitted from one auscultatory area to another. Because of this, the predominant breath sound heard in the peripheral lung fields is bronchovesicular. The thin chest wall also makes the newborn's xiphoid process more prominent than that of an older child or adult.

Abnormal findings. Coughing, stridor, grunting, sternal or supraclavicular retractions, and nasal flaring are abnormal findings that indicate the infant is in respiratory distress. Any one of these findings warrants immediate medical attention because infants with respiratory distress tire and become hypoxic quickly. Stridor is a high-pitched sound that is primarily heard during inspiration. It occurs secondary to upper airway narrowing or obstruction. Stridor may result in the infant's inspiratory phase being three or four times longer than the expiratory phase. Respiratory grunting is a mechanism by which the infant tries to prolong expiration to prevent end-expiratory alveolar collapse. Sternal, intercostal, and supraclavicular retractions and nasal flaring are indications of respiratory distress. Clinically this may be observed as "see-saw" type of breathing with alternating movements of the chest and abdomen. If any of these signs are observed, they indicate that the infant is working very hard to try to maintain adequate breathing and require immediate intervention.

Heart and Peripheral Vascular System

Procedure. Assessing the cardiovascular system of a newborn or infant usually follows the same sequence as for an adult. The apical pulse of the newborn normally is felt in the fourth or fifth intercostal space (ICS) just medial to the midclavicular line. Examine the heart within the first 24 hours of birth and again at 2 to 3 days to assess changes from fetal to extrauterine circulation. The heart must be auscultated when the infant is quiet and for 1 full minute. The stethoscope used must have a small diaphragm and bell to detect specific cardiac sounds of the newborn or infant. Palpate the femoral and brachial pulses and assess capillary refill. Pulse oximetry is conducted as a mandatory part of newborn screening within the first 24 hours after birth for critical congenital heart defects (CHDs); low levels of oxygen in the blood can be a sign of CHD.[12]

Expected findings. Normally the heart rate of infants is faster when they are awake and slower when they are asleep. Infant heart rate may increase during inspiration and decrease during expiration. Systolic murmurs are common in infants up to 48 hours after birth due to closure of fetal shunts (ductus arteriosus and foramen ovale). Capillary refill in infants is very rapid (i.e., <1 second after the first day of life). Acrocyanosis (cyanosis of hands and feet) in the newborn without central cyanosis is of little concern and usually disappears within hours to days of birth.

Abnormal findings. Central cyanosis may indicate CHDs. Notice if cyanosis increases with crying or feeding. Severe cyanosis that appears shortly after birth may indicate transposition of the great vessels, tetralogy of Fallot, a severe septal defect, or severe pulmonic stenosis. Cyanosis that appears after the first month of life suggests pulmonic stenosis, tetralogy of Fallot, or large septal defects. Infants with murmurs that are unusually loud, diastolic, persist after 3 days, or are accompanied by other abnormal cardiovascular findings such as thrills, lifts, increased precordial activity, cyanosis, and increased or decreased pulses must be referred for further evaluation. A pneumothorax shifts the apical impulse away from the area of the chest where the pneumothorax is located. The infant's heart may be shifted to the right by a diaphragmatic hernia commonly found on the left. Dextrocardia (location of the heart in the right hemithorax) causes the apical pulse to shift toward the right side. Bounding pulses may indicate a patent ductus arteriosus creating a left-to-right shunt (when blood from the left side of the heart flows to the right side). Weak or thin peripheral pulses may be associated with decreased cardiac output or peripheral vasoconstriction. Coarctation of the heart is suspected when the femoral pulses are diminished or absent or there is a difference in pulse amplitude between upper and lower extremities.

Abdomen and Gastrointestinal System

Procedure. The abdominal examination is straightforward, with the infant lying supine on an examining table. Follow the same procedure for examining the abdomen as for adults, although percussion is not ordinarily performed.

Expected findings. On inspection, the abdomen of a newborn or infant should be symmetric, soft, and rounded. There is synchronous abdominal and chest movement with breathing. Diastasis rectus (a gap between the rectus muscles) may be noted during crying. Visible pulsations in the epigastric areas are common.

Inspect the umbilicus in the newborn. Immediately after the umbilical cord is cut, two arteries and one vein should be noted. After the cord is clamped, it slowly changes from white to black as it dries; it should dry in 5 days and fall off spontaneously in 7 to 14 days. Active bowel sounds can be auscultated several hours after birth. The abdomen of a newborn should be soft and nondistended on palpation. The edge of the infant's liver may be up to 1 to 2 cm below the right costal margin. The spleen is generally not palpable, although the tip may be felt in the left upper quadrant (far left costal margin). Both kidneys may be noted with deep palpation, especially in newborns. Deep or rigorous kidney palpation should not be performed in toddlers especially if asymmetry or enlargement is detected. A cancerous tumor that occurs with relative frequency in toddlers is a Wilms tumor, also known as nephroblastoma. Deep palpation of the kidneys increases the risk of rupturing this encapsulated tumor, which could cause the cancerous cells to spread to other areas in the body.

Abnormal findings. Notice distention or masses as well as concave, sunken, or flat appearance, or abdominal wall defects. A scaphoid-shaped abdomen suggests diaphragmatic hernia. Additional abnormal findings may include discharge, odor, or redness around the umbilicus; a protrusion or nodular appearance of the umbilicus; and a thin or green-stained umbilical cord. Absence of bowel sounds may indicate a bowel obstruction. An enlarged liver 3 cm or more below the margin, palpable spleen, masses near the kidneys, and enlarged kidneys are considered abnormal findings.

Musculoskeletal System

Procedure. Examine the infant undressed and lying supine. Shortly following birth newborns should have a neuromuscular examination called a Ballard Assessment that is routinely completed by nurses caring for newborns. This assessment is completed to assess a newborn's neuromuscular maturity in comparison with the gestational age. In newborns palpate clavicles for evidence of fractures, a common birth injury. Inspect the arms and legs and notice any abnormalities of fingers or toes. Extend both arms and legs to compare muscle tone and length. Inspect the back and spine for alignment, tufts of hair, bulges, or obvious malformations. Assess hip stability by performing the Barlow and Ortolani maneuvers. These maneuvers should be performed regularly until 3 months of age, with special attention paid to breech-birth newborns. With the infant supine, the nurse flexes the infant's knees, holding his or her thumbs on the inner midthighs and fingers outside on the hips touching the greater trochanters. Adduct the legs, exerting downward pressure (Barlow maneuver) (Fig. 19.25A). Then abduct them, moving the knees apart and down toward the table and applying upward pressure with the fingers on the greater trochanter (Ortolani maneuver) (Fig. 19.25B). The Allis sign is another assessment for hip dislocation. With the infant supine, flex the knees with the feet flat on the table and align

the femurs. Observe for even height of the knees. Assess the feet for shape and position. Observe the lateral and medial borders of the foot. If the borders are not straight, assess flexibility of the forefoot by gently moving it to a neutral position. Notice the relationship of the forefoot to the hindfoot.

Expected findings. Stable and smooth clavicles without crepitus are expected. Arms and legs should have spontaneous, equal movement and be of equal length. The feet should be flexible. The hindfoot aligns with the lower leg, and the forefoot may turn inward slightly. The Barlow and Ortolani maneuvers should feel smooth and produce no clicks or clunks. When both knees are the same height, an Allis test is negative. The spine should be flexible and straight without curvatures, dimples, or masses.

Abnormal findings. Abnormal muscle tone is noted as hypotonia or hypertonia. Limited shoulder or arm range of motion and deformity may indicate a fractured clavicle or humerus. Erb palsy (paralysis of shoulder and upper arm muscles) may be noticed. Asymmetry of extremities, limited movement, syndactyly (fused digits), and polydactyly (extra digits) are also abnormal findings. Metatarsus adductus (an inward curve of the forefoot) or talipes equinovarus (clubfoot) may be noted. Hip dislocation (hip dysplasia) may be identified by four procedures. A positive Barlow, Ortolani, or Allis sign indicates hip instability; when one knee is lower than the other, the Allis sign is positive (Fig. 19.26). Uneven skinfolds are another sign that suggests hip dislocation (Fig. 19.27). Any asymmetric spinal curve, masses (hair tufts, dimples), or abnormal posture may indicate underlying spinal or vertebral malformations.

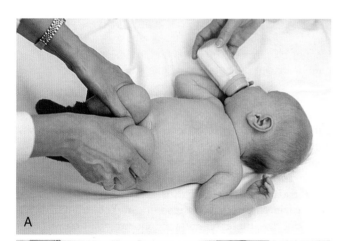
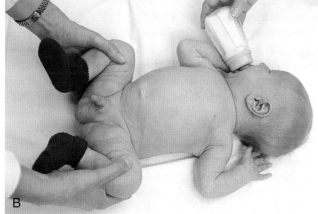

FIG. 19.25 Barlow and ortolani maneuvers to detect hip dislocation. (A) Phase I, adduction. (B) Phase II, abduction. This is a negative finding because no dislocation is found.

⊕ ETHNIC, CULTURAL, AND SPIRITUAL VARIATIONS

Hip Dislocation

Navajo Indians and Canadian Eskimos are among the cultures with the highest incidence of hip dislocation. In these cultures, newborns are tightly wrapped in blankets or strapped to cradle boards. Hip dislocation is virtually unknown in cultures in which infants are carried on their mother's backs or hips in the widely abducted straddle position such as in the Far East and Africa.

Neurologic System

Procedure. Observe spontaneous motor activity for symmetry. Assessments of head size and fontanelles are discussed under general assessment of the head but must also be considered a part of any infant's neurologic assessment. Additional neurologic assessment includes quality of cry and infant's response to touch. Determine the presence of the newborn reflexes (Moro, tonic neck, rooting, sucking, palmar grasp, Babinski, and plantar) as applicable. Primitive reflexes that should be evident in the newborn are shown in Table 19.4. CNs are assessed by observing eye movements and blinking (CNs III, IV, and VI), sucking (CN V),

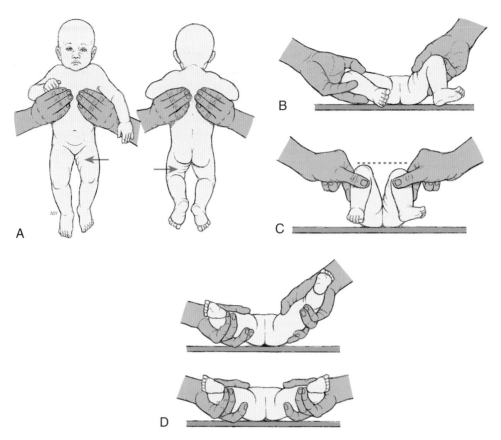

FIG. 19.26 Signs of developmental dysplasia of the hip. (A) Asymmetry of gluteal and thigh folds with shortening of the thigh (Galeazzi sign). (B) Limited hip abduction, as seen in flexion (Ortolani test). (C) Apparent shortening of the femur, as indicated by the level of the knees in flexion (Allis sign). (D) Ortolani test with femoral head moving in and out of acetabulum (in infants 1 to 2 months old). (From Hockenberry et al., 2013.)

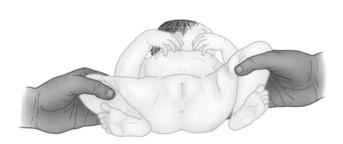

FIG. 19.27 Sign of hip dislocation. The three skinfolds on the left upper leg and limited abduction indicate left hip dysplasia.

wrinkling of the forehead (CN VII), turning the head toward a sound (CN VIII), and swallowing (CN IX). With the infant supine, pull to a sitting position holding the hands; observe head control. Evaluate resting posture for muscle tone.

Expected findings. Expected development of the infant by month is outlined in Table 18.3. Expected findings include fontanelles that are open, soft, and flat (posterior fontanelle closes by 2 months and anterior fontanelle closes by 18 months). The primitive reflexes are present but disappear during the first year as the infant's nervous system matures. The

Babinski reflex is an exception; it disappears by 18 months. Some head lag normally is present up to 4 months of age. Spontaneous movement should be smooth and symmetric, and appropriate tone is demonstrated with resistance to passive range of motion. Postural reflexes develop after birth and are associated with balance, posture, and coordination. Assessment for these reflexes and documentation of their appearance is an important component of an infant's neurologic status.

Abnormal findings. Fontanelles that feel full and distended or close prematurely are abnormal. Lethargy, irritability, shrill cry, weakness, and "sunset eyes," are all abnormal neurologic findings. An abnormally large head circumference may indicate hydrocephalus (see Fig. 19.55 later in the chapter). An abnormally small head size (microcephaly) is also an abnormal finding. Motor activity abnormalities indicating neurologic damage include hypotonia, as evidenced by poor head control and limp extremities; hypertonia; stiff legs; jittery arm movements; and tightly flexed hands. An arched back (opisthotonos) with a stiff neck and extension of extremities may indicate meningitis. Any asymmetric posture is also abnormal. Notice any spasticity, which may be an early sign of cerebral palsy. If present, the legs quickly extend and adduct, possibly even in a scissoring pattern.

TABLE 19.4 INFANTILE REFLEXES

REFLEX	TECHNIQUE FOR EVALUATION	AGE APPEARS AND DISAPPEARS	NORMAL RESPONSE
Reflexes to Evaluate Position and Movement			
Moro	Startle infant by making loud noise, jarring examination surface, or slightly raising infant off examination surface and letting him or her fall quickly back onto examining table	Appears: Birth Disappears: 1–4 months	Infant abducts and extends arms and legs; index finger and thumb assume C position; then infant pulls both arms and legs up against trunk as if trying to protect self
Palmar grasp	Touch object against ulnar side of infant's hand; then place finger in palm of hand	Appears: Birth Disappears: 3–4 months	Infant grasps finger; grasp should be tight, and nurse may be able to pull infant into sitting position by infant's grasp
Tonic neck	Infant supine; rotate head to side so chin is over shoulder	Appears: Birth to 6 weeks Disappears: 4–6 months	Arm and leg extend on side to which head turns; opposite arm and leg flex; infant assumes fencing position (some normal infants may never show this reflex)
Plantar grasp	Touch object to sole of infant's foot	Birth	Toes flex tightly downward in attempt to grasp
Babinski	Stroke lateral surface of infant's sole, using inverted J curve from sole to great toe (see Fig. 15.22F).	Appears: Birth Disappears: 18 months	Infant response: positive response showing fanning of toes
Step in place	Infant in upright position, feet flat on surface	Appears: Birth Disappears: 3 months	Paces forward using alternating steps

Continued

TABLE 19.4 INFANTILE REFLEXES—cont'd

REFLEX	TECHNIQUE FOR EVALUATION	AGE APPEARS AND DISAPPEARS	NORMAL RESPONSE
Clonus	Dorsiflex foot; pinch sole of foot just under toes (see Fig. 15.22G)	Appears: Birth Disappears: 4 months	May get clonus movement of foot (not always present)
Feeding Reflexes			
Rooting response (awake)	Brush infant's cheek near corner of mouth	Appears: Birth Disappears: 3–4 months	Infant turns head in direction of stimulus and opens mouth slightly
Sucking	Touch infant's lips	Appears: Birth Disappears: 10–12 months	Sucking motion follows with lips and tongue

Breasts

Procedure. The examination of the newborn's and infant's breasts generally requires inspection only.

Expected findings. Neonates of both genders may have full, slightly enlarged breasts secondary to the mother's estrogen level before the infant was born. Maternal hormones are also responsible for the production of a small amount of watery or milky nipple discharge (sometimes referred to as *witch's milk*) during the first month of life in approximately 5% of neonates.[13] The nipples normally are located slightly lateral to the midclavicular line between the fourth and fifth ribs; the nipple should be flat and surrounded by a slightly darker pigmented areola.

Reproductive System and Perineum

Female Examination

Procedure. During infancy the examination is limited to an evaluation of the external genitalia. The infant is placed on the examination table in frog-leg position (hips flexed with the soles of the feet together and up to the buttocks). Using gloved hands, place both thumbs on either side of the labia majora and gently move the tissue laterally and down. This should permit visualization of the genitalia, the urethra, the clitoris, the hymen, and possibly the vaginal opening.

Expected findings. Secondary to maternal hormones, the newborn's genitalia may appear somewhat engorged, with edematous labia majora and prominent and protruding labia minora. The clitoris also looks relatively large, and the hymen may appear thick and protrude through the introitus; the vaginal opening may be difficult to see. A mucoid, white, or slightly bloody vaginal discharge may be observed during the early period following birth but should disappear by 1 month.

Abnormal findings. Fused labia (termed labial adhesions), markedly enlarged clitoris, or the lack of a vaginal opening may be signs of ambiguous genitalia.

Male Examination

Procedure. Inspect the penis, foreskin, and scrotum. If the infant is circumcised, the urinary meatus will be visible.

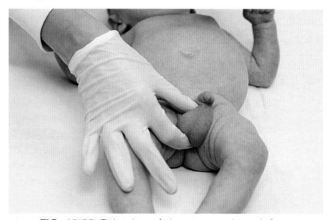

FIG. 19.28 Palpation of the scrotum in an infant.

In uncircumcised males the urinary meatus may not be visible because of the tight foreskin. Do not attempt to retract the foreskin. Force may tear the prepuce from the glans, which in turn could cause binding adhesions to form between the prepuce and the glans.

Palpate the scrotum to determine presence of the testes (Fig. 19.28). If a mass other than a testicle or spermatic cord is palpated in the scrotum, transillumination is indicated to determine the presence of fluid (hydrocele) or mass (possible hernia) in the testicle.

Expected findings. If the infant is uncircumcised, the foreskin should cover the glans. The foreskin has little mobility in infants. The foreskin should permit unobstructed urinary stream. The urinary meatus should be centered at the tip of the glans penis. If possible, observe the infant's urine stream. It should be full and strong. The full-term infant has a pendulous scrotum with deep rugae; the size of the scrotum usually appears large when compared with the penis. The scrotum appears pink in light-skinned infants and dark brown in dark-skinned infants. A testis should be palpable in each scrotum. If one or both testicles are not palpable, gently place a finger over the upper inguinal ring and gently push downward toward the scrotum. If the testicle can be pushed into the scrotum, it is considered descended even though it retracts into the inguinal canal.

Abnormal findings. A weak stream with dribbling is an abnormal finding and may indicate stenosis of the urethral meatus or a tight foreskin. Enlargement of the scrotum may indicate a hydrocele or a hernia. A hydrocele is a collection of fluid and transilluminates (glows when a light source is applied). It is a common abnormal finding in an infant (especially among premature infants) and often resolves spontaneously. A mass such as a hernia, a protrusion of bowel into the scrotum, will not transilluminate and should be referred as it may require surgical repair. Undescended testes (cryptorchidism) should resolve by 3 months of age, and if the teste(s) do not descend, the child should be referred for further evaluation.

Perianal Examination

Procedure. The perianal examination is performed routinely with comprehensive assessment; however, a rectal exam is not routinely performed in infants. In the newborn inspect the perineum and anus for lesions, fissures, and inflammation. If stool is present when the diaper is removed, notice characteristics including color and consistency.

Expected and abnormal findings. The perineal and perianal skin and buttocks should be free of lesions, inflammation, or rash. Mongolian spots are a common variation as are some birthmarks. An imperforate anus is an abnormal finding and should be assessed at the first newborn exam. A tuft of hair or dimpling in the pilonidal (sacrococcygeal) area may indicate a lower spinal deformity or sinus tract.

EXAMINATION OF TODDLERS AND CHILDREN

If the young child is cooperative and does not appear to be fearful, the nurse can proceed with the physical examination in the same sequence as the adult examination, although examination of the ears and mouth are best left to the end of the examination in this age group. Allow the child to sit on the parent's lap when possible to reduce fear or anxiety. Showing the equipment to the child, explaining the procedure, and allowing the child to use the equipment (e.g., a stethoscope) on a doll or teddy bear helps to enlist his or her cooperation (Fig. 19.29). Having the child blow bubbles or "blow out" the light of the otoscope or penlight before and during the examination may also help elicit his or her cooperation.

Skin, Hair, and Nails

No special procedure is necessary when examining the skin, hair, and nails other than keeping the young child warm during the examination.

Skin

Expected findings. The skin should be smooth with consistent color and no lesions. Although bruising is common on the lower legs as the toddler becomes mobile, information about the bruising from the caregiver is important. When skin is assessed for turgor, it should move easily when lifted and return to place immediately when released.

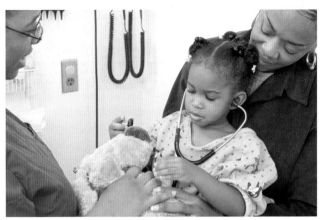

FIG. 19.29 Allow the child to touch examination equipment to reduce fear.

Abnormal findings. The most common abnormal lesions found in the young child are associated with communicable diseases such as roseola, fifth disease, tinea corporis (ringworm), impetigo, pediculosis corporis (body lice), and scabies. Eczema is also commonly found in toddlers and preschool children. This is usually a chronic and/or intermittent disorder. Less commonly, infants and children who are not fully immunized may present with varicella (chickenpox), rubella, and rubeola. Recently, there has been a significant increase in the incidence of rubeola (measles) related to lack of vaccination. Evidence of bruising that may be inconsistent with the child's developmental level or in an unusual area is cause for concern. Bruising in unusual areas (e.g., upper arms, back, buttocks, and abdomen) or multiple or large bruises should be investigated further to rule out abuse.[14] Likewise a child who is seriously dehydrated (more than 3% to 5% of body weight) and has skin that appears "tented" after the abdominal skin is pinched warrants further investigation.

Hair and Nails

Expected and abnormal findings. The young child should have very little body or facial hair. Nails should be intact and smooth. Common problems associated with the scalp and hair of the young child include alopecia (hair loss), which may be secondary to hair pulling, twisting, or head rubbing; and lice, nits, and scabies. Nail biting is an abnormal behavior and finding. Evidence of cyanosis of the nail bed or nail clubbing requires careful evaluation because they may indicate a cardiac or respiratory disease.

Head, Eyes, Ears, Nose, and Throat
Head

Examination and findings of the head are similar to those of the adult. The anterior fontanelle should be closed by 18 months of age.

Eyes

Procedure. Most of the examination of children's eyes is the same as that for adults. The assessment of vision and eyes should be appropriate for the developmental stage and age of the child. Traditionally, visual acuity screening in 2½- to 3-year-old children (pre-literate) has included the use of LEA Symbols or HOTV letters. To complete this assessment, show the large cards with pictures to the child up close to be sure that the child can identify them. Then present each picture at the appropriate distance (as directed per card instructions) from the child. Use a Snellen "E" chart for children 3 to 6 years of age (see Chapter 10). Have children point their fingers in the direction of the "arms" of the E. Begin using the standard Snellen chart, as described for adults when the child is 7 to 8 years of age. Begin by testing both eyes, then test each eye separately with and without glasses as appropriate. Be sure to screen children two separate times before referring them. Test for color vision once between ages 4 and 8. The red and green lines on a Snellen chart can be used as a gross screening tool for color blindness, to be followed with the Ishihara Color Blind test as needed. Ask the child to identify each pattern seen in the cards. The ocular alignment of very young children also should be regularly assessed.[15] A cover-uncover test can be used to assess this, although an instrument-based photoscreening assessment has been developed as a smartphone application. This assessment application has been found to be feasible, with high levels of sensitivity and specificity for amblyopia (otherwise known as "lazy eye").[16]

Prepare children for the ophthalmoscope examination by showing them the light, explaining how it shines in the eye, and explaining why the room must be darkened. Eliciting a bilateral red reflex using the ophthalmoscope is important. Perform the corneal light reflex or Hirschberg at a distance of about 12 inches from the child's eyes (see Chapter 10 for specific instructions). Complete the cover/uncover test regularly. Have the child fixate on the light of the ophthalmoscope. If the child is uncooperative, ask him or her fixate on a toy. Use one hand to cover the eye and observe the uncovered eye for fixation on the object. Screen for nystagmus by inspecting the movement of the eyes to the six cardinal fields of gaze. The nurse may need to stabilize the child's chin with his or her hand to prevent the entire head from moving.

Expected findings. The normal visual acuity for children between the ages of 3 and 5 is 20/40 or better.[17] For ages 6 to 7 normal visual acuity is 20/30 or better, and children 8 years or older should have 20/20 vision.[18] A child with normal color vision sees the number or pattern embedded in the Ishihara test. A symmetric corneal light reflex is an expected finding (Fig. 19.30) as is a clear and symmetric red reflex.

Abnormal findings. Lack of tears in a toddler or preschooler is the first sign of dehydration and should be documented. A referral to an ophthalmologist is necessary for children with less than expected visual acuity. Additionally, a two-line difference between eyes, even within the passing range, warrants referral. A child who is color-blind is unable to recognize the number or pattern in the Ishihara test. Children who are found to have strabismus (eyes going in different directions) need to be referred to an ophthalmologist, as early recognition and treatment can restore binocular vision.

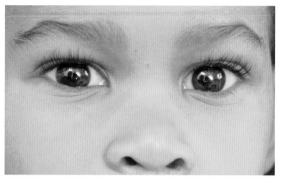

FIG. 19.30 Corneal light reflex.

Diagnosis of strabismus after age 6 is difficult to treat and has poor long-term outcomes.

Ears

Procedure. Examining the auditory canal and TM of the young child is often challenging due to his or her lack of cooperation. The best way to position a child for ear assessment is to have the child straddle their parent's lap facing them and asking the parent to place a hand on the child's forehead as their head is turned sideways (see Fig. 19.19A). Restraining the young child in either the supine or prone position as discussed previously with the infant may be necessary (see Fig. 19.19B). Inadequate restraint can result in pain to the child and also may cause injury to the ear canal. If the child is fearful, screaming, or uncooperative, the nurse should place his or her hand against the child's head to protect the ear canal from sudden movement or jolt. Because the otoscopic examination may be perceived by a young child as traumatic, it may be deferred until the last procedure of the examination and allow the child to touch and play with the examination light and tools. If the child becomes upset during the examination, be sure to quickly return him or her to the parent for comforting.

The nurse should take the time to elicit the child's cooperation during the examination as he or she gets older. If the nurse has any question regarding the child's ability to hold perfectly still during the otoscope examination, the parent or adult who is with the child should assist in restraining the child to ensure his or her safety.

The procedure for examination proceeds as previously discussed for the infant. If the child is younger than 1 year of age, the pinna should be pulled down and back during the examination as described for the infant. If the child is older, the pinna should be pulled up and backward as for the adult. Hearing screening may be indicated for children, particularly if risk factors were identified during infancy.

Expected findings. The findings of the examination of the ears do not differ significantly for children from those of the adult.

Abnormal findings. Foreign bodies, which are commonly found in the ears of children, need to be removed by a physician or advanced practice registered nurse. Small polyethylene tubes in the TM of a child who has recently had a myringotomy

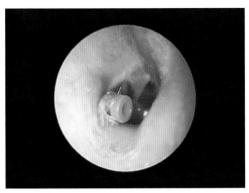

FIG. 19.31 Tympanotomy tube protruding from the right tympanic membrane. (From Bingham, Hawke, and Kwok, 1992.)

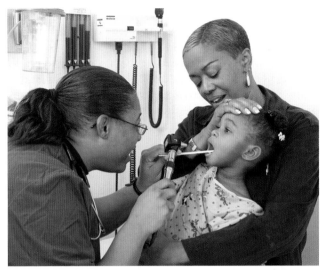

FIG. 19.32 Technique for immobilizing a young child's head for examination.

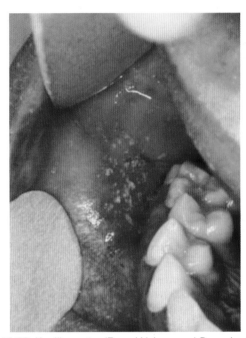

FIG. 19.33 Koplik spots. (From Weisse and Papania, 2016.)

may be observed (Fig. 19.31). These are surgically placed through the TM to relieve middle ear pressure and permit the drainage of fluid or material collected behind the TM. They are commonly put in the ears of young children because of recurrent ear infections. Usually the tubes spontaneously extrude (work their way out) from the TM within 6 to 12 months after insertion.

Hearing evaluation of the young child is necessary if the parent or nurse perceives a lag in his or her development. Behavioral manifestations that may indicate hearing impairment include delay in verbal skills; speech that is monotone, garbled, or difficult to understand; inattentiveness during conversation; facial expressions that appear strained or puzzled; withdrawal and lack of interaction with others; frequently asking "What?" or asking for statements to be repeated; or having frequent earaches.

Nose and Mouth

Procedure. A toddler or young child will probably tolerate the mouth and nose examination better while sitting on the parent's lap with his or her back to the parent. The parent may then restrain the child's legs by placing them between the adult's legs. The parent then has both hands free. One hand should be used to reach around the child's body to restrain his or her arms and chest. The other hand may be used to assist the nurse by restraining the child's head (Fig. 19.32). Once the child becomes too large for the parent's lap, he or she can be examined in a supine position on the examination table.

The young child's nose should be assessed in the same manner as that of the infant. Use a thumb to lift the tip of the nose to improve visualization inside the nares. Palpation of the sinuses can be done after ages 7 or 8. When examining the teeth, notice the eruption sequence; the timing, condition, positioning, and hygiene of the teeth; and the presence of debris or decay around the teeth or gum line.

Expected findings. The presence of a transverse crease at the bridge of the nose is called an *allergic salute,* which occurs when a child has a frequent runny nose or allergies and wipes the nose with an upward sweep of the palm of the hand. The buccal mucosa should be pink, moist, and without lesions. The child's tonsils are larger than an adult's but should not

interfere with swallowing or breathing. They should be dark pink and without vertical reddened lines, general erythema, edema, or exudate. Tooth eruption depends on the age of the child.

Abnormal findings. Abnormal findings may include a foul odor and unilateral discharge from a nostril caused by a foreign body. Dryness, flaking, or cracking corners of the mouth may indicate excess licking of the lips, vitamin deficiency, or infection such as impetigo. Lesions such as Koplik spots (as seen in measles) or candidiasis (thrush) may be observed (Fig. 19.33). An excessively dry mouth may indicate dehydration or fever. Excessive salivation may indicate gingivostomatitis or multiple dental caries. Excessive drooling after 12 months of age may indicate a neurologic disorder.

Flattened edges on the teeth may indicate teeth grinding (bruxism). Darkened, brown, or black teeth may indicate decay or staining from oral iron therapy. Mottled or pitted teeth may result from tetracycline therapy during tooth development or exposure in utero. If the mouth has a fetid or musty smell, hygiene practices, local or systemic infections, or sinusitis should be investigated further.

Neck

Procedure. Examining the neck of the child is the same as for the adult. The thyroid examination in young children may be deferred. When assessed, use the same techniques as for the adult.

Expected findings. Normally lymph nodes up to 3 mm may be palpable in children and may reach 1 cm in the cervical areas; but they are mobile and nontender. The term *shotty* may be used to describe small, firm, and mobile nodes occurring as a normal variation in children. Enlarged postauricular and occipital nodes in children younger than 2 years of age are a normal variation. Likewise, cervical and submandibular nodal enlargements are more frequent in older children. While occipital lymph nodes are often a normal finding, when palpated, the nurse should also palpate the child's head for inflammation or infection (i.e., fungus, bacterial).

Abnormal findings. Nodes that are tender, fixed, or greater than 1 cm are abnormal. Enlarged, tender nodes may occur with upper respiratory infection.[9] An enlarged thyroid at any age requires further investigation.

Lungs and Respiratory System

Procedure. The examination procedure for the lungs and respiratory system of the child is the same as those for the adult. By age 2 or 3 years, the child may be cooperative during the respiratory examination (Fig. 19.34). If the nurse takes the time to develop a relationship with the child, his or her cooperation can usually be obtained.

If performing chest palpation, the nurse should adjust the number of fingers used to palpate the chest wall to be appropriate for the size of the child's chest. For example, if the child is small, the nurse may use only two or three fingers. On the other hand, if the child is large, three or four fingers may be used. Percussion is performed infrequently until the child is at least 10 years of age.

Expected findings. By age 5 or 6 the rounded thorax of the child approximates the 1:2 ratio of anteroposterior-to-lateral diameter of the adult. By ages 6 or 7 the child's breathing pattern should change from primarily nasal and abdominal to thoracic in girls and abdominal in boys. The child's respiratory rate should gradually slow as he or she becomes older (see Table 19.2). Depending on the size of the child and the musculature of the chest, slight variations in auscultation may be found. Findings for a small or young child with undeveloped chest musculature may include more bronchovesicular breath sounds in the peripheral lung areas and, because of the small chest size and underdeveloped musculature, a blending of breath sounds may occur. If the child is larger and has started to develop more, the breath sounds are

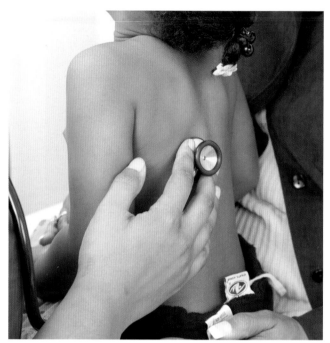

FIG. 19.34 Auscultation of lungs on a young child.

equivalent to those of the adult (vesicular in the peripheral lung fields). Palpation findings for the child are the same as those for the adult.

Abnormal findings. Increased respiratory rate, retractions (which may be accompanied with grunting and flaring), and adventitious sounds such as crackles, rhonchi, or wheezing are abnormal findings. If the child's chest proportion remains rounded, it may be an outward indication of a significant problem such as asthma or cystic fibrosis.

Heart and Peripheral Vascular System

Procedure. The child may sit on the exam table or the caregiver's lap for examination of the heart. The nurse should inspect and palpate the chest noticing size, shape, and abnormal pulsations. The child's heart is auscultated in the same areas as that of the adult (Fig. 19.35). The chest should be visible, and auscultation should be performed with a pediatric stethoscope in contact with the child's skin and not through clothing. If an irregular rhythm is noted, have the child hold his or her breath so only heart sounds are heard. Auscultate with the bell of the stethoscope over the right supraclavicular space at the medial end of the clavicle along the anterior border of the sternocleidomastoid muscle for a venous hum (Fig. 19.36). A venous hum is a vibration heard over the jugular vein caused by turbulent blood flow; it has a continuous, low-pitched sound that is louder during diastole. It may be stopped by gentle pressure between the trachea and the sternocleidomastoid muscle at the level of the thyroid cartilage. Assessment of the peripheral vascular system is the same as the adult. Pulses should be felt using the tips of the nurse's fingers directly against the pulse points and not through clothing. Notice differences (such as rate and amplitude) between pulses, particularly the radial and femoral.

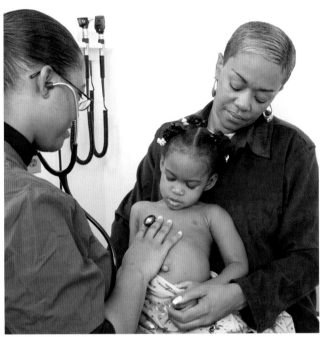

FIG. 19.35 Auscultation on a young child.

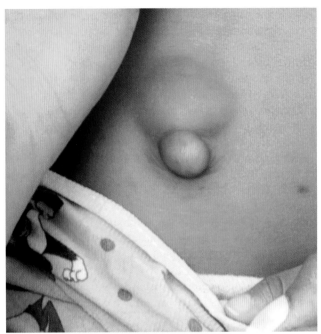

FIG. 19.37 Umbilical hernia on a toddler.

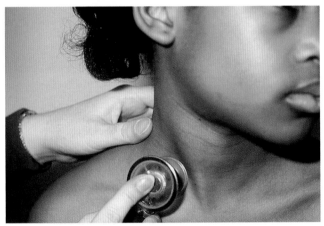

FIG. 19.36 Auscultation for venous hum. (From Seidel et al., 2003.)

Notice color of nailbeds and assess capillary refill. Any edema of the legs and arms should be noted.

Expected findings. Changes in heart rates in children are listed in Table 19.2. A venous hum in the jugular vein is considered a normal variation. A child's pulse may normally increase on inspiration and decrease on expiration. Nailbeds should be pink with rapid capillary refill.

Abnormal findings. Record the abnormal findings observed during the child's activities. Squatting may be a compensatory position for a child with a congenital heart defect. Cyanosis or pallor may indicate poor perfusion. Notice if there is more cyanosis with crying and if there is facial (particularly periorbital edema) or ankle edema. Notice signs of poor feeding and reports of caregiver that the child stops eating to get his or her breath, which may indicate a heart problem. Labored respirations could indicate a cardiovascular problem. Weak or absent femoral pulses may indicate coarctation of the aorta.

Abdomen and Gastrointestinal System

Procedure. Children may resist abdominal palpation because they are ticklish. Assessment of children is generally the same as that of adults, with the exception of the areas noted in the normal and abnormal findings.

Expected findings. Toddlers normally exhibit a rounded (potbelly) abdomen while both standing and lying down. School-age children may show this rounded appearance until about 13 years of age when standing; when lying, the abdomen should be flat. An umbilical hernia is a common variation in children, more so in African American children (Fig. 19.37). Most resolve spontaneously in early childhood.

Notice movement of the abdomen during respiration. Until about age 7 children are abdominal breathers. Diastasis recti abdominis (two rectus muscles fail to approximate one another) is common in African American children but should disappear during the preschool years.[9] The lower edge of the liver may be palpable in young children 1 to 2 cm below the right costal margin. Normally the liver descends during inspiration. It may not be palpable in older children.

Abnormal findings. Abdominal pain is always considered an abnormal finding. Generalized distention is an abnormal finding. A hernia that is not easily reducible is an abnormal finding at any age. Hernias that persist past the school age years require further evaluation. Other abnormal findings include liver or spleen enlargement and abdominal masses. If an enlarged spleen is suspected, the nurse must discontinue palpation in order to avoid rupturing the spleen.

Musculoskeletal System

Procedure. When evaluating children, compare data with tables of normal age and sequence of motor development. (Chapter 18 discusses expected motor development for children.)

Observe the gait for steadiness. The back exam begins with the nurse standing behind the child and inspecting the shoulders, scapula, and iliac crest for symmetry. Then, the nurse instructs the child to bend and touch his/her toes in order to visualize the spine for any curvature. All joints and muscle groups are examined for range of motion, tone, and strength.

Expected findings. Toddlers have a wide stance and a wide-waddle gait pattern, which tends to disappear by age 24 to 36 months. The gait should become progressively stronger, steadier, and smoother as the child matures. The spine should be straight. By 12 to 18 months the lumbar curve develops as the child learns to walk; lumbar lordosis is common in toddlers; after 18 months the cervical spine is concave, the thoracic spine is convex (although less than that of adults), and the lumbar spine is concave (similar to that of adults). There should be no bulges or dimpling along the spine. Lordosis is seen more frequently in African American children but should not be seen in children over 6 years of age. The knees should be in a direct straight line between the hip, the ankle, and the great toe. Valgus (outward) rotation of the lower extremities (medial malleoli greater than 2.5 cm apart with knees touching) is normal in children 2 to 3.5 years of age and may be present up to 12 years of age. Varus (inward) rotation of the lower extremities (medial malleoli touching, with knees greater than 2.5 cm apart) requires further evaluation for tibial torsion; it may be normal until 18 to 24 months of age. Full active and passive range of motion of all joints is expected as well as symmetric and firm muscles with 5/5 strength bilaterally (see Table 14-1), and adequate, symmetric muscle tone.

Abnormal findings. Any deviation from the developmental pattern or a history of increasing falls or balance problems should be considered abnormal. Any asymmetry of the shoulders, scapula, or iliac crest is abnormal. These findings, as well as any curvature of the spine, require further evaluation. Any asymmetry of tone, or limits in range of motion or strength, requires further evaluation.

Neurologic System

Procedure. Follow the same sequence of evaluation as for adults when dealing with children. Observe the child carefully during spontaneous activity because he or she may not be able to cooperate with requests as an adult would. Making the examination a game helps in data collection. Observe the child for achievement of expected developmental milestones for fine- and gross-motor, social-adaptive, and language skills described in Tables 18.4 and 18.5. Evaluate the child's general behavior while he or she is at play, interacting with parents, and cooperating with parents and with the nurse.

In testing cranial nerves, sense of smell usually is not tested; if it is, use a scent familiar to the child such as an orange. In testing visual fields and gaze (CNs II, III, IV, and VI), gently immobilize the head so the child cannot follow objects with the whole head but only with the eyes. When testing CN VII, approach it like a game, asking the child to make "funny faces" as the nurse models them (Fig. 19.38).

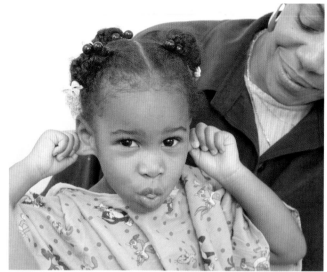
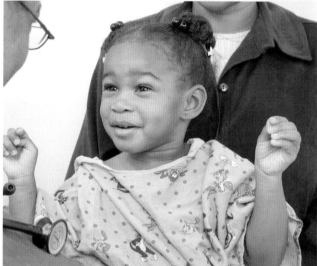

FIG. 19.38 Ask the child to make a "funny face" to assess cranial nerve VII.

Using an appropriate developmental approach, assess fine-motor coordination in children under 6 years of age. For children older than 6 years, use the finger-to-nose test, with the nurse's finger held 2.5 to 5 cm away from the child's nose.

Sensory function is not normally tested before age 5. Carefully explain what is being done when children are tested and use descriptions that the child can understand such as "this will feel like a tickle." Use simple numbers (such as 0, 7, 5, 3, or 1) for graphesthesia testing and X and O for younger children.

The screening for neurologic "soft" signs in school-age children is used to describe vague and minimal dysfunction signs such as clumsiness, language disturbances, motor overload, mirroring movement of extremities, or perceptual development difficulties (Table 19.5).

Typically, deep tendon reflexes (DTRs) are not tested in young children unless they present with neurologic symptoms (i.e., muscle weakness, dizziness). However, if it is warranted, perform the DTR test in the same manner as in the adult examination.

TABLE 19.5 SCREENING ASSESSMENT OF NEUROLOGIC "SOFT" SIGNS

INSTRUCTIONAL TECHNIQUE	IMPORTANT OBSERVATIONS	VARIABLES AND CONSIDERATIONS
Evaluation of Fine-Motor Coordination		
Observe child during:		
a. Undressing, unbuttoning	Note child's general coordination	
b. Tying shoe	Note general coordination	
c. Rapidly touching alternate fingers with thumb	Note if similar movement on other side	For items c to e and h and i, movement of other side noted as associated motor movements, adventitious overflow movements, or synkinesis
d. Rattling imaginary doorknob	Note if similar movement on other side	
e. Unscrewing imaginary light bulb	Note if similar movement on other side	
f. Grasping pencil and writing	Note excessive pressure on pen point; fingers placed directly over point, or placed greater than 2.5 cm up shaft	May indicate difficulty with fine-motor coordination
g. Moving tongue rapidly	Note general coordination	
h. Demonstrating hand grip	Note if similar movement on opposite side	
i. Inverting feet	Note if similar movement on opposite side	
j. Repeating several times "pa, ta, ka" or "kitty, kitty, kitty"	Accurate reproduction of these sounds indicates auditory coordination	
Evaluation of Special Sensory Skills		
a. Dual simultaneous sensory tests (face-hand testing): First demonstrate technique, then instruct child to close eyes; nurse performs simultaneously: (1) Touch both cheeks (2) Touch both hands (3) Touch right cheek and right hand (4) Touch left cheek and right hand (5) Touch left cheek and left hand (6) Touch right cheek and left hand	Failure to perceive hand stimulus when face is simultaneously touched is referred to as *rostral dominance*	Approximately 80% of normal children able to perform this test by age 8 years without rostral dominance
b. Finger localization test (finger agnosia test): Touch two spots on one finger or two fingers simultaneously; child has eyes closed; ask, "How many fingers am I touching, one or two?"	Evaluate number of correct responses with four trials for each hand Six out of eight possible correct responses is a pass	Approximately 50% of all children able to pass test by age 6 years Approximately 90% of all children able to pass test by age 9 Reflects child's orientation in space, concept of body image, sensation of touch, and position sense
Evaluation of Child's Laterality and Orientation in Space		
a. Imitation of gestures: Instruct child to use same hand as nurse and imitate the following movements ("Do as I do"): (1) Extend little finger (2) Extend little and index fingers (3) Extend index and middle fingers (4) Touch two thumbs and two index fingers together simultaneously (5) Form two interlocking rings—thumb and index finger of one hand, with thumb and index finger of other hand (6) Point index finger of one hand down toward cupped finger of opposite hand held below	Note difficulty with fine finger movements, manipulation, or reproduction of correct gesture Note any marked right-left confusion regarding nurse's right and left hands	Helps to evaluate child's finger discrimination; awareness of body image; and right, left, front, back, and up and down orientation Especially important after age 8 years if there continues to be marked right-left confusion

Continued

TABLE 19.5 SCREENING ASSESSMENT OF NEUROLOGIC "SOFT" SIGNS—cont'd

INSTRUCTIONAL TECHNIQUE	IMPORTANT OBSERVATIONS	VARIABLES AND CONSIDERATIONS

b. Following directions: ask child to:
  (1) Show me your left hand
  (2) Show me your right eye
  (3) Show me your left elbow
  (4) Touch your left knee with your left hand
  (5) Touch your right ear with your left hand
  (6) Touch your left elbow with your right hand
  (7) Touch your right cheek with your right hand
  (8) Note any difficulty with following
      sequence of directions
  (9) Point to my left ear
  (10) Point to my right eye
  (11) Point to my right hand
  (12) Point to my left knee
	Note any incorrect response
	
	Note any difficulty with following
	  sequence of directions
		Items 1 through 7 mastered by approx-
		  imately age 6 years
		
		Items 8 through 11 mastered by age
		  8 years

Expected and abnormal findings. Expected findings should generally be the same as those for adults. Soft neurologic signs may be considered normal in the young child; but, as the child matures, the signs should disappear.

Abnormal findings are the same as those for the adult. Spasticity; paralysis; or impaired vision, speech, or hearing may indicate neurologic abnormalities. The identification of soft signs as the child matures indicates failure of the child to perform age-specific activities (see Table 19.5), and the child should be referred to a health care professional for further evaluation. Inattention, motor restlessness, and easy distractibility may indicate attention-deficit/hyperactivity disorder.

Breasts

Procedure. The examination of the child generally requires only inspection. The child's chest should be exposed.

Expected and abnormal findings. The nipples normally are located slightly lateral to the midclavicular line between the fourth and fifth ribs. For the prepubescent child the nipple should be flat and surrounded by a slightly darker pigmented areola. As the female reaches prepubertal age, sometimes as young as age 8, her breasts show prepubertal budding. Precocious development of breasts in females before age 8 should be investigated further.

Reproductive System and Perineum

Female Examination

Procedure. The extent of the genitalia examination in children depends on their age and the report of problems during the history, but typically the examination is limited to inspection of the external genitalia to determine if the structures are intact and without obvious abnormalities. In many cultures, children are taught at a very early age that the genitalia should not be exposed or touched. An inspection of a young girl's external genitalia should be included with each routine examination. If this examination is performed consistently, the child may experience less anxiety and embarrassment in later years. Internal examination in the prepubertal girl is not indicated.

The nurse must take the time to gain the cooperation and understanding of the child; how this is done depends largely on the age of the child and previous experiences. Whenever possible, reassure the child that she is growing up normally. By the time a child is 4 to 6 years of age, she must be reassured that the exam procedure involves only looking at her genitalia and touching her on the outside. Approach the child in a matter-of-fact manner, informing her about the procedure and what to expect. The child may have difficulty understanding the difference between a permissible genitalia examination by a nurse and inappropriate touching by others. The parent's involvement in this discussion is important.

When nurses examine younger children, they can invite the parents to participate by helping to position the child. In all cases ensure privacy for the child. She should participate in the decision about whether or not the parent should be present in the room during the examination. Some girls may want a parent present, whereas the preteen child may not. Confer with the child before the examination and, if appropriate, ask the parent to wait outside.

Position the child on her back and place her legs in a frog-leg position (hips flexed with the soles of the feet together and up to her buttocks), with the head slightly elevated so she can observe the nurse. The techniques of the external genitalia examination are the same as for the infant. Using gloved hands, gently spread the labia so the genitalia may be inspected.

Occasionally, situations warrant a more complete examination. The decision to do this is usually based on external examination findings or the history. For example, if the child has a history of urinary tract infections; vaginal discharge or irritation; or complaints of itching, rash, or pain, a more complete examination is necessary. A complete examination is also necessary if there is any indication of sexual abuse or mishandling of the child. In this case such an examination is performed by a sexual assault nurse examiner or other qualified health care provider. A rectal examination may be necessary if there is any suspected history of abuse, the possibility of a foreign body in the rectum, or specific rectal symptoms. Internal inspection is considered an advanced skill and should only be attempted by nurses who have received adequate training for this type of examination.

Expected and abnormal findings. Until approximately age 7, the labia majora are flat, the labia minora are thin, and the clitoris is relatively small. Usually the hymen membrane has a visible opening, although there are a number of normal variations in the appearance of the hymen. In older girls the labia majora and minora appear thicker, and evidence of pubic hair may be seen by the time the child reaches pubescence—usually between ages 8 and 11. There should be no vaginal discharge, vaginal odor, or evidence of bruising.

Male Examination

Procedure. The procedure for examining the male child's genitalia are the same as those for the infant. The major difference in the examination is the approach. In many cultures, children are taught at a very early age that the genitalia should not be exposed or touched. In the presence of the child's parent, reassure him that his genitalia must be examined just as all of his other body areas. Asking the parent to reassure the child that he needs to be examined to make sure that he is healthy is important. Whenever possible, reassure the child that he is growing up normally.

The examination can be performed with the child sitting or standing. If the child is sitting, he should be in a slightly reclining position with his knees flexed and heels near the buttocks (Fig. 19.39) or sitting with his knees spread and ankles crossed. If the child has not been circumcised, do not force the foreskin to be retracted. Wearing gloves, retract the foreskin only to the point of tightness. Then evaluate whether it is retracted far enough to permit adequate urination and cleaning. Determine if the child has any discharge, crusting, or lesions around or under the foreskin. In addition, examine the scrotum for shape, size, and color, and palpate to determine the presence of testicles in the scrotum. Evidence of pubic hair may be seen by the time the child reaches pubescence.

Expected and abnormal findings. The findings for children are the same as those for the infant. By ages 3 to 4 the

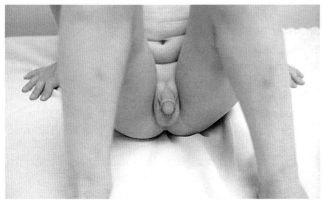

FIG. 19.39 Position of young child for examination of genitalia. (From Ball et al., 2015.)

foreskin can be retracted easily. A scrotum with well-formed rugae indicates that the testes have descended into the scrotum. A small, flat, and underdeveloped scrotum is considered abnormal and may indicate cryptorchidism (undescended testes). If the nurse is unable to palpate one or both testicles, then an exam by either a physician or advanced practice registered nurse is required.

Perianal Examination

Procedure. Inspection of the perianal area is routinely performed during a comprehensive assessment. For the external examination, be sure to respect the child's modesty and apprehension; take the time to explain what is going to happen and what the child can expect. Children should be positioned so the perianal area is adequately exposed and the child is comfortable. The child should be positioned either in a knee-chest position or on the left side with the hips and knees flexed toward the abdomen (the same positioning as for the adult).

Internal rectal examination is not performed in children unless there are specific symptoms such as severe abdominal pain, constipation, or injury. If an internal rectal examination is warranted, the nurse should use the little finger to perform the examination. Even when this is done, there may occasionally be slight rectal bleeding. The parent should be told about this possibility before the examination. The procedure for the internal examination is the same as that for the adult.

Expected and abnormal findings. The findings for external examination are the same for the child as for the adult. The findings for the internal examination are the same as for the adult, with the exception that the prostate in the small child is not palpable. Variations are based on developmental maturity. Redness or irritation may be an indication of a bacterial or fungal infection or pinworms. Assess for signs of physical or sexual abuse such as bruising, anal tearing, anal dilation, or extreme or inappropriate apprehension from the child. If there is suspicion of child abuse or assault, report the findings to the appropriate child protective services.

EXAMINATION OF ADOLESCENTS

The sequence of examination for the adolescent is the same as for the adult. As children enter their teen years, they should be given a choice about whether a parent is present during the physical examination. This ensures privacy and encourages teens to begin assuming responsibility for their health care.

Skin, Hair, and Nails

Although the examination of the skin, hair, and nails is straightforward, maturational changes and body hair development often make the adolescent more sensitive than children or adults. Provide adequate privacy and be sensitive to the patient's concerns during the examination.

Skin

Expected findings. As the child becomes an adolescent, the skin undergoes significant changes. The skin texture takes on more adult characteristics. In addition, there is increased perspiration, oiliness, and acne secondary to an increase in sebaceous gland activity.

Abnormal findings. The most common abnormal finding in the adolescent is acne, which may appear as young as 7 to 8 years of age but peaks in adolescence at approximately 16 years of age. Although most acne appears on the face, it may also be prevalent on the chest, back, and shoulders. Acne may appear as blackheads (open comedones) or whiteheads (closed comedones),[19] pustules, or cysts (Fig. 19.40). Inflamed lesions of acne can be mild or severe. These lesions are painful and are of concern to the patient because of the appearance (Fig. 19.41).

Hair and Nails

Expected and abnormal findings. The presence and characteristics of facial hair in males and body hair in both males and females change significantly throughout adolescence. By the end of adolescence there is an adult hair distribution

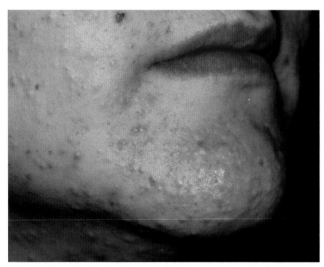

FIG. 19.40 Comedonal acne. (Courtesy Lemmi and Lemmi, 2013.)

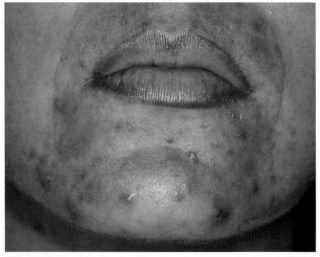

FIG. 19.41 Acne vulgaris. (Courtesy Lemmi and Lemmi, 2013.)

pattern (see Chapter 17). The expected findings are the same as those for the adult. Persistent nail biting may be a habit, indicating a coping mechanism for dealing with stress. The nurse should take the time to evaluate why nail biting persists.

Head, Eyes, Ears, Nose, and Throat

The procedure as well as expected and abnormal findings for the adolescent are the same as for the adult.

Lung and Respiratory System

The procedure, as well as expected and abnormal findings, for the adolescent are the same as for the adult. The nurse should be sensitive to the modesty of the female adolescent and provide a drape for the breasts while the anterior chest is being assessed.

Heart and Peripheral Vascular System

The procedure, as well as expected and abnormal findings, for the cardiovascular assessment are the same as for the adult.

Abdomen and Gastrointestinal System

The procedure, as well as expected and abnormal findings, for the gastrointestinal assessment are the same as for the adult.

Musculoskeletal System

Procedure. Examination of the adolescent is the same as that of the adult. Observe the adolescent's posture. Adolescents are screened for scoliosis, kyphosis, and lordosis.

Expected and abnormal findings. The expected findings for the adolescent are the same as those for the adult. Assessment of the spine is of particular importance in adolescence. Scoliosis is suggested by visual curvature of the spine or an asymmetric "rib hump" (see Fig. 19.54, later in this chapter). Referral to an orthopedic physician specializing in scoliosis for further evaluation is necessary to determine the degree of curvature, its progression, and treatment. Poor posture, regardless of the cause (e.g., low self-esteem or heavy backpack), contributes to kyphosis. Postural kyphosis is almost always accompanied by a compensatory lordosis (i.e., an abnormally concave lumbar curvature).

Neurologic System

The procedure, as well as expected and abnormal findings, for the adolescent are the same as for the adult.

Breasts

Procedure. The key breast assessment relates to sexual maturity staging and progression of puberty; this involves inspection only. A complete breast exam is not routinely performed unless there is a specific complaint. When performed, the technique is the same as in the adult.

Expected and abnormal findings: Female. Breast development occurs in five stages over an average of 4 years (Fig. 19.42).[20] Menarche coincides with stage 3 or 4 breast

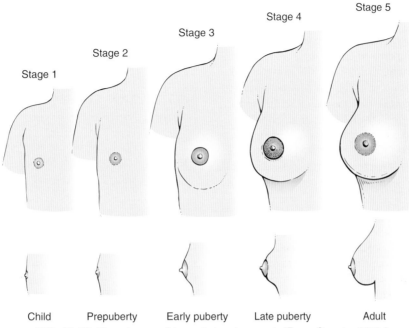

FIG. 19.42 Five stages of breast development. (From Swartz, 2010.)

Stage 1   Stage 2   Stage 3   Stage 4   Stage 5

Child   Prepuberty   Early puberty   Late puberty   Adult

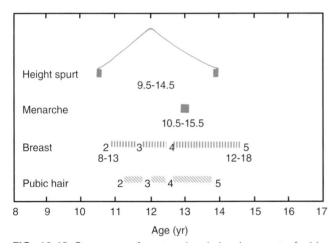

FIG. 19.43 Summary of maturational development of girls. The numbers 2 to 5 refer to the stage of development. (From Marshall and Tanner, 1969.)

Height spurt — 9.5-14.5
Menarche — 10.5-15.5
Breast — 2 3 4 5; 8-13, 12-18
Pubic hair — 2 3 4 5
Age (yr) 8 9 10 11 12 13 14 15 16 17

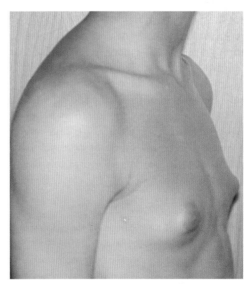

FIG. 19.44 Prepubertal gynecomastia. (Courtesy Wellington Hung, MD, Children's National Medical Center, Washington, DC.)

development, usually just after the peak of the adolescent growth spurt, which is approximately age 12 in most females (Fig. 19.43). However, the nurse should consider the development stages as a general guideline, because there is variability in age of breast development across racial/ethnic groups. For example, Harlan found that African American girls developed secondary sex characteristics earlier than Caucasian girls of the same age.[21] The right and left breasts may develop at different rates. When this difference is found, reassuring the patient that this is common and that in time the development may equalize is important. The breast tissue in the adolescent female should feel firm and elastic throughout both breasts. By age 14 most females have developed breasts that resemble those of the adult female. Abnormal findings include a lack of breast development, lesions, lumps, and nipple drainage.

Expected and abnormal findings: Male. Male adolescents, especially obese males, may have transient unilateral or bilateral subareolar masses (Fig. 19.44). These firm and sometimes tender masses may be of great concern to the patient. Reassure the young adolescent that they are generally transient and should disappear within a year or so. Gynecomastia, on the other hand, is an unexpected enlargement of one or both breasts in the male. It may be caused by hormonal or systemic disorders; however, it is commonly a result of adipose tissue associated with obesity or the body change transition that occurs during early puberty.[9] Most adolescent males with gynecomastia are very self-conscious of this finding.

Reproductive System

Female Examination

Procedure. If a parent is present, the adolescent should be given a choice to be examined alone, and she should be assured of privacy and confidentiality. The nurse must take time to develop a relationship with the patient and reassure her in a matter-of-fact manner that the examination of the genitalia is an essential part of a complete examination. Reassure the patient that the changes her body is undergoing are normal. Because many preadolescents and adolescents are becoming interested in their own bodies and the changes that are taking place, they may want to take an active part in the examination. This may be a perfect opportunity to teach the patient about her anatomy and the changes that she will experience. A mirror may be used during the examination for instruction.

The positioning and techniques for examination of the external genitalia are the same as for the adult. A pelvic examination should be performed beginning at age 21 or at any time the patient has signs of genital or vaginal irritation or infection. The procedure to be followed is the same as for an adult woman, but additional time must be taken to explain the procedure, show the equipment, and tell the patient exactly what she may expect.

Expected and abnormal findings. Sexual maturity is assessed through a gradual emergence of pubic hair (from straight, downy hair to curly, coarse, and thick hair) that gradually covers the pubic area to the inner thighs. The expected and abnormal findings for the adolescent are the same as for the adult with careful attention to the sequence of pubertal changes. Notice if the physical attributes are early, late, or if the sequence does not follow the expected maturational development for girls (see Fig. 19.43) as this may denote a significant endocrine issue.

Male Examination

Procedure. Genital assessment of the adolescent male is important to ensure that the maturational development is progressing and because testicular cancer occurs in this age group. This is also the time when modesty is at its peak. The nurse must take time to develop a relationship with the patient and reassure him in a matter-of-fact manner that the examination of the genitalia is an essential part of a complete

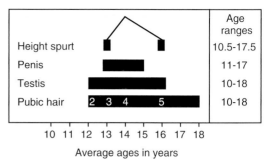

FIG. 19.45 Development of male genitalia and pubic hair associated with height spurt and age. (From Tanner, 1962.)

examination. Ensuring privacy and adequate draping when the genitalia are not being examined is important. Deferring the genitalia assessment to the last procedure of the examination is usually best. The process of examination is essentially the same as previously discussed for the adult.

Expected and abnormal findings. Expected findings for the young adolescent male depend on the maturational stage of the patient. Maturational changes include a height spurt, gradual development of pubic hair, and gradual growth of the penis and scrotum (Fig. 19.45). In the preadolescent male there is an absence of pubic hair, and enlargement of penis and scrotum has not begun. The first signs of maturation include the emergence of long and straight pubic hair, slight enlargement of the penis, and enlargement of the testes and scrotum with a darkening of the skin. As maturation continues, hair growth increases and becomes thick and coarse, the penis enlarges in both length and diameter, and the scrotum enlarges, with a darkening skin tone. Alterations in maturational sequencing should be noted. Findings for the older adolescent are essentially the same as previously discussed for the adult. Abnormal findings include testicular pain or masses, varicoceles, or signs suggestive of sexually transmitted infections (e.g., discharge or lesions).

Perianal Examination

Rectal examinations are not performed routinely unless warranted by symptoms (e.g., rectal bleeding). The prostate examination is not performed routinely in adolescent males. If performed, the procedure and findings for the adolescent are the same as for the adult.

COMMON PROBLEMS AND CONDITIONS

SKIN CONDITIONS

Atopic Dermatitis

Atopic dermatitis is a chronic superficial inflammation of the skin with an unknown cause. It may be associated with allergies and asthma, and it is thought to be familial. It is commonly seen in infancy and childhood. **Clinical Findings:** Red, weeping, crusted lesions may appear on the face, scalp, extremities, and diaper area. In older children lesion characteristics include erythema, scaling, and lichenification. The

lesions are usually localized to the hands, feet, arms, and legs (particularly at the antecubital fossa and popliteal space) and are associated with intense pruritus (Fig. 19.46).

Diaper Dermatitis

One of the most common causes of irritant contact dermatitis, diaper dermatitis, is an inflammatory reaction to urine, feces, moisture, or friction. It is common among infants between 4 and 12 months of age. **Clinical Findings:** This dermatitis is characterized by a primary irritant rash involving

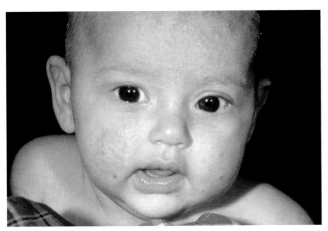

FIG. 19.46 Atopic dermatitis. (From Lemmi and Lemmi, 2013.)

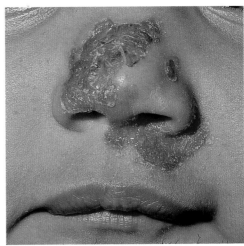

FIG. 19.48 Impetigo. (From Weston, Lane, and Morelli, 1996.)

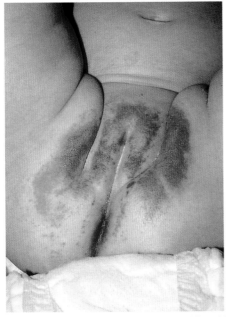

FIG. 19.47 Severe diaper rash. (From White, 2004.)

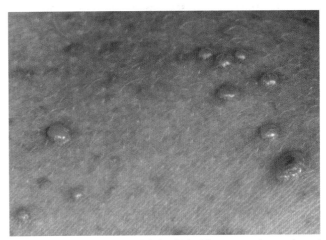

FIG. 19.49 Chickenpox (Varicella). (Courtesy Lemmi and Lemmi, 2013.)

skin areas in contact with soiled diaper surfaces. The rash is composed of red macules and papules that may be raised and confluent in severe cases (Fig. 19.47).

Impetigo

This is a common and highly contagious bacterial infection caused by staphylococcal or streptococcal pathogens. It is most prevalent in children, especially among those in crowded conditions such as school or child care settings.[22] It commonly occurs in mid-to-late summer, with the highest incidence in hot, humid climates. **Clinical Findings:** This infection appears as an erythematous macule that becomes a vesicle or bulla and finally a honey-colored crust after the vesicles or bullae rupture (Fig. 19.48).

Herpes Varicella (Chickenpox)

This is a highly communicable viral infection spread by droplets that often occurs during childhood. **Clinical Findings:** The

lesions first appear on the trunk and then spread to the extremities and the face. Initially the lesions are macules; they progress to papules and then vesicles, and finally the old vesicles become crusts. The lesions erupt in crops over a period of several days. For this reason, lesions in various stages are seen concurrently (Fig. 19.49).

EAR AND EYE CONDITIONS

Acute Otitis Media

This infection of the middle ear may appear with the presence of middle ear effusion that can be viral or bacterial in origin. It is one of the most common of all childhood infections. **Clinical Findings:** The major symptom associated with acute otitis media (AOM) is ear pain (otalgia). Infants, unable to verbally communicate pain, demonstrate irritability, fussiness, crying, lethargy, and pulling at the affected ear. Associated manifestations may include fever, vomiting, and decreased hearing. On inspection in the early stages, the TM appears inflamed—it is red and may be bulging and immobile (Fig. 19.50). Later stages may reveal discoloration (white

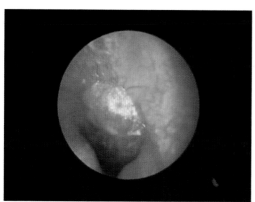

FIG. 19.50 Acute otitis media of the left ear with redness and edema of the pars flaccida. (From Bingham, Hawke, and Kwok, 1992.)

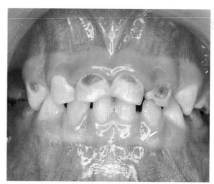

FIG. 19.51 Dental caries. (From Zitelli and Davis, 2007.)

or yellow drainage) and opacification to the TM. Purulent drainage from the ear canal with a sudden relief of pain suggests perforation of the TM.

Conjunctivitis

An inflammation of the palpebral or bulbar conjunctiva is termed *conjunctivitis*. It is caused by local infection of bacteria or virus and by an allergic reaction, systemic infection, or chemical irritation. **Clinical Findings:** The conjunctiva and sclera appear red (injected), and there may be thick, sticky discharge on the eyelids.

MOUTH AND THROAT CONDITIONS

Dental Caries

Dental caries is a significant problem in children and may be caused by prolonged exposure to sweetened liquids or poor oral hygiene. **Clinical Findings:** An erosion of the tooth enamel leads to dark or blackened teeth. Gingival irritation is also commonly seen (Fig. 19.51).

Tonsillitis

Tonsillitis is one of the most common oropharyngeal infections among children. It can be viral or bacterial in origin; common bacterial pathogens include beta-hemolytic streptococci. **Clinical Findings:** The classic presentation of tonsillitis includes sore throat, pain with swallowing (odynophagia), fever, chills, and tender cervical lymph nodes. Some children may also complain of ear pain and have swollen anterior cervical lymph nodes. On inspection the tonsils appear enlarged and red and may be covered with white or yellow exudates (Fig. 19.52).

Cleft Lip and Cleft Palate

Cleft lip and cleft palate are incomplete fusion of the maxillary process and/or the secondary palate during fetal development. These conditions are the most common congenital craniofacial defects and the fourth most common congenital defects seen in the United States. **Clinical Findings:** Usually diagnosed before or at birth, the defects are characterized by

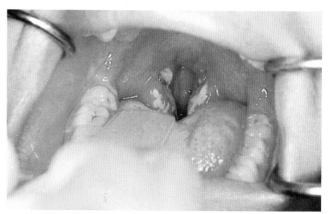

FIG. 19.52 Tonsillitis and pharyngitis. (Courtesy Dr. Edward L Applebaum, Head, Department of Otolaryngology. University of Illinois Medical Center.)

a defect in the upper lip or a complete separation extending to the floor of the nostril. This can be unilateral or bilateral (Fig. 19.53). A subtle finding may be incomplete bony closure of the upper palate, which can be detected by palpation with a gloved finger of a bifid uvula.

RESPIRATORY CONDITIONS

Cystic Fibrosis

This is an autosomal-recessive genetic disorder of the exocrine glands. It is a multisystem disease affecting most body systems but especially the lungs, pancreas, and sweat glands. Respiratory system dysfunction develops because of abnormally thick mucus production, which leads to a chronic, diffuse, obstructive pulmonary disease. Symptoms commonly appear before the age of 4, although a milder form of disease may delay diagnosis until late childhood or early adolescence. **Clinical Findings:** The classic symptom of cystic fibrosis (CF) is the production of thick, sticky mucus. Stools of children with CF are often frothy, foul smelling, and greasy (steatorrhea). Respiratory signs and symptoms include a chronic moist productive cough with frequent respiratory infections. As the disease progresses, children develop a barrel chest (see Fig. 11.15) and finger clubbing (see Fig. 9.10 and Fig. 12.23).

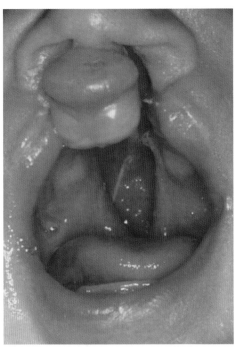

FIG. 19.53 Bilateral cleft lip and complete cleft palate. (From Zitelli, McIntire, and Nowalk, 2012.)

Childhood Asthma

This chronic respiratory disorder is characterized by airway obstruction and inflammation caused by multiple factors, including environmental exposures, viral illnesses, allergens, and genetic predisposition. Although it can occur anytime during childhood, most children develop symptoms in early childhood. **Clinical Findings:** The most common finding is a persistent cough that is worse at night. Exacerbations may present with increased respiratory rate with prolonged expiration, audible wheeze, shortness of breath, tachycardia, anxious appearance, possible use of accessory muscles, and cough (see Fig. 11.28).

Croup Syndromes

The term *croup* describes a wide range of upper-airway illnesses that result from edema of the epiglottis and larynx that often extends into the trachea and bronchi. The three most common conditions—laryngotracheobronchitis, epiglottitis, and tracheitis—affect the greatest number of children across all age groups (although it is most common in young children). **Clinical Findings:** The classic findings include inspiratory stridor, a barking-like cough, hoarseness, and a cherry red epiglottis. Related findings may include fever and runny nose. In severe cases the child may display respiratory distress, including rapid, labored breathing with retractions and lethargy. The child may assume a position of comfort to ease respirations, and profuse drooling due to an inability to swallow secretions may occur. If these findings exist, an oral examination should not be done because it could trigger airway obstruction.

CARDIOVASCULAR CONDITIONS

Congenital Heart Defects

The most common congenital heart defects involve an abnormal connection between the left and right side of the heart (septal defects) or between the great arteries (patent ductus arteriosus). Large defects are typically diagnosed before or shortly after birth, whereas smaller defects may be undiagnosed until the preschool years. **Clinical Findings:** Among infants and children, poor feeding and poor weight gain are often seen; elevations in heart and respiratory rates may be observed with feeding. A murmur is often auscultated, and splitting heart sounds may be noted. Children fatigue easily and may assume a squatting position to relieve cyanotic spells. Signs associated with congestive heart failure may be observed with larger defects.

MUSCULOSKELETAL CONDITIONS

Muscular Dystrophies

This is a group of inherited diseases characterized by progressive muscle wasting caused by degeneration of muscle fibers. The most common form in childhood is Duchenne muscular dystrophy. **Clinical Findings:** In infancy, sucking and swallowing difficulties may be observed. In early childhood, weakness involving the lower extremities becomes evident with frequent tripping or toe walking. The muscle weakness progresses to muscle wasting; eventually the child loses the ability to walk.

Myelomeningocele

This neural tube defect is characterized by a posterior vertebral anomaly. Types of myelomeningocele range from a defect in posterior vertebra only to protrusion of the spinal cord through the vertebral defect. These defects occur within the first month of gestation. **Clinical Findings:** At birth, a saclike protrusion may be noted on the infant's back along the spine, or there may be no obvious signs. These defects can occur anywhere from the upper thoracic to the sacral spine. A wide range of impairments (e.g., motor impairment, sensory impairment of the lower extremities, and possibly sensory loss involving the anus and genitalia) are also noted.

Scoliosis

An S-shaped deformity of the vertebrae, referred to as *scoliosis*, creates deformity of three planes, usually involving lateral curvature, spinal rotation causing rib asymmetry, and thoracic kyphosis (Fig. 19.54). The most common form of scoliosis in children is idiopathic, although it is thought to have a genetic link. This condition can occur in early childhood but is commonly seen in children over age 10 at about the time of puberty. **Clinical Findings:** Scoliosis produces uneven shoulders and hip levels. A curvature less than 10% is considered a normal variation, and curves between 10% and 20% are considered mild. Rotation deformity also may cause a rib hump and flank asymmetry on forward flexion.

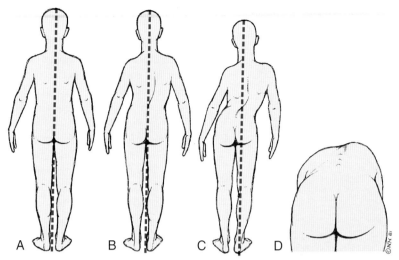

FIG. 19.54 Scoliosis. (A) Normal Spine. (B) Mild. (C) Severe. (D) Rib hump and flank asymmetry seen in flexion. (Redrawn from Hilt & Schmitt, 1975).

Depending on the severity of the curve, physiologic function of lungs, spine, and pelvis may be compromised.

NEUROLOGIC CONDITIONS

Hydrocephalus

An abnormal accumulation of cerebrospinal fluid (CSF) is called hydrocephalus. In infants, it is usually a result of an obstruction of the drainage of CSF from the ventricles. **Clinical Findings:** In infants, a gradual increase in intracranial pressure occurs, leading to an actual enlargement of the head (Fig. 19.55). As the head enlarges, the facial features appear small in proportion to the cranium, the fontanelles may bulge, and the scalp veins dilate.

Cerebral Palsy

This is a group of motor function disorders caused by permanent, nonprogressive brain lesions that occur during fetal development or near the time of birth. Classifications of cerebral palsy are spastic, accounting for 50% of cases; dyskinetic (athetoid, 20%); ataxic (10%); and mixed (20%). **Clinical Findings:** Deficits may include spasticity; seizures; muscle contractions; delayed motor development; and impaired vision, speech, and hearing. Cognitive impairment may be a related finding.

Attention Deficit Hyperactivity Disorder

Attention deficit hyperactivity disorder (ADHD is a condition that begins in childhood characterized by inattentiveness,

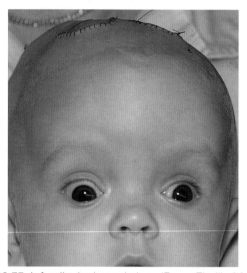

FIG. 19.55 Infantile hydrocephalus. (From Zitelli, McIntire, and Nowalk, 2012.)

impulsivity, and hyperactivity that are developmentally inappropriate. ADHD is diagnosed nearly three times more often in boys than girls.[23] **Clinical Findings:** The manifestations may be numerous or few, mild or severe, and vary with the developmental level of the child. An important clinical manifestation is distractibility. The child seems to have selective attention and often does not seem to listen or follow through.

CLINICAL APPLICATION AND CLINICAL JUDGMENT

See Appendix B for answers to exercises in this section.

CASE STUDY

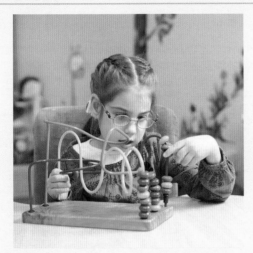

Megan Grady is an 8-year-old girl with cerebral palsy who is being treated for seizures.

Interview Data

Megan's mother states that Megan was at home watching television when she started "shaking and jerking all over." The seizure occurred several hours ago but lasted longer than 20 minutes. The mother is concerned because her daughter has never had a seizure that lasted this long. Megan denies recent headaches or problems with balance; she takes primidone 125 mg twice a day.

Examination Data

- *Vital Signs:* Blood pressure, 110/68 mm Hg; pulse, 84 beats/min; respiratory rate, 18 breaths/min; temperature, 98.6°F (37°C).
- *Cognition:* She is a cooperative, alert child with flat affect. She communicates slowly but appropriately.
- *Neurologic:* She has voluntary, symmetric, coordinated movement of all extremities with full range of motion; muscle strength is 5 bilaterally. DTRs are 2+ bilaterally. Sensation is present in arms and legs to vibration, cotton, and pinprick bilaterally.

Clinical Judgment

1. What cues do you recognize that suggest deviations from normal, suggesting a need for further investigation?
2. For which additional information should the nurse ask or assess?
3. Based on the data, which risk factors for injury does Megan have?
4. With which health care team members would you collaborate to meet this patient's needs?

REVIEW QUESTIONS

1. Which finding on a 2-month-old baby is considered abnormal and requires further follow-up?
   1. The anterior fontanelle is not palpable.
   2. The thyroid gland cannot be palpated.
   3. The head circumference is slightly greater than the chest circumference.
   4. Head lag is observed when the shoulders are lifted off the examination table.

2. A nurse is palpating the lymph nodes of an 18-month-old toddler and finds enlarged postauricular and occipital nodes. What is the significance of this finding?
   1. This is a normal finding for a toddler.
   2. The toddler may have an ear infection.
   3. The toddler may have an inflammation of the scalp.
   4. The toddler needs to be referred to a pediatrician.

3. While examining the ear of an infant with an otoscope, the nurse pulls down on the ear for which reason?
   1. Increases the depth that the otoscope can be inserted
   2. Stabilizes the ear to avoid injury if the infant moves the head suddenly
   3. Enhances visualization of the tympanic membrane by straightening the ear canal

   4. Facilitates drainage of cerumen from the ear canal, allowing better visualization of inner ear structures

4. What is an expected finding of the newborn's vision that the nurse teaches the parents?
   1. Binocular vision is normally achieved at this age.
   2. Peripheral sight does not develop until age 3 or 4 months.
   3. The newborn can only distinguish the colors of blue and green.
   4. The newborn is nearsighted and cannot see items unless they are close.

5. Which disorder, if any, does a nurse screen for when examining a healthy adolescent?
   1. Muscle weakness
   2. Limited joint range of motion
   3. Curvature of the spine
   4. No screening is needed.

6. Which is an expected finding of a newborn's respiratory assessment?
   1. Thoracic breathing
   2. A 1:2 ratio of anteroposterior-to-lateral diameter

3. Flaring of the nares noted on inspiration
4. Bronchovesicular breath sounds in peripheral lung fields

7. Which finding of a preschooler is abnormal during a cardiovascular system examination?
   1. Heart rate of 106 beats/min
   2. Failure to gain weight because of fatigue while eating
   3. Continuous low-pitched vibration heard over the jugular vein
   4. Pulse increasing on inspiration and decreasing on expiration

8. How does a nurse respond to parents of a 5-year-old who are worried that their child has a protruding abdomen?
   1. Assesses the child to differentiate a normal "potbelly" from a hernia
   2. Suggests that the parents administer an appropriate dose of a laxative at bedtime
   3. Refers the parents to a nutritionist to develop an appropriate weight-loss diet for the child
   4. Informs the parents that a protruding abdomen is always an abnormal finding in this age group

9. Which position is ideal when examining the genitalia of a 3-year-old boy?
   1. Prone position with legs flexed in a frog-leg position
   2. Supine position with knees spread and ankles spread apart
   3. Lithotomy position with knees and ankles spread apart
   4. Sitting position with knees spread and ankles crossed

10. On assessment of the neurologic status of a 4-month-old infant, the nurse notes which finding as abnormal?
    1. The infant abducts and extends arms and legs when startled.
    2. When the infant's sole is touched, the toes flex tightly in an attempt to grasp.
    3. When stroking the infant's foot from sole to great toes, there is fanning of the toes.
    4. The infant steps in place when held upright with feet on a flat surface.

Assessment of the Pregnant Patient

evolve

http://evolve.elsevier.com/Wilson/assessment

Assessment of the pregnant patient warrants special attention because of the multiple hormonal, structural, and physiologic changes associated with pregnancy. This chapter builds on previous chapters regarding obtaining a health history and conducting an examination.

Ideally the pregnant woman is seen on a regular basis throughout pregnancy. Prenatal visits are recommended every 4 weeks up to 28 weeks, every 2 weeks from 28 to 36 weeks, and weekly after 36 weeks; more frequent visits may occur at the discretion of the provider or at a patient's request. The initial prenatal visit includes a comprehensive history and examination; follow-up visits are more limited in scope, monitoring the progress of the pregnancy and assessing for complications while providing patient education appropriate for week of gestation.

ANATOMY AND PHYSIOLOGY

Maternal physiologic adaptations during pregnancy result from hormonal changes and mechanical pressures caused by the enlarging uterus and changes in other tissues. These changes protect the woman's physiologic functioning, allow adaptation to the metabolic demands associated with pregnancy, and provide a protective environment for the growing fetus. Box 20.1 presents selected changes associated with pregnancy.

SIGNS OF PREGNANCY

A combination of laboratory tests and the clinical findings is used to determine the presence of a pregnancy. Laboratory tests used to determine pregnancy detect an antigen-antibody reaction between human chorionic gonadotropin (hCG) hormone and an antiserum within the urine or blood. Many physiologic changes are recognized as signs and symptoms of pregnancy. Some of these findings are categorized as: (1) presumptive symptoms (i.e., symptoms experienced by the woman); (2) probable signs (i.e., changes observed by the nurse); and (3) positive signs (i.e., findings that prove the presence of a fetus). Table 20.1 lists the signs of pregnancy by category and when they may become evident.

HEALTH HISTORY

COMPONENTS OF PRENATAL HEALTH HISTORY

A comprehensive history should be obtained at the first prenatal visit to establish baseline data; it can then be updated as needed during subsequent visits. The history is similar to that of the adult (see Chapter 2) but with a special emphasis on collecting data that could affect pregnancy outcomes. Factors affecting pregnancy outcome should include considerations of family history, genetic history, nutritional status, folic acid intake, environmental exposures, and teratogens. Additionally, psychosocial screening is recommended at least once each trimester to identify issues that may require further evaluation, intervention, or outside referral.[1]

Reason for Seeking Care

The pregnant woman may be seeing her health care provider for routine prenatal care or for a specific problem that may or may not directly relate to the pregnancy. Prenatal visits are needed to monitor the health of the mother and the growth

BOX 20.1 SELECTED ANATOMIC AND PHYSIOLOGIC CHANGES ASSOCIATED WITH PREGNANCY

Integumentary System
- Increased estrogen increases vascularity to the skin, causing itching and a reddened appearance of the hands and feet.
- Increased secretion of melanotropin causes pigmentation changes to the skin, including chloasma (mask of pregnancy; see Fig. 20.1); linea nigra (dark-pigmented line on abdomen); and increased pigmentation to nipples, areolae, axillae, and vulva.
- Increasing size of breasts and abdomen contribute to striae gravidarum (stretch marks) over abdomen and breasts.
- Increased hair or nail growth is reported by some individuals.

Respiratory System
- Uterine enlargement pushes up on the diaphragm, causing periodic shortness of breath.
- Respiratory rate may increase slightly; tidal volume (amount of air inhaled in a normal breath) increases; breathing becomes more thoracic than abdominal; thoracic cage widens.

Cardiovascular System
- Blood volume increases by 1500 mL to meet the need of an enlarged uterus and fetal tissue, causing increased cardiac workload (increased heart rate and blood volume).
- Uterine enlargement pushes up on the heart, causing it to shift upward and forward.
- Enlarged uterus increases pelvic pressure, causing decreased venous return, which results in varicosities and edema in lower extremities.

Gastrointestinal System
- Rise in human chorionic gonadotropin early in pregnancy causes nausea and vomiting (morning sickness).
- Uterine enlargement results in displacement of intestines and decreased peristalsis, causing heartburn and constipation, respectively.
- Increased pelvic pressure and vascularity cause hemorrhoids.
- Increased estrogen increases vascularity and tissue proliferation of gums, resulting in swollen and bleeding gums.

Urinary System
- Increased pressure of the growing uterus on the bladder in early pregnancy and the fetal head exerting pressure on the bladder in late pregnancy result in nocturia and urinary frequency.

Musculoskeletal System
- Increased size of uterus and growing fetus results in the center of gravity moving forward, causing lordosis (see Fig. 20.5) and back discomfort; waddling gait and balance problems may occur.
- Abdominal wall muscles stretch and lose tone, which may lead to separation of abdominal muscles (diastasis recti) in the third trimester.

Reproductive System
- Uterus enlarges, and fundus becomes palpable because of the growing fetus.
- Vagina, vulva, and cervix take on a bluish color caused by increased vascularity.

Breasts
- Breasts become full and tender early in pregnancy.
- Breasts enlarge as pregnancy progresses.
- Nipples and areolae are more prominent and deeply pigmented.
- Increased mammary vascularization causes veins to become engorged; visible under skin surface.

TABLE 20.1 SIGNS AND SYMPTOMS OF PREGNANCY

CATEGORY	SIGN	TIME OF OCCURRENCE (WEEKS OF GESTATION)
Presumptive signs and symptoms	Breast fullness/tenderness	3–4
	Amenorrhea	4
	Nausea, vomiting	4–12
	Urinary frequency	6–12
	Quickening (fetal movement)	16–20
Probable signs	Chadwick sign (violet-blue color to cervix)	6–8
	Goodell sign (softening of cervix)	5
	Hegar sign (softening of lower uterine segment)	6–12
	Positive pregnancy test (hCG):	
	Serum	4–12
	Urine	6–12
	Ballottement (presence of a floating object)	16–28
Positive signs	Visualization of fetus by ultrasound	5–6
	Auscultation of fetal heart tones:	
	Doppler	8–17
	Fetoscope	17–19
	Palpation of fetal movements	19–22
	Observable fetal movements	Late pregnancy

hCG, Human chorionic gonadotropin.

of the fetus, and to educate the mother and family about the care of mother and family about the care of mother and neonate during the delivery process and neonatal period.

Present Health Status

Data collected are the same as those discussed in Chapter 2. Data specific to the pregnant woman include her present general physical and psychosocial well-being. In addition, determining which medications the patient uses is essential, because many pregnant women assume that the use of over-the-counter medications and dietary supplements are safe and are not aware of the potentially harmful effects on the fetus.[2,3]

Past Health History

Data collected in this section are the same as those discussed in Chapter 2. Document any chronic illness (such as diabetes mellitus, thyroid or cardiovascular conditions, renal disease, and depression) and other current risk factors that the pregnant patient may have.

Gynecologic and Obstetric History

The past health history includes the gynecologic and obstetric history. General information regarding the reproductive system (e.g., problems with menstruation, infections, cervical treatments, infertility, painful intercourse, and sexual patterns) should also be included (see Chapter 17).

The obstetric history includes information regarding the current and past pregnancies. On the first prenatal visit, ask the patient the exact date of the last menstrual period (LMP) to calculate the estimated date of delivery (EDD) (Box 20.2). Starting at approximately the 20th week of pregnancy, ask the patient about fetal movement, including frequency and time of day.

An obstetric history includes gravidity (G) (number of pregnancies, including current pregnancy); the number of full-term births (T); the number of preterm births (P); the number of abortions (A), which can be specifically identified as spontaneous abortion (SAB) or miscarriage, and elective abortion (EAB); and the number of living children (L). The acronym GTPAL may be of help in remembering this system of documentation (Table 20.2).

The obstetric history also includes specific data regarding each pregnancy. Document the following information:

- The course of each pregnancy (including the duration of gestation, date of delivery, and significant problems or complications)

BOX 20.2 ESTIMATED DATE OF DELIVERY

Nägele's Rule

To calculate the estimated date of delivery (EDD), determine the first day of the last menstrual period (LMP), subtract 3 months, and then add 7 days. Example:

First day of LMP = November 1

−3 months = August 1

+7 days = August 8 EDD

Note: Most women give birth during the period extending from 7 days before to 7 days after the EDD.

- The process of labor (including manner in which labor was started [i.e., spontaneous or induced], length of labor, and complications associated with labor)
- The delivery (presentation of the infant, method of delivery [i.e., vaginal or cesarean section], and pain management strategies used for delivery, if any)
- Condition of the infant at birth (including weight)
- Postpartum course (including any maternal or infant problems)
- Fertility interventions necessary to achieve pregnancy (e.g., in vitro fertilization)

Family History

In addition to the family history described in Chapter 2, a pregnant woman's family history should specifically address the childbearing history of her mother and sister(s), including multiple births, chromosome abnormalities, genetic disorders, congenital disorders, and chronic illnesses, e.g., diabetes mellitus, renal disease, cancer.

Personal and Psychosocial History

Attitude Toward the Pregnancy

Inquire how the woman feels about her pregnancy. Was the pregnancy intended/unintended? Wanted/unwanted? Would she like to explore her options regarding continuation of the pregnancy? Is her partner aware of the pregnancy and involved? Who is her support system? What kind of expectations does she have regarding being pregnant, the process of labor, childbirth, and parenthood? Explore if the patient has any fear (such as fear of pain) regarding the pregnancy and delivery process (Box 20.3). Adjustments to parenthood, such as role changes within the family, should also be explored. Assessment of the patient's emotional stability is performed; this includes questions about things such as the incidence of excessive crying, social withdrawal, or decisions related to infant care.

Diet/Nutritional History

A woman's nutritional status prior to and during pregnancy affects maternal and fetal health. An understanding of the woman's usual dietary practices and use of vitamins and supplements is essential for nutritional assessment. Sufficient folic acid intake prior to conception is associated with decreased risk of a neural tube defect (spina bifida and anencephaly) in the newborn; folic acid supplementation is routinely recommended throughout pregnancy. Anemia is a common problem during pregnancy because of the high fetal demand for iron, and an iron supplement is often recommended, along with a prenatal vitamin.[4] Culturally sensitive considerations should be taken into account when exploring and providing education about dietary practices. Patients should be interviewed regarding food allergies or intolerance as well as individual dietary preferences (such as vegetarian). Development of an individualized dietary plan may be necessary to ensure that nutritional needs are met, particularly if the patient must avoid particular foods.

TABLE 20.2 DETERMINING GRAVIDITY AND PARITY USING A FIVE-DIGIT (GTPAL) SYSTEM

	G	T	P	A	L
CONDITION	GRAVIDA	TERM BIRTH	PRETERM BIRTH	ABORTIONS	LIVING CHILDREN
Woman who is pregnant for the first time	1	0	0	0	0
Woman who has carried her first pregnancy to term and the infant survived	1	1	0	0	1
Woman who is currently pregnant for the second time; has one child from the first pregnancy born full term	2	1	0	0	1
Woman who has been pregnant twice; has one child who was born preterm and had one miscarriage	2	0	1	1	1
Woman who has been pregnant once and delivered full-term twins	1	1	0	0	2

Modified from Lowdermilk DL, Perry SE, Cashion MC, Alden KR: *Maternity and women's health care*, ed 10, St Louis, 2012, Mosby.

BOX 20.3 CLINICAL NOTE

Most women have some concerns about pain during the childbirth process. The discomfort and pain associated with childbirth are unique not only to each woman but also as a pain experience in itself. Compared with other known painful events or experiences, the potential for achieving satisfactory pain relief is high because of the uniqueness of this pain experience. Unique points include the following:

- The woman knows that the pain will happen.
- The woman knows approximately when (within a week or so) the pain will happen.
- The woman knows that there will be a predictable pattern to the pain.
- The woman knows that there is a time limit to the pain experience (hours as opposed to days or weeks) and that it will end.
- The woman knows that there is a tangible end product associated with the birth (i.e., the birth of her child).

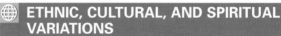

ETHNIC, CULTURAL, AND SPIRITUAL VARIATIONS

Dietary Beliefs During Pregnancy

Cultural diversity should be considered with dietary assessment. An understanding of how different foods are viewed is important. Specific foods may be considered healthful or harmful during pregnancy and lactation by some cultures. For example, in some cultures, eating hot foods is believed to provide warmth for the fetus and enable the baby to be born into a warm, loving environment. In addition, many cultural groups believe that certain cravings for foods should be met while pregnant to avoid harm to the baby.

Dietary assessment should also include questions regarding ingestion of nonnutritive substances known as pica. Clay, starch, baking soda, and dirt are some of the reported cravings during pregnancy.[5] To assess the potentially harmful effects of eating nonnutritive substances, determine what is being ingested, the quantity, and the frequency.

Tobacco, Alcohol, and Illicit Drug Use

Universal screening for substance use during the perinatal period is essential in providing optimal care. Personal habits such as the use of tobacco, cannabis, alcohol, and illicit drugs are modifiable risk factors during pregnancy and thus a focus of assessment and intervention for the pregnant woman. Screening, brief intervention, and referral to treatment (SBIRT) is an evidenced-based approach to managing substance abuse and can readily be integrated into prenatal care.[6] Screening tools that are brief, reliable, and easy to use (such as the CAGE and AUDIT described in Chapter 7) and interventions to reduce or eliminate the use of tobacco, alcohol, and other drugs have been found to be effective.

Smoking tobacco during pregnancy is associated with a wide range of negative consequences, both maternal and neonatal. Some women will switch from smoking to "vaping" using an e-cigarette, believing it to be safer; however, they must be taught that nicotine exposure via tobacco carries the same risk to health regardless of delivery method (smoking, vaping, chewing).[7] Tobacco use correlates with an increased risk of infertility, preterm delivery, stillbirth, low birth weight, and sudden infant death syndrome; maternal smoking can result in adverse respiratory, behavioral, and neurocognitive effects in children. While the impacts of smoking cannabis (marijuana) are less clear, it has been linked to maternal anemia, low birth weight (although less of an influence than tobacco), and small-for-gestational-age (SGA) infants.[8]

The incidence of co-use of tobacco and cannabis has increased significantly in the past decade and may be associated with additive adverse health effects, relative to the use of tobacco only. In addition, maternal co-use of tobacco and cannabis has been linked with the likelihood of engagement in additional high-risk behaviors during pregnancy.[9]

There are no safe amounts of alcohol or safe times for its use during the perinatal period; pregnant females should be advised to avoid alcohol consumption altogether. Alcohol is a teratogen, and its consumption can result in miscarriage, still birth, and a wide range of disabilities known as fetal alcohol spectrum disorders (FASDs).[10] The use of SBIRT has been shown to be effective in modifying the behaviors of tobacco and alcohol consumption, specifically; the motivation for behavior change is high for many expectant mothers.[6]

Illicit drug use, which includes the use of illegal drugs (street drugs, i.e., cocaine, amphetamines, opioids) and/or misuse of prescription medications, is known to impact fertility and maternal and infant health. In addition to the deleterious effects of direct exposure to a substance, illicit drug use is also associated with limited prenatal care, polysubstance use, environmental stressors, and alterations in parenting behaviors.[11] The use of SBIRT in the perinatal period can potentially minimize the negative impact of substance use and abuse on maternal-child health.[6]

RISK FACTORS

High-Risk Pregnancy

Maternal Characteristics
- Age: Under 16 or over 35 years of age
- Marital status: Single (or lack of supporting relationship) (M)
- Short stature: Less than 5 feet (150 cm) tall
- Weight: Less than 100 lb (45 kg) or more than 200 lb (91 kg) (M)
- Socioeconomic: Poverty, low education level (M)
- Lives at a high altitude (M)

Maternal Habits
- Alcohol consumption (M)
- Illicit drug use (M)
- No early prenatal care (M)
- Smoking (M)
- High-risk sexual behaviors (M)
- Poor diet (M)

Obstetric History
- Previous birth to infant weighing less than 2500 g
- Previous birth to infant weighing more than 4000 g
- Previous pregnancy ending in perinatal death
- More than two previous spontaneous abortions
- Birth to infant with congenital or perinatal disease
- Birth to infant with isoimmunization or ABO incompatibility

Current Medical Problems
- Chronic illnesses, including diabetes mellitus, thyroid disorder, heart disease, hypertension, pulmonary disease, renal failure, anemia, sickle cell disease
- Sexually transmitted disease
- Infectious disease (e.g., rubella or cytomegalovirus)

Problems With Current Pregnancy
- Bleeding
- Pregnancy-induced hypertension
- Eclampsia or preeclampsia
- Fetal position breech or transverse at term
- Polyhydramnios (excessive amniotic fluid)
- Multiple fetus (e.g., twins, triplets)
- Postmaturity (gestation >40 weeks)
- Premature rupture of membranes
- Weight gain that is inadequate or excessive

M, Modifiable risk factor.

Environment

Pregnant women should be questioned about safety issues, including activities at work and in the home, routine safety practices such as the use of seat belts while in a car, and the presence of physical abuse and violence in the home. Pregnant women are advised to limit exposure to cat litter and feces to avoid a parasite infection known as toxoplasmosis.[12] Further assessment may include questions regarding potential exposure to chemicals including lead, mercury, asbestos, solvents, pesticides, and phthalates, which are commonly found in plastics.[13]

Problem-Based History

The health history includes questions related to the function of body systems. The following is an outline of common problems organized by body systems. Conduct a symptom analysis using the mnemonic OLD CARTS that includes *O*nset, *L*ocation, *D*uration, *C*haracteristics, *A*ggravating factors, *R*elated symptoms, *T*reatment measures, and *S*everity (see Box 2.6).

Skin, Hair, Nails
- Skin marks, lines, varicosities
- Pruritus

Nose and Mouth
- Nose bleeding or stuffiness
- Gum bleeding or swelling

Ears
- Changes in hearing
- Sense of fullness in ears

Eyes
- Excessive dryness
- Visual changes

Respiratory System
- Shortness of breath

Cardiovascular System
- Palpitations
- Edema of extremities
- Orthostatic hypotension (dizziness when standing up)

Breasts
- Enlargement, engorgement, tenderness
- Nipple discharge

Gastrointestinal System
- Nausea, vomiting (morning sickness), loss of appetite, food aversions
- Heartburn (gastric reflex), epigastric pain (second and third trimesters)

- Constipation (second and third trimesters)
- Hemorrhoids (second and third trimesters)

Genitourinary System

- Urinary pain, frequency, and urgency
- Vaginal discharge or bleeding

Musculoskeletal System

- Backache
- Leg cramps

Neurologic System

- Headaches

HEALTH PROMOTION FOR EVIDENCE-BASED PRACTICE

Maternal-Infant Health

Prenatal care can contribute to reductions in maternal and perinatal illness, disability, and death by identifying and minimizing potential risks and helping women address behavioral factors such as smoking and alcohol use, which contribute to poor outcomes. Major maternal complications of pregnancy include hemorrhage, ectopic pregnancy, pregnancy-induced hypertension, embolism, and infection. The maternal mortality rate among African American women has consistently been three to four times that of Caucasian women. Prematurity and low birth weight (LBW) are among the leading causes of neonatal death. LBW is also associated with long-term disabilities.

Recommendations to Reduce Risk (Primary Prevention)

- Counsel pregnant women about eating a healthy diet; encourage all women who are planning or capable of pregnancy to take daily multivitamins with folic acid to reduce the risk of neural tube defects.
- Encourage healthy body weight during pregnancy.
- Encourage regular exercise while pregnant.
- Counsel patients regarding the need to abstain from smoking, drug use, and alcohol use while pregnant. Remind patients that over-the-counter medications are potentially harmful and to consult with their health care provider.
- Counsel patients to avoid exposure to chemicals while pregnant.

Screening Recommendations (Secondary Prevention)

- *Ultrasound:* The benefit of performing an ultrasound examination of the fetus in the second trimester in low-risk pregnant women is unknown. Routine third-trimester ultrasound examination is not recommended.
- *Preeclampsia:* Screening for preeclampsia with blood pressure measurement in all pregnant women at first prenatal visit and throughout pregnancy is recommended.
- *Rh incompatibility:* Rh typing and antibody screening for all pregnant women at the first prenatal visit is recommended. Repeat screening is recommended at 24–28 weeks of gestation for unsensitized Rh-negative women.
- *Down syndrome:* Offering amniocentesis or chorionic villus sampling for chromosome studies for pregnant women age 35 or older and those at high risk for having a Down syndrome infant is recommended.
- *Neural tube defects:* Offering screening for neural tube defects by maternal serum alpha fetoprotein measurement at 16–18 weeks of gestation is recommended.
- *Anemia:* Screening for anemia among all pregnant women is recommended.
- *Sexually transmitted infection:* Screening for hepatitis B, human immunodeficiency virus, and syphilis among all pregnant women, and for gonorrhea and chlamydial infections for pregnant women who are at high risk, is recommended.

From American College of Obstetricians and Gynecologists' website, available at www.acog.org; *U.S. Preventive Services Task Force Recommendations,* available at www.uspreventiveservicestaskforce.org.

EXAMINATION

Positioning the pregnant patient for an examination is the same as discussed in previous chapters, with one exception: Do not position the pregnant woman flat on her back for an extended length of time after the 20th week gestation.

The examination follows the same general process as a head-to-toe approach, although many nurses examine the abdomen just before the genitalia.

Routine techniques

MEASURE temperature, blood pressure, pulse, and respiration.
MEASURE height and weight.
INSPECT and PALPATE hands and nails.
INSPECT and PALPATE lower extremities.
INSPECT head and face.
INSPECT eyes and TEST vision.
INSPECT ears, nose, and mouth.
INSPECT and PALPATE the neck.
INSPECT, PALPATE, and AUSCULTATE the anterior, lateral, and posterior chest.
INSPECT and PALPATE the breasts.
INSPECT and PALPATE the nipples.
INPSECT and PALPATE the spine, extremities, and joints.
INSPECT posture and gait.
EXAMINE for neurologic changes.

INSPECT the abdomen.
PALPATE the abdomen.
MEASURE fundal height.
AUSCULTATE the abdomen.

PALPATE fetal position.
INSPECT external genitalia.
PALPATE the cervix.
INSPECT and PALPATE the anus and rectum.

Equipment needed

- Thermometer • Watch or clock with second hand • Stethoscope • Sphygmomanometer • Weight and height scale • Reflex hammer
- Tape measure • Doppler ultrasound stethoscope (ultrasonic gel) or Fetoscope • Examination gloves

PROCEDURES WITH EXPECTED FINDINGS

ABNORMAL FINDINGS

PERFORM hand hygiene.

VITAL SIGNS AND BASELINE MEASUREMENTS

MEASURE temperature, blood pressure, pulse, and respiration.

Vital signs are measured with every visit.

Pulse: The heart rate increases as much as 10 to 15 beats/min.

Respiration: Respiratory rate may increase slightly, especially during the third trimester; the patient may also experience shortness of breath.

Excessive shortness of breath and dyspnea are of concern and may indicate pulmonary complications such as embolus.

Blood pressure: Document blood pressure trends throughout pregnancy. Blood pressure (BP) should remain fairly consistent during pregnancy. It may decrease slightly in the second trimester and then return to the usual level during the third trimester. The approach to BP measurement should be consistent throughout pregnancy for accurate comparisons over time. Specifically, use the same arm, with an appropriate size cuff, with the patient in a sitting position.

Preexisting hypertension in pregnancy significantly increases the risk of preterm delivery and infant mortality. Pregnancy-induced hypertension (PIH), also known as gestational hypertension, is a serious disorder that requires prompt and close medical management. It is characterized by systolic blood pressure of at least 140 mm Hg, a rise of 30 mm Hg or more above the usual level in two readings 6 hours apart, diastolic blood pressure of 90 mm Hg or more, or a rise of 15 mm Hg above baseline in two readings done 6 hours apart.

MEASURE height and weight.

Height should be measured on the first visit. Weight should be measured with every visit. Prepregnancy weight may give the nurse insight into the woman's nutritional status. On the initial visit, complete a weight-for-height assessment or body mass index (BMI) to determine an appropriate weight gain goal for pregnancy. Women with a normal prepregnancy BMI and those who meet appropriate weight gain goals are healthier and have healthier children.[14]

A prepregnancy BMI more than 29 increases the risk of both inadequate and excessive weight gain during pregnancy.[15] A rapid increase in weight could indicate multiple gestation, preeclampsia, or diabetes associated with pregnancy. If a woman gains more than 2 lb (0.9 kg) in any 1 week, or more than 6 lb (2.7 kg) in 1 month, preeclampsia should be suspected.[16]

PROCEDURES WITH EXPECTED FINDINGS

TABLE 20.3 EXPECTED WEIGHT GAIN DURING PREGNANCY

PREPREGNANCY CATEGORY	PREPREGNANCY BMI	SUGGESTED WEIGHT GAIN
Underweight	Less than 18.5	28–40 lb
Normal weight	18.5–24.9	25–35 lb
Overweight	25–29.9	15–25 lb
Obese	30 and over	11–20 lb

BMI, Body mass index.
From Institute of Medicine: *Weight gain during pregnancy: reexamining the guidelines,* Washington, DC, 2009, National Academy of Sciences Press.

Evaluate the rate of weight change at each prenatal visit in addition to assessment of overall weight change. Expected patterns of weight gain are based on prepregnancy weight category from BMI calculations.[17] Target weight gain is presented in Table 20.3. Generally, a total weight gain of 25–35 lb (11.4–16 kg) is associated with a positive pregnancy outcome for women with normal prepregnancy weight. Underweight women should gain more weight, whereas overweight women should gain somewhat less weight.

EXTREMITIES

INSPECT the hands and nails for color, surface characteristics, and movement; PALPATE for edema and sensation.

Pinkish-red blotches or diffuse mottling of the hands caused by an increase in estrogen is termed *palmar erythema* and is considered an expected finding. The patient's nails may become thin and brittle. Women who take prenatal vitamins may report fast-growing, strong nails. Movement and sensation of fingers and hands should remain the same as previously discussed for the adult.

INSPECT the lower extremities for surface characteristics and redness; PALPATE for edema and tenderness.

Edema in the lower extremities is seen almost universally during the later stages of pregnancy. Typically, women notice it late in the day or after long periods of standing. Palpating the legs helps to determine the extent of the edema (see Fig. 12.18). Vascular spiders or varicosities may appear on the lower legs and thighs and are considered normal findings. The legs should be free from redness and tenderness.

HEAD, EYES, EARS, NOSE, AND THROAT

INSPECT the head and face for skin characteristic pigmentation, and edema.

Blotchy, brownish pigmentation of the face (i.e., chloasma, or the mask of pregnancy) is an expected finding (Fig. 20.1). There should be no facial edema. Fine, lanugo-type hair may be observed on the face and is an expected finding.

ABNORMAL FINDINGS

During the first trimester, a weight loss of up to 5 lb (2.3 kg) may be caused by nausea and vomiting. Poor weight gain or weight loss may be associated with a small-for-gestational age (SGA) infant or more serious complications such as placental dysfunction or fetal death in utero. Low-birth-weight (LBW) infants have more health problems than normal-weight infants; in one study, LBW infants were 37 times more likely to die than normal-birth-weight infants.[18]

Although some edema is considered normal, excessive edema (particularly if noted on the hands, face, and lower extremities) is considered pathologic and may be an indication of PIH. Some pregnant patients may periodically report numbness of the fingers caused by a brachial plexus traction syndrome (caused by drooping shoulders associated with increased breast size and weight). Carpal tunnel syndrome caused by compression of the median nerve in the wrist and the hand may lead to symptoms of numbness, tingling, burning, and impaired finger movement.

Edema not associated with preeclampsia or normal lower-extremity swelling should be evaluated for adequate protein intake. Redness in the legs, particularly if accompanied by tenderness, may be an indication of thrombophlebitis.

Facial edema is considered an abnormal finding and should be reported.

PROCEDURES WITH EXPECTED FINDINGS

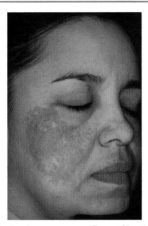

FIG. 20.1 Mask of pregnancy. (From Sheth, et al. 2010.)

INSPECT the eyes and TEST vision for acuity.

The eye examination should proceed as discussed in Chapter 10. Findings generally remain the same as previously discussed for the adult; however, the eyelids of some women may darken from melanin pigment. Visual acuity should be tested with the first visit to establish a baseline. Visual checks should be repeated if the patient verbalizes a change in vision during the pregnancy. Contact lenses may be uncomfortable to wear because of increased dryness. Both eyesight and the corrective prescription may change.

INSPECT the ears, nose, and mouth.

The examination of the ears, nose, and mouth should proceed as discussed in Chapter 10. Findings generally are the same as previously discussed for the adult. However, the nurse may notice an increase in vascularization of the external ear, the auditory canal, and the tympanic membrane. Changes of the nose and mouth of the pregnant woman are also associated with an increase in vascularization, causing redness in the nose, pharynx, and gums; the gums become edematous and spongy and may bleed easily. A normal variation seen in many women toward the end of the third trimester is an epulis. An epulis is hypertrophied gum tissue that presents as a small painless raised nodule.

INSPECT and PALPATE the neck for skin characteristics, presence of lumps and masses.

The examination of the neck and thyroid should proceed as discussed in Chapter 10. Findings generally are the same as previously discussed. There may be transient thyroid enlargement that makes the thyroid more easily palpable, but this disappears following delivery.

ANTERIOR, LATERAL, AND POSTERIOR CHEST

INSPECT, PALPATE, and AUSCULTATE the anterior, lateral, and posterior chest.

The examination of the anterior, lateral, and posterior chest proceeds as discussed in Chapters 11 and 12. The findings are the same as in the adult female except for the lateral shift of the heart (see Fig. 20.2). If the patient is near term or has difficulty breathing when lying down, perform chest examination when she is in a sitting position.

The breathing pattern changes from abdominal to costal or lateral; likewise, it may be shallow with an increased respiratory rate. A wide thoracic cage and increased costal angle may be noted.

ABNORMAL FINDINGS

Pale conjunctivae may indicate anemia. PIH may cause blurred vision. Chromatopsia may be noted, characterized by unusual color perception, seeing spots, or blindness in the lateral visual field. This requires immediate follow-up. Retinal arteriole constriction, disc edema, and retinal detachment (which is an emergency) are concerns; these may be caused by PIH.

Some women develop a pregnancy-induced tumor in the mouth. With the exception of hypertrophied gum tissue, any growth in the mouth is an abnormal finding.

Excessive or asymmetric enlargement of the thyroid gland or nodules on the thyroid gland is an abnormal finding.

Abnormal findings as discussed in Chapters 11 and 12 also apply to the pregnant patient. Dyspnea, orthopnea, fatigue, and palpitations may be attributed to the pregnancy but should be evaluated for other causes. Preexisting cardiac conditions may have pronounced symptoms because of the increased blood volume. Notice any signs of heart failure. Notice elevations in blood pressure, especially in the third trimester.

PROCEDURES WITH EXPECTED FINDINGS	ABNORMAL FINDINGS

The heart shifts laterally in response to the positions of the uterus and diaphragm (Fig. 20.2). The point of maximum impulse also shifts upward and rotates slightly to the left. Murmurs, splitting of S_1 and S_2, and the presence of S_3 may be heard after the twentieth week of gestation.

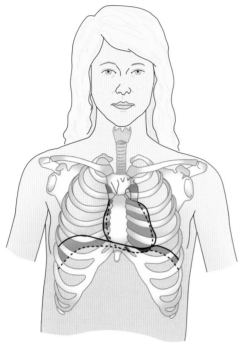

FIG. 20.2 Changes in the position of heart, lungs, and thoracic cage during pregnancy. *Broken line,* nonpregnant; *solid line,* changes during pregnancy. (From Lowdermilk, Perry, and Cashion, 2010.)

BREASTS

INSPECT the breasts for surface characteristics and PALPATE for tissue characteristics.

Examine the breasts as described in Chapter 16. During the first trimester, the breasts become fuller and have transient tenderness. As the pregnancy advances the breasts increase in size, and striae may develop. A subcutaneous venous pattern may be seen as a network of blue tracings across the breasts (Fig. 20.3). Palpation of the breasts reveals fullness and coarse nodularity. Following delivery, breast engorgement peaks at approximately the third to fifth day. Engorged breasts may be very uncomfortable and painful. This is more pronounced in women who are not breastfeeding.

Notice any asymmetry, bulging, or retraction of either breast. Abnormal findings during the breast palpation include masses or isolated areas of tenderness or pain.

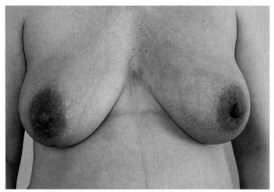

FIG. 20.3 Enlarged breasts in pregnancy with venous network and darkened areolae and nipples.

PROCEDURES WITH EXPECTED FINDINGS

INSPECT the nipples for surface characteristics and shape; PALPATE for discharge.

During the first trimester, the nipples may become somewhat flattened or inverted. As pregnancy progresses, the areolae become darker and Montgomery tubercles may appear. The nipples often protrude (Fig. 20.4). Press on the nipple just behind the areola to express any discharge and notice whether the nipple protracts or inverts. Following the first trimester, colostrum may be expressed from the breast (a yellowish discharge).

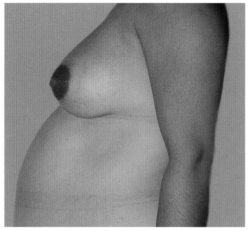

FIG. 20.4 Full-term pregnancy. Note enlargement of breasts, darkening of nipples, and lordotic curve. (Courtesy Lemmi and Lemmi, 2013.)

MUSCULOSKELETAL SYSTEM

INSPECT and PALPATE the spine, extremities, and joints. INSPECT posture and gait.

Examination of the musculoskeletal system proceeds as described in Chapter 14. Changes that are expected during pregnancy include progressive lordosis, anterior cervical flexion, kyphosis, and slumped shoulders (Fig. 20.5). A characteristic "waddling" gait develops at the end of pregnancy.

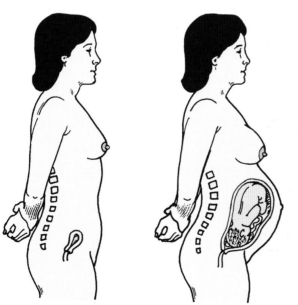

FIG. 20.5 Lordosis during pregnancy. (From Lowdermilk, Perry, and Cashion, 2010.)

ABNORMAL FINDINGS

Thickening of the nipple tissue, a mass, and loss of elasticity are signs consistent with malignancy. Nipple discharge is considered an abnormal finding (except for expression of colostrum as described).

Exaggerated posture or excessive activity can cause muscle strain. Preexisting musculoskeletal conditions (e.g., chronic back pain) may become worse during the pregnancy and after delivery. Muscle cramps, numbness, and weakness of the extremities are considered abnormal findings.

PROCEDURES WITH EXPECTED FINDINGS

NEUROLOGIC SYSTEM

EXAMINE for neurologic changes.

Examine the patient as described in Chapter 15. Although the examination proceeds as for other adults, balance may be altered by pregnancy. Assessment of deep tendon reflexes may also provide valuable data if eclampsia is suspected.

ABDOMEN

INSPECT the abdomen for surface characteristics and fetal movement.

Common changes to the skin on the abdomen are linea nigra (Fig. 20.6), striae gravidarum, and venous patterns. After the twenty-eighth week, fetal movements may be observed.

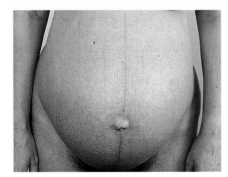

FIG. 20.6 Linea nigra on abdomen. (From Ball et al., 2015.)

PALPATE the abdomen for fetal movement and uterine contraction.

The mother should report fetal movements (also known as quickening) by approximately 20 weeks of gestation. Fetal movement and uterine contraction can be evaluated by placing the hands directly on the abdomen.

MEASURE the fundus for height.

Enlargement of the uterus results in significant abdominal protrusion. Measure fundal height from the top of the symphysis pubis to the top of the fundus (Fig. 20.7). From the twentieth to thirty-sixth week of gestation, the expected pattern of uterine growth is an increase in fundal height of approximately 1 cm per week (Fig. 20.8). Uterine size should correlate roughly with gestational age. Measurement of fundal height is an estimate and may vary among nurses by 1 to 2 cm.

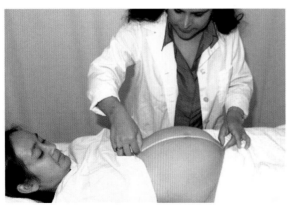

FIG. 20.7 Measuring fundal height. (Courtesy Chris Rozales, San Francisco, CA. In Perry et al., 2010.)

ABNORMAL FINDINGS

Seizures or increased frequency of seizures associated with pregnancy is abnormal. Other abnormal findings are signs of carpal tunnel syndrome (burning, pain, tingling in hand, wrist, or elbow), or hand numbness as a result of brachial plexus traction. These conditions return to the prepregnant state after delivery. Hyperreflexia is an abnormal finding that may indicate eclampsia.

Absence of fetal movement could indicate fetal demise.

The absence of palpable fetal movement after 22 weeks is an abnormal finding.

Any discrepancy greater than 2 cm between fundal height and the estimate of gestational age (based on last menstrual period) should be evaluated further. A uterus that is larger than expected may be caused by inaccurate dating of the pregnancy, more than one fetus, gestational diabetes, or polyhydramnios (excessive fluid in the uterus). A uterus that is smaller than expected for gestational age may be caused by inaccurate dating of the pregnancy or growth retardation of the fetus.

| PROCEDURES WITH EXPECTED FINDINGS | ABNORMAL FINDINGS |

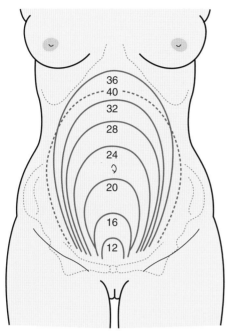

FIG. 20.8 Changes in fundal height during pregnancy. Weeks 1 through 12, the uterus is within the pelvis. Weeks 36 through 40, fundal height drops as the fetus begins to engage in the pelvis (lightening). (From Perry et al., 2010.)

AUSCULTATE the abdomen for fetal heart sounds.

Auscultation of fetal heart tones is performed by use of a Doppler ultrasonic stethoscope after 10 to 12 weeks of gestation or with a fetoscope after 17 to 19 weeks (Fig. 20.9). The fetal heart rate is usually heard over the lower abdomen for fetuses that are in a head-down position. The expected fetal heart rate ranges between 120 and 160 beats/min. (The Doppler and fetoscope are discussed in Chapter 3.)

Increases and decreases in fetal heart rate can be caused by multiple factors stressing the fetus. A fetal heart rate of more than 160 beats/min or below 120 beats/min requires further investigation. Absence of fetal heart tones is always abnormal and usually indicates fetal demise.

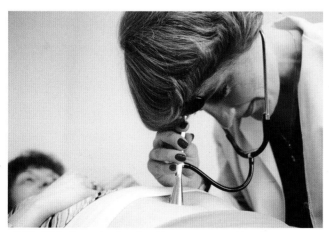

FIG. 20.9 Auscultating fetal heart tones with a fetoscope.

| **PROCEDURES WITH EXPECTED FINDINGS** | **ABNORMAL FINDINGS** |

PALPATE fetal position for fetal lie and presentation, position, and attitude.

The outline of the fetus can be determined after 26 to 28 weeks through a technique known as Leopold's maneuvers (Fig. 20.10A–D). The patient should be lying supine, with head slightly elevated and knees flexed slightly. The fetal lie, presentation, position, and attitude can be determined through these maneuvers (Table 20.4).

Fundal palpation: This is done to determine which part of the fetus is at the fundus. Typically, the feet or buttocks are at the fundus. The buttocks feel firm, but not hard, and slightly irregular. If the head is at the fundus, you will palpate a firm, movable part (see Fig. 20.10 A).

Lateral palpation: Palpate the sides of the uterus to identify the spine of the fetus. It is smooth and convex compared with the irregular feel on the other side of the fetus (i.e., the hands, elbows, knees, and feet) (see Fig. 20.10 B).

Inability to palpate the fetal position could be associated with polyhydramnios. A fetus with breech presentation or a transverse lie before delivery is of concern because of higher risks during the labor and delivery process.

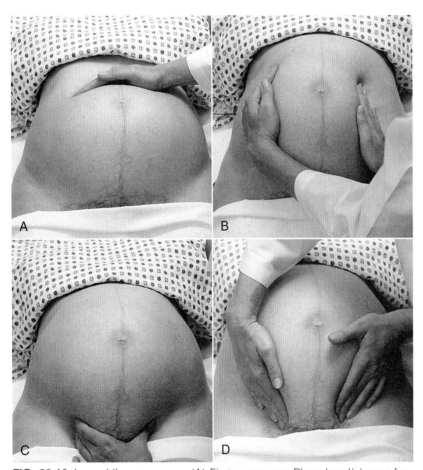

FIG. 20.10 Leopold's maneuvers. (A) First maneuver. Place hand(s) over fundus and identify the fetal part. (B) Second maneuver. Use palmar surface of one hand to locate the back of the fetus. Use other hand to feel the irregularities such as hands and feet. (C) Third maneuver. Use thumb and third finger to grasp presenting part over the symphysis pubis. (D) Fourth maneuver. Use both hands to outline the fetal head. With a head presenting deep in the pelvis, only a small portion may be felt. (Modified from Ball et al., 2015.)

TABLE 20.4 FETAL ASSESSMENT TERMS

TERM	ILLUSTRATION
Fetal Lie The lie is the relationship of the long axis of the fetus to the long axis of the uterus. **A,** Longitudinal lie. **B,** Oblique lie. **C,** Transverse lie.	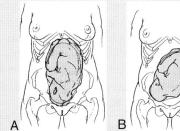 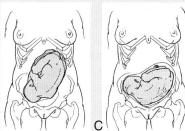
Presentation The presentation is determined by the fetal lie and by the body part of the fetus that enters the pelvic passage first. The presentation may be vertex, brow, face, shoulder, or breech. **A,** Vertex. **B,** Brow. **C,** Face. **D,** Shoulder. **E,** Breech.	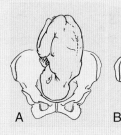 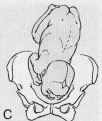 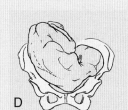 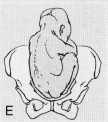
Position Position refers to the relationship of the landmark on the presenting fetal part to the front, sides, or back of the maternal pelvis. The landmark on the fetal presenting part is related to four imaginary quadrants of the pelvis: left anterior, right anterior, left posterior, and right posterior. These quadrants indicate whether the presenting part is directed toward the front, back, left, or right of the pelvic passage. **A,** Left occiput anterior. **B,** Left occiput transverse. **C,** Left occiput posterior.	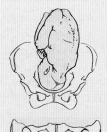 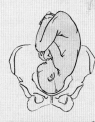 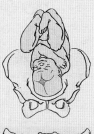 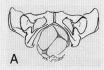 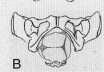
Attitude The attitude is the relationship of the fetal head and limbs to the body. **A,** Fully flexed. **B,** Poorly flexed. **C,** Extended.	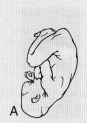 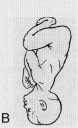 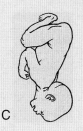

Illustrations from Barkauskas VH et al: *Health and physical assessment*, ed 3, St Louis, 2002, Mosby.

PROCEDURES WITH EXPECTED FINDINGS

Symphysis pubis palpation: This is done to assess which part of the fetus is in or just above the pelvic inlet, and helps to determine if the presenting part is engaged. Gently grasp the presenting anatomic part over the symphysis pubis using your dominant hand. If the head is the presenting part, it feels very smooth, round, and firm. If it is movable from side to side and you are able to palpate all the way around it, the head is not engaged in the pelvis. If engaged, the head is not movable and is below the level of the symphysis, preventing palpation all the way around the head. The presenting part could also be the buttocks. The buttocks feel softer and irregular (see Fig. 20.10C).

Deep pelvic palpation: If the head is the presenting part, palpation allows you to determine the position and attitude (see Fig. 20.10D). Use both hands to identify the outline of the fetal head. Depending on the fetal position, the cephalic prominence can be either the forehead or the occiput.

GENITALIA, RECTUM, AND ANUS

INSPECT the external genitalia for general appearance and discharge.

Follow the guidelines described in Chapter 17. By the second month of pregnancy there is slight increase in vaginal secretions.

PALPATE the cervix to determine length (effacement) and dilation.

During the last 4 weeks, the cervix shortens (known as effacement) as the fetal head descends. Palpating for effacement and dilation is a regular assessment technique performed by nurses near the expected date of delivery and once labor begins.

Don examination gloves to palpate the cervix. The cervix should not efface until approximately the 36th week. The cervical os should remain closed until near delivery. The cervical os softens and is pulled upward, becoming incorporated into the isthmus of the uterus. As the cervix shortens, it also begins to dilate. Cervical dilation is measured in centimeters from 0 cm when completely closed to 10 cm when completely open. The effacement and dilation of the cervix are estimated by palpation.

INSPECT and PALPATE the anus and rectum.

The perianal and rectal examination should be carried out in the pregnant woman as described in Chapter 17. The rectum and anus are commonly examined while the patient is in the lithotomy position with her legs up in stirrups. Early during pregnancy, the patient should have minimal difficulty attaining and maintaining the position for the examination. However, later in pregnancy, positioning for the rectal examination could be uncomfortable.

The presence of hemorrhoids, a common variation, is usually considered normal with pregnancy. The patient may not have hemorrhoids during the early phase of pregnancy, but toward the last trimester the hemorrhoids may appear secondary to pressure on the pelvic floor or possible constipation with straining when having a bowel movement. The hemorrhoids may be either internal in the lower segment of the rectum or prolapsed as external hemorrhoids.

ABNORMAL FINDINGS

Notice the presence of infection of genitalia, including lesions or vaginal discharge with a foul odor. Leakage of watery fluid may be associated with preterm labor. During early pregnancy, slight bleeding may occur for unknown reasons and be of no consequence, or it could indicate an impending abortion. During late pregnancy, bleeding could be caused by abruptio placentae or placenta previa (discussed later in this chapter). Bleeding should never be considered a normal finding in pregnancy and should always be investigated thoroughly.

Effacement and dilation of the cervix before the thirty-sixth week may result in premature delivery. Failure of the cervical os to efface and dilate impedes the progression of labor. If the cervix has inadequate effacement and dilation at the onset of delivery, trauma to the cervix often results.

Presence of lesions or rectal bleeding is considered an abnormal finding.

COMMON PROBLEMS AND CONDITIONS

Abruptio Placentae

The premature separation of the implanted placenta before the birth of the fetus is referred to as abruptio placentae (Fig. 20.11). This usually occurs during the third trimester, but it could occur as early as 20 weeks. The most important risk factor for abruptio placentae is maternal hypertension.[19] Because it is the most common cause of intrapartum fetal death, abruptio placentae is considered an obstetric emergency. The prevalence ranges from 0.4% to 1% of pregnancies.[20] **Clinical Findings:** Bleeding, abdominal pain, and uterine contractions are the three classic findings of this complication. The blood is usually described as dark red, and the pain can range from mild to excruciating.

Placenta Previa

A placenta attachment in the lower uterine segment near or over the cervical os (as opposed to a more typical attachment higher in the uterus) is referred to as placenta previa (Fig. 20.12A, B, and C). This condition, which occurs in 0.5% of all pregnancies in the United States, is often associated with premature rupture of membranes, preterm birth, anemia, infections, and postpartum hemorrhage.[19] **Clinical Findings:** The classic finding is painless vaginal bleeding, commonly during the third trimester; however, bleeding can occur any time after 24 weeks. In a small percentage of women, the bleeding is accompanied by mild uterine contractions. On palpation, the uterus is typically soft and nontender.

Hydramnios (Polyhydramnios)

An excessive quantity of amniotic fluid is referred to as *hydramnios* and occurs in 1% to 2% of pregnancies; approximately half of the cases are idiopathic.[21] This is common in pregnancies with more than one fetus. In single-fetus pregnancies, it is associated with fetal malformation of the central nervous system and gastrointestinal tract. Hydramnios may result in perinatal death from premature labor and fetal abnormalities. **Clinical Findings:** Excessive uterine size, tense uterine wall, difficulty palpating fetal parts, and difficulty hearing fetal heart tones are common findings associated with this condition. The woman may also experience dyspnea, edema, and discomfort caused by pressure on the surrounding organs.

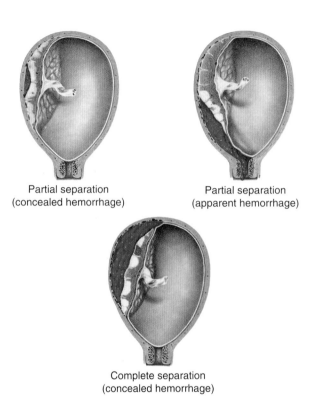

Partial separation
(concealed hemorrhage)

Partial separation
(apparent hemorrhage)

Complete separation
(concealed hemorrhage)

FIG. 20.11 Abruptio placentae. Premature separation of normally implanted placenta. (From Lowdermilk, Perry, and Cashion, 2010.)

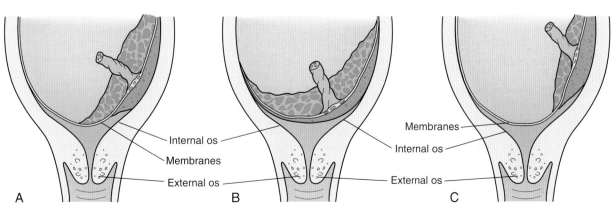

A   B   C

Internal os
Membranes
External os

Membranes
Internal os
External os

FIG. 20.12 Types of placenta previa after onset of labor. (A) Low-lying placenta in second trimester. (B) Placenta previa. (C) Marginal placenta previa. (From Perry et al., 2010.)

Pregnancy-Induced Hypertension

PIH involves a group of hypertensive conditions during pregnancy in a previously normotensive patient. *Preeclampsia* refers to a condition of PIH with proteinuria and edema. *Eclampsia* is the occurrence of seizures precipitated by PIH in a preeclamptic patient. Hypertension occurs in 5% to 8% of all pregnancies.[22] **Clinical Findings:** Hypertension in pregnancy is defined as follows: Systolic blood pressure is 140 mm Hg or higher, *or* there is an increase of more than 30 mm Hg of systolic blood pressure from baseline in the first half of pregnancy; *or* diastolic blood pressure is more than 90 mm Hg, *or* there is an increase of more than 15 mm Hg of diastolic blood pressure from baseline.[19]

Premature Rupture of Membranes

A spontaneous rupture of uterine membranes before the onset of labor is referred to as *premature rupture of membranes (PROM)*. It can occur at any time during the pregnancy but is usually seen with term pregnancy. This situation is associated with a high risk of perinatal and maternal morbidity and mortality, occurring in approximately 3% of all pregnancies.[23] The cause of PROM is not known, although infection and hydramnios are thought to be related factors. **Clinical Findings:** PROM manifests as passage of amniotic fluid from the vagina before labor.

CLINICAL APPLICATION AND CLINICAL JUDGMENT

See Appendix B for answers to exercises in this section.

CASE STUDY

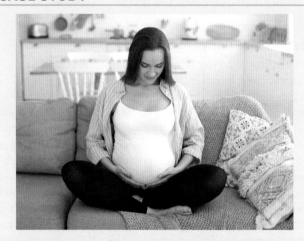

Kristin Walters is a 17-year-old pregnant patient (G_1, T_0, P_0, A_0, L_0) who is in her thirtieth week of pregnancy. She comes to the clinic for a routine prenatal visit. The following data are collected by the nurse.

Interview Data

Ms. Walters tells the nurse, "I've been feeling pretty good the last few weeks; but I've noticed that my feet, hands, and face are getting so puffy. I feel like I'm full of water." When asked about other symptoms or problems, Kristin responds, "I have a backache sometimes." Ms. Walters indicates that she feels the baby move "all the time now." She conveys to the nurse that she is excited about the baby but is very worried about how bad the labor pain will be. "My friend Shawna told me that the pain is so bad that I'll want to be knocked out when it's time to have the baby."

Examination Data

- *Vital signs:* BP, 154/96 mm Hg (prepregnancy BP reading, 114/70 mm Hg—within normal limits up until this visit); pulse, 92 beats/min; respiration rate, 18 breaths/min; temperature, 98.3°F (36.8°C).
- *Weight:* 152 lb (69 kg) (prepregnancy weight, 116 lb [52.7 kg]). She has had an increase of 10 lb (4.5 kg) in last month.
- *Fundal height:* 31 cm.
- *Urine dipstick:* 3+ protein.

Clinical Judgment

1. What cues do you recognize that suggest deviation from normal findings, suggesting a need for further investigation?
2. For which additional information should the nurse ask or assess?
3. Based on the data, which risk factors for high-risk pregnancy does this patient have?
4. With which additional health care professionals should you consider collaborating to meet her health care needs?

REVIEW QUESTIONS

1. What does the nurse assess for during each prenatal visit?
   1. Blood pressure
   2. Hemorrhoids
   3. Personal habits (smoking, alcohol consumption)
   4. Visual acuity

2. During an initial prenatal visit, the nurse identifies which factor as consistent with a high-risk pregnancy?
   1. Patient is 18 years old.
   2. Patient height is 5 feet 4 inches.
   3. Birth weight of infant with last pregnancy was 2800 g.
   4. Patient smokes one-half pack of cigarettes a day.

3. A patient with a missed menstrual period and nausea has which signs and symptoms of pregnancy?
   1. Questionable
   2. Presumptive
   3. Probable
   4. Positive

4. What is the nurse assessing when measuring from the patient's symphysis pubis to the top of the fundus?
   1. Fetal development
   2. Fetal lie and position
   3. Attitude of the fetus
   4. Gestational age

5. Which finding is considered abnormal during late pregnancy?
   1. Watery vaginal discharge
   2. Hemorrhoids
   3. Lordosis
   4. Abdominal striae

Assessment of the Older Adult

evolve

http://evolve.elsevier.com/Wilson/assessment

Aging is a normal developmental process that begins at conception. There is no specific age at which one becomes old: everyone ages at a different rate. Biologic, social, and functional ages are more important than chronologic age. Approximately 16% of the population of the United States is age 65 years and older, and the percentage will increase to 20% by 2030.[1] The 85 and over population is projected to more than double from 6.5 million in 2017 to 14.4 million in 2040 (a 123% increase).[2] A suggested classification based on age is shown below.[3]

- Young-old: 65 to 74 years
- Middle-old: 75 to 84 years
- Old-old: 85 to 100

- Centenarians: 100 to 104 years
- Semisupercentenarians: 105 to 109 years
- Supercentenarians: 110 to 119 years

Being physically, mentally, and socially active into the 100s is considered normal. Conditions such as high blood pressure, pain, urinary incontinence, and severe memory loss are not a part of healthy aging, although the incidence of chronic health problems does increase with advanced age. Therefore nurses must know the difference between healthy aging and disease and not assume that clinical manifestations of disease are caused by age alone. Healthy lifestyle behaviors such as nutrition, regular exercise, and sleep are very important and can be implemented at any age.

ANATOMY AND PHYSIOLOGY

As adults grow older, they experience gradual changes in every body system; thus nurses must recognize the expected anatomic and physiologic changes of older adults and understand how these expected changes may alter the functioning of people in these age groups. Box 21.1 presents some of the expected changes associated with older adults.

HEALTH HISTORY

Nurses interview patients to collect subjective data about their present health status, past health history, and personal and psychosocial history. The health history for older adults is similar to that presented in Chapter 2. The most common and important differences that may be noted on assessment of older people are presented in this chapter.

When obtaining a health history from an older adult, seek information directly from the patient first, if possible, rather than from relatives who may accompany the patient (Fig. 21.1). During the interview, maintain eye contact so the patient can see the movements of the mouth, which helps if there is a hearing problem. Observe for hearing or vision deficits that may affect data collection.

COMPONENTS OF THE GERIATRIC HEALTH HISTORY

Present Health Status

Data collected are the same as described in Chapter 2.

Common chronic illnesses among older adults include diabetes mellitus, osteoarthritis, as well as cardiovascular and neurologic conditions. Review all medications that the patient is taking. Older adults often take many medications prescribed by more than one health care provider. Specifically ask about allergies and adverse effects with the medications and if the patient has problems getting access to the drugs (because of financial or transportation restraints). Also ask about recent immunizations

BOX 21.1 SELECTED ANATOMIC AND PHYSIOLOGIC CHANGES ASSOCIATED WITH OLDER ADULTS

Skin, Hair, and Nails
- Decreased sebaceous and sweat gland activity causes dry skin and less perspiration.
- The dermis loses elasticity and collagen, causing sagging and wrinkling.
- Loss of subcutaneous fat impairs heat regulation related to hypothermia.
- Decreased melanin production tends to produce gray hair; reduced hormonal functioning causes thinning of scalp, axillary, and pubic hair.
- The nails become thicker, brittle, hard, and yellowish; they also develop ridges and are prone to splitting into layers.

Head, Eyes, Ears, Nose, and Throat
- Pupillary response to light is decreased.
- Corneal sensitivity is often diminished so older adults may be unaware of infection or injury.
- Loss of lens elasticity results in presbyopia[4]
- Night vision and depth perception are decreased because less light passes through the eye.
- Adaptation of light declines, requiring more time to adjust when moving from dark room to light room and vice versa.
- The lens becomes more yellow, which creates a difficulty seeing blue, violet, and green.
- A decrease in active sebaceous glands causes the cerumen to become very dry; it may completely obstruct the external auditory canal, resulting in diminished hearing.
- Both conductive and sensorineural hearing losses occur with aging due to degeneration of cochlear structures. *Presbycusis* is the term for gradual hearing loss, which first occurs with high-frequency sounds and progresses to lower-frequency tones.
- Decreased saliva production contributes to a dry mouth.
- Taste perception may diminish due to a decreased number of papillae and taste buds.
- Muscle weakness may result in chewing and swallowing difficulties.
- Increased concave cervical curvature causes forward and downward positioning of the head.
- Lymph nodes may decrease in both size and number with advanced age.

Lungs and Respiratory System
- Diminished strength of the respiratory muscles results in diminished breath sounds in the bases. Kyphoscoliosis, a common finding associated with aging, causes the thorax to shorten and the anteroposterior diameter to increase.
- As the alveoli become less elastic and more fibrous, dyspnea on exertion becomes more frequent.

Heart and Peripheral Vascular System
- Increased arterial resistance contributes to hypertension.
- Reduced elasticity of arteries impairs peripheral blood flow.
- Orthostatic hypotension may contribute to falls.

Abdomen and Gastrointestinal System
- Motility of the entire gastrointestinal system is slowed, causing a decrease in transit time through the intestines.
- Decreased motility and lower esophageal pressure increase likelihood of regurgitation.
- Bacterial flora in the intestines become less biologically active, contributing to food intolerance and impaired digestion.
- Decrease in internal sphincter tone and sensation may contribute to occasional fecal incontinence.
- The bladder decreases in size, shape, and muscle tone, which can cause more frequent urination and increase likelihood of stress incontinence.

Musculoskeletal System
- A decrease in bone mass increases the risk for stress fractures. Intervertebral disk space narrows, which results in a loss of height.
- Posture becomes more flexed, which, in turn, changes the center of gravity.
- Tendons and muscles decrease in elasticity and tone, with the muscles losing both mass and strength.

Neurologic System
- Speed of fine-motor movement decreases.
- Impaired balance increases risk of falling.
- Functional changes in sensory and motor function, memory, cognition, and proprioception occur at different rates. Short-term memory (e.g., of names and recent events) may decline with age, but long-term memory is usually maintained.

Reproductive System
Female Genitourinary System
- The vaginal introitus may diminish in size, with a shortening and narrowing of the vagina and a thinning and drying of the vaginal mucosa.

Male Genitourinary System
- Hyperplasia of the prostate is associated with aging.

Breasts
- After menopause, the glandular tissue in the breast continues to atrophy and is replaced by fat and connective tissue.
- Changes to the breast tissue and the relaxation of the suspensory ligaments result in a tendency for the breast to hang more loosely from the chest wall, giving it a flattened appearance.

Data from Cavanaugh JC, Blanchard-Fields F: *Adult Development and Aging*, ed 8, Boston, 2019, Cengage; Touhy T, Jett K, editors: *Ebersole and Hess' Toward Healthy Aging: Human Needs & Nursing Response*, ed 9, St Louis, 2015, Elsevier; Jett K: Biological theories of aging and age-related physical changes. In Touhy TA, Jett K: *Ebersole and Hess' Gerontological Nursing & Healthy Aging*, ed 5, St Louis, 2018, Elsevier, pp. 22–39.

the patient has had such as influenza, pneumococcal, and varicella vaccines.

Past Health History

Data collected in this section are the same as those described in Chapter 2. Obviously, the time span included in the past

health history is longer, and the patient's memory may affect accuracy.

Family History

Although the family history provides data about illnesses and the causes of death of relatives, the value of this

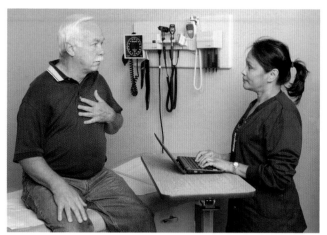

FIG. 21.1 During the interview, maintain eye contact and give the patient time to explain symptoms.

information for an older adult is questionable. A genogram is not used routinely to document the family history for an older adult.

Personal and Psychosocial History

Many of the aspects of personal and psychosocial history are the same as those previously described for the younger adult. However, a shift in focus in this section reflects changes in roles and perceptions during the retirement years.

Personal Status

Ask the older adult for a general statement of feelings about self. Ask about current living arrangements and satisfaction with these living arrangements. Explore areas of potential concern including work/retirement, reduced/fixed income, moving/selling home, living alone, and role changes.

Family and Social Relationships

Ask about sufficient and satisfactory access to family and friends, presence of a pet in the home, participation in family activities and family decisions, presence of conflict with family members, and problems in relationship with the spouse.

Diet/Nutrition

Ask about any decrease in appetite, changes in the taste of food, decrease in saliva, and difficulty chewing or swallowing. One validated tool for assessing nutritional status of older adults is the Mini Nutritional Assessment-Short Form (MNA-SF), which has six questions about food intake, weight loss, mobility, recent psychological stress or acute disease, dementia or depression, and body mass index (BMI).[7]

Functional Ability

Assessing functional ability focuses on a person's ability to perform in two areas. The first area is performing self-care activities or *activities of daily living (ADLs)*, which include skills such as dressing, toileting, bathing, eating, and ambulating. The second area is called *instrumental activities of daily living (IADLs)*, consisting of skills that enable the patient to function independently and include preparation of meals, shopping, safe use of medications, management of finances, and ability to travel within the community.[8] Ask the patient (or other family member) to describe his or her ability (independent, partially independent, or dependent) to perform these activities. Indicators of IADL are listed in Box 21.2.

Mental Health

Emotional experiences of sadness, grief, response to loss, and temporary "blue" moods are expected responses in older adults. While an estimated 25% of older adults experience a mental disorder, these disorders are not an expected part of aging. Anxiety, depression, dementia, and delirium are the most prevalent mental health diagnoses in older adults.

Anxiety is a normal human reaction and is rational within reason. It becomes problematic when the anxiety is prolonged, exaggerated, and interferes with function. Anxiety disorders are not part of the normal aging process, but the changes and challenges for older adults may contribute to the development of anxiety symptoms. Older adults may deny psychological symptoms and attribute anxiety-related symptoms to physical illness.[9] One anxiety disorder unique to older adults is the fear of falling (FOF), which results in keeping individuals at home, therefore restricting their activities.[3] When being assessed for anxiety, older adults may not consider their distress to be the result of anxiety; thus nurses ask questions such as "Do you have a hard time putting thoughts out of your mind?" Asking what the patient was doing when experiencing symptoms of anxiety, such as worrying,

BOX 21.2 INDICATORS OF INSTRUMENTAL ACTIVITIES OF DAILY LIVING

For each category indicate the description that most closely resembles the patient's highest functional level (either 0 or 1)

- Ability to use the telephone (look up numbers, make calls)   0   1
- Ability to shop for necessities (alone even if needs someone to provide transportation)   0   1
- Ability to prepare meals (plan and prepare full meals safely)   0   1
- Ability to do housework   0   1
- Ability to do laundry   0   1
- Ability to travel (alone [e.g., drive] or with another)   0   1
- Ability to self-administer medication (the right drug at the right time)   0   1
- Ability to manage money (e.g., write checks, pay bills)   0   1

Summary of score ranges from 0 (low function, dependent) to 8 (high function, independent) for women and 0 through 5 for men to avoid potential gender bias.

Graf C: The Lawton Instrumental Activities of Daily Living (IADL) Scale, *Am J of Nursing* 108(4):52-62, 2008.

experiencing insomnia, or having difficulty concentrating, provides a better understanding of the patient's anxiety in relation to time and situation. Also determining the circumstances of the patient's worries may help differentiate typical or expected worries from pathologic ones.[5]

Depression may be overlooked because older adults are less willing to talk about feelings of sadness or grief, or they may show less obvious symptoms. The risk for suicide for men increases with age, particularly for white men ages 65 and older whose risk is six times higher than females the same age.[3] Among males, the suicide rate is highest for those aged 65 and older (31.0 per 100,000).[10] Early identification of risk factors and treatment for depression are key interventions for suicide prevention. Some protective factors include spiritual beliefs, being married, personal resilience, perception of social/family support, and having children.[3]

Delirium often accompanies physical illness in older adults. Both dementia and delirium are described in Chapter 7.

Sleep

Many people believe that poor sleep is a normal part of aging, but it is not. Older adults need about the same amount of sleep as younger adults – approximately 7 to 9 hours per night. Older adults with good general health, positive moods, and participation in more active lifestyles and meaningful activities report better sleep. Ask about any bedtime rituals, such as reading, watching television, or listening to music, which are essential to that person's ability to fall asleep. Ask about the quality of sleep and any problems that interfere with sleep, e.g., pain, chronic illness, urinary urgency,

medications, alcohol use, depression, or anxiety. Interrupted sleep at night may require the older adult to nap during the day. Poor sleep may lead to a number of problems such as depressed mood, attention and memory problems, or excessive daytime sleepiness.[11]

Alcohol Use

Ask about the type, amount, and frequency of alcohol consumed. Adults over age 65 who are healthy and do not take medications should not have more than seven drinks weekly. Aging can lower the body's tolerance for alcohol. Older adults generally experience the effects of alcohol more quickly than when they were younger. Also, since the amount of water in the body is less in older adults, the blood alcohol level stays higher longer than when they were younger. Alcohol can interfere with the actions of medication.[12]

Environment

Data on environmental safety and comfort should be gathered, with a specific focus on problems unique to older adults.

- Hazards in the home: Inadequate heating or cooling, stairs to climb (stairs without handrails, steep stairs), fear of falling, gait or balance problems, slippery or irregular surfaces in the home (including throw rugs), inadequate space for maneuvering walker or wheelchair, inadequate lighting in dark hallway/stairs, statement by the patient related to abuse or neglect
- Hazards in the neighborhood: Noise, water, and air pollution; safety concerns; heavy traffic on surrounding streets; overcrowding; isolation from neighbors

Review of Systems

Specific components of a Review of Systems commonly associated with older adults are described below.

Pain

Questions asked in the pain assessment are the same as those described for the younger adult. Some older adults may perceive pain as an expected aspect of aging that they must endure. Determining how the pain is affecting their function, sleep, appetite, activity, mood, and relationships with others is essential to the assessment. Asking how the pain feels helps determine the source and type of pain. For example, neuropathic pain is almost always described as "burning," "tingling," or "shooting," rather than aching or stabbing.[13] One valid and reliable pain intensity scale appropriate for older adults is the Iowa Pain Thermometer (IPT), a numeric rating scale that is vertically oriented (Fig. 21.2). Other valid and reliable tools include the Faces Pain Scale – revised (FPS-r) and the Numeric Rating Scale (NRS) (see Fig. 6.2).[14]

Skin, Hair, and Nails

- *Skin:* Excessive dryness or thinning of skin that tears easily
- *Hair:* Changes in texture or distribution
- *Nails:* Become thicker

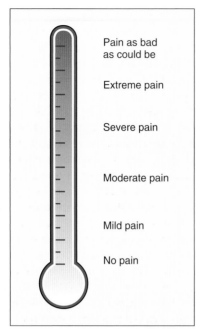

FIG. 21.2 Vertical pain scale. (Used with permission of Keela Herr, PhD, RN, AGSF, FAAN, The University of Iowa.)

Head, Eyes, Ears, Nose, and Throat

- *Vision:* Recent changes in or problems with near, distant, and peripheral vision and problems with night vision or the ability to recognize colors. Dry or irritated eyes are a frequent symptom experienced by older adults because of the decrease in quantity of tears.
- *Hearing:* Difficulty hearing conversations, doorbell, or telephone; ringing in the ears (tinnitus); date of last ear and hearing exam. Tinnitus may be caused by an adverse effect of medications, ear wax blocking the ear canal, or other health conditions.[6]
- *Nose and mouth:* Dry nose and mouth may be an adverse effect of many medications.
- Use of prosthetic devices (dentures) and date of last dental examination. Ask specifically if the patient is experiencing difficulty chewing and swallowing. These problems may be caused by a number of things (e.g., ill-fitting dentures, dental pain, neuromuscular conditions, and esophageal motility) and can lead to inadequate nutritional intake aspiration.

Respiratory System

- *Fatigue, shortness of breath, cough:* Ask about these symptoms of respiratory disorders. The incidence of chronic respiratory disease is higher in older adults.

Cardiovascular System

- *Dizziness, blackouts, fainting, palpitations:* Atherosclerosis may interfere with blood flow to the brain, causing confusion, dizziness, or fainting.

- *Chest pain, fatigue, shortness of breath with exertion or at night, edema in the legs or feet:* These symptoms may be associated with coronary artery disease or heart failure; risk of heart disease increases with age.
- *Pain, discoloration, coldness, chronic wounds in legs or feet:* These symptoms may indicate poor peripheral circulation or heart disease and are more common among older adults.

Gastrointestinal System

- *Abdominal pain:* Older adults often have nonspecific signs and symptoms of abdominal pain. Frequent manifestations of abdominal disorders may be low-grade fever, tachycardia, and vague abdominal discomfort.
- *Constipation:* Constipation is a common problem of older adults that may not be reported voluntarily. Ask about frequency of bowel movements and consistency of stool.

Urinary System

- *Urgency, frequency, and incontinence:* Ask about urine leakage since patient may be reluctant to report it. Ask when the leakage occurs. Leakage that occurs when sneezing, lifting, or laughing suggests stress incontinence, whereas a strong urge to void more often than every 2 hours suggests urge incontinence. Ask how long the leakage has been experienced.[15] A bladder diary can be helpful. The National Institute of Diabetes and Digestive and Kidneys Diseases (NIDDK) has a printable diary that includes type and amount of fluids consumed, number of trips to the bathroom, accidental leaks, feeling of urgency, and activity at the time of the leaks.[16]
- *Difficulty starting urinary stream:* Enlargement of the prostate, which is a common condition among older men, may cause hesitancy, weak urinary stream, and incomplete bladder emptying.

Musculoskeletal System

- *Changes in muscle strength, joint pain:* Independence in activities of daily living may be interrupted by muscle weakness or joint pain.
- *Mobility, gait, balance, use of assistive devices (walker, cane, wheelchair):* The degree, ease, and confidence related to mobility and assistive devices provide information about how patients maintain independence or suggest ways that these devices could be used. Mobility aids can prevent falls and improve independence.
- *Recent falls and fall prevention, use of assistive devices in home (such as grab bars):* Discussing fall prevention with older adults is important. Inquire about potential hazards in the environment such as steps, throw rugs, inadequate light, and curbs.
- Synthesize data from musculoskeletal, mental status, elimination, and medication assessment to determine risk for falls.

RISK FACTORS
Falls in Older Adults

- Muscle weakness, especially in the legs
- Problems with balance or gait
- Postural hypotension, dizziness
- Slower reflexes
- Visual problem: poor depth perception
- Mental status: confusion or disorientation
- Adverse effect of medications
- Environment: loose rugs, clutter on floor or stairs, no stair railing or grab bars (M)

M, Modifiable risk factor.
Data from National Institute on Aging: Prevent falls and fractures.
Available at https://www.nia.nih.gov/health/prevent-falls-and-fractures.

Neurologic System

The review of systems for the neurologic system is the same as described in Chapter 15.

Reproductive System

- *Sexual activity:* Sexual activity is normal at any adult age. Ask about any concerns or questions the patient has about fulfilling sexual needs. Also ask how the patient's sexual relationship with the partner has changed with age. If the patient reports physical difficulties that interfere with sexual activity, the nurse assesses what they are, how much they interfere, and what the patient or partner has done to resolve the difficulty. Intercourse may be painful for women because of vaginal dryness secondary to hormonal changes. Older adults may welcome the opportunity to discuss sexual issues; this can be a time of education and encouragement. Some drugs depress sexual function (e.g., antihypertensives, sedatives, tranquilizers, and alcohol).
- *Women:* Vaginal itching or dryness: Physiologic changes may cause a decrease in vaginal fluids.
- *Women:* Vaginal bleeding: Postmenopausal bleeding may have many causes, from friable vaginal tissue to cancer of the uterus. If the patient has postmenopausal bleeding, she should be referred to a health care provider for further evaluation.

EXAMINATION

An examination of an older adult proceeds as described for the younger adult. The nurse assesses the patient's level of comfort in different positions needed for the examination. The examination description that follows highlights expected and abnormal findings of the older adult. As with all examinations, perform hand hygiene before you begin.

Equipment needed: Thermometer, watch with second hand, stethoscope, blood pressure cuff, weight and height scale, ophthalmoscope, Snellen chart, handheld vision screener (Rosenbaum or Jaeger), cover card (opaque), tuning fork, audioscope, otoscope, penlight, nasal speculum, tongue blade, examination gloves, 4 × 4 gauze, and reflex hammer.

VITAL SIGNS AND BASELINE MEASUREMENTS

Vital signs are measured with every visit. The procedures for assessing vital signs are the same as for the younger adult.

Temperature

The expected temperature is usually lower for older adults (97.2°F, 36.2°C) because of decreased metabolism and less physical activity. Older adults are especially prone to hypothermia. If the patient's expected oral temperature is 94°F (34.4°C), a temperature of 98°F (36.6°C) may indicate a fever.

Heart and Respiratory Rates

These rates are assessed for the same qualities as in the younger adult. Pulse rates do not differ from those of younger adults unless the patient has heart or peripheral vascular disease. Determine the pulse rate, rhythm, amplitude, and contour of the radial pulse. Unless the patients have a lung disorder, their respiratory rates do not differ from those of other adults, although breathing may be more shallow and rapid.

Blood Pressure

Use the appropriate-size blood pressure cuff for an accurate reading (see Chapter 4).

Expected blood pressure values are the same as for younger adults unless the patient has hypertension or heart disease. Although blood pressure elevations frequently occur in older adults, they are not considered a normal variation. Isolated systolic hypertension (>140 mm Hg) is frequently seen in older adults as a result of atherosclerotic changes.

Height and Weight

Height and weight are measured in the same manner as described for the younger adult. If the scale does not have a handle close by to hold on to, stand close to the scale because some older people may have a problem standing on a small surface off the floor. The height and weight are used to determine the BMI (see Chapter 8).

Expected and abnormal findings. *Height:* Most older adults experience a decrease in height due to shortening of the vertebrae and thinning of the vertebral disks. Decreases in height may occur more often in women because of osteoporosis. *Weight:* For those in their eighties and beyond, body weight may decrease because of muscle wasting or chronic diseases. The total body water declines, which contributes to weight loss. Subcutaneous fat distribution shifts from the face and extremities to the abdomen and hips.

SKIN, HAIR, AND NAILS

Procedures for assessing skin, hair, and nails of an older adult are the same as those described in Chapter 9 (Fig. 21.3).

Skin

Two common concerns with the skin of an older adult are sun exposure and signs of abuse. Inspect the sun-exposed areas such as nose, lips, and ears for color and lesions. The American Medical Association recommends screening all older-adult patients for mistreatment.[17] Notice indications of abuse such as bruising or lacerations, fractures inconsistent with functional ability, pressure ulcers, dehydration, and poor hygiene, which may be indications of mistreatment.[6]

Expected findings. As skin thins it takes on a parchment-like appearance, especially over bony prominences, the dorsal surfaces of the hands and feet, the forearms, and the lower legs (Fig. 21.4). The skin hangs loosely on the frame, secondary to a loss of adipose tissue and elasticity. The skin may be cool because of impaired circulation. Skin tears may occur as a result of thin, fragile texture. Normal variations in the skin of the older adult include findings such as the following:

- *Solar lentigo (liver spots):* Irregularly shaped, flat, deeply pigmented macules that may appear on body surface areas having repeated exposure to the sun (see Fig. 21.4).
- *Seborrheic keratoses:* Pigmented, raised, warty-appearing lesions that may be seen on the face or trunk (Fig. 21.5). Differentiate these benign lesions from similar-appearing actinic keratoses, which are premalignant lesions.
- *Acrochordon (skin tag):* Small, soft tag of skin that generally appears on the neck and upper chest (Fig. 21.6). These tags may or may not be pigmented.

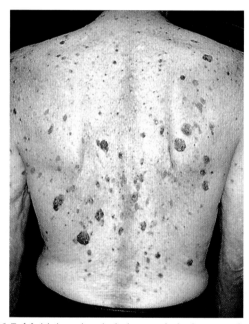

FIG. 21.5 Multiple seborrheic keratosis lesions on the trunk. (From Goldstein and Goldstein, 1997. Courtesy Department of Dermatology, Medical College of Georgia.)

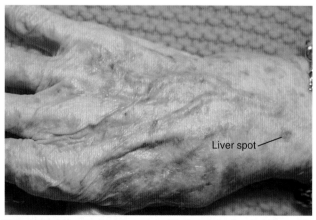

FIG. 21.3 After inspection, palpate the skin for texture, temperature, moisture, mobility, turgor, and thickness.

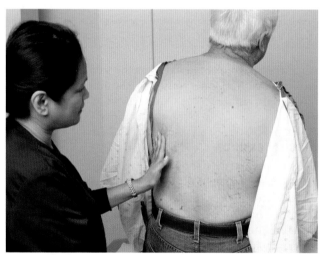

Liver spot

FIG. 21.4 Hands of older adult. Notice prominent veins, thin appearance of the skin, and solar lentigo (liver spots). (From Ignatavicius and Workman, 2016.)

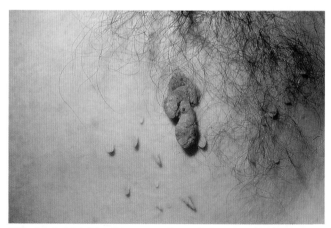

FIG. 21.6 Multiple skin tags. (From Goldstein and Goldstein, 1997. Courtesy Department of Dermatology, University of North Carolina at Chapel Hill.)

Abnormal findings. of the skin are the same as those discussed for adults. Dry skin may indicate dehydration or malnutrition. Tenting of the skin is no longer a reliable indicator of dehydration due to loss of subcutaneous tissue.[18] Edema may indicate fluid retention from cardiovascular or renal disease. Bruising, lacerations, and pressure ulcers require additional follow-up. Refer to Chapter 9 for descriptions of squamous cell and basal cell cancers and malignant melanoma.

Hair

The hair may be thin, gray, and coarse in texture. Symmetric balding may occur in men; a decrease in the amount of body, pubic, and axillary hair occurs in both men and women. Men have an increase in the amount and coarseness of nasal and eyebrow hair, and women may develop coarse facial hair.

Nails

Nails may be thick and brittle, especially the toenails.

HEAD, EYES, EARS, NOSE, AND THROAT

Procedure for assessing the head, eyes, ears, nose, and throat of the older adult are the same as those described in Chapter 10.

Eyes and Vision

Eyes

Expected findings. Pseudoptosis, or relaxed upper eyelid, may be seen, with the lid resting on the lashes. Orbital fat may have decreased so the eyes appear sunken or may herniate, causing bulging on the lower lid or inner third of the upper lid. Brown spots may appear near the limbus as a normal variation. Bulbar conjunctiva may appear dry, clear, and light pink without discharge or lesions. The cornea is transparent, clear, often yellow; arcus senilis (a gray-white circle around the limbus) is common but not associated with any pathologic condition (Fig. 21.7).

Abnormal findings. include ectropion, in which the lower lid drops away from the globe (Fig. 21.8), or entropion, in which the lower lid turns inward (Fig. 21.9). Gradual loss of central vision may be caused by macular degeneration resulting from changes in the retina. The difficulty or inability to visualize the internal structures of the eye may denote cataracts.

Vision

Expected and abnormal findings. Central and peripheral vision may decrease after age 70. Acuity of 20/20 or 20/30 with corrective lenses is common. Accommodation takes longer. Color perception of blue, violet, and green may be impaired. Presbyopia is decreased near vision, which usually occurs after age 40 and is treated with corrective lenses.

Ears and Hearing

Expected and abnormal findings. When the patient wears a hearing device, his or her ear should be carefully assessed for skin irritation or sores that may be secondary to the molded device. There may be the presence of or an increase in wiry hair in the opening of the auditory canal, and the tympanic membrane may appear whiter, opaque, and thickened. If the patient wears a hearing device, there is an increased likelihood of cerumen impaction. Presbycusis is hearing loss associated with aging. The ability to hear high-frequency sounds diminishes first, making high-pitched sounds such as "s" and "th" difficult to hear and tell apart. The speech of others seems mumbled or slurred.

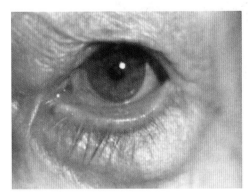

FIG. 21.8 Ectropion. (Courtesy Dr. Ira Abrahamsom, Jr, Cincinnati, Ohio. From Stein, Slatt, and Stein, 1988.)

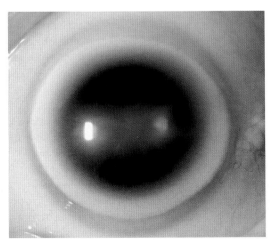

FIG. 21.7 Arcus senilis (a Gray-white circle around the limbus). (From Paley and Krachmer, 1997.)

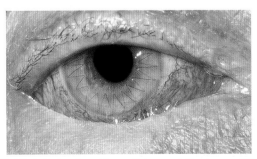

FIG. 21.9 Entropion. (From Paley and Krachmer, 1997.)

Mouth

Patients with dentures should have an examination with the dental appliance both in and out.

Expected and abnormal findings. The surface of the lips may be marked with deep wrinkling. Aging causes the gum line to recede secondary to bone degeneration, causing the teeth to appear longer. The teeth may be darkened or stained. Abnormal findings include fissures at the corners of the mouth (perlèche), which may be associated with overclosure of the mouth or vitamin deficiency. The older patient is at higher risk for squamous cell carcinoma of the lip, especially if he has been a longtime pipe smoker. The gums may be more friable and bleed with slight pressure. Many older adults may have caps or bridges; some may be edentulous. Dental occlusion surfaces may be markedly worn down. Malocclusion of the teeth may be common secondary to the migration of teeth after tooth extraction. A red, edematous tongue with erosions in the corners of the mouth may indicate iron deficiency anemia.

Neck

Procedure. To avoid causing dizziness on movement, assess the range of motion of the neck with one movement at a time rather than a full rotation of the neck. Note any pain, crepitus, dizziness, or limited movement.

Expected and abnormal findings. Flexion, hyperextension, lateral bending, and rotation of the neck are expected, but the range may be less than the younger adult. A stiff neck in the older adult may indicate cervical arthritis.

LUNGS AND RESPIRATORY SYSTEM

Procedures for assessing an older adult are the same as those described in Chapter 11.

Expected and abnormal findings. The thorax and scapulae should be symmetric. The anteroposterior diameter of the chest should be approximately one half the lateral diameter. Older adults may have decreased elasticity and ability to clear the air passages. Breath sounds are the same as for younger adults. Abnormal findings may include kyphoscoliosis, which is formed by an anteroposterior and a lateral curvature of the spine. It may alter the chest wall configuration and make adequate lung expansion more difficult. It may also increase the anteroposterior diameter, which may result in shallow breathing.

HEART AND PERIPHERAL VASCULAR SYSTEM

Procedures for assessing an older adult are the same as those described in Chapter 12 (Fig. 21.10).

Expected and abnormal findings. Occasional ectopic beats are common and may or may not be significant. The S_4 heart sound is common in older adults and may be associated with decreased left ventricular compliance. Abnormal findings may include carotid bruits, indicating arteriosclerosis. Cool feet and weak pedal pulses may be found because of peripheral arterial disease.

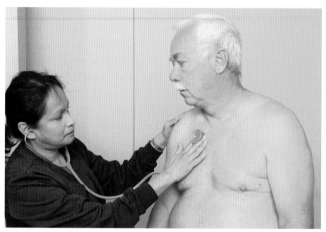

FIG. 21.10 Auscultate for heart sounds using the same procedure as with the younger adult.

ABDOMEN AND GASTROINTESTINAL SYSTEM

Procedures for assessing an older adult are the same as those described in Chapter 13.

Expected and abnormal findings. Older adults may have increased fat deposits over the abdominal area, even with decreased subcutaneous fat over the extremities. The abdomen may feel soft because of decreased abdominal muscle tone. Abnormal findings may include abdominal distension due to fluid or gas, asymmetry from hernias, constipation or bowel obstruction, or hypoactive bowel sounds.

MUSCULOSKELETAL SYSTEM

Procedures for assessing an older adult are generally the same as those described in Chapter 14. Assess balance and gait when indicated.

Expected and abnormal findings. Muscle mass is decreased compared to findings in younger adults (Fig. 21.11). Muscles that are not equal bilaterally may indicate muscle atrophy. Common findings include osteoarthritis changes in joints, which may result in decreased range of motion in affected joints. Many joints may not have the expected degree of movement or range of motion seen in younger adults. Abnormal findings may include unsteady balance and gait that may increase the risks of falls.

NEUROLOGIC SYSTEM

Procedures for assessing an older adult are the same as those described in Chapter 15. Cranial nerves are assessed during the examination of the head, eyes, ears, nose, and throat.

Expected and abnormal findings. For indications of the patient's ability to perform ADLs, notice his or her personal hygiene, appearance, and dress. Be aware that some older adults have slowed responses, move more slowly, or show a decline in function (e.g., the sense of taste). Other expected changes with aging may include deviation of gait from

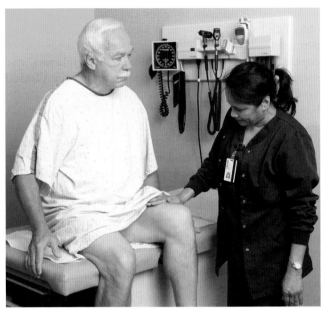

FIG. 21.11 Muscle mass of older adults may be decreased compared with findings in younger adults.

midline, difficulty with rapidly alternating movements, and some loss of reflexes and sensations (e.g., the knee-jerk or ankle-jerk reflexes). Abnormal findings may include resting tremor of the hands that is reduced with purposeful movement, dizziness or vertigo, or hemiparesis of upper or lower extremities.

BREASTS

Procedures for assessing an older adult are the same as those described in Chapter 16. Postmenopausal women and older men should continue to have regular breast examinations.

Expected findings. The breasts in postmenopausal women may appear flattened and elongated or pendulous secondary to a relaxation of the suspensory ligaments. A normal variation found when palpating the breasts in the older adult is a granular feeling of the glandular tissue of the breast. If the woman had cystic disease earlier in life, her breasts are now more likely to feel smoother and less cystic. The inframammary ridge thickness may now be more prominent, and the nipples may be smaller and flatter.

REPRODUCTIVE SYSTEM AND PERIANAL AREA

Female Reproductive System

Procedures for assessing an older adult are the same as those described in Chapter 17.

Expected findings. The labia and clitoris of the older woman are small and pale. The skin may appear dry and have a shiny appearance. The pubic hair may be sparse, patchy, or absent. Because of pelvic musculature relaxation, the patient may have prolapse of the vaginal walls or uterus.

Male Reproductive System

Procedures for assessing an older adult are the same as those described in Chapter 17.

Expected and abnormal findings. Pubic hair tends to be finer and less abundant, sometimes leading to pubic alopecia. The scrotal sac of the patient may appear elongated or pendulous. The testes may feel slightly smaller and softer than in the younger patient. The patient may have injury or excoriation of the scrotal sac surface secondary to sitting on the scrotum.

Perianal Area

Procedures for assessing an older adult are the same as those described in Chapter 17. The patient may need assistance getting into an adequate position for the examination. If lying on the back on the examination table, the patient may need assistance turning to a left lateral lying position.

Expected and abnormal findings. The examination findings for the older adult are the same as those for the adult. The prostate may feel smooth and rubbery; the median sulcus may or may not be palpable. The nurse may also note a relaxation of the patient's perianal muscles and decreased sphincter control when the older adult bears down. Prostate hyperplasia is a common abnormal finding.

COMMON PROBLEMS AND CONDITIONS

A list of common problems and conditions of older adults follows. Most of these have been discussed in previous chapters; the chapter number is included beside the category. Those not previously discussed (in *italics*) are described (i.e., macular degeneration, Alzheimer disease, and urinary incontinence).

Skin, Hair, and Nails—See Chapter 9
   Skin cancer
Vision—See Chapter 10
   Cataracts
   Macular degeneration
   Glaucoma
   Diabetic retinopathy
Hearing—See Chapter 10
   Conductive hearing loss
   Sensorineural hearing loss
Respiratory System—See Chapter 11
   Asthma
   Chronic obstructive pulmonary disease
   Pneumonia
Cardiovascular System—See Chapter 12
   Hypertension

Angina
Myocardial infarction
Valvular heart disease
Heart failure
Peripheral arterial disease
Anemia
Gastrointestinal System—See Chapter 13
Gastrointestinal reflux disease
Constipation
Musculoskeletal System—See Chapter 14
Osteoporosis
Fractures
Osteoarthritis
Gout
Neurologic System—See Chapter 15
Alzheimer disease
Cerebrovascular accident (stroke)
Parkinson disease
Genitourinary System—See Chapters 13 and 17
Urinary tract infections—Chapter 13
Urinary incontinence
Benign prostatic hyperplasia—Chapter 17

Macular Degeneration

The macula is an oval yellow spot in the center of the retina that helps provide central vision. As the maculae degenerate, central visual is impaired. Risk factors are age older than 50 years, Caucasian, smoking, hypertension, and cardiovascular disease. **Clinical Findings:** Loss of central vision, decline in visual acuity, a dark spot in the center of vision, and straight lines appear crooked or wavy (Fig. 21.12).[5]

Alzheimer Disease

A decline in memory is a common first indication of Alzheimer Disease (AD), an incurable, progressive neurologic disorder. AD is the most common cause of dementia among older adults. An estimated 5.5 million Americans have dementia caused by this disorder. Dementia is the loss of cognitive functioning such as thinking, remembering, and reasoning, which interferes with a person's daily life. **Clinical Findings:** This progressive disease begins with early symptoms that progress to mild, moderate, and then severe AD. The first symptoms vary, but for many non-memory aspects of cognition are noted such as word-finding, vision/spatial issues, and impaired reasoning or judgment. Mild AD is noted when people experience greater memory loss and have problems such as wandering and getting lost, trouble with money, repeating questions, taking longer to complete usual daily tasks, and personality changes. People are often diagnosed at this stage. In moderate AD, the memory loss and confusion become worse and people have difficulty recognizing family members and friends. Also, hallucinations, delusions, and paranoia occur, and the person may act impulsively. People with severe AD cannot communicate and are completely dependent on others.[19]

Urinary Incontinence

This common urinary disorder occurs when the person is unable to control urination associated with relaxation of the bladder and/or urinary sphincter. Risk factors include multiple pregnancies, abdominal wall weakness, obesity, urinary tract infections, cerebrovascular accident, or multiple sclerosis. **Clinical Findings:** The person may report feeling an immediate urge to void (urge incontinence); leaking of urine when laughing, coughing, or sneezing (stress incontinence); a continuous leakage of urine; or a leakage of urine during sleep (nocturnal enuresis). Consequences of incontinence are skin breakdown, risk for falls, social isolation, and feelings of embarrassment.

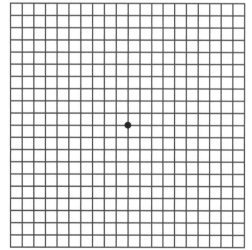 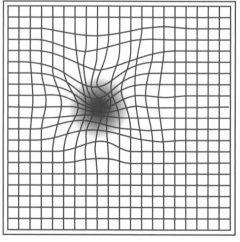

FIG. 21.12 Amsler grid used to evaluate central vision as occurs in macular degeneration. (Available at www.macular.org/Amsler-chart.)

CLINICAL APPLICATION AND CLINICAL JUDGMENT

See Appendix B for answers to exercises in this section.

CASE STUDY

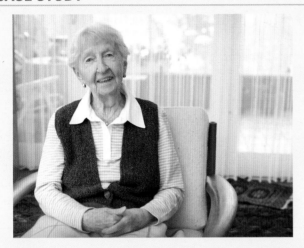

Sara Reinarz is an 80-year-old woman who recently developed confusion and urinary incontinence. She lives with her daughter, Megan, who reports that her mother has fallen several times at home. She is admitted to the hospital for assessment for possible fractures and confusion.

Interview Data

The daughter reports that her mother has fallen several times going to the bathroom. This is the first time Sara reported pain after the fall. Megan is concerned about her mother's confusion. Two weeks ago, Ms. Reinarz was independent and caring for herself at home. Megan recalled that last year her mother became confused and was diagnosed with a urinary tract infection at the same time. As soon as the urinary tract infection was treated, her mother's confusion stopped. Ms. Reinarz has no allergies to food or medications. She takes calcium with vitamin D for osteoporosis, and thyroid hormone for hypothyroidism. She does not smoke or drink alcohol.

Examination Data

Vital signs: Blood pressure, 141/86 mm Hg; pulse, 88 beats/min; respiration rate, 22 breaths/min; temperature, 98.3°F (36.8°C). *Weight:* 152 lb. (69 kg.). Patient confused, but oriented to person. Appears anxious. Bruise on her right hip and thigh. Full range of motion of right leg, but movement painful. Muscle strength 4/5. Pedal pulses 1+ and symmetric.

Clinical Judgment

1. What cues do you recognize that suggest deviations from normal findings, suggesting a need for further investigation?
2. For which additional data should the nurse ask or assess?
3. Based on the data, which risk factors for falls does Ms. Reinarz have?
4. With which health team member would the nurse collaborate to help meet this patient's needs?

REVIEW QUESTIONS

1. During inspection of the mouth of a 72-year-old male patient, the nurse notices a red lesion at the base of his tongue. What additional information does the nurse obtain from this patient?
   1. Alcohol and tobacco use
   2. Date of his last dental examination
   3. How well his dentures fit
   4. A history of gum disease

2. On inspection of the eyes of an 82-year-old woman, the nurse notes which finding as expected?
   1. Opaque coloring of the lens
   2. Clear cornea with a gray-white ring around the limbus
   3. Dilated pupils when looking at an item in her hand
   4. Impaired perception of the colors yellow and red

3. The nurse notes which finding as abnormal during a thoracic assessment of an older adult?
   1. A skeletal deformity affecting curvature of the spine
   2. Shortness of breath on exertion
   3. An increase in anteroposterior diameter
   4. Bronchovesicular sounds in the peripheral lung fields

4. When assessing the mood of older adult patients, a nurse documents which finding as abnormal?
   1. Sadness and grief after returning from the funeral of a long-time friend
   2. Depression that interferes with the ability to perform activities of daily living
   3. Frustration about rearranging the day's schedule to attend a grandson's birthday party
   4. Crying about the unexpected death of a pet that had been with the family 12 years

5. Which would be an abnormal finding during an abdominal examination of an older adult?
   1. Report of incontinence when sneezing or coughing
   2. Loss of abdominal muscle tone
   3. Bowel sounds every 15 seconds in all quadrants
   4. Silver-white striae and a very faint vascular network

6. Which finding is an expected age-related change for a woman 80 years old?
   1. Kyphosis
   2. Back pain
   3. Loss of height
   4. Depression

CHAPTER

22

Conducting a Head-to-Toe Examination

evolve

http://evolve.elsevier.com/Wilson/assessment

Now that you have studied and practiced examining each body system separately, you are ready to put everything together. Although you began with knowledge and procedures specific for each system, you perform a physical examination by viewing the patient as a whole person. You must organize your procedures to examine the entire person, literally from "head to toe." Therefore when you begin with the head, you should examine the facial characteristics (i.e., skin, hair, eyes, ears, mouth, throat, and range of motion of the neck) in a systematic, organized manner that incorporates neurologic, integumentary, musculoskeletal, visual, and auditory systems within the head, neck, nose, and mouth regions. You then move on to the next region of the body. After examining all body regions, you document your findings by body system.

Each nurse's approach to a head-to-toe examination is unique, just as each patient is unique. As a student you determine which sequence works best for you. Use a systematic method so you do not omit any data. When performing other types of assessment (focused, episodic, shift, or screening), you refer only to regions based on the patient's chief complaint and additional data gathered during the history.

GUIDELINES FOR ADULT HEAD-TO-TOE EXAMINATION

Use the following sequence only as a guide. It was developed to demonstrate how examination of one body system is integrated with other body systems to permit a comprehensive regional assessment. Notice in the following example that all relevant body systems in one region are examined before moving to the next body system. For example, when examining the patient's anterior chest, the nurse must consider the other body systems in that region that must be assessed simultaneously and incorporate them into an integrated assessment. These body systems would include skin; respiratory, lymphatic, cardiovascular, musculoskeletal systems; and breasts. Procedures for a routine examination are listed, along with additional procedures that may be indicated for that patient.

Tips for success:
- Be organized.
- Develop a routine. This helps with consistency.
- Before you begin the actual examination, have a clear picture in your mind of what you plan to do and in what order.
- Practice, practice, practice so you learn to become systematic and inclusive.
- Imagine yourself as the patient, and consider how you would want a nurse to be prepared if he or she were to assess you.

Exactly how the examination proceeds depends on the purpose, the needs of the patient, the nurse's ability, and the policies of the facility where the examination is conducted. Equipment for an examination is listed in Box 22.1.

Getting Started
- The patient should be placed in an examination room (or space with privacy) wearing an examination gown.
- Perform hand hygiene.
- Introduce yourself, and ask the patient what name he or she prefers to be called.
- Tell the patient what to expect during the history and examination.

Obtain a History
Take the patient's history including the components in Box 22.2. Notice the following about the patient during introductions and history taking:
- Level of consciousness and mental status
- Facial expression

484

BOX 22.1 EQUIPMENT FOR HEALTH EXAMINATION IN SUGGESTED ORDER OF USE

- Writing surface for nurse
- Scale with height measurement
- Thermometer
- Watch with second hand
- Vision charts—Snellen or Jaeger card
- Sphygmomanometer
- Stethoscope with bell and diaphragm
- Patient gown
- Drape sheet
- Examination table (with stirrups for female patients)
- Otoscope with pneumatic bulb
- Tuning fork
- Audioscope
- Ophthalmoscope
- Nasal speculum
- Tongue blade
- Penlight
- Gauze pads
- Nonsterile examination gloves
- Ruler and tape measure
- Marking pen
- Goniometer
- Aromatic items
- Cotton balls
- Items to assess sharp and dull perception
- Objects for stereognosis such as a key or comb
- Percussion hammer
- Lubricant
- Gooseneck light

BOX 22.2 COMPONENTS OF A HEALTH HISTORY

Biographical data
Reason for seeking care
History of present illness
Present health status
Past health history
Family history
Personal and psychosocial history
Review of systems

- Speech for articulation and voice quality
- Comprehension of verbal communication
- Ability to see, hear, and speak
- Mood or affect
- Personal hygiene and dress
- Skin color
- Posture/position
- Mobility and balance
- Breathing effort

Assess Vital Signs and Other Baseline Measurements

Stand in front of patient who is seated.
- Measure the temperature, radial pulse, respirations, and blood pressure. (Fig. 22.1)
If indicated,
- Take the blood pressure in both arms.
Assess the height, weight, and body mass index.

Examine Hands

Inspect the skin surface of the hands for characteristics and color.

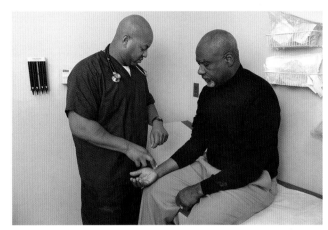

FIG. 22.1 Palpating the right radial pulse.

Inspect the hands for symmetry.
Inspect the nails for shape, contour, color, thickness, and cleanliness.
Palpate the nails for firmness.
Assess capillary refill of the fingers.

Examine Head and Face

Inspect the head for size, shape, and position and hair for distribution, quantity, and color.
Inspect the skin and scalp for surface characteristics.
Palpate the scalp and hair for surface characteristics and texture.
If indicated,
- palpate the skull for symmetry, tenderness, and intactness.
- palpate the scalp for tenderness and intactness.
- palpate the temporal pulses for pulsation, texture, and tenderness.
- auscultate the temporal pulses for sounds.
Inspect the facial structures for size, symmetry, movement, skin characteristics, and facial expressions (CN V and VII).
Inspect the skin for color and lesions.
If indicated,
- palpate the bony structures of the face and jaw, noting jaw movement and tenderness.
- observe the symmetry as patient clenches eyes tightly; wrinkles forehead; smiles; sticks out tongue; and puffs out cheeks (CN VII).
- assess the sensation of forehead, cheeks, and chin to light touch (CN V).
- palpate each temporomandibular joint for movement, pain, and sounds.
- assess range of motion of the temporomandibular joint.

Examine Eyes

Assess distant, near, and peripheral vision (CN II).
Inspect the eyebrows, eyelashes, and eyelids for symmetry, skin characteristics, and discharge.
Inspect each conjunctiva for color, drainage, and lesions.
Inspect each corneal light reflex for symmetry.
Inspect each sclera for color and surface characteristics.
Inspect each cornea for transparency and surface characteristics.

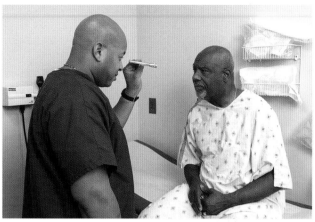

FIG. 22.2 Examining pupillary response, consensual reaction, corneal light reflex, and accommodation.

Inspect each iris for shape and color.

Inspect the pupils for size, shape, reaction to light, consensual reaction, and accommodation (Fig. 22.2).

If indicated,

- assess the extraocular eye movements in six cardinal field of gaze (CN III, IV, VI).
- perform the cover-uncover test.
- palpate the eyes, eyelids, and lacrimal puncta for firmness, tenderness, and discharge.
- evert the upper eyelids to inspect the conjunctiva.
- assess each corneal reflex.
- inspect each anterior chamber for transparency, iris surface, and chamber depth.
- inspect the intraocular structures of each eye:
  - inspect red reflex, disc margins, shape, size, color and physiologic cup.
  - inspect retinal vessels for color, arteriolar light reflex, artery-to-vein ratio, and arteriovenous crossing changes.
  - inspect the retinal background for color, presence of microaneurysms, hemorrhages, and exudates.
  - inspect the macula for color and surface characteristics.

Examine Ears

Inspect external ear for alignment, position, size, symmetry, skin color, skin intactness, and deformities.

Inspect each external auditory canal for discharge or lesions.

If indicated,

- palpate each external ear and mastoid process for characteristics, tenderness, and edema.
- inspect the auditory canals and tympanic membranes.
- inspect the ear canals for cerumen, odor, edema, erythema, discharge, and foreign bodies.
- inspect the tympanic membranes for landmarks, color, contour, translucence, and fluctuation.
- assess auditory function (CN VIII):
  - whispered voice test to evaluate gross hearing (CN VIII).
  - finger-rubbing test to evaluate gross hearing.
  - Weber test to evaluate lateralization of sound.
  - Rinne test to evaluate bone and air conduction.
  - audioscope to measure the degree of hearing loss.

Examine Nose

Inspect the external nose for appearance, symmetry, and discharge.

If indicated,

- evaluate the sense of smell (CN I).
- palpate the nose for tenderness and to assess patency.
- inspect the nasal cavity for surface characteristics, lesions, erythema, discharge, and foreign bodies.
- palpate the frontal and maxillary sinus areas for tenderness.
- transilluminate the sinuses for signs of congestion.

Examine Mouth

Inspect the lips for color, symmetry, moisture, and texture.

Inspect the teeth and gums for color, surface characteristics, condition, and alignment.

Assess the tongue for movement, symmetry, color, surface characteristics, and strength (CN XII).

Inspect the buccal mucosa and anterior and posterior pillars for color, surface characteristics, and odor.

Inspect the palate, uvula, posterior pharynx, and tonsils for texture, color, surface characteristics, and movement.

If indicated,

- palpate the teeth, inner lips, and gums for condition, stability, and tenderness with gloved hands.
- palpate the tongue for texture with gloved hands.
- inspect the oropharynx for gag reflex (CN IX) and movement of soft palate (cranial nerve X).
- assess the tongue for taste (CN VII).

Examine Neck

Inspect the neck position in relationships to the head and trachea.

Inspect the neck for skin characteristics, presence of lumps, and masses.

Palpate the neck muscles for tone and pain.

Assess range of motion of the neck (cervical spine).

Assess the neck muscles for strength.

If indicated,

- palpate the neck for anatomic structures (tracheal rings, cricoid cartilage, and thyroid cartilage) and trachea.
- palpate the thyroid gland for size, consistency, tenderness, and presence of nodules.
- palpate the regional lymph nodes for size, consistency, mobility, and tenderness: preauricular, parotid, postauricular, occipital, retropharyngeal (tonsillar), submandibular, submental, anterior and posterior cervical chain, and supraclavicular.
- test the shoulders and neck muscles for strength, movement, and symmetry (CN XI).

Palpate the carotid pulses for amplitude.

If indicated,

- auscultate the carotid arteries for bruits.

Inspect the jugular veins for pulsations.

Examine Upper Extremities

Inspect the shoulders and shoulder girdle for equality of height, symmetry, and contour.

Palpate the shoulders and upper arms for firmness, fullness, symmetry, and pain.

Inspect the arms for skin surface characteristics, symmetry, and color and for hair distribution, quantity, and texture.

Palpate the skin for surface characteristics, moisture, skin integrity, turgor, and temperature.

Inspect the joints of the wrists and hands for symmetry, alignment, and number of digits.

Palpate the elbows, wrists, and fingers for surface characteristics and pain.

Palpate the pulses for presence and amplitude (brachial and radial).

If indicated,

- palpate the epitrochlear lymph nodes for size, consistency, mobility, tenderness, and warmth.
- palpate the ulnar pulses for presence and amplitude.

Assess range of motion of the shoulders, elbows, wrists, and fingers.

Assess muscle tone of the upper and lower arms.

Assess muscle strength of the upper and lower arms (Fig. 22.3).

Assess the arms for deep tendon reflexes (triceps, biceps, and brachioradialis) (Fig. 22.4).

If indicated,

- assess the arms for coordination.
- assess the arms for sensory function.

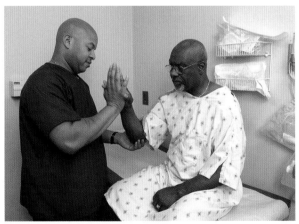

FIG. 22.3 Assessing muscle strength of the right arm.

Examine Posterior and Lateral Thorax

Move behind patient who is seated; gown is lowered to waist for men, open in back for women.

Inspect the posterior and lateral chest for shape, muscular development, and scapular placement.

Observe the respiratory movement for symmetry, depth, and rhythm of respirations.

Inspect the skin for color, intactness, lesions, and scars.

If indicated,

- percuss the kidneys for costovertebral angle pain.
- palpate the posterior thorax and muscles for tenderness and symmetry.
- palpate the posterior thorax for expansion.
- palpate the posterior thoracic wall for fremitus.

Auscultate the posterior and lateral thoraxes for breath sounds (Fig. 22.5).

Examine Anterior Thorax

Move to front of patient who is seated with gown lowered to waist.

Inspect the skin for color, intactness, lesions, and scars.

Inspect the anterior thorax for shape, symmetry, muscle development, and costal angle.

Inspect the anterior thorax for anteroposterior to lateral diameter.

If indicated,

- palpate the anterior thorax and muscles for tenderness and symmetry.
- palpate the anterior thoracic wall for expansion.
- palpate the anterior thoracic wall for fremitus.

Female patients may replace gown over the upper body.

Palpate the left anterior thorax to locate point of maximum impulse (PMI).

Auscultate the anterior thorax for breath sounds.

Auscultate the heart for rate, rhythm, intensity, splitting of S_1 or S_2 or presence of S_3, S_4, or murmurs (Fig. 22.6).

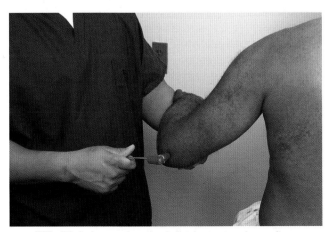

FIG. 22.4 Assessing the left triceps tendon reflex.

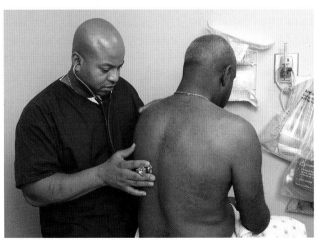

FIG. 22.5 Auscultating the left posterior thorax.

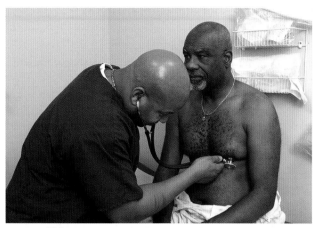

FIG. 22.6 auscultating the apical heart rate.

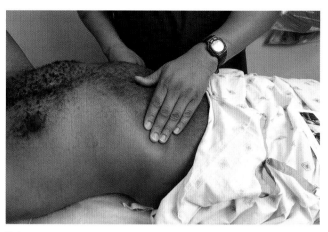

FIG. 22.7 Lightly palpating the right upper quadrant of the abdomen.

Examine Breasts

Female patient

Inspect the breasts for size, symmetry, and shape.

Inspect the skin of the breast for surface characteristics, color, and venous patterns.

Inspect the areolae for color, shape, and surface characteristics.

Inspect the nipples for position, symmetry, surface characteristics, lesions, bleeding, and discharge.

Inspect the breasts in various positions for bilateral pull, symmetry, and contour.

Inspect the axilla for rashes or lesions.

Palpate the axillae for enlarged lymph nodes, lesions, and masses.

Assist the patient to a supine position.

Palpate the breasts for tissue characteristics.

Palpate the nipples for surface characteristics and discharge.

Male patient

Inspect the breasts and nipples for symmetry, color, size, shape, rash, and lesions.

Palpate the breasts, nipples, and areolar for surface characteristics, tenderness, size, and masses.

Palpate the axillae for enlarged lymph nodes, rash, lesions, and masses.

Examine Abdomen

Assist the patient to a supine position with abdomen exposed.

Inspect the abdomen for skin color, surface characteristics, venous patterns, contour, and surface movements.

Auscultate the abdomen for bowel sounds and arterial and venous sounds.

Palpate lightly all quadrants for tenderness and muscle tone (Fig. 22.7).

Palpate all quadrants for pain, masses, and aortic pulsation.

If indicated,

- percuss the abdomen for tones.
- percuss the liver to determine span and descent.
- percuss the spleen for size.
- palpate the liver for lower border and pain.
- palpate the gallbladder for pain.

- palpate the spleen for border and pain.
- palpate the inguinal region for femoral pulses and bulges that may be associated with hernia.
- palpate the inguinal lymph nodes for size, consistency, mobility, tenderness, and warmth.
- palpate the kidneys for contour and pain.
- measure the blood pressure with the patient supine to compare earlier reading with patient sitting.

Examine Lower Extremities

Patient remains supine; legs exposed, abdomen and chest should be covered.

Inspect the knees, legs, ankles, and feet for symmetry, skin integrity, skin color, surface characteristics, vascular sufficiency, hair distribution, number of digits, and deformities.

Palpate the hips for stability and pain.

Palpate the lower legs for temperature, skin turgor, pain, numbness, and edema.

Palpate the skin of legs for texture, moisture, and thickness.

Palpate the pulses for presence and amplitude (popliteal, posterior tibial, and dorsalis pedis pulses) (Fig. 22.8).

Palpate the knees for contour.

Assess capillary refill of the toes.

Inspect the nails for shape, contour, color, and thickness.

Palpate the nails for firmness.

If indicated,

- calculate the ankle-brachial index.
- measure the circumference of each thigh and calf.

Assess range of motion of the hips and knees.

Assess muscle tone of the legs.

Assess muscle strength of the legs (Fig. 22.9).

If indicated,

- assess the legs for sensory function.
- assess the legs for coordination.
- assess for nerve root compression.

The patient moves to a seated position.

Assess range of motion of the ankles, feet, and toes.

Assess the legs for deep tendon reflexes (patellar, Achilles, plantar, and ankle clonus).

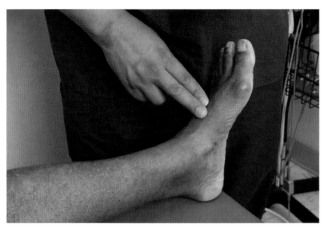

FIG. 22.8 Palpating the left dorsalis pulse.

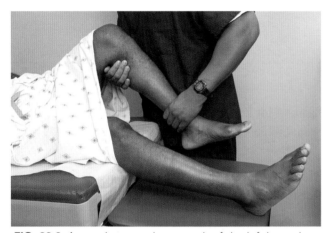

FIG. 22.9 Assessing muscle strength of the left lower leg.

Ask the patient to stand, while you move behind.

Inspect the shoulders and cervical, thoracic, and lumbar spine for alignment and symmetry.

Inspect the hips for symmetry.

Palpate the posterior neck, spinal processes, and paravertebral muscles for alignment and pain.

Observe the gait for conformity, rhythm, and symmetry as patient walks away and returns.

Observe hyperextension of the hips (patient may need to hold on to a table to maintain balance).

With patient bending forward from the waist, assess range of motion of the thoracic and lumbar spine and symmetry of spine

If indicated,
- test for balance.

Examine Genitalia, Perianal Area, and Rectum
Male patient

Patient is lying and adequately draped.

Don examination gloves.

Inspect the pubic hair for distribution and skin for surface characteristics.

Inspect the penis for surface characteristics and color.

Palpate the penis for tenderness and discharge.

Inspect the scrotum for color, texture, surface characteristics, and position.

If indicated,
- palpate the scrotum for surface characteristics and tenderness.

Position patient lying on left side with right hip and knee flexed.

Inspect the sacrococcygeal areas for surface characteristics.

Palpate the sacrococcygeal areas for tenderness.

Inspect the perianal area and anus for pigmentation and surface characteristics.

If indicated,
- palpate the anus for sphincter tone with a gloved finger.
- palpate the anal canal and rectum for surface characteristics with lubricated gloved finger.
- examine stool for characteristics and presence of occult blood when the gloved finger is removed.

Patient is standing.

Inspect the inguinal region and the femoral area for bulges.

If indicated,
- palpate the testes, epididymides, and vas deferens for location, consistency, tenderness, and nodules.

Patient resumes a seated position.

Female patient

Patient should be lying in lithotomy position.

Don examination gloves.

Inspect the pubic hair and skin over the mons pubis and inguinal area for distribution and surface characteristics.

Inspect the labia majora, labia minora, and clitoris for pigmentation.

Palpate the labia majora, labia minora, and clitoris for surface characteristics.

Inspect the urethral meatus, vaginal introitus, and perineum for positioning and surface characteristics.

Inspect the sacrococcygeal areas for surface characteristics.

Palpate the sacrococcygeal areas for tenderness.

If indicated,
- palpate the Skene and Bartholin glands for surface characteristics, discharge, and tenderness.
- palpate the vaginal wall for tone.

Inspect the perianal area and anus for color and surface characteristics.

If indicated,
- palpate the rectal wall for surface characteristics.
- assess the anal sphincter for muscle tone.
- examine stool for characteristics and presence of occult blood.

Patient resumes seated position.

evolve

http://evolve.elsevier.com/Wilson/assessment

At the completion of a health assessment, the nurse documents the data to use in providing nursing care and to share with other health care professionals. The health record serves as a legal document and permanent record of the patient's health status at the time of the nurse-patient interaction. Recorded data should be accurate, concise, and without bias or opinion.

A variety of formats to document assessment findings are used in various health care settings. The amount of information documented reflects the depth and scope of the health assessment. The purpose of this chapter is to provide you with an example of documentation of a comprehensive history and examination for a well patient. At the end of the documentation, the nurse forms a problem list, which provides the basis for determining the plan of care, including the education needs of the patient.

HEALTH HISTORY

Biographic Data

Name: Maria S. Griego
Gender: Female
Address: 1000 1st Street, Angus, TX 87123
Telephone numbers: (111) 999-9999, home; (111) 444-4444, work
Email address: msgriego@gmail.com
Birth date: 10-13-63
Birthplace: Houston, Texas
Race/ethnicity: Hispanic
Religion: Catholic
Marital status: Married, 36 years
Occupation: Counselor in a high school
Contact person: Christopher Griego, spouse
Source of interview data: Patient

Reason for Seeking Care

"I am here for an exam—it has been a while since I have had a checkup."

History of Present Illness

Not applicable.

Present Health Status

Overall health described as "good." *Chronic illnesses*: None. *Medications:* Takes no prescription drugs; does not use herbal preparations; takes one multivitamin each morning. *Allergies:* Reports allergy to penicillin; "gives me hives"; no known food allergies.

Past Health History

Childhood illnesses: Measles, mumps, rubella, chickenpox, streptococcal throat, otitis media. *Surgeries and hospitalizations:* 1982 appendectomy; vaginal deliveries 1985 and 1987. *Accidents/injuries*: Denies. *Immunizations:* Childhood immunizations for school, tetanus immunization unknown. *Last examinations*: Physical and Papanicolaou (Pap) test 5 years ago. *Dental:* 1 year ago. *Vision:* 6 months ago. *Mammogram:* 2 years ago. *Obstetric history:* G2, P2. Both vaginal deliveries without complication.

Family History

Maternal grandmother deceased age 70, hypertension and heart failure; maternal grandfather deceased age 72, colon cancer; paternal grandmother deceased age 84, "old age"; paternal grandfather deceased age 81, prostate cancer; mother, age 83, hypertension, arthritis, dementia; father, deceased age 62, myocardial infarction. Patient has no brothers or sisters. Denies family history of stroke, diabetes mellitus, kidney disease, mental disorders, or seizure disorders. Both children in good health.

Personal and Psychosocial History

Personal Status

Patient states that she feels good about herself most of the time. Her cultural affiliation is self-described as middle-class Hispanic female. She has a master's degree in counseling and has been a high school counselor with the same school for 25 years. Overall, she enjoys her job but experiences frustration with the social issues of her students. Hobbies include playing piano and gardening.

Family and Social Relationships

Patient lives with husband and mother in a four-bedroom home in a suburban area; both sons live in the same community and remain close. Both sons are married; three grandchildren. The patient considers relationship with husband as close; she also speaks of two other very close female friends. Mother is elderly and has moderate dementia and occasional falls, requiring increasing supervision. Patient expresses concerns about meeting her mother's needs in the future and the ongoing physical demands.

Diet/Nutrition

Describes appetite as excellent; no changes in appetite or weight. Reports balanced food intake. 24-hour recall: *Breakfast:* muffin, 1% milk, fruit juice, coffee; *Lunch:* spaghetti, green beans, salad, tea; *Dinner:* chicken, mashed potatoes, apple sauce, roll, tea, chocolate cake for dessert; *Snack:* crackers with peanut butter; *Fluid:* 4 glasses of water, 2 cups coffee, and 2 glasses tea daily.

Functional Ability

Activities include maintaining a home, working full time, and caring for her mother.

Mental Health

Patient verbalizes frequent episodes of frustration and despair in meeting her mother's needs. She does not feel that her husband is supportive of this situation, which has caused some conflict. She counts on her friends to help her "talk through" stress periods. The patient and her spouse have had marriage counseling on two different occasions, which she believes were beneficial. Also verbalizes stress at work regarding issues with students and administration. Recently, she has not been able to find time to exercise, but when she can, she finds this helpful in coping with the stress. She has had no previous psychiatric or mental health counseling.

Tobacco, Alcohol, and Illicit Drug Use

Denies drug use; 1 glass of wine daily; previously a smoker with a 7 pack-year history; has not smoked for 15 years.

Health Promotion Activities

Reports walking 1 mile two to three times per week to stay fit but has not been able to maintain this routine recently. Wears seat belt when in a car.

Environment

Believes that her home and neighborhood environments are safe and without hazards.

Review of Systems

General Symptoms

Considers herself in "good health" but frequently feels fatigued because of obligations of caring for her mother and working full time.

Skin, Hair, and Nails

Skin: Denies lesions, masses, discolorations, or rashes to skin. *Hair:* Denies texture changes or loss, uses hair color monthly to cover gray; no scalp irritation reported from hair coloring. *Nails:* Denies changes in texture, color, shape. *Health promotion:* Uses sunscreen "occasionally" when outside.

Head, Eyes, Ears, Nose, Throat

Denies headache, vertigo, syncope. *Eyes:* Wears multi-focal glasses; is being monitored for cataracts by ophthalmologist. Denies discharge, pruritus, pain, visual disturbances. *Ears:* Denies pain, discharge, tinnitus. *Nose:* Denies nasal discharge, epistaxis, olfactory deficit, snoring. *Mouth:* Denies sore throat, lesions, gum irritation, chewing or swallowing difficulties, hoarseness, voice changes. *Neck:* Denies tenderness or range-of-motion difficulties. *Health promotion:* Brushes teeth twice daily, sees dentist and ophthalmologist each year.

Breasts

No tenderness; denies lumps, masses, or nipple discharge. *Health promotion:* Mammogram 2 years ago.

Cardiovascular System

Denies chest pain, shortness of breath, and palpitations; feet frequently feel cold; denies discoloration or peripheral edema. *Health promotion:* Uses a fitness tracker. Until recently has walked 1 mile two to three times a week; has trouble finding time to do this recently.

Respiratory System

Denies breathing difficulties, cough, shortness of breath.

Gastrointestinal System

Denies eating and digestion problems or abdominal pain. Daily bowel movement formed, brown; does not use stool softener or laxatives; denies hemorrhoids.

Urinary System

Describes urine as yellow and clear; voiding frequency four to five times daily; denies problems with voiding, changes in urinary pattern, or pain.

Musculoskeletal System

Denies muscular weakness, twitching, and pain; gait difficulties; and extremity deformities. States that she has occasional joint stiffness but has not experienced pain, edema, or crepitus.

Neurologic System

Denies changes in cognitive function, coordination, and sensory deficits.

Reproductive System

Went through menopause at age 51. States that she is sexually active with husband and satisfied with sexual relationship, although often experiences painful intercourse because of vaginal dryness; denies genital lesions or discharge; denies history of sexually transmitted disease.

PHYSICAL EXAMINATION

General Survey

Cooperative, oriented, alert woman; sitting with erect posture; maintains eye contact; appropriately groomed and dressed. *Vital signs:* blood pressure 110/78; pulse 78; R 14; temperature 98°F (36.7°C); weight 137 lb (62 kg); height 5 ft 3 inches; body mass index 24.3.

Skin, Hair, and Nails

Smooth, soft, moist, tanned, warm, intact skin with elastic turgor; hair brown with female distribution, soft texture; nails smooth, rounded, manicured, nail base angle 160 degrees.

Head

Skull symmetric; scalp intact; face and jaw symmetric. Temporal arteries palpable bilaterally with regular rhythm, amplitude 2+, smooth contour.

Eyes

Vision 20/20 in both eyes with glasses; near vision, able to read magazine at 13 inches with contacts, horizontal and color perceptions intact. Peripheral vision present; EOM intact; brows, lids, and lashes symmetric; lacrimal ducts pink and open without discharge. Palpebral fissures equal bilaterally, and eyelid color appropriate for race. Eyelid margins pale pink and cover top of the brown iris. Eyelid closure complete, with frequent, bilateral, and involuntary blinking. Conjunctiva clear; sclera white, moist, and clear; cornea smooth and transparent; iris transparent and flat, PERRLA, consensual reaction present. Corneal light reflex symmetric. Eyeballs indent with slight pressure, no tenderness of eyelids. Irises clear, with no shadow noted. *Ophthalmic examination:* Red reflex present; disc margins distinct, round, yellow; artery-to-vein ratio 2:3, retina red uniformly; macula and fovea slightly darker.

Ears

Hearing intact as noted in general conversation; pinna aligned with eyes, ears symmetric, earlobes pierced once. Upper part of ear firm, flexible, and soft without discomfort; ears symmetric. Cerumen in auditory canal, TM pearly gray, cones of light reflex present.

Whispered words repeated correctly, tone heard bilaterally in Weber test, AC:BC = 2:1.

Nose

Septum midline, nasal passages patent; turbinates pink with no drainage. No pain with sinus palpation.

Mouth

Temporomandibular joint moves without difficulty; no halitosis. Lips symmetric, moist, smooth; 28 white, smooth, and aligned teeth; fillings noted in all lower molars. Mucous membranes pink and moist, symmetric pillars, clear saliva. Tongue symmetric, pink, moist, and movable. Hard palate smooth, pale; soft palate smooth, pink, and rises; uvula midline; posterior pharynx pink, smooth; tonsils pink with irregular texture.

Neck

Trachea midline; thyroid smooth, soft, size of thumb pad; full range of motion (ROM) of neck; no palpable lymph nodes.

Chest and Lungs

Breathing quiet and effortless. AP: lateral diameter 1:2; Thorax symmetric, with ribs sloping downward at approximately 45 degrees relative to the spine. Muscle development of thorax equal bilaterally, without tenderness. Thoracic expansion symmetric. Tactile fremitus equal anteriorly and posteriorly. Spinous processes in alignment; scapulae symmetric. Lungs clear to auscultation throughout lung fields, with vesicular breath sounds heard over most lung fields, bronchovesicular breath sounds in the posterior chest over the upper center area of the back and around the sternal border, and bronchial breath sounds heard over the trachea.

Breasts

Moderate size, even color, bilaterally symmetric and hang equally with smooth contour. R slightly >L; no dimpling present. Granular consistency bilaterally but more pronounced in outer quadrants, without tenderness, lumps, or nodules; areolae round, symmetric; nipples protruding, soft, pliable, smooth, and intact without discharge; symmetric venous pattern; no palpable axillary lymph nodes.

Heart

Apical pulse palpated at fifth LICS, MCL; no lifts, heaves, or thrills or abnormal pulsations, No carotid bruit heard. S_1 low-pitched, louder at the apex, and S_2 high-pitched, louder at the base, regular rate and rhythm, no splitting or murmurs present.

Peripheral Vascular

Distal pulses palpable, smooth contour; amplitude 2+ in all pulses; no jugular distention noted; lower extremities warm and pink with symmetric hair distribution, no edema or tenderness; elastic turgor, capillary refill less than 1 second in all fingers, nail beds pink with angle 160 degrees. Thigh circumferences equal. ABI = 1.2.

Abdomen

Rounded, striae noted; skin smooth; faint 4 inches (10 cm) scar to right lower quadrant, umbilicus midline; bowel sounds present with no vascular sounds; abdomen soft, no tenderness, masses, or aortic pulsations noted with light or deep abdominal palpation. Umbilical ring feels round with no irregularities or bulges. Tympany tones over abdomen and spleen; dullness over suprapubic area. Liver spans 3 inches (7.5 cm) at midclavicular line, lower border descends downward 1 inch (2.5 cm). No CVA tenderness, no inguinal lymphadenopathy. Liver border smooth. Gallbladder, spleen, and kidneys not palpable.

Musculoskeletal

Full ROM in all joints without pain; muscles symmetric and firm with 5/5 strength bilaterally, adequate muscle tone, extremities aligned and symmetric, vertebral column straight; coordinated smooth gait.

Neurologic

Oriented to time, place, person; speech understandable and of sufficient volume; cranial nerves I to XII grossly intact; peripheral sensation intact. Balanced gait, movement coordinated bilaterally. Deep tendon reflexes 2+ bilaterally. No clonus present.

Genitalia

Pubic hair in female distribution; labia smooth and soft; urethral meatus midline; perineum smooth and without lesions; two small hemorrhoids noted on anus.

PROBLEM LIST

- Education regarding health promotion: immunizations, exercise
- Dyspareunia
- Concerned about providing care for mother

CHAPTER
24
Adapting Health Assessment

evolve
http://evolve.elsevier.com/Wilson/assessment

In the previous chapters you learned which questions to ask to obtain a history and which techniques to use when performing a head-to-toe assessment. When learning health assessment, you practice on relatively healthy people, often other students. This chapter presents examples of people whose medical treatment requires nurses to adapt the assessment. What follows are photos of 13 patients who have had different procedures performed that require adaptations of the usual assessment procedures.

ADAPTING ASSESSMENT OF THE SKIN

Intravenous Infusion Site

Patient 1 has an intravenous (IV) catheter in the forearm for the administration of fluids and medications. Inspect the skin around the insertion site for redness, edema, and drainage. Palpate the site to assess for pain. The skin surrounding the IV catheter should be without redness, edema, or drainage. A dressing should cover the insertion site, and the IV should be secured. Fig. 24.1 is an example of how an IV insertion site appears.

Surgical Incision

Patient 2 has a surgical incision of the left leg (Fig. 24.2). Inspect the incision for redness, edema, drainage, and intact skin. This incision is described as well approximated because the edges are close together. The incision may be measured. Additional data you may collect are the patient's rating of pain and the extent to which the incision interferes with activities.

Open Wound

Patient 3 has a wound with edges that are not approximated (Fig. 24.3). Inspect the wound for color, size, and drainage. This wound has red-to-pink granulation tissue, indicating healing of tissue. The lines show how the width and depth of this wound are measured for documentation. Notice the type of drainage in the wound, if present, or on the dressing. In

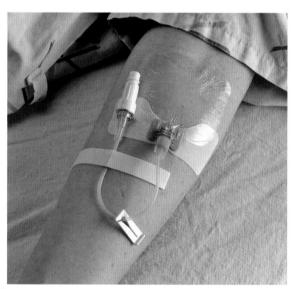

FIG. 24.1 Inspect the intravenous site for redness and edema. (From Ignatavicius and Workman, 2010.)

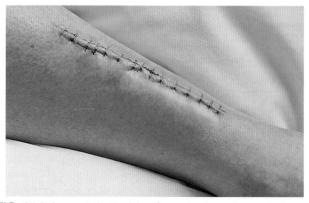

FIG. 24.2 Inspect the incision for redness, edema, drainage, and intact staples and measure the length of the incision. (From Perry, Potter, and Elkin, 2012.)

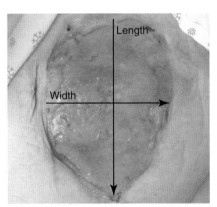

FIG. 24.3 Describe the color of the wound and measure the length and width to document healing. (From Perry, Potter, and Elkin, 2012.)

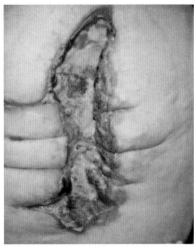

FIG. 24.4 When assessing a dehisced wound, describe the wound and drainage and measure the width, length, and depth. (From Perry, Potter, and Elkin, 2012.)

this case, serous drainage is observed. Photographs provide valuable documentation of wounds to monitor healing. Because this patient has an open wound, a nutritional assessment may be indicated (see Chapter 8).

Infected Incision

Patient 4 had an abdominal surgical procedure, but the wound became infected and the suture line dehisced (rupture of a surgical incision) (Fig. 24.4). Assessment of this wound includes describing the wound and its drainage and measuring the width, length, and depth. A cotton-tipped applicator is placed at various locations in the wound to measure the depth. The location of four previous retention sutures can be seen. There is a small amount of dark necrotic tissue at the lower left side of the incision approximately at the 7 o'clock location using a clock reference. Some granulation (red) tissue and yellow and white exudate are noted within the wound.

ADAPTING ASSESSMENT OF THE LUNGS AND RESPIRATORY SYSTEM

Nasal Cannula

Patient 5 requires oxygen therapy that is delivered by a nasal cannula (Fig. 24.5). In addition to the usual assessment data, notice the patient's respiratory effort and the oxygen saturation. Ask the patient about any cough, including the color and amount of sputum expectorated. Ask if the cough is interfering with self-care activities and sleep. Inspect the skin of the nares and behind the helix of her ears for redness and signs of pressure from nasal prongs and oxygen tubing, respectively.

Oxygen Mask

Patient 6 requires oxygen therapy using a Venturi mask (Fig. 24.6). Notice the patient's use of accessory muscles to breathe or tripod sitting. Inspect the skin of his face for redness or indentation from the facemask and behind the helix of his ears for signs of pressure from the oxygen tubing.

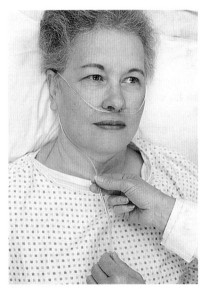

FIG. 24.5 Inspect the nares and behind the ears for pressure from the nasal cannula. (From Perry, Potter, and Elkin, 2012.)

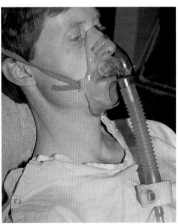

FIG. 24.6 Inspect the face and ears for pressure from the venturi mask. (From Perry, Potter, and Elkin, 2012.)

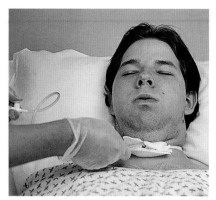

FIG. 24.7 Inspect the skin around the tracheostomy tube and the neck for redness. (From Perry, Potter, and Elkin, 2012.)

Tracheostomy Tube

Patient 7 has a tracheostomy tube that the nurse is suctioning to remove secretions (Fig. 24.7). This tube is inserted into the trachea as an artificial airway and is held in place by ties that are secured around the patient's neck. Tracheostomy tubes are used for administration of mechanical ventilation, relief of airway obstruction, or clearing of secretions. Patients who have tracheostomy tubes are unable to speak because the air passes through the tube rather than the vocal cords. They may be able to mouth words or write notes to communicate. The collar over the tracheostomy tube delivers humidified oxygen to warm and humidify the air the patient inhales since the nose is bypassed. Assessment includes respiratory effort and the amount and color of secretions suctioned from the tracheostomy tube. Also inspect the skin around the tracheostomy tube and the neck for redness, excoriation, or skin breakdown.

Chest Tube

Patient 8 had a thoracotomy (incision into the thoracic cavity) to remove a tumor from the right lung (Fig. 24.8). A chest tube was placed in the pleural space to drain blood and secretions after surgery. The chest tubes initially are attached to a drainage system that works with gravity or suction. In addition to the usual physical assessment data collected, assess this patient's pain from the surgical site, especially when inhaling deeply. When suction is used, it may create a sound that can be heard during chest auscultation, making auscultation more difficult. The sound from the suction may be mistaken for abnormal lung sounds. The dressing around the chest tube is inspected; it should be dry and intact. This dressing is not removed until the surgeon is ready to remove the chest tubes. The color and amount of drainage from the chest tube that collects in the bedside drainage container are noted.

ADAPTING ASSESSMENT OF THE ABDOMEN AND GASTROINTESTINAL SYSTEM

Nasogastric Tube

Patient 9 has a nasogastric (NG) tube (Fig. 24.9) used to provide a liquid diet, water, and medications. Inspect the skin of

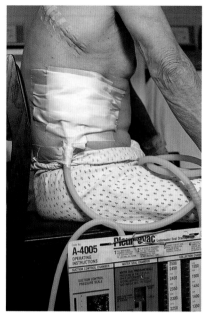

FIG. 24.8 Assess patency of pleural chest tubes attached to suction. (From Elkin, Perry, and Potter, 2008.)

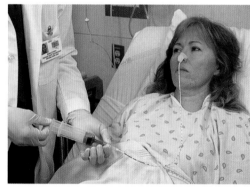

FIG. 24.9 Notice which naris contains the nasogastric tube and inspect the skin of the naris for irritation from the pressure of the tube. (From Perry, Potter, and Elkin, 2012.)

the naris containing the NG tube for redness from pressure, and inspect the tape attaching the NG tube to the patient's nose to make sure that it is secure. Expected findings include skin of nares intact without redness.

Gastrostomy Tube

Patient 10 has a gastrostomy tube (G tube) that has been inserted through the abdominal wall into the stomach (Fig. 24.10). The tube is used to provide a liquid diet, water, and medications. Assessment includes inspecting the oral mucous membranes for moisture because he is unable to take fluids orally. Also inspect the skin around the G tube for redness, edema, and drainage. The gingiva and oral mucous membranes should be pink and moist, and the skin around the G tube should be consistent with adjacent abdominal tissue.

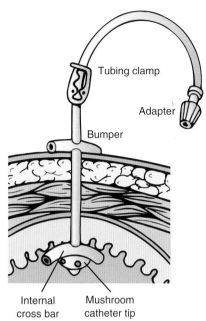

FIG. 24.10 A gastrostomy tube (G tube) is surgically placed through the abdominal wall into the stomach. (From Perry, Potter, and Elkin, 2012.)

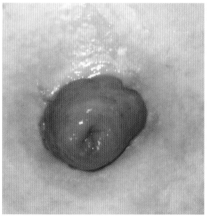

FIG. 24.11 Describe the appearance of the stoma and the skin surrounding it. (From Perry, Potter, and Elkin, 2012.)

Ostomy

Patient 11 had the descending and transverse colon removed (partial colectomy). The remaining colon was brought to the abdominal wall to create an artificial anus called a *colostomy,* shown in Fig. 24.11. The colostomy allows stool to be evacuated from the colon into the pouch shown in Fig. 24.12. Assessment includes inspection of the stoma, the skin around the stoma, the character of the stool, and the colostomy appliance. The stoma should appear red and moist. The skin around the stoma and under the ostomy appliance should appear intact without lesions, irritation, or areas of excoriation. Describe the color and characteristics of the output from the colostomy. A newly created colostomy will not have stool draining from it until the patient starts eating. If the patient has had a transverse (upper colon) level colostomy,

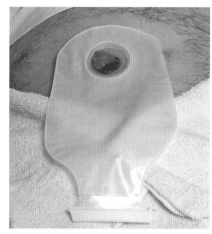

FIG. 24.12 A pouch attached around the stoma. (From deWit, 2009.)

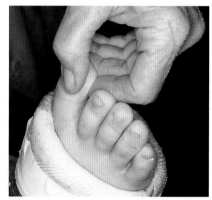

FIG. 24.13 Assess capillary refill to determine arterial circulation to the right toes. (From Perry, Potter, and Elkin, 2012.)

the stool is mushy. If the patient's colostomy is in the area of the descending or sigmoid (lower) colon, the stool is more solid. When the entire colon is removed, the distal ileum is brought to the abdominal wall to form an ileostomy. The contents from the ileostomy, which contain digestive enzymes from the small intestine, are a thick liquid consistency and are secreted continuously.

ADAPTING ASSESSMENT OF THE MUSCULOSKELETAL SYSTEM

Cast

Patient 12 has a cast on the right leg (Fig. 24.13). Assessing circulation, movement, and sensation of the toes distal to the cast is critical. Because of the cast location of this patient, the dorsalis pedis pulse is not accessible to palpation. Thus circulation is determined by assessing capillary refill in the toes and noting the temperature and color of the skin. Ask the patient to move the right toes to assess movement. Place your hand adjacent to the toes so the patient cannot see which toe you touch. Ask him or her to identify which toe you are touching to assess sensation. Expected findings are capillary refill 2 seconds or less and warm temperature and color consistent with the uninjured foot with movement and sensation present.

External Fixator

Patient 13 has an injury to his left hand requiring an external fixator to hold the bones in place while they heal (Fig. 24.14). Assessment includes determining presence of circulation, movement, and sensation of the fingers. Assess capillary refill of the fingers and the radial pulse. Ask the patient to move the fingers to assess motion. Use the same procedures to test sensation as used with Patient 12. Because the external fixator penetrates the skin, the insertion sites are inspected for evidence of infection (i.e., redness, edema, and drainage). Expected findings are radial pulse 2+, capillary refill less than 2 seconds, and movement and sensation of fingers present. Fingers are edematous with clean, dry dressing of the third finger. Insertion sites of external fixator are clean without redness.

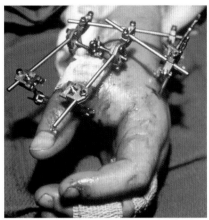

FIG. 24.14 Assess circulation, movement, sensation, and the skin at insertion sites. (From Perry, Potter, and Elkin, 2012.)

SUMMARY

The patient descriptions in this chapter provide a few examples of adaptations needed to complete a physical assessment when patients are receiving treatment for a common problems and conditions. The knowledge and skills you have gained in your study of health assessment form a foundation for future practice.

ABBREVIATIONS

ABI	ankle-brachial index		LSB	left sternal border
AMI	acute myocardial infarction		LUQ	left upper quadrant
ANS	autonomic nervous system		MCL	midclavicular line
AOM	acute otitis media		mg/dL	milligram per deciliter
AP	anteroposterior		MGF	maternal grandfather
AV	atrioventricular		MGM	maternal grandmother
AWS	alcohol withdrawal syndrome		min	minute
BMI	body mass index		mL	milliliter
BP	blood pressure		mm	millimeter
BPH	benign prostatic hyperplasia		mm Hg	millimeters of mercury
BRCA1, BRCA2	symbols for breast cancer genes		MSM	men who have sex with men
C	Celsius		OME	otitis media with effusion
CC	chief complaint		P	pulse
cm	centimeter		PAD	peripheral arterial disease
CN	cranial nerve		Pap	Papanicolaou
CNS	central nervous system		PCM	protein calorie malnutrition
COPD	chronic obstructive pulmonary disease		PE	pulmonary embolism
CSF	cerebrospinal fluid		PERRLA	pupils equal, round, react to light, and
CVA	costovertebral angle; cerebrovascular accident			accommodation
DBW	desired body weight		PID	pelvic inflammatory disease
DT	delirium tremors		PIH	pregnancy-induced hypertension
DVT	deep vein thrombosis		PGF	paternal grandfather
ECG, EKG	electrocardiogram; electrocardiograph		PGM	paternal grandmother
EOM	extraocular movement		PMI	point of maximal impulse
F	Fahrenheit		PMS	premenstrual syndrome
ft	feet		PPE	personal protective equipment
g, G	gram		PROM	premature rupture of membranes
GCS	Glasgow Coma Scale		PTSD	posttraumatic stress disorder
GI	gastrointestinal		R	right, respirations
HEENT	head, eyes, ears, nose, and throat		RA	rheumatoid arthritis
HIV	human immunodeficiency virus		RICS	right intercostal space
HPV	human papilloma virus		RLQ	right lower quadrant
HSV	herpes simplex virus		RMCL	right midclavicular line
Ht	height		ROM	range of motion
HTN	hypertension		RSB	right sternal border
Hz	Hertz		RUQ	right upper quadrant
ICS	intercostal space		S_1	first heart sound
in	inch		S_2	second heart sound
kcal	kilocalorie		S_3	third heart sound
kg	kilogram		S_4	fourth heart sound
km	kilometer		SGA	small for gestational age
L	left		STD	sexually transmitted disease
lb	pound		STI	sexually transmitted infections
LBW	low birth weight		T	temperature
LED	light-emitting diode		TIA	transient ischemic attack
LICS	left intercostal space		TM	tympanic membrane
LLQ	left lower quadrant		TMJ	temporomandibular joint
LMCL	left midclavicular line		UBW	usual body weight
LMP	last menstrual period		UTI	urinary tract infection

Symbols

<	less than
>	greater than
°	degree

APPENDIX

B

Answer Key

CHAPTER 1: INTRODUCTION TO HEALTH ASSESSMENT

Case Study 1

1. *Subjective data:* Abdominal pain in right abdomen. Pain feels like a knife and goes to her shoulder. Patient reports nausea, feels exhausted, and has not slept for three nights; pain keeps her awake. Patient hurts too much to move.
2. *Objective data:* Dark circles under eyes. Vital signs: blood pressure, 132/90 mm Hg; pulse, 104 beats/min; respiratory rate 22 breaths/min; temperature, 101.8°F (38.8°C). Elevated white blood cell count. Patient lying in fetal position.

Case Study 2

1. **Pain** *Subjective data:* Complains of pain in right leg. Pain medication helps only a little bit, and "butt hurts" because he can't move around. *Objective data:* Patient has complex fractured femur. Right leg is in immobilizer. Taking ibuprofen 400 mg every 4 to 6 hours; oxycodone 1 or 2 by mouth every 4 to 6 hours as needed for pain.
2. **Altered elimination** *Subjective data:* No bowel movement for 3 days. Stool looked like "hard, dry rabbit turds." Usual bowel elimination daily. *Objective data:* Limited mobility as a result of immobilizer. Fluid intake average ≤1000 mL/day. Eating 30% of meals. Abdomen slightly distended. Active bowel sounds. Taking ibuprofen and oxycodone for pain, has taken two oxycodone pills every 6 hours over last 2 days.
3. **Risk for skin breakdown** *Subjective data:* "My butt hurts because I can't move around." "The food is horrible." *Objective data:* Patient has limited mobility because of immobilizer. Fluid intake average ≤1000 mL/day. Eating 30% of meals. Red area over sacrum 2-inch (5 cm) diameter, (skin intact).

Review Questions

1. 1
2. 2
3. 2
4. 3
5. 1

CHAPTER 2: OBTAINING A HEALTH HISTORY

Genogram

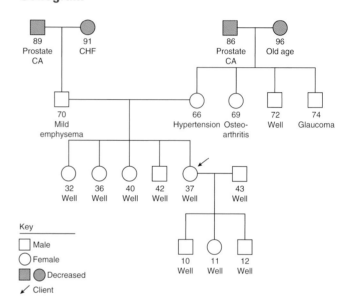

Review Questions

1. 2
2. 4
3. 3
4. 1
5. 4
6. 3
7. 2

CHAPTER 3: TECHNIQUES AND EQUIPMENT FOR PHYSICAL ASSESSMENT

Review Questions

1. 4
2. 1
3. 3
4. 1
5. 2
6. 4
7. 2
8. 3

CHAPTER 4: GENERAL INSPECTION AND MEASUREMENT OF VITAL SIGNS

Review Questions

1. 2
2. 2
3. 1
4. 3
5. 4
6. 1
7. 3

CHAPTER 5: CULTURAL COMPETENCE

Review Questions

1. 2
2. 2
3. 1
4. 1
5. 4
6. 3
7. 3

CHAPTER 6: PAIN ASSESSMENT

Case Study

The patient's description of pain suggests some sort of acute problem, which indicates a need to search for the source of the problem.

1. Data that deviate from expected are signs and symptoms consistent with acute pain. The signs are elevated heart and respiratory rates and diaphoresis. The symptoms are his reports of pain at 12 (on a scale of 10) and nausea.
2. Ask if the pain radiates to any other site and if there are any symptoms associated with urination such as blood in the urine or pain with urination. Ask the patient if he has ever had pain like this before. If yes, ask him to describe it. Ask if he has noticed anything that reduces the intensity or if he has taken any medications or tried any self-treatment. Ask him about his past experiences with pain.
3. The health care team member most helpful in this case is the physician who can prescribe pain medication and perform diagnostic tests to determine the cause of the pain and order treatment.

Review Questions

1. 4
2. 2
3. 3
4. 1
5. 2

CHAPTER 7: MENTAL HEALTH ASSESSMENT

Case Study

1. Unkempt general appearance; crying behavior; excessive sleeping; self-deprecating, slow speech with flat affect.
2. Ask about the onset of symptoms and current stressors. Ask about recent changes in her life, and identify coping mechanisms. Ask about interpersonal relationships with friends and boyfriend. Ask her if she takes any medications.
3. Risk factors for depression: Gender: She is female. Age: Late adolescence. Personal characteristics: She may have a distorted perception of her parent's reaction to her performance in school and a pessimistic outlook.
4. Collaborate with a psychiatric advanced practice registered nurse, counselor, or psychologist.

Review Questions

1. 2
2. 1
3. 3
4. 2
5. 1
6. 4

CHAPTER 8: NUTRITIONAL ASSESSMENT

Case Study

1. *Subjective data:* Fatigue. Shortness of breath. Change in diet. Weight loss. Patient's perception of health. *Objective data:* Height for weight. Scaling of skin. Hair is thin, dull, and easily plucked. Cracks in corner of mouth. Pale conjunctiva.
2. Ask about other symptoms that she may be experiencing; if her appetite has been affected; if weight loss has been intentional; her usual body weight (UBW) and if she has a history of weight loss. Assess her knowledge regarding a vegetarian diet. Calculate the body mass index (BMI), the desired body weight (DBW), her percent of DBW, and the percent weight change in 4 months from her UBW.
3. Risk factors for nutritional problems: Lack of money to buy food. New vegetarian diet.
4. Collaborate with a physician and dietitian.

Review Questions

1. 1
2. 2
3. 4
4. 3
5. 2

CHAPTER 9: SKIN, HAIR, AND NAILS

Case Study

1. Foul-smelling odor; loss of appetite; flat affect; 6 feet 2 inches, 153 pounds; skin breakdown; minimal activity.
2. Ask the patient if he is aware of the skin breakdown. Ask about recent weight loss with reduced activity. Assess ulcers to determine stage and presence of infection. Assess other pressure areas for evidence of skin breakdown. Perform a nutritional assessment.

3. Risk factors for pressure ulcers: He has impaired mobility and no sensation below his level of spinal cord injury. He may be poorly nourished, which may also contribute to skin breakdown.
4. Collaborate with a physician, wound care nurse, and dietitian.

Review Questions

1. 3
2. 4
3. 1
4. 1
5. 2
6. 4
7. 4
8. 3

CHAPTER 10: HEAD, EYES, EARS, NOSE, AND THROAT

Case Study

1. Fever; complaints of ear pain; presence of drainage in ear canal; tympanic membrane perforation; reduction of hearing in left ear; quiet affect; limited talking.
2. Ask the patient what treatment she has received for the ear pain in the past. Ask if she has ever seen drainage from the ear with past problems. Hearing assessment using an audiometer is indicated.
3. Risk factors for hearing loss: perforated tympanic membrane, multiple ear infections.
4. Collaborate with a physician or advanced practice registered nurse.

Review Questions

1. 1
2. 1
3. 4
4. 2
5. 1
6. 4
7. 3
8. 2
9. 4
10. 3
11. 1
12. 4

CHAPTER 11: LUNGS AND RESPIRATORY SYSTEM

Case Study

1. History of shortness of breath; limitation in activity; interrupted sleep (requires two pillows); smoking history; labored breathing with tachypnea; presence of cyanosis; underweight/protruding ribs; increased anteroposterior (AP) diameter; reduced chest wall movement; adventitious and diminished breath sounds.
2. Ask about chest pain with shortness of breath and about the presence of a cough. Ask how old the patient was when she started smoking and how long she has been smoking as much as she currently is. Assess oxygen saturation, body weight, and rhythm of breathing pattern. Assess for presence of retraction. Count how many words she can say without taking a breath to assess dyspnea.
3. Risk factor for lung cancer: Her smoking.
4. Collaborate with a physician, a respiratory therapist, and a dietitian.

Review Questions

1. 2
2. 4
3. 3
4. 1
5. 3
6. 4
7. 1
8. 1
9. 2
10. 4

CHAPTER 12: HEART AND PERIPHERAL VASCULAR SYSTEM

Case Study

1. Complaint of shortness of breath, fatigue that interferes with routine activities, and sleeping difficulty; labored breathing with elevated respiratory rate, pulse rate, and blood pressure; pitting edema in lower extremities; frothy-looking phlegm.
2. Complete a symptom analysis on the shortness of breath and fatigue. Ask the patient if he has symptoms associated with chest pain, cough, or nocturia. Perform an assessment, including inspection, palpation, and auscultation.
3. Risk factors for coronary artery disease: Age, gender, and family history.
4. Collaborate with physician, dietitian, and cardiac rehabilitation personnel.

Review Questions

1. 4
2. 2
3. 3
4. 2
5. 3
6. 2
7. 3
8. 1
9. 4
10. 3

CHAPTER 13: ABDOMEN AND GASTROINTESTINAL SYSTEM

Case Study

1. Abdominal pain (progressively worse); loss of appetite and nausea; guarded position; hot skin, possibly indicating fever; absence of bowel sounds; pain on palpation and guarding of RLQ.
2. Ask if vomiting accompanies her nausea. Ask about her last menstrual period (LMP) and about the possibility of pregnancy. Ask her about bowel elimination (last bowel movement) and appearance of stool. Check vital signs (of particular interest is temperature). Auscultate for arterial bruits and venous hums. Percuss kidney for costovertebral angle (CVA) tenderness.
3. Risk factors (for most cancers of the gastrointestinal system): Smoking.
4. Collaborate with the physician and dietitian.

Review Questions

1. 4
2. 1
3. 3
4. 1
5. 3
6. 2
7. 4
8. 4
9. 2
10. 3

CHAPTER 14: MUSCULOSKELETAL SYSTEM

Case Study

1. Significant joint pain; limitations in self-care activities; limitations in socialization; difficulty with posture and gait; deformities to joints; tender, inflamed joints with palpation; subcutaneous nodules at the ulnar surface of the elbows.
2. Ask the patient if she is using any nonpharmaceutical therapies. Ask if she uses any assistive devices and if she receives any assistance with self-care activities. Document range of motion (ROM) in various joints. Use of a goniometer would be particularly helpful.
3. Risk factors for osteoporosis: Age, gender, race (Asian), family history, medication to treat her rheumatoid arthritis.
4. Collaborate with physician, physical therapist, and occupational therapist.

Review Questions

1. 1
2. 4
3. 2
4. 4
5. 1

6. 1
7. 3
8. 2
9. 4
10. 3

CHAPTER 15: NEUROLOGIC SYSTEM

Case Study

1. The patient was diagnosed with right cerebrovascular accident (CVA); he had a headache preceding incident. He is unable to talk, has absence of sensation and trace-to-no muscle strength on the left arm and leg, requires assistance for mobility, and avoids eye contact and cries.
2. Ask the patient if he feels he can swallow normally and whether he has any pain or discomfort. Ask the patient's wife about medical and family history and medications he may be taking currently. Ask her if her husband lost consciousness or had a seizure with this incident. Assess gag reflex. Test deep tendon reflexes. Assess for drooling.
3. Risk factors for CVA: Age, gender, race, and history of diabetes mellitus, hypertension, and smoking.
4. Collaborate with a physician, physical therapist, occupational therapist, speech therapist, and discharge planner.

Review Questions

1. 2
2. 4
3. 3
4. 1
5. 4
6. 3
7. 1
8. 4
9. 2
10. 2

CHAPTER 16: BREAST AND AXILLA

Case Study

1. Patient has a history of nontender breast lump, noticeable for approximately 9 months; mass has increased in size over 9 months; palpable lump is present in left upper outer quadrant; dimpling is noted on left breast; left nipple is slightly retracted; bloody discharge is noted from nipple when squeezed.
2. Ask about personal or family history of breast disease. Ask patient if she has ever had a mammogram. Ask about the location of the lump, whether it is tender now, and whether she has noticed nipple discharge. Ask about changes in the lump size in relation to menstrual cycle. Inspect the areolae. Besides location, the following characteristics must be assessed with a breast mass: size, shape, consistency, tenderness, mobility, and borders. Palpate the axilla for evidence of enlarged lymph nodes. Noting any lumps or masses in the left axilla is especially important.

3. Risk factors for breast cancer: Age, early onset of menarche, and no children.
4. Collaborate with a physician or advanced practice registered nurse.

Review Questions

1. 3
2. 4
3. 3
4. 2
5. 1

CHAPTER 17: REPRODUCTIVE SYSTEM AND THE PERINEUM

Case Study

1. The history suggests some type of acute inflammation. It also suggests multiple sex contacts, and the primary partner has multiple sex contacts. Vaginal mass with inflammation, discharge, and extreme pain on palpation need further evaluation.
2. Discussion is needed regarding past sexual history and associated medical problems, if any. Identification of protection (or lack of it) is also important to discuss. Obtain a culture of the discharge for evaluation. If patient is too uncomfortable for internal examination, it may need to be delayed until the inflammation has resolved. Use of protection from STDs is unknown. Data are unclear about how many sex partners the patient has.
3. The risk factors for sexually transmitted diseases (STDs): sexual activity and being in a nonmonogamous sexual relationship.
4. Collaborate with a physician or advanced practice registered nurse.

Review Questions

1. 2
2. 1
3. 4
4. 2
5. 1
6. 3
7. 1
8. 3
9. 3
10. 2

CHAPTER 18: DEVELOPMENTAL ASSESSMENT THROUGHOUT THE LIFE SPAN

Case Study

1. *Subjective data:* Patient recently lost spouse (5 months ago). Son says that his mother has "gone downhill." He indicates that patient is no longer keeping her house clean and is not cooking appropriate meals. He reports significant change in patient's personal hygiene habits (loss of interest in getting hair done or getting dressed for the day). He reports that patient becomes angry when he talks about other living options; patient states, "You think I'm helpless and want to lock me away."
2. *Objective data:* 78-year-old woman; sits quietly during conversation. Overall hygiene—patient appears clean; hair matted; clothes do not match and are badly wrinkled. Speech clear. Overall affect dull; makes no eye contact with her son or nurse. Age-consistent findings with physical examination; no overt physical problems identified.
3. This patient is in Erikson stage of ego integrity versus despair.
4. She may be struggling with the following developmental tasks: dealing with the death of her spouse; adapting to living arrangements; adjusting to relationships with adult children and grandchildren; adjusting to slower physical and intellectual responses; managing leisure time and remaining active; maintaining physical and mental health; finding the meaning of life.
5. Additional assessment data needed include her ability to perform activities of daily living and assessment for depression since the death of her husband.

Review Questions

1. 2
2. 3
3. 1
4. 3
5. 4

CHAPTER 19: ASSESSMENT OF THE INFANT, CHILD, AND ADOLESCENT

Case Study

1. Reported seizure, "shaking all over" lasted 20 minutes. History of seizures, but length of seizure atypical (according to mother).
2. Ask if there was a loss of consciousness; how long ago since the last seizure. Ask if there were any warning signs before the seizure. Ask about change in medication, dose, or adherence. Ask about recent changes (e.g., in health status or appetite, excessive fatigue).
3. Risk for falls, musculoskeletal injury, or head injury.
4. Collaborate with a physician or advanced practice registered nurse.

Review Questions

1. 1
2. 1
3. 3
4. 4
5. 3
6. 4
7. 2
8. 1
9. 4
10. 4

CHAPTER 20: ASSESSMENT OF THE PREGNANT PATIENT

Case Study

1. *Subjective data:* Symptoms of puffiness to hands and feet. Backache. Fear of excessive labor pain. *Objective data:* Increase in blood pressure. Sudden, excessive increase in weight. 3+ protein in urine.
2. Assess fetal heart tones; palpate fetal movement. Assess the extent of the edema, including how far up on the legs and the degree of edema, if pitting. Check her visual acuity. Conduct a neurologic assessment, particularly to check deep tendon reflexes. Ask her about her diet, specifically sodium intake, because this may be contributing to the edema. Get more information about the back discomfort; do a symptom analysis. Determine her knowledge level of the labor and delivery process; assess pain experiences.
3. Risk factors for high-risk pregnancy: pregnancy-induced hypertension (PIH), excessive weight gain, and evidence of preeclampsia (proteinuria and edema).
4. Collaborate with a physician or advanced practice registered nurse and dietitian.

Review Questions

1. 1
2. 4
3. 2
4. 4
5. 1

CHAPTER 21: ASSESSMENT OF THE OLDER ADULT

Case Study

1. The patient is confused, disoriented, and incontinent. She has a history of urinary tract infection (UTI) that has contributed to her confusion. Moving her right hip is painful because of the fall and bruise on right hip and thigh.
2. Assess adequacy of her diet. Assess her vision. Assess neurologic status. Assess for depression.
3. Risk factors for falls: confusion, but a complete fall risk assessment needs to be completed.
4. Collaboration with a physician or advanced practice registered nurse and perhaps a physical therapist.

Review Questions

1. 1
2. 2
3. 4
4. 2
5. 1
6. 3

A

abduction: Movement of a limb away from the body.

accommodation: The adjustment of the eye to variations in distance.

adduction: Movement of a limb toward the body.

adnexa: General term meaning adjacent or related structures. *Example:* The ovaries and fallopian tubes are adnexa of the uterus.

adventitious sounds: Breath sounds that are not normal.

affect: Observable behaviors that indicate an individual's feelings or emotions.

air trapping: An abnormal respiratory pattern seen in patients with chronic obstructive pulmonary disease; characterized by rapid inspirations with prolonged forced expirations.

alopecia: Absence or loss of hair.

alveolar ridge: Bony prominences of the maxilla and mandible that support the teeth; in edentulous patient, these structures support dentures.

amenorrhea: Absence of menstruation.

anesthesia: Partial or complete loss of sensation.

angina pectoris: Paroxysmal chest pain often associated with myocardial ischemia; pain patterns and severity vary among individuals.

angle of Louis: Visible and palpable angulation between the sternum and manubrium; also referred to as the *manubriosternal junction.*

ankylosis: Fixation of a joint, often in an abnormal position.

annular: Type of lesion that forms a ring around a center of normal skin.

annulus: Dense fibrous ring surrounding the tympanic membrane.

anosmia: Absence or impairment of the sense of smell.

anterior: Referring to the front.

anterior triangle (of the neck): Landmark area for palpating chains of lymph nodes; sectioned by the anterior surface of the sternocleidomastoid muscle, the mandible, and an imaginary line running from the chin to the sternal notch.

anuria: Complete absence of urine production.

anxiety: A feeling of uneasiness or discomfort experienced in varying degrees, from mild anxiety to panic; anxiety is a response to no specific source or actual object.

apathy: Lack of emotional expression; indifference to stimuli or surroundings.

aphakia: Absence of the crystalline lens of the eye.

aphasia: A neurologic condition in which language function is absent or severely impaired.

aphthous ulcer (canker sore): Painful ulcer on the mucous membrane of the mouth.

apical: Refers to the top portion (apex) of an organ or part.

apnea: Absence of breathing.

apocrine sweat glands: Secretory dermal structures located in the axillae, nipples, areolae, scalp, face, and genital area.

arcus senilis: Gray ring composed of lipids deposited in the peripheral cornea; commonly seen in older adults. Also called *arcus cornealis.*

areola: Circular, darkly pigmented area around the nipple of the breast.

arteriosclerosis: General term denoting hardening and thickening of the arterial walls.

ascites: Accumulation of serous fluid in the peritoneal cavity.

assessment: First step in the nursing process involving collection of data pertinent to the patient's health or situation.

astigmatism: Visual distortion resulting from an irregular corneal curvature that prevents light rays from being focused clearly on the retina.

ataxia: Inability to coordinate muscular movement.

atelectasis: Shrunken, airless alveoli or collapse of lung tissue.

atherosclerosis: Formation of plaques within arterial walls that results in thickening of the walls and narrowing of the lumen.

atrophy: Wasting or decrease in size or physiologic activity of a part of the body because of disease or other influences.

auricle: The external ear; also called the *pinna.*

auscultatory gap: Temporary silent interval between systolic and diastolic sounds that may cover a range of 40 mm Hg.

B

balano: Prefix that denotes the glans penis. *Example: Balanitis* means inflammation of the glans penis.

ballottement: Technique of palpating a floating structure in the abdomen by bouncing it gently and feeling it rebound.

Bartholin glands: Two mucus-secreting glands located within the posterolateral vaginal vestibule.

bilateral: Relating to or referring to two sides.

blepharitis: Inflammation of the eyelid.

body mass index (BMI): Method to evaluate height-weight ratio.

borborygmi: Abdominal sounds produced by hyperactive intestinal peristalsis that is audible at a distance.

boutonniere deformity: Common deformity of the hands seen in patients with rheumatoid arthritis; involves flexion of the proximal interphalangeal joint and hyperextension of the distal interphalangeal joint.

bradycardia: Abnormally slowed heart rate, usually under 60 beats/min.

bradykinesia: Abnormal slowness of movement.

bradypnea: Breathing that is abnormally slow.

bronchial breath sounds: High-pitched breath sounds normally heard over the trachea and the area around the manubrium.

bronchitis: Inflammation of the bronchi.

bronchophony: An abnormality in vocal resonance. When lungs are auscultated, the patient says "ninety-nine" or "one, two, three" indicating lung consolidation.

bronchovesicular breath sounds: Refers to breath sounds at a moderate pitch heard in the posterior chest over the outer center of the back on either side of the spine between the scapulae and in the anterior chest around the sternal border.

bruise: Swelling, discoloration, and pain without a break in the skin.

bruit: Audible murmur (a blowing sound) heard when auscultating over a peripheral vessel or an organ.

buccal: Pertaining to the inside of the cheek, the surface of a tooth, or the gum beside the cheek.

bulbar conjunctiva: Thin, transparent mucous membrane that covers the sclera and adjoins the palpebral conjunctiva, which lines the inner eyelid.

bulla: Elevated, circumscribed, fluid-filled lesion greater than 1 cm in diameter.

bursa: Fibrous, fluid-filled sac found between certain tendons and the bones beneath them.

bursitis: Inflammation of a bursa.

C

cachexia: Severe malnutrition and wasting of muscles associated with a chronic illness such as cancer.

callus: Hyperkeratotic area caused by pressure or friction; usually not painful.

canthus: Outer or inner angle between the upper and lower eyelids.

carpal tunnel syndrome: Painful disorder of the wrist and hand induced by compression of the median nerve between the inelastic carpal ligament and other structures within the carpal tunnel.

cataract: Opacity of the crystalline lens of the eyes.

cauliflower ear: Thickened, disfigured ear caused by repeated trauma such as blows to the ear.

cellulitis: Diffuse spreading infection of the skin or of subcutaneous or connective tissue.

cerumen: Waxy secretion of the glands of the external acoustic meatus; earwax.

chalazion: Small, localized swelling of the eyelid caused by obstruction and dilation of the meibomian gland.

Cheynes-Stokes: An abnormal breathing pattern characterized by intervals of apnea interspersed with a deep and rapid breathing pattern.

chromatopsia: Unusual color perception, seeing spots, or blindness in the lateral visual field.

circumduction: Circular movement of a limb.

circumoral: Pertaining to the area around the mouth.

circumscribed: Well-defined, limited, and encircled.

clonus: Abnormal pattern of neuromuscular functioning characterized by rapidly alternating involuntary contraction and relaxation of skeletal muscles.

clubbing: Broadening and thickening of the fingernails or toenails associated with an increased angle of the nail greater than 180 degrees; associated with chronic hypoxia.

coarctation: Stricture or narrowing of the wall of a vessel as the aorta.

cochlea: Conical bony structure of the inner ear; perforated by numerous apertures for passage of the cochlear division of the acoustic nerve.

cognitive function: An individual's perception of his or her intellectual awareness, potential for growth, and recognition by others for his or her mental skills and contributions.

compulsive behavior: Repetitive act that usually originates from an obsession.

condyloma acuminatum (wart): Soft, warty, papillomatous projection that appears on the labia and within the vaginal vestibule.

condyloma latum: Slightly raised, moist, flattened papules that appear on the labia or within the vaginal vestibule.

confluent: Describes lesions that run together.

consensual reaction: The constriction of the iris and pupil of one eye when a light is shone in the opposite eye.

consolidation: Increasing density of lung tissue caused by pathologic engorgement.

Cooper ligaments: Suspensory ligaments of the breast.

corn: Hyperkeratotic, slightly raised, circumscribed lesion caused by pressure over a bony prominence.

costal angle: Costal margin angle formed on the anterior chest wall at the base of the xiphoid process where the ribs separate.

crackles: Abnormal respiratory sound heard during auscultation, characterized by discontinuous bubbling sounds; heard over distal bronchioles and alveoli that contain serous secretions; formerly called *rales.*

crepitus: Dry, crackling sound or sensation heard or felt as a joint is moved through its range of motion.

cricoid cartilage: Lowermost cartilage of the larynx.

crust: Dried serum, blood, or purulent exudate on the skin surface.

cryptorchism: Failure of one or both of the testicles to descend into the scrotum.

cyanosis: Bluish-gray discoloration of skin and mucous membranes caused by an excess of deoxygenated hemoglobin in the blood.

cycloplegia: Paralysis of the ciliary muscle resulting in a loss of accommodation and a dilated pupil.

cystocele: Bulging of the anterior vaginal wall caused by protrusion of the urinary bladder through relaxed or weakened musculature.

D

darwinian tubercle: Blunt point projecting up from the upper part of the helix of the ear.

database: Collection or store of information.

deciduous teeth: Twenty teeth that appear normally during infancy: four incisors, two canines, and four molars in the upper and lower jaw.

delirium: An acute, reversible organic mental disorder characterized by confusion, disorientation, restlessness, anxiety, and excitement.

delusion: Persistent belief or perception that is illogical or improbable.

dementia: Broad term that indicates impairment of intellectual functioning, memory, and judgment.

depression: An abnormal mood state in which a person characteristically has a sense of sadness, hopelessness, helplessness, worthlessness, and despair resulting from some personal loss or tragedy.

desquamation: Sloughing process of the cornified layer of the epidermis.

diaphoresis: Sweating.

diaphragmatic excursion: Extent of movement of the diaphragm with maximum inspiration and expiration.

diarthrotic joint: Joint that permits relatively free movement; types of diarthrotic joints include hinge joints, pivot joints, condyloid joints, ball-and-socket joints, and gliding joints.

diastole: Period of time within the cardiac cycle in which ventricles are relaxed and filling with blood.

diffuse: Spread out, widely dispersed, copious.

diplopia: Double vision.

distal: Refers to the area farthest away from a point of reference.

dizziness: Sensation of faintness.

dorsal: Refers to the back or posterior part of an anatomic structure. *Example:* Dorsal aspect of the hand.

dorsiflexion: Upward or backward bending or flexion of a joint.

dyskinesia: Refers to a reduced ability to perform voluntary movements.

dysmenorrhea: Abnormal pain associated with the menstrual cycle.

dyspareunia: Pain associated with sexual intercourse.

dysphagia: Difficulty swallowing.

dysphasia: A neurologic condition in which language function is absent or severely impaired.

dysphonia: Difficulty in controlling laryngeal speech sounds; can be a normal event such as male vocal changes occurring at puberty.

dyspnea: Breathing that is labored or difficult.

dysuria: Difficulty, pain, or burning sensation associated with urination.

E

ecchymosis: Discoloration of skin or a mucous membrane caused by leakage of blood into the subcutaneous tissue; can also be a bruise.

eccrine sweat glands: Secretory dermal structures distributed over the body that secrete water and electrolytes and regulate body temperature.

ectopic: An event that occurs away from its usual location such as a premature ventricular contraction.

ectropion: Abnormal outward turning of the margin of the eyelid.

eczematous: Superficial inflammation characterized by scaling, thickening, crusting, weeping, and redness.

edema: Excessive accumulation of fluid within the interstitial space.

effacement: The shortening of the vaginal portion of the cervix and the thinning of its walls as it is stretched and dilated by the fetus during labor.

egophony: Abnormality in vocal resonance; when lungs are auscultated, the patient says "e-e-e," but the nurse hears "a-a-a"; suggests pleural effusion.

embolus: Foreign object (composed of air, fat, or clustered cellular elements) that circulates through the blood and usually lodges in a vessel, causing some degree of occlusion.

emesis: Vomit.

emphysema: Chronic pulmonary disease characterized by permanent enlargement of air spaces caused by destruction of alveolar walls.

enophthalmos: Abnormal backward placement of the eyeball.

entropion: Abnormal inward turning of the margin of the eyelid.

enuresis: Any involuntary urination, especially during sleep.

epicondyle: Round protuberance above the condyle (at the end of a bone).

epididymitis: Inflammation of the epididymis.

epiphysis: End of a long bone that is cartilaginous during early childhood and becomes ossified during late childhood.

epispadias: Congenital defect in which the urinary meatus opens on the dorsum of the penis.

epistaxis: Bleeding from the nose.

epulis: Hypertrophied gum tissue that appears as a small, painless raised nodule and is a normal variation at the end of the third trimester of pregnancy.

erosion: Wearing away or destruction of the mucosal or epidermal surface; often develops into an ulcer.

erythematous: Redness (of the skin).

erythroplakia: Red lesion of the oral mucous membrane that may be precancerous.

eschar: Scab or dried crust that results from trauma, such as a thermal or chemical burn, infection, or excoriating skin disease.

euphoria: Sense of elation or well-being; can be a normal feeling or exaggerated to the extent of distorting reality.

eustachian tube: Tube lined with mucous membrane that joins the nasopharynx and the tympanic cavity.

eversion: Outward turning as with a foot, or an inside-out position as with an eyelid.

exacerbation: Increase in intensity of signs or symptoms.

excoriation: Scratch or abrasion on the skin surface.

exophthalmos: Abnormal forward placement of the eyeball.

extension: Movement that brings a joint into a straight position.

external rotation: Turning a limb outward or away from the midline of the body.

F

fasciculation: Localized, uncoordinated, uncontrollable twitching of a single muscle group innervated by a single motor nerve fiber.

fissure: Linear crack in the skin.

flaccid: Referring to muscles that lack tone.

flail chest: Unstable, flapping chest wall caused by fractures of the sternum and ribs.

flank: Part of the body between the bottom of the ribs and the upper border of the ilium; it overlies the kidneys.

flatulence: Presence of excessive amounts of gas in the stomach or intestines.

flexion: Movement that brings a joint into a bent position.

fontanel: Unossified space or soft spot lying between the cranial bones of an infant.

fornix (plural: fornices): General term designating a fold or an archlike structure.

fourchette: Small fold of membrane connecting the labia minora in the posterior part of the vulva.

frenulum (lingual): Band of tissue that attaches the ventral surface of the tongue to the floor of the mouth.

friction rub: Sound produced by the rubbing of the pleura around the lung or the pericardium around the heart.

G

gingiva: Pertaining to the gum.

glaucoma: Eye disease characterized by abnormally increased intraocular pressure.

glossitis: Inflammation of the tongue.

goiter: Hypertrophy of the thyroid gland, usually evident as a pronounced increase in its size.

gout: Metabolic disease associated with abnormal uric acid metabolism that is a form of acute arthritis; marked by inflammation of the joints.

graphesthesia: Ability to recognize symbols, numbers, or letters traced on the skin.

gravida: Denotes number of pregnancies.

guarding: Protective withdrawal or positioning of a body part during an injury.

gynecomastia: Abnormally large mammary glands in the male.

H

hallucination: Sensory perception that does not arise from an external stimulus; can be auditory, visual, tactile, gustatory, or olfactory.

heave: Palpable, diffuse, sustained lift of the chest wall or a portion of the wall.

helix: Margin of the external ear.

hemangioma: Benign tumor consisting of a mass of blood vessels.

hematuria: Presence of blood in the urine.

hemoptysis: Coughing up blood or referring to bloody sputum.

hernia: Abnormal opening in a muscle wall or cavity that permits protrusion of its contents.

herpetiform: Describes a cluster of vesicles resembling herpes lesions.

hirsutism: Excessive body hair, usually in a masculine distribution.

hordeolum (stye): Infection of a sebaceous gland at the margin of the eyelid.

hydramnios: Excess formation of amniotic fluid during pregnancy.

hydrocele: Nontender, serous fluid mass located within the tunica vaginalis (layered, hollow membrane adjacent to the testis).

hymenal remnants: Small, irregular, fleshy projections that are remnants of a ruptured hymen.

hyoid: U-shaped bone suspended from the styloid process of the temporal bone.

hyperesthesia: Abnormally increased sensitivity to sensory stimuli such as touch or pain.

hyperextension: Refers to the extension of a body part beyond normal limits of extension.

hyperkinesis: Hyperactivity or excessive muscular activity.

hyperopia (farsightedness): Refractive error in which light rays focus behind the retina.

hyperplasia: Increase in the number of cells of a body part that results from an increased rate of cellular metabolism.

hyperresonance: Sound elicited by percussion; very loud intensity and very low pitch with a booming quality; heard over lungs when air is trapped in emphysema.

hypertension: Refers to abnormally high blood pressure.

hyperventilation: An abnormal respiratory pattern characterized by increased rate and depth of breathing.

hypoesthesia: Decreased or dulled sensitivity to stimulation.

hyposmia: Decreased sense of smell.

hypospadias: Congenital defect in which the urinary meatus opens on the ventral aspect of the penis.

hypotension: Refers to abnormally low blood pressure.

hypovolemic: Pertaining to decreased blood volume; usually refers to a state of shock resulting from massive blood loss and inadequate tissue perfusion.

hypoxemia: Abnormal reduction of oxygen content in the arterial blood.

hypoxia: Abnormal reduction of oxygen delivery to body tissue.

I

illusion: Perceptual distortion of an external stimulus. *Example:* A mirage in a desert.

incus: One of three ossicles in the middle ear; resembling an anvil.

induration: Hardening of the skin, usually caused by edema or infiltration by a neoplasm.

infarct: Localized area of tissue necrosis caused by prolonged anoxia.

infection: Redness, heat, edema, and fever secondary to pathogenic microorganisms.

inferior: Lower surface of an organ; refers to a position that is lower in relation to another.

intermittent claudication: Pain in the legs that occurs while walking but that can be relieved by rest.

internal rotation: Inward turning of a limb.

introitus: General term denoting an opening or the orifice of a cavity or hollow structure.

inversion: Turning inside out or upside down.

ischemia: Diminished supply of blood to a body organ or surface; characterized by pallor, coolness, and pain.

J

jaundice: A yellow discoloration of the skin, mucous membrane, and sclera.

K

keloid: Hypertrophic scar tissue; prevalent in nonwhite races.

keratosis: Overgrowth and thickening of the cornified epithelium.

kinesthetic sensation: Ability to detect muscle movement and position.

Koplik spots: Lesions that appear in the prodromal stage of measles; they appear as small bluish-white lesions with irregular borders on the buccal mucosa opposite the molar teeth.

Korotkoff sounds: Sounds heard during the taking of blood pressure.

Kussmaul respiration: Rapid deep respiration often associated with ketoacidosis.

kyphosis: Abnormal convexity of the posterior curve of the spine.

L

labile emotions: Unpredictable, rapid shifting of expression of feelings.

labyrinth: Complex structure of the inner ear, containing receptors for hearing and balance.

lateral: Referring to the side; position away from the middle.

Leopold's maneuvers: Series of palpation techniques used to determine fetal presentation, position, and lie.

lesion: A pathologically or traumatically altered area of tissue.

leukoplakia: Thickened, white, well-circumscribed patch that can appear on any mucous membrane; sometimes precancerous.

leukorrhea: White vaginal discharge.

lichenification: Thickening of the skin characterized by accentuated skin markings; often the result of chronic scratching.

light reflex: Triangular landmark area on the tympanic membrane that most brightly reflects the nurse's light source.

lordosis: Abnormal anterior concavity of the spine.

lower motor neurons: Nerve cells that originate in the anterior horn cells of the spinal column and travel to innervate the skeletal muscle fibers.

lymphadenopathy: Enlargement of lymph nodes greater than 1.5 cm.

lymphedema: Swelling caused by obstruction of the lymphatic system and accumulation of interstitial fluid.

lymphoma: General term for the growth of new tissue in the lymphatic area; generally refers to malignant growth.

M

macule: Flat, circumscribed lesion of the skin or mucous membrane that is 1 cm or less in diameter.

malleus: Innermost ossicle of the middle ear; resembling a hammer.

mastitis: Inflammation of the breast.

mastoid process: Conical projection of the temporal bone extending downward and forward behind the external auditory meatus.

medial: Referring to the middle; the median plane of the body.

mediastinum: Space within the thoracic cavity positioned behind the sternum, in front of the vertebral column, and between the lungs.

menarche: Onset of menstruation.

menopause: The period that marks the cessation of menstrual cycles.

menorrhagia: Abnormally heavy or extended menstrual periods.

metrorrhagia: Menstrual bleeding at irregular intervals, sometimes prolonged, but of expected amount.

midaxillary line: Vertical line extending downward from the midaxillary fold; used in assessment as an anatomic reference point.

midclavicular line: Vertical line extending downward from the middle of the clavicle.

miosis: Condition in which the pupil is constricted.

Montgomery tubercles: Small sebaceous glands located on the areola of the breast.

Murphy's sign: Pain elicited during abdominal palpation indicating gallbladder disease.

myalgia: Tenderness or pain in the muscle.

mydriasis: Condition in which the pupil is dilated.

myoclonus: Twitching or clonic spasm of a muscle group.

myopia (nearsightedness): Refractive error in which light rays focus in front of the retina.

N

nabothian cyst (retention cyst): Small white or purple firm nodule that commonly appears on the cervix.

nares (singular: naris): Nostrils; anterior openings of the nose.

necrosis: Localized death of tissue.

neonate: Newborn infant during the first 28 days of life.

neurosis: Ineffective or troubled coping mechanism stemming from anxiety or emotional conflict.

nevus: Congenital pigmented area on the skin. *Example:* Mole, birthmark.

nicking: Abnormal condition showing compression of a vein at an arteriovenous crossing; visible through an ophthalmoscope during a retinal examination.

nociceptor: Free nerve endings that are located at the ends of nerve fibers and initiate an action potential.

nocturia: Excessive urination during the night.

nodule: Solid skin elevation that extends into the dermal layer and that is 1 to 2 cm in diameter.

nystagmus: Involuntary rhythmical movement of the eyes; oscillations may be horizontal, vertical, rotary, or mixed.

O

objective data: Data obtained from examination, measurements, or diagnostic tests; observable by the nurse.

obsession: Persistent thought or idea that preoccupies the mind; not always realistic and may result in compulsive behavior.

obsessive-compulsive disorder: An anxiety disorder that develops when the patient tries to resist an obsession or compulsion.

odynophagia: A severe sensation of burning, squeezing pain while swallowing.

oligomenorrhea: Abnormally light or infrequent menstruation.

oliguria: Inadequate production or secretion of urine (usually less than 400 mL in a 24-hour period).

orchi: Combining form that denotes the testes. *Example: Orchitis* means inflammation of one or both of the testes.

orthopnea: Difficulty breathing in any position other than an upright one.

osteoarthritis: Form of arthritis in which one or many of the joints undergo destruction of cartilage.

otalgia: Pain in the ear.

P

palmar: Relating to the palm of the hand.

palpebral conjunctiva: Thin, transparent mucous membrane that lines the inner eyelid and adjoins the bulbar conjunctiva, which covers the sclera.

palpebral fissure: Opening between the upper and lower eyelids.

palpitation: Sensation of pounding, fluttering, or racing of the heart; can be a normal phenomenon or caused by a disorder of the heart.

papilla: General term for a small projection; dorsal surface of the tongue is composed of a variety of forms of papillae that contain openings to the taste buds.

papule: Solid, elevated, circumscribed, superficial lesion 1 cm or less in diameter.

paradoxical pulse: Diminished pulse amplitude on inspiration with increased amplitude on expiration.

paralysis: Loss of muscle function, loss of sensation, or both.

paranoia: Sense of being persecuted or victimized; suspicion of others.

paraphimosis: Condition characterized by the inability to pull the foreskin forward from a retracted position.

paresis: Motor weakness.

paresthesia: Abnormal sensation such as numbness or tingling.

parity: Denotes the number of viable births.

paronychia: Inflammation of the skinfold that adjoins the nail bed.

paroxysmal nocturnal dyspnea (PND): Periodic acute attacks of shortness of breath that awaken a person, usually after several hours of sleep in a recumbent position.

pars flaccida: Small portion of the tympanic membrane between the mallear folds.

pars tensa: Larger portion of the tympanic membrane.

patch: Flat, circumscribed lesion of the skin or mucous membrane that is more than 1 cm in diameter.

peau d'orange: Dimpling of the skin that resembles the skin of an orange.

pectoralis major muscle: One of the four muscles of the anterior upper portion of the chest.

pectus carinatum: Abnormal prominence of the sternum.

pectus excavatum: Abnormal depression of the sternum.

perception of pain: The third phase in the pain process that occurs when the parietal lobe is stimulated, causing a conscious experience of pain.

periodontitis (pyorrhea): Inflammation and deterioration of the gums and supporting alveolar bone.

peristalsis: Alternating contraction and relaxation of the smooth muscles of the intestinal tract to propel contents forward.

perlèche (cheilosis, cheilitis): Fissures at the corners of the mouth that become inflamed.

petechiae: Tiny, flat purple or red spots on the surface of the skin resulting from minute hemorrhages within the dermal or submucosal layers.

phimosis: Tightness of the foreskin that results in an inability to retract it.

phobia: Uncontrollable and often unreasonable intense fear of a specific object or event.

photophobia: Ocular discomfort caused by exposure of the eyes to bright light.

pinna: Auricle or projected part of the external ear.

pitch: The quality of a tone or sound dependent on the perception of the rapidity of the vibrations by which it is produced. Pitch may be used to describe heart sounds as producing a low-pitch or high-pitch.

plantar: Referring to the bottom surface of the foot.

plantar flexion: A toe-down motion of the foot at the ankle.

plaque: Solid, elevated, circumscribed, superficial lesion more than 1 cm in diameter.

plaque (dental): Film that accumulates on the surface of the teeth.

pleximeter: Finger placed on the skin surface to receive the taps from the percussion hammer or plexor; used in percussion.

point of maximum impulse (PMI): Specific area of the chest where the heartbeat is palpated strongest; usually the apical impulse, located in the fourth or fifth intercostal space along the midclavicular line.

polyuria: Excessive urine excretion.

posterior: Referring to the back.

posterior triangle (of neck): Landmark area for palpating chains of lymph nodes located along the anterior border by the sternocleido-mastoid muscle, the posterior border by the trapezius muscle, and the bottom by the clavicle.

precipitating factor: Event or entity that hastens the onset of another event.

precordium: Area of the chest that overlies the heart and adjacent great vessels.

predisposing factor (risk factor): Event or entity that contributes to the cause of another event. *Example:* A family history of obesity increases a patient's risk for obesity.

presbycusis: Impairment of hearing in older adults that involves loss of hearing sensitivity and reduction of the clarity of speech.

presbyopia: Loss of accommodation (ability to focus on near objects) associated with older adults.

problem list: Compilation of findings that appear at the end of a database; may be diagnoses (medical or nursing), clusters of interrelated findings, or isolated findings.

pronate: To turn the forearm so the palm faces downward or to rotate the leg or foot inward.

proprioception: Awareness of body posture, movement, and changes in equilibrium.

pruritus: Itching.

psychosis: Any major mental disorder char-acterized by greatly distorted perceptions and severe disorganization of the personality.

ptosis: Drooping of the upper eyelid.

ptyalism: Excessive salivation.

pudendum: Collective term denoting the external genitalia.

pulse deficit: Discrepancy between the ventricular rate auscultated over the heart and the arterial rate palpated over the radial artery.

pulse pressure: Difference between systolic and diastolic pressures.

pulsus alternans: Alternating pulse; abnor-mal pulse characterized by a regular rhythm in which a strong beat alternates with a weaker one.

purpura: Hemorrhage into the tissue, usually circumscribed; lesions may be described as petechiae, ecchymoses, or hematomas, ac-cording to size.

pustule: Vesicle or bulla that contains pus.

pyramidal tract: Bundle of upper motor neurons that coordinate voluntary move-ments originating in the motor cortex of the brain; nerve fibers travel from the frontal lobe through the brainstem and the spinal cord, where they synapse with anterior horn cells.

pyrosis: Burning sensation in the epigastric and sternal region; also called *heartburn*.

pyuria: Presence of white cells (pus) in the urine.

R

rebound tenderness: Sign of inflammation in the peritoneum in which pain is elicited by a sudden withdrawal of a hand pressing on the abdomen.

rectocele: Bulging of the rectum and posterior vaginal wall through relaxed or weakened musculature of the vagina.

red reflex: Red glow over the pupil created by light illuminating the retina.

refraction: Deviation of light rays as they pass from one transparent medium into another of different density.

remission: Disappearance or diminishment of signs or symptoms.

respiratory stridor: A harsh, high-pitched sound associated with breathing.

reticular: Describes a netlike pattern or structure of veins on a tissue surface.

retraction: Shortening or drawing the skin backward.

rhino: Combining form that denotes the nose.

rhonchus: Loud, low-pitched, coarse sound similar to a snore heard on auscultation of an obstructed airway.

rigidity: An increase in muscle tone that may result from neuromuscular disorders.

Romberg test: Test of cerebellar function that evaluates an individual's ability to maintain a given position when standing erect with feet together and eyes closed.

S

scale: Small, thin flake of epithelial cells.

scoliosis: Lateral curvature of the spine.

scotoma: Defined area of blindness within the visual field; can involve one or both eyes.

sebaceous glands: Secretory dermal struc-tures that produce sebum, an oily substance.

seborrhea: Group of skin conditions charac-terized by noninflammatory, excessively dry scales or excessive oiliness.

shifting dullness: Change in the dull sounds heard with percussion; at first the dull sound is heard in one location and then in a differ-ent location.

shotty node: Small lymph node that feels hard and nodular; generally movable and nontender.

sign: Objective finding perceived by the nurse.

Skene glands: Mucus-secreting glands that lie just inside the urethral orifice of women; not visible during examination.

slough: Tissue that has been shed.

smegma: Secretion of sebaceous glands, especially the cheesy, foul-smelling secretion sometimes found under the foreskin of the penis and at the base of the labia minora near the glans clitoris.

spasticity: Increased tone or contractions of muscles causing stiff and awkward movements.

spermatocele (epididymal cyst): Painless, fluid-filled epididymal mass that contains spermatozoa.

spinothalamic tract: Sensory nerve tract that carries impulses of pain, pressure, and tem-perature from the spinal cord to the thalamus.

spondylitis: Inflammation of one or more of the spinal vertebrae; usually characterized by stiffness and pain.

sprain: Traumatic injury to the tendon.

stapes: One of the ossicles in the middle ear.

stereognosis: Ability to recognize objects by the sense of touch.

sternocleidomastoid muscle: Major muscle that rotates and flexes the head.

stoma: General term that means opening or mouth.

strabismus: Condition in which the eyes are not directed at the same object or point.

strain: Temporary damage to the muscles usually caused by excessive physical effort.

striae: Streaks of linear scars that often result from rapidly developing tension in the skin; also called *stretch marks*.

stridor: Shrill, harsh sound heard during inspiration.

subjective data: Data obtained from a health history or provided to the nurse by the patient.

subluxation: Partial or incomplete dislocation of a joint.

superior: Upper surface of an organ; also refers to a position that is higher in relation to another.

supernumerary nipple: Extra nipple.

supinate: To turn the forearm so the palm faces upward or to rotate the foot and leg outward.

symptom: Subjective indicator or sensation perceived by the patient.

syncope: Sudden, temporary loss of con-sciousness; fainting.

systole: Period of time within the cardiac cycle in which the ventricles contract.

T

tachycardia: Rapid heart rate (more than 100 beats/min).

tachypnea: Rapid breathing; a respiratory rate that is faster than 20 breaths/min.

tactile fremitus: Vibratory sensations of the spoken voice felt through the thoracic wall on palpation.

tail of Spence: Upper outer tail of the breast that extends into the axillary region.

telangiectasia: Dilation of a superficial capillary or network of small capillaries that produces fine, irregular, red lines on the skin surface.

tendinitis: Inflammation of a tendon.

thrill: Palpable murmur.

thrombophlebitis: Inflammation of a vein.

thrombus: Blood clot attached to the inner wall of a vessel.

tic: Spasmodic muscular contraction most commonly involving the face, head, neck, or shoulder muscles.

tinnitus: Tinkling or ringing sound heard in one or both ears.

tophi: Deposits of uric acid in subcutaneous tissue associated with gout.

torsion (of spermatic cord): Twisting of the spermatic cord that results in an infarction of the testis.

tragus: Cartilaginous projection in front of the exterior meatus of the ear.

trapezius muscle: Major muscle that rotates and extends the head.

tremor: Continuous involuntary trembling movement of a part or parts of the body.

trimester: Refers to a period of time during pregnancy. There are three trimesters during pregnancy; each trimester lasts a period of 3 months.

tumor: Solid skin elevation that extends into the dermal layer and is more than 1 cm in diameter.

turbinates: Extensions of the ethmoid bone located along the lateral wall of the nose.

turgor: Expected resiliency of the skin.

two-point discrimination: Ability to identify being touched by two sharp objects simultaneously.

tympany: Low-pitched note heard on percussion of a hollow organ such as the stomach.

U

ulcer: Circumscribed crater on the surface of the skin or mucous membrane that results from necrosis.

umbo: Central depressed portion of the concavity of the lateral surface of the tympanic membrane; marks the spot where the malleus is attached to the inner surface.

unilateral: Relating to or referring to one side.

urinary frequency: Excreting urine often in small amounts.

urinary incontinence: Inability to control urination.

urinary urgency: Sudden, almost uncontrollable need to urinate.

urticaria (hives): Pruritic wheals; often transient and allergic in origin.

uvula: A small, cone-shaped tissue suspended midline from the soft palate.

V

vaginitis: Inflammation of the vaginal vault.

valgus: Turning outward.

varicocele: Abnormal tortuosity and dilation of spermatic veins; spermatic cord is described as feeling like a bag of worms.

varus: Turning inward.

vellus hair: Soft nonpigmented hair that covers the body.

vermilion border: Demarcation point between the mucosal membrane of the lips and the skin of the face.

vertigo: Sensation of moving around in space (whirling motion; subjective vertigo) or of objects moving about themselves (objective vertigo).

vesicle: Fluid-filled, elevated, superficial lesion 1 cm or less in diameter.

vesicular breath sounds: Expected breath sounds heard over most of the lungs.

vestibule: Middle part of the inner ear located behind the cochlea and in front of the semicircular canals.

vocal fremitus: Vibratory sensations of the spoken voice felt through the chest wall on palpation; also known as tactile fremitus.

vulva: External female genitalia; also referred to as the *pudendum.*

W

wheal: Elevated, solid, transient lesion; often irregularly shaped but well demarcated; an edematous response.

wheeze: High-pitched, musical noise that sounds like a squeak; heard during auscultation of a narrowed airway.

whispered pectoriloquy: Transmission of whispered words through the chest wall, heard during auscultation.

X

xerostomia: Dryness of the mouth.

400 Self-assessment picture tests in clinical medicine, 1984. By permission of Mosby International.

Ali NS, Sartori-Valinotti JC, Bruce AJ: Periodic fever, aphthous stomatitis, pharyngitis, and adenitis (PFAPA) syndrome, *Clin Dermatol* 34[4], 482–486, 2016. Copyright © 2016 Elsevier Inc

Allan PL, Baxter GM, Weston MJ: *Clinical Ultrasound*, ed 3, © 2011, Elsevier Limited. All rights reserved.

American Cancer Society: *Cancer facts & figures 2020*, Atlanta, 2020, American Cancer Society; United States Preventive Services Task Force: Skin Cancer Prevention: Behavioral Counseling, 2018.

American Cancer Society: *Cancer facts and figures 2019*, Atlanta, 2019, American Cancer Society

American College of Asthma, Allergy, and Immunology. https://acaai.org/allergies/types/food-allergy; Nordqvist C: What is a food intolerance? *Medical News Today*. Medi-Lexicon, Intl., December 20, 2017

American College of Obstetricians and Gynecologists. FAQ009: *How to prevent sexually transmitted infections*, 2017

American College of Rheumatology: *Clinical slide collection of the rheumatic diseases,* Atlanta, 1991, 1995, 1997, American College of Rheumatology.

American Heart Association: Pediatric Advanced Life Support Provider Manual, 2015 and Whelton PK, Carey RM, Aronow WS, et al: 2017 ACC/AHA/AAPA/ABC/ACPM/ AGS/ APhA/ASH/ASPC/ NMA/PCNA guideline for the prevention, detection, evaluation, and management of high blood pressure in adults: executive summary: a report of the American College of Cardiology/American Heart Association Task Force on Clinical Practice Guidelines. *Hypertension* 71:1269–1324, 2018.

©Andy Dean Photography/Shutterstock.com

Angel CA: *Circumcision. Emedicine.medscape.com*, 2018.

Applegate E: *The Anatomy and Physiology Learning System,* ed 4, St. Louis, 2011, Saunders.

©auremar/Shutterstock.com

Ball JW, et al.: *Seidel's guide to physical examination,* ed 8, St Louis, 2015, Mosby.

Baran R, Dawber RR, Levene GM: *Color atlas of the hair, scalp, and nails,* St Louis, 1991, Mosby.

Barber and Sharma, 2019

Barkauskas VH et al.: *Health and physical assessment,* ed 3, St. Louis, 2002, Mosby.

Beaven DW, Brooks SE: *Color atlas of the nail in clinical diagnosis,* ed 2, London, 1994, Times Mirror International Publishers.

Bedford MA: *Color atlas of ophthalmological diagnosis,* ed 2, London, 1986, Wolfe.

Belcher AE: *Cancer nursing,* St Louis, 1992, Mosby.

Bingham, Hawke, and Kwok: *Atlas of clinical otolaryngology,* St. Louis, 1992, Mosby.

Black J, Hawks J: *Medical-surgical nursing,* ed 7, St Louis, 2005, Saunders.

Blazer D, Domnitz S, Liverman C: *Hearing health care for adults: priorities for improving access and affordability,* 2016, National Academy of Sciences

Bluestone C, et al.: *Pediatric otolaryngology,* ed 4, Philadelphia, 2003, Saunders.

Bohadana A, Izbicki G, Kraman SS: Fundamentals of lung auscultation, *N Engl J Med* 370(8):744, 2014

Bolognia JL, Jorizzo JL, Schaffer JV: *Dermatology,* ed 3, © 2012, Elsevier Limited. All rights reserved.

Bonewit-West K: *Clinical procedures for medical assistants,* ed 8, 2012, Saunders.

Bowden VP, et al.: *Children and their families: the continuum of care,* Philadelphia, 1998, Saunders.

Brinster et al., Statis Dermatitis. In: Brinster et al., *Dermatopathology High Yield Pathology*, Saunders, 2011, Philadelphia

Canobbio MM: *Cardiovascular disorders,* St Louis, 1990, Mosby.

Cavanaugh JC, Blanchard-Fields F: *Adult Development and Aging,* ed 8, Boston, 2019, Cengage

Centers for Disease Control: What are the Risk Factors for Skin Cancer? 2020. Available at www.cdc.gov/cancer/skin/basic_info/risk_factors.htm

Centers for Disease Control and Prevention: *Core curriculum on tuberculosis: what clinicians should know,* ed 6, Atlanta, GA, 2013.

Centers for Disease Control and Prevention: *Latent tuberculosis infection: a guide for primary health care providers,* Atlanta, GA.

Centers for Disease Control and Prevention: *Screening and diagnosis of hearing Loss,* 2018

Centers for Disease Control and Prevention: Sexually transmitted disease treatment guidelines 2015, *MMWR* 64(3) 1–137

Centers for Disease Control and Prevention: Osteoarthritis. www.cdc.gov/arthritis/basics/osteoarthritis.htm. Last reviewed January 10, 2019.

Centers for Disease Control: What are the risk factors for breast cancer? 2018. Retrieved from: https://www.cdc.gov/cancer/breast/basic_info/risk_factors.htm

Childhood and Society by Erik H. Erikson. © 1950, © 1963 by W.W. Norton & Company, Inc., renewed © 1978, 1991 by Erikson

Chipps EM, Clanin NJ, Campbell VG: *Neurologic disorders,* St Louis, 1992, Mosby.

Christensen B, Kockrow E: *Adult health nursing,* ed 6, St Louis, 2011, Mosby.

Cohen, Atlas of pediatric dermatology, London, 1993, Mosby.

Copstead LC, Banasik J: *Pathophysiology,* ed 5, St. Louis, 2013, Saunders. Macular Degeneration Network. Available at www.macular-degeneration.org/.

Copyright © iStock/XiXinXing

Copyright © iStock/monkeybusinessimagesCopyright 1983, Wong-Baker FACES ® Foundation, www.WongBakerFACES.org

Coronary artery disease—coronary heart disease. Available at https://www.heart.org/en/health-topics/heart-attack/

understand-your-risks-to-prevent-a-heart-attack?s=q%3D risk%2520factors%2520for%2520coronary%2520artery% 2520disease%26sort%3Drelevancy. Accessed June 30, 2016

Coulson I, Lebwohl MG, Berth-Jones J, Heymann WR: Herpes zoster. In Nawas Z, Hatch MM, Tyring SK, editors: *Treatment of Skin Disease: Comprehensive Therapeutic Strategies*, 2017, Elsevier, pp 340-343, Chapter 105. © 2018, Elsevier Limited. All rights reserved

Cummings NH, Stanley-Green S, Higgs P: *Perspectives in athletic training*, St Louis, 2009, Mosby.

Cutaneous squamous cell carcinoma. Elsevier Point of Care. Released August 20, 2019. Copyright Elsevier BV. All rights reserved.

deWit SC: *Fundamental Concepts and Skills for Nursing*, ed 3, St. Louis, 2009, Saunders.

Dinulos, JGH: Vascular tumors and malformations. In Dinulos JGH, editor: *Skin disease: diagnosis and treatment*, ed 4, Elsevier. © 2018, Elsevier Inc.

Doughty DB, Jackson DB: *Gastrointestinal disorders*, St Louis, 1993, Mosby.

Drake RL, Vogl W, Mitchell AWM: *Gray's anatomy for students*, ed 2, Philadelphia, 2010, Churchill Livingstone.

Dr. Ira Abrahamsom, Jr, Cincinnati, Ohio. From Stein, Slatt, and Stein, 1988.)

Dr. Edward L Applebaum, Head, Department of Otolaryngology. University of Illinois Medical Center

Dr. Richard A. Buckingham, Clinical Professor, Otolaryngology, Abraham Lincoln School of Medicine, University of Illinois, Chicago. From Barkauskas et al., 2002

Duderstadt K: *Pediatric physical examination: an illustrated handbook*, St. Louis, 2006, Mosby.

Duvall EM, Miller BC: *Marriage and family development*, ed 6, New York, 1985, Harper & Row

Elkin MK, Perry AG, Potter PA: *Nursing interventions and clinical skills*, ed 4, St Louis, 2008, Mosby.

Evans, RC: *Illustrated Orthopedic Physical Assessment*, ed 3, 2009, Mosby.

Farrar WE, et al.: *Infectious diseases: text and color atlas*, ed 2, London, 1992, Gower.

Frisancho AR: New norms of upper limb fat and muscle areas for assessment of nutritional status, *Am J Clin Nutr* 34:2540–2545, 1981

Forbes CD, Jackson WF: *Color atlas and text of clinical medicine*, ed 3, St Louis, 2003, Elsevier.

Fortunato N, McCullough SM: *Plastic and reconstructive surgery*, St Louis, 1998, Mosby.

Francis CC, Martin AH: *Introduction to human anatomy*, ed 7, St Louis, 1975, Mosby.

Frazier M, Drzymkowski J: *Essentials of human diseases and conditions*, ed 4, St Louis, 2008, Saunders.

Gallager HS, et al.: *The breast*, St Louis, 1978, Mosby.

Goldstein BG, Goldstein AO: *Practical dermatology*, ed 2, St Louis, 1997, Mosby.

Gould B, Dyer R: *Pathophysiology for the health professions*, ed 4, St Louis, 2011, Saunders.

Graf C, The Lawton Instrumental Activities of Daily Living (IADL) Scale, *Am J of Nursing* 108 (4): 52-62, 2008

Grimes DE: *Infectious diseases*, St Louis, 1991, Mosby.

Grodner, M. Nutritional foundations and clinical applications, ed 5, St. Louis, 2012, Elsevier; Center for Disease Control, Fact Sheet: Health Disparities in Obesity, 2015, available from: http://www.cdc.gov/minorityhealth/reports/CHDIR11/FactSheets/Obesity.pdf

Gunton KB, Wasserman BN, DeBenedictis C: Strabismus, *Prim Care Clin Office Pract* 42[3]:393–407, 2015 Copyright © 2015 Elsevier Inc. Credits source as: Courtesy Kammi Gunton, MD

Habif TP: *Clinical dermatology: a color guide to diagnosis and therapy*, ed 5, St Louis, 2010, Mosby.

Habif TP: *Clinical dermatology: a color guide to diagnosis and therapy*, ed 3, Philadelphia, 1996, Mosby.

Haies CM, Carroll MD, Fryar CD, Ogden, CL: *Prevalence of Obesity Among Adults and Youth, United States, 2015–2016*. NCHS Data Brief, No. 288, October 2017. Retrieved from: https://www.cdc.gov/nchs/data/databriefs/db288.pdf

Halter M: *Varcarolis' Foundations of psychiatric mental health nursing: a clinical approach*, ed 8, St Louis, 2018, Elsevier.

Harkreader H, Hogan M, Thobaben M: *Fundamentals of nursing: caring and clinical judgment*, ed 3, St Louis, 2007, Mosby.

Herlihy B: *The human body in health and illness*, ed 4, St Louis, 2011, Mosby.

Hill MJ: *Skin disorders*, St Louis, 1994, Mosby.

Hockenberry MJ, et al.: *Wong's nursing care of infants and children*, ed 7, St Louis, 2003, Mosby.

Hockenberry MJ, et al.: *Wong's nursing care of infants and children*, ed 9, St Louis, 2011, Mosby.

Hockenberry MJ, Wilson D: *Wong's essentials of pediatric nursing*, ed 9, St. Louis, 2013, Mosby.

Hockenberry MJ, Wilson D, editors: *Wong's nursing care of infants and children*, ed 11, St Louis, 2018, Elsevier/Mosby, pp 243

Huether S, McCance K: *Understanding pathophysiology*, ed 4, St Louis, 2008, Mosby.

Ignatavicius D, Workman ML: *Medical-surgical nursing: Patient-centered collaborative care*, ed 7, Philadelphia, 2010, Saunders.

Ignatavicius D, Workman ML: *Medical-surgical nursing: Patient-centered collaborative care*, ed 8, Philadelphia, 2016, Saunders.

Institute of Medicine: *Weight gain during pregnancy: reexamining the guidelines*, Washington, DC, 2009, National Academy of Sciences Press

Jachmann-Jahn U: *Clinical symptoms guide to differential diagnosis*, 2009, Urban and Fischer.

James WD, Berger T, Elston D: *Andrews' disesases of the skin*, ed 11, St. Louis, 2011, Elsevier.

James WD, Elston DM, McMahon PJ: Contact dermatitis and drug eruptions. In *Andrews' Diseases of the Skin Clinical Atlas*, 65–85, Chapter 6, Philadelphia, 2018, Elsevier.

Jellinek MS, et al.: Screening 4- and 5-year-old children for psychosocial dysfunction: a preliminary study with the pediatric symptom checklist, *J Dev Behav Pediatr* 15:191, 1994.

Jett K: Biological theories of aging and age-related physical changes. In Touhy TA, Jett K: *Ebersole and Hess' Gerontological Nursing & Healthy Aging*, ed 5, St Louis, 2018, Elsevier, pp. 22–39.

Jennings JJ, Shaffer AD, Stapleton AL: Pediatric nasal septal perforation, *Int J Pediatr Otorhinolaryngol* 118, 15–20. Copyright © 2019 Elsevier B.V.

Joseph P. Fiorellini, Hector L. Sarmiento, David M. Kim and Yu-Cheng Chang Newman and Carranza's Clinical Periodontology, Chapter 18, 248–255.e4 Newman and Carranza's Clinical Periodontology Thirteenth Edition Copyright © 2019 by Elsevier, Inc

Kabashima-Kubo R1, Nakamura M, Sakabe J, et al. A group of atopic dermatitis without IgE elevation or barrier impairment shows a high Th1 frequency: possible immunological state of the intrinsic type, *J Dermatol Sci* 67[1]:37-43, 2012. Copyright © 2012 Japanese Society for Investigative Dermatology, *Journal of Dermatological Science* Volume 67, Issue 1

Kamal A, Brocklehurst JC: *Color atlas of geriatric medicine*, London, 1991, Wolfe.

Katz S et al.: Progress in development of eh index of ADL, *Gerontologist* 10(1):20-30, 1970.

Keela Herr, PhD, RN, AGSF, FAAN, The University of Iowa

Kirnbauer R, Lenz P: Human papillomaviruses. In Kirnbauer R, Lenz P, editors: *Dermatology*, ed 4, Elsevier, pp 1383-1399, Chapter 79. All rights reserved

Kirton C: Assessing edema, *Nursing 96* 26(7):54, 1996.

Know your risk factors for high blood pressure. Available at https://www.heart.org/en/health-topics/high-blood-pressure/why-high-blood-pressure-is-a-silent-killer/know-your-risk-factors-for-high-blood-pressure. Accessed December 31, 2017.

Krachmer JH, Palay DA: *Conjunctivitis*, ed 3, Cornea Atlas, Chapter 7, 62–85. Copyright © 2014, Elsevier Inc

LaFleur Brooks M, LaFleur Brooks D: *Exploring Medical Language*, ed 8, St. Louis, 2012, Mosby.

LaFleur Brooks M, LaFleur Brooks D: *Exploring Medical Language*, ed 7, St. Louis, 2009, Mosby.

Linton D: *Introduction to medical surgical nursing*, ed 4, St. Louis, 2008, Saunders.

Lemmi F, Lemmi C: *Physical assessment findings CD-ROM*, Philadelphia, 2013, Saunders.

Lemmi F, Lemmi C: *Physical assessment findings CD-ROM*, Philadelphia, 2000, Saunders.

Lewis SL, et al.: *Medical-surgical nursing: assessment and management of clinical problems*, ed 9, St. Louis, 2014, Mosby.

Lewis SL, et al.: *Medical-surgical nursing: assessment and management of clinical problems*, ed 8, St Louis, 2011, Mosby.

Lewis SL, Heitkemper MM, Dirksen SR: *Medical-surgical nursing: assessment and management of clinical problems*, ed 7, St Louis, 2007, Mosby.

Lewis SM, et al.: *Medical-surgical nursing: assessment and management of clinical problems*, ed 6, St. Louis, 2004, Mosby.

Lloyd-Davies RW, et al.: *Color atlas of urology*, ed 2, London, 1994, Wolfe.

Lowdermilk DL, Perry SE, Cashion MC: *Maternity nursing*, ed 8, St Louis, 2011, Mosby.

Lowdermilk DL, Perry SE, Cashion MC, Alden KR: *Maternity and women's health care*, ed 10, St Louis, 2012, Mosby.

Mahan LK, Escott-Stump S: *Krause's food & nutrition therapy*. ed 12, Philadelphia: Saunders; 2008.

Mahnaz Fatahzadeh DMD Robert A. Schwartz MD, MPH: Human herpes simplex virus infections: Epidemiology, pathogenesis, symptomatology, diagnosis, and management, *J Am Acad Dermatol* 57[5], 737–763, 2007. Copyright © 2007 American Academy of Dermatology, Inc.

Mangels AR: Malnutrition in older adults. *Am J Nursing* 118(3); 34–41, 2018

Mansel R, Bundred N: *Color atlas of breast disease*, St Louis, 1995, Mosby-Wolfe.

Marshall WA, Tanner JM: Variations in pattern of pubertal changes in girls, *Arch Dis Child* 44:291, 1969.

Marx J, et al.: *Rosen's emergency medicine*, ed 7, Philadelphia, 2010, Mosby.

McCance KL, Huether SE: *Pathophysiology: the biologic basis for disease in adults and children*, ed 4, St Louis, 2002, Mosby.

McCance KL, Huether SE: *Pathophysiology: the biologic basis for disease in adults and children*, ed 6, St Louis, 2010, Mosby.

McEwen M: Spiritual nursing care: state of the art. *Holistic Nurs Pract* 19:161–168, 2005

McKenry LM, Salerno E: *Mosby's pharmacology in nursing*, ed 21, St Louis, 2003, Mosby.

McLaren DS: *A colour atlas and text of diet-related disorders*, ed 2, St Louis, 1992, Wolfe.

Melzack R, Katz J: Pain measurement in persons with pain. In Wall PD, Melzack R, editors: *Textbook of pain*, ed 3, New York, 1994, Churchill-Livingstone.

Minkin MJ, Reiter S, Maamari R: Prevalence of postmenopausal symptoms in North America and Europe, *Menopause* 22(11):1231–1238, 2015

Moon RY: SIDS and other sleep-related infant deaths: expansion of recommendations for a safe infant sleeping environment, *Pediatrics* 128(5):e1341–e1367, 2011

Monahan F, et al.: *Phipps' medical-surgical nursing*, ed 8, St Louis, 2007, Mosby.

Monahan FD, Drake DT, Neighbors M, editors: *Medical-surgical nursing: Foundations for clinical practice*, ed 2, Philadelphia, 1998, Saunders–Elsevier.

Monteleone JA: *Recognition of child abuse for the mandated reporter*, ed 2, London, 1996, GW Medical Publishing.

Mourad LA: *Orthopedic disorders*, St Louis, 1991, Mosby.

Narayan M: Culture's effects on pain assessment and management, *AJN* 110:40, 2010

Nassif N, Berlucchi M, Redaelli de Zinis LO: Tympanic membrane perforation in children: Endoscopic type I tympanoplasty, a newly technique, is it worthwhile? *Int J Pediatr Otorhinolaryngol*;79[11]:1860–1864, 2015. Copyright © 2015 Elsevier Ireland Ltd

National Eye Institute, National Institutes of Health: https://nei.nih.gov/

National Institute on Aging: Prevent falls and fractures available at https://www.nia.nih.gov/health/prevent-falls-and-fractures. Content reviewed March 15, 2017

National Institute on Alcohol Abuse and Alcoholism (NIAAA), Helping patients who drink too much: A clinician's guide, 2005, Patient Education Materials, What's a standard Drink. www.niaaa.nih.gov. Accessed September 7, 2011.

National Institutes of Health/National Heart, Lung, and Blood Institute: *Clinical guidelines on the identification, evaluation, and treatment of overweight and obesity in adults: the evidence report,* June 1998. NIH Publication 98-4093. Available at www.nhlbi.nih.gov/guidelines/obesity/ob_gdlns.pdf.

National Institutes of Health, National Heart, Lung, and blood Institute https://www.nhlbi.nih.gov/health-topics/stroke, February, 2020

National Osteoporosis Foundation. Are you At Risk? www.nof.org/preventing-fractures/general-facts/bone-basics/are-you-at-risk/.

National Pressure Ulcer Advisory Panel (NPUAP). All photographs displayed are reprinted with permission of the copyright holder, Gordian Medical, Inc. dba American Medical Technologies. www.npuap.org.

Newell FW: *Ophthalmology: principles and concepts,* ed 7, St Louis, 1992, Mosby.

Newell FW: *Ophthalmology: principles and concepts,* ed 8, St Louis, 1996, Mosby.

NIH. Osteoporosis Overview. www.bones.nih.gov/health-info/bone/osteoporosis/overview. Last reviewed October, 2018

Ogueta CI, Ramírez PM, Jiménez OC, Cifuentes MM: Geographic tongue: What a dermatologist should know, *Actas Dermosifiliogr* 110(5), 341–346, 2019. Copyright © 2019 Elsevier España, S.L.U. and AEDV Dermatology

Pagana KD, Pagana TJ, Pagana TN: Mosby's diagnostic and laboratory test reference, ed 13, St Louis, 2017, Mosby; and National Cancer Institute Short Dietary Assessment Instruments. 2014. http://appliedresearch.cancer.gov/diet/screeners/

Pasero C, McCaffery M: *Pain assessment and pharmacologic management,* St Louis, 2011, Mosby.

Patton KT, Thibodeau GA, Douglas MM: *Essentials of Anatomy and Physiology,* ed 1, St. Louis, 2012, Mosby.

Patton KT, Thibodeau GA: *Anatomy & physiology,* ed 7, St Louis, 2010, Mosby.

PDQ® Screening and Prevention Editorial Board: *PDQ Ovarian, Fallopian Tube, and Primary Peritoneal Cancer Prevention,* Bethesda, MD, 2019, National Cancer Institute

Pinkering TG, Hall JE, Appel LJ, et al.: Recommendations for blood pressure measurement in humans and experimental animals. Part 1: Blood pressure measurement in humans, *Hypertension* 45:142–161, 2005

Perry AG, Potter PA, Elkin MK: *Nursing interventions and clinical skills,* ed 5, St Louis, 2012, Mosby.

Perry S, Hockenberry M, Lowdermilk D, Wilson D: *Maternal-child nursing care,* ed 4, St. Louis, 2010, Mosby.

Pfenninger JL, Fowler GC: *Pfenninger and Fowler's Procedures for Primary Care,* ed 3, St. Louis, 2011, Saunders.

Potter PA, et al.: *Fundamentals of nursing,* ed 8, St Louis, 2013, Mosby.

Potter PA, Perry AG: *Basic nursing: essentials for practice,* ed 6, St Louis, 2006, Mosby.

Potter PA, Perry AG: *Basic nursing: theory and practice,* ed 2, St Louis, 1991, Mosby.

Potter PA, Perry AG: *Fundamentals of nursing,* ed 7, St Louis, 2009, Mosby.

Prior, Silberstein, and Stang, Physical diagnosis: the history and examination of the patient, ed 6, St. Louis, 1981, Mosby.

Purnell L: *Transcultural health care: A culturally competent approach,* ed 4, Philadelphia, 2012, F.A. Davis.

Rafferty J: Ensuring comprehensive care and support for transgender and gender-diverse children and adolescents, *Pediatrics* 142 (4), October, 2018

Rafferty J: Gender identity development in children. Retrieved from https://www.healthychildren.org/English/ages-stages/gradeschool/Pages/Gender-Identity-and-Gender-Confusion-In-Children.aspx. Last updated September 18, 2018

Rakel R, Bope E: *Conn's current therapy 2004,* Philadelphia, 2004, Saunders.

Regezi JA, Sciubba JJ, Jordan RC: *Oral pathology: clinical pathologic correlations,* ed 6, Philadelphia, 2012, Saunders.

Regezi JA, Sciubba JJ, Jordan RCK: *Oral pathology,* ed 7, Elsevier, pp xiv-lxxxix. Copyright © 2017, by Elsevier, Inc. All rights reserved

Report of the US Preventive Services Task Force: Guide to clinical preventive services, ed 2, US Department of Health and Human Services, 1996, Washington, DC.

©Rob Marmion/Shutterstock.com

Robb PJ, Williamson I: Otitis media with effusion in children: current management, *Pediatric Child Health* 22, 9–12, 2012. Copyright © 2015 Elsevier Ltd Paediatrics and Child Health Volume 26, Issue 1 Copyright © 2015 Elsevier Ltd

Roberts J, Hedges J: *Clinical procedures in emergency medicine,* ed 5, Philadelphia, 2009, Saunders.

Rosen T, Stern ME, editors: Abuse and neglect of the geriatric patient. In *Rosen's emergency medicine: concepts and clinical practice,* ed 9, Elsevier, 2341-2348.e1, Chapter 186. Copyright © 2018 by Elsevier, Inc. All rights reserved

Ross Products Division, Abbott Laboratories. In Seidel HM et al: *Mosby's guide to physical examination,* ed 7, St Louis, 2011, Mosby

Saks M, Nisbet B: Symmetric skin lesions in an Asian male with flu-like symptoms, *J Emerg Med* 2:21–22, 2016. Copyright © 2015 Elsevier Inc.)

Salt Lake City/County STD Clinic Book Chapter: Herpes Simplex Virus Infection John D. Kriesel and Christopher M. Hull 23, 110–116. Netter's Infectious Diseases Copyright © 2012 by Saunders, an imprint of Elsevier Inc

Salvo SG: *Mosby's pathology for massage therapists,* ed 2, St Louis, 2009, Mosby.

Sanders M: *Mosby's paramedic textbook,* ed 3, St Louis, 2007, Mosby.

Schuster C, Ashburn S: The process of human development: a holistic life-span approach, Boston, 1992, Lippincott.

Scully C, Welbury R: *Color atlas of oral diseases in children and adolescents,* London, 1994, Wolfe.

Seeley RR, Stephens TD, Tate P: *Anatomy and physiology,* ed 3, St Louis, 1995, Mosby.

Seidel HM, et al.: *Mosby's guide to physical examination*, ed 5, St Louis, 2003, Mosby.

Seidel HM, et al.: *Mosby's guide to physical examination*, ed 6, St Louis, 2006, Mosby.

Seidel HM, et al.: *Mosby's guide to physical examination*, ed 7, St Louis, 2011, Mosby.

Shade BR, et al.: *Mosby's EMT- intermediate textbook for the 1999 national standard curriculum,* ed 3, St. Louis, 2012, Mosby/JEMS.

Sorrentino SA, Gorek B: *Mosby's textbook for long term care assistants,* ed 5, St Louis, 2007, Mosby.

Spagrud LJ, Piira T, von Baeyer CL: Children's self-report of pain intensity: The Faces Pain Scale—Revised, *Am J Nurs* 03[12]:62–64, 2003

Stenchever M, et al.: *Comprehensive gynecology,* ed 4, St Louis, 2001, Mosby.

Stoy W, et al.: *Mosby's EMT-basic textbook,* ed 2, St Louis, 2012, Mosby.

Swartz MH: *Textbook of physical diagnosis: history and examination,* ed 5, Philadelphia, 2006, Saunders.

Swartz MH: *Textbook of physical diagnosis: history and examination,* ed 6, Philadelphia, 2010, Saunders.

Swartz MH: *Textbook of physical diagnosis: history and examination,* ed 7, Philadelphia, 2014, Saunders.

Symonds EM, MacPherson MBA: *Color atlas of obstetrics and gynaecology,* London, 1994, Mosby-Wolfe.

Tanner C: Thinking like a nurse: A research-based model of clinical judgment in nursing, *J Nurs Educ* 45:204-211, 2006.

Tanner JM: *Growth at adolescence,* ed 2, Oxford, England, 1962, Blackwell Scientific Publications.

Taylor PK: Diagnostic picture tests in sexually transmitted diseases, London, 1995, Mosby.

U.S. Department of Agriculture, http://www.choosemyplate.gov/

The Joint Committee on Infant Hearing: Year 2007 position statement: principles and guidelines for early hearing detection and intervention programs, *Pediatrics* 120(4):898–921, 2007

Thibodeau GA, Patton KT: *Anatomy & physiology,* ed 3, St Louis, 1996, Mosby.

Thibodeau GA, Patton KT: *Anatomy and physiology,* ed 4, St Louis, 1999, Mosby.

Thibodeau GA, Patton KT: *Anatomy and physiology,* ed 6, St Louis, 2007, Mosby.

Thibodeau GA, Patton KT: *The human body in health and disease,* ed 5, St Louis, 2010, Mosby.

Thibodeau GA, Patton KT: *Structure & Function of the Body,* ed 14, St. Louis, 2012, Mosby.

Thompson JM, et al.: *Mosby's clinical nursing,* ed 3, St Louis, 1993, Mosby.

Thompson JM, et al.: *Mosby's clinical nursing,* ed 5, St Louis, 2002, Mosby.

Topham D, Ware D: Quality improvement project: Replacing the Numeric Rating Scale with a Clinically Aligned Pain Assessment (CAPA) tool, *Pain Management Nursing* 18(6):363–371, 2017

Totonchi A, Armijo B, Guyuron B: Plastic Surgery: Volume 2: Aesthetic Surgery, 18, 487–501.e2 Fourth Edition © 2018, Elsevier Inc

Townsend CM, et al.: *Sabiston textbook of surgery,* ed 18, Philadelphia, 2008, Saunders.

Townsend CM, et al.: *Sabiston textbook of surgery,* ed 19, Philadelphia, 2012, Saunders.

Touhy T, Jett K, editors: *Ebersole and Hess' Toward Healthy Aging: Human Needs & Nursing Response,* ed 9, St Louis, 2015, Elsevier

Urden LD, Stacy KM, Lough ME: *Critical care nursing: diagnosis and management,* ed 6, St Louis, 2010, Mosby.

U.S. Department of Agriculture, www.choosemyplate.gov/

U.S. Preventive Services Task Force, Final Recommendation Statement: *Breast Cancer Screening, 2016*

U.S. Preventive Services Task Force: *Guide to clinical preventive services, 2014.* AHRQ Pub. No. 14-05158.

U.S. Preventive Services Task Force: *Tobacco smoking: Cessation in adults, including pregnant women: behavioral and pharmacotherapy interventions.* Released September, 2015

U.S. Preventive Services Task Force: *Weight Loss to Prevent Obesity-Related Morbidity and Mortality in Adults: Behavioral Interventions,* 2018

Vitale SA, Prashad T: Cultural awareness: coining and cupping, *International archives of Nursing and Health Care* 3(3), 2017

Walker BR, Colledge NR, Ralston SH, Penman I: *Davidson's Principles and Practice of Medicine,* ed 22, Churchill Livingstone, 2014, Elsevier Limited.

Wellington Hung, MD, Children's National Medical Center, Washington, DC

Welsh O, Vera-Cabrera L, Welsh E: Onychomycosis, *Clin Dermatol* 28 [2]: 151-159, 2010. Copyright © 2010 Elsevier Inc

Welton PK, Carey RM, Aronow WS, et al: ACA/AHA/AAPA/ABC/ACPM/AGS/APhA/ASH/ASPC/NMA/PCNA guideline for the prevention, detection, evaluation, and management of high blood pressure in adults: executive summary, *Hypertension* 71:1269–1324, 2018.

Weston WL, Lane AT, Morelli JG: *Color textbook of pediatric dermatology,* ed 2, St Louis, 1996, Mosby.

Weston WL, Lane AT, Morelli JG: *Color textbook of pediatric dermatology,* ed 3, St Louis, 2002, Mosby.

Wroblewska-Seniuk KE, Dabrowski P, Szyfter W, Mazela J: University newborn hearing screening: methods and results, obstacles, and benefits, *Pediatr Res Mar* 81(3):415–422, 2017

White GM, Cox N: *Diseases of the skin: a color atlas and text,* St Louis, 2000, Mosby.

White GM, Cox N: *Diseases of the skin: a color atlas and text,* ed 2, St Louis, 2006, Mosby.

White GM: *Color atlas of regional dermatology,* St Louis, 1994, Mosby-Wolfe.

White G: *Color atlas of dermatology,* ed 3, Edinburgh, 2004, Elsevier.

Yanoff M, Duker JS: *Ophthalmology*, ed 3, St Louis, 2009, Mosby.

Yesavage JA, Brink TL: Development and validation of a geriatric depression screening scale: a preliminary report, *J Psychiatr Res* 17: 37-49, 1983. Copyright 1983 Elsevier Science. Reprinted Journal of Psychosomatic Research with permission Elsevier Science.

Yoost BL, Crawford LR: *Fundamentals of Nursing,* ed 1, St. Louis, 2016, Mosby.

Young AP: *Kinn's the administrative medical assistant*, ed 7, St Louis, 2011, Saunders.

Zitelli Bj, et al. Zitelli and Davis' Atlas of Pediatric Physical Diagnosis, ed 7, St. Louis, 2018, Elsevier.

Zitelli BJ, Davis HW: *Atlas of pediatric physical diagnosis*, ed 5, St. Louis, 2007, Mosby.

Zitelli BJ, McIntire SC, Nowalk AJ: *Zitelli and Davis' atlas of pediatric physical diagnosis*, ed 6, 2012, Mosby.

CHAPTER 1: INTRODUCTION TO HEALTH ASSESSMENT

1. American Nurses Association: *Nursing: scope and standards of practice,* ed 3, Silver Springs, MD, 2015, American Nurses Association.
2. Institute of Medicine: *Health professions education: a bridge to quality,* Washington, DC, 2003, National Academies Press.
3. Munroe B, Curtis K, Considine J, Buckly T: The impact of structured patient assessment formats has on patient care: an integrative review, *J Clin Nurs* 22:2991–3005, 2013.
4. HealthIT.gov: *What is an electronic health record?* 2018. HealthIT.gov. https://www.healthit.gov/faq/what-electronic-health-record-ehr.
5. Giddens JF: A survey of physical assessment techniques performed by RNs: lessons for nursing education, *J Nurs Educ* 46:83–87, 2007.
6. Anderson B, Nix E, Norman B, McPike H: An evidence-based approach to undergraduate physical assessment practicum course development, *Nurse Educ Pract* 14: 242–246, 2014.
7. Birks M, James A, Chung C, et al: The use of physical assessment skills by registered nurses in Australia: issues for nursing education, *Collegian* 20(1):27–33, 2013.
8. Secrest JA, Norwood BR, duMont PM: Physical assessment skills: a descriptive study of what is taught and what is practiced, *J Prof Nurs* 21(2):114–118, 2005.
9. Barbarito C, Carney L, Lynch A: Refining a physical assessment course, *Nurse Educ* 22:6, 1997.
10. Douglas C, Windsor C, Lewis P: Too much knowledge for a nurse? Use of physical assessment by final-semester nursing students, *Nurs Health Sci* 17(4):492–499, 2015.
11. Zambus SI: Purpose of the systematic physical assessment in everyday practice: critique of a "sacred cow," *J Nurs Educ* 49:305–310, 2010.
12. Hoffman KA, Aitken LM, Fuffield C: A comparison of novice and expert nurses' cue collection during clinical decision making: verbal protocol analysis, *Int J Nurs Stud* 46:1335–1344, 2009.
13. Fennessey A, Whittmann-Price RA: Physical assessment: a continuing need for clarification, *Nurs Forum* 46: 45–50, 2011.
14. Tanner C: Thinking like a nurse: a research-based model of clinical judgment in nursing, *J Nurs Educ* 45:204–211, 2006.
15. Dickison P, Haerling KA, Lasater K: Integrating the National Council of State Boards of Nursing Clinical Judgement Model into nursing education frameworks, *J Nurs Educ* 58(2):72-78, 2019.
16. Pender NJ, Murdaough CL, Parsons MA: *Health promotion in nursing practice,* ed 7, Upper Saddle River, NJ, 2015, Pearson.

CHAPTER 2: OBTAINING A HEALTH HISTORY

1. Munroe B, Curtis K, Considine J, Buckly T: The impact of structured patient assessment formats has on patient care: an integrative review, *J Clin Nurs* 22:2991–3005, 2013.
2. Institute of Medicine: *Crossing the quality chasm: a new health system for the 21st century,* Washington, DC, 2001, National Academies Press.
3. Epstein RM, Street R: The values and value of patient-centered care, *Ann Fam Med* 9(2):100–103, 2011.
4. Calvillo E, Clark L, Ballantyne JE, et al: Cultural competency in baccalaureate nursing education, *J Transcult Nurs* 20:137–145, 2009.
5. Campinha-Bacote J: *The process of cultural competence in the delivery of healthcare services: the journey continues,* ed 5, Cincinnati, 2007, Transcultural C.A.R.E Associates.
6. Reisner S: *Meeting the health care needs of transgender people,* Boston, MA, 2012, The Fenway Institute. http://www.lgbthealtheducation.org/wp-content/uploads/Sari-slides_final1.pdf.
7. GenderSpectrum: *Understanding gender,* 2018. https://www.genderspectrum.org/quick-links/understanding-gender/.
8. Alborn J, McKinney KC: Use of and interaction with medical interpreters, *Am J Health-Syst Parm* 71:1044–1048, 2014.
9. DeMartino E, Dudzinski DM, Doyle CK, et al: Who decides when a patient can't? Statues on alternate decision makers, *N Engl J Med* 376(15):1478–1482, 2017.
10. Fortin AH, Dwarnena FC, Frankel RM, Smith RC: *Smith's patient-centered interviewing: an evidence-based method,* ed 3, New York, 2012, McGraw Hill.
11. Washburn J: What nurses need to know about human trafficking, *J Christ Nurs* 35(1):18–25, 2018.
12. American Nurses Association: *Genetics/genomics nursing: scope and standards of practice,* ed 2, Silver Springs, MD, 2016, American Nurses Association.
13. Olson LM, Radecki L, Frintner MP, et al: At what age can children report dependably on their health status? *Pediatrics* 119:e93–e102, 2007.

CHAPTER 3: TECHNIQUES AND EQUIPMENT FOR PHYSICAL ASSESSMENT

1. Agency for Healthcare Research and Quality: *Quality indicators: patient safety indictors technical specifications updates,* 2018. https://www.qualityindicators.ahrq.gov/Modules/PSI_TechSpec_ICD10_v2018.aspx.
2. Centers for Disease Control and Prevention: *Standard precautions for all patient care,* 2017. https://www.cdc.gov/infectioncontrol/basics/standard-precautions.html.
3. Centers for Disease Control and Prevention: *Hand hygiene in healthcare settings,* 2018. https://www.cdc.gov/handhygiene/index.html.

4. The Joint Commission: *Update citing observations of hand hygiene noncompliance,* 2017. https://www.jointcommission.org/assets/1/18/Update_Citing_Observations_of_Hand_Hygiene_Noncompliance.pdf.

5. Centers for Disease Control and Prevention: *Hand hygiene in healthcare settings: clean hands for healthcare providers,* 2018. https://www.cdc.gov/handhygiene/providers/index.html.

6. Siegel JD, Healthcare Infection Control Practices Advisory Committee: *2007 Guideline for isolation precautions: preventing transmission of infectious agents in healthcare settings,* 2007. http://www.cdc.gov/hicpac/pdf/isolation/Isolation2007.pdf.

7. Centers for Disease Control and Prevention: *Sequence for donning and removing personal protective equipment,* n.d. https://www.cdc.gov/hai/pdfs/ppe/PPE-Sequence.pdf.

8. Centers for Disease Control and Prevention: *Respiratory hygiene/cough etiquette in healthcare settings,* 2012. https://www.cdc.gov/flu/professionals/infectioncontrol/resphygiene.htm.

9. Centers for Disease Control and Prevention: *One and only campaign,* n.d. http://www.oneandonlycampaign.org/.

10. National Institute for Occupational Safety and Health (NIOSH): *NIOSH alert preventing allergic reactions to natural rubber latex in the workplace,* NIOSH pub no 97-135, Cincinnati, OH, 1997, NIOSH.

11. Wu M, Mcintosh J, Liu J: Current prevalence rate of latex allergy: why it remains a problem? *J Occup Health* 58(2):138–144, 2016.

12. Turner S, McNamee R, Agius R, et al: Evaluating interventions aimed at reducing occupational exposure to latex and rubber glove allergens, *Occup Environ Med* 69(12):925–931, 2012.

13. Singler K, Thomas B, Heppner H, et al: Diagnostic accuracy of three different methods of temperature measurement in acutely ill geriatric patients, *Age Ageing* 42:740–746, 2013.

14. Titus MO, Hulsey T, Heckman J, Losek JD: Temporal artery thermometry utilization in pediatric emergency care, *Clin Pediatr* 48:190–193, 2009.

15. Fletcher T, Whittam A, Simpson R, et al: Comparison of non-contact infrared skin thermometers, *J Med Eng Technol* 42(2):65–71, 2018.

16. Niven DJ, Gaudet JE, Laupland KB, et al: Accuracy of peripheral thermometers for estimating temperature: a systematic review, *Ann Intern Med* 163(10):768–777, 2015.

17. Morgensen CB, Vihelmsen MB, Jepsen JB, et al: Ear measurement of temperature is only useful for screening for fever in adult emergency department, *BMC Emerg Med* 18(1):51, 2018.

18. Mogensen CB, Wittenhoff L, Fruerhoj G, et al: Forehead or ear temperature measurement cannot replace rectal measurements except for screening purposes, *BMC Pediatr* 18(1):15, 2018.

19. Bijur PE, Shah PD, Esses D: Temperature measurement in the adult emergency department: oral, tympanic membrane, and temporal artery temperatures versus rectal temperature, *Emerg Med J* 33(12):843–847, 2016.

20. Oguz F, Yidiz I, Varkal, MA, et al: Axillary and tympanic temperature measurement in children and normal values for ages, *Pediatr Emerg Care* 34(3):169–173, 2018.

21. Editorial Staff: Digital stethoscope gets FDA clearance, *Health Data Manag* 23(8), 2015.

22. Swarup S, Makaryus A: Digital stethoscope: technology update, *Med Devices* 11:29–36, 2018.

23. Armstrong RS: Nurses' knowledge of error in blood pressure measurement technique, *Int J Nurs Pract* 8:118–126, 2002.

24. Anderson, DJ, Anderson MA, Hill P: Location of blood pressure measurement, *Medsurg Nurs* 19(5):287–294, 2010.

25. American Heart Association: *Monitoring your blood pressure at home,* 2017. https://www.heart.org/en/health-topics/high-blood-pressure/understanding-blood-pressure-readings/monitoring-your-blood-pressure-at-home#.WOU_jBLyv-Z\.

26. Bell AL, Rodes E, Keller LC: Childhood eye examination, *Am Fam Physician* 88(4):241–248, 2013.

CHAPTER 4: GENERAL INSPECTION AND MEASUREMENT OF VITAL SIGNS

1. Lockwood C, Conroy-Hiller T, Page T: Vital signs, *JBI Rep* 2:207–230, 2004.

2. Braun CA: Accuracy of pacifier thermometers in young children, *Pediatr Nurs* 32:413–418, 2006.

3. Lawson L, Bridges EJ, Ballou I, et al: Accuracy and precision of non-invasive temperature measurement in adult intensive care patients, *Am J Crit Care* 16:485–496, 2007.

4. Titus MO, Hulsey T, Heckman J, Losek JD: Temporal artery thermometry utilization in pediatric emergency care, *Clin Pediatr* 48:190–193, 2009.

5. Jensen B, Jensen FS, Madsen SN, Løssl K: Accuracy of digital tympanic, oral, axillary and rectal thermometers compared with standard rectal mercury thermometers, *Eur J Surg* 166:848–851, 2002.

6. Thomas K, Burr R, Wang SY, et al: Axillary and thoracic skin temperatures poorly comparable to core body temperature circadian rhythm: results from 2 adult populations, *Biol Res Nurs* 5:187–194, 2004.

7. Sund-Levander M, Grodzinsky E: Assessment of body temperature measurement options, *Brit J Nurs* 22(15):880–889, 2013.

8. Singler K, Thomas B, Heppner H, et al: Diagnostic accuracy of three different methods of temperature measurement in acutely ill geriatric patients, *Age Ageing* 42:740–746, 2013.

9. Allegaert K, Casteels K, van Gorp I, Bogaert G: Tympanic infrared skin, and temporal artery scan thermometers compared with rectal measurement in children: a real-life assessment, *Curr Ther Res Clin Exp* 76:34–38, 2014.

10. Prasad B: High altitude and respiratory system, *Med Update* 2(56):256–266, 2017. http://www.apiindia.org/pdf/medicine_update_2017/mu_056.pdf.

11. Moore C, Dobson A, Kinagi M, Dillon B: Comparison of blood pressure measured at the arm, ankle and calf, *Anaesthesia* 63:1327–1331, 2008.

12. Schell K, Lyons D, Bradley E, et al: Clinical comparison of automatic, noninvasive measurements of blood pressure in the forearm and upper arm with the patient supine or with the head of the bed raised 45°: a follow-up study, *Am J Crit Care* 15:196–205, 2006.

13. Whelton PK, Carey RM, Aronow WS, et al: 2017 ACC/AHA/AAPA/ABC/ACPM/AGS/APhA/ASH/ASPC/NMA/PCNA Guideline for the prevention, detection, evaluation, and management of high blood pressure in adults: executive summary: a report of the American College of Cardiology/American Heart Association Task Force on Clinical Practice Guidelines, *Hypertension* 71:1269–1324, 2018.

14. Pickering TG, Hall JE, Appel LJ, et al: Recommendations for blood pressure measurement in humans and experimental animals. Part 1: blood pressure measurement in humans, *Hypertension* 45:142–161, 2005.

15. Bern L, Brandt M, Mbelu N, et al: Differences in blood pressure values obtained with automated and manual methods in medical inpatients, *MedSurg Nurs* 16:356–361, 2007.

16. Heinemann M, Sellick K, Rickard C, et al: Automated versus manual blood pressure measurement: randomized crossover trial, *Int J Nurs Pract* 14:296–302, 2008.

17. The Joint Commission: *Pain management standards—hospital*, 2018. https://www.jointcommission.org/topics/pain_management_standards_hospital.aspx.

CHAPTER 5: CULTURAL COMPETENCE

1. American Nurses Association: *Scope and standards of practice*, ed 3, Silver Springs, MD, 2015, Author.

2. United States Census: *Older people projected to outnumber children for first time in U.S. history*, 2018. https://www.census.gov/newsroom/press-releases/2018/cb18-41-population-projections.html.

3. Tutwiler SW: *Mixed-race and schooling: the fifth minority*, New York, 2016, Rutledge.

4. US Census Bureau. *Demographic turning points for the United States: population projections from 2020 to 2060*, 2020. https://www.census.gov/library/publications/2020/demo/p25-1144.html.

5. Campinha-Bacote J: *The process of cultural competence in the delivery of healthcare services: a culturally competence model of care*, ed 4, Cincinnati, OH, 2003, Transcultural C.A.R.E. Associates.

6. Spector RE: *Cultural diversity in health and illness*, ed 7, Upper Saddle River, NJ, 2009, Pearson Prentice Hall.

7. Galanti G: *Caring for patients from different cultures*, ed 5, Philadelphia, PA, 2015, University of Pennsylvania Press.

8. Purnell L, Paulanka B: *Guide to culturally competent care*, Philadelphia, 2005, FA Davis.

9. Koenig H: *Spirituality in patient care: why, how, when and what*, ed 2, Philadelphia, PA, 2007, Templeton Foundation Press.

10. Sessanna L, Finnell D, Jezewski MA: Spirituality in nursing and health-related literature: a concept analysis, *J Holistic Nurs* 25(4):252–262, 2007.

11. Puchalski CH, Ferrell B: *Making health care whole: integrating spirituality into patient care*, West Conshohocken, PA, 2010, Templeton Press.

12. Blankinship L: Providing culturally sensitive care of Islamic patients and families, *J Christ Nurs* 35(2):94–99, 2018.

13. Reisner S: *Meeting the health care needs of transgender people*, Boston, MA, 2012, The Fenway Institute. http://www.lgbthealtheducation.org/wp-content/uploads/Sari-slides_final1.pdf.

14. Tracy, JK, Schluterman NH, Greenberg DR: Understanding cervical cancer screening among lesbians: a national survey, *BMC Public Health*, May 4, 2013. https://www.ncbi.nlm.nih.gov/pmc/articles/PMC3693978/.

15. HHS.gov: *The national CLAS standards*, 2018. https://minorityhealth.hhs.gov/omh/browse.aspx?lvl=2&lvlid=53.

16. Squires A: Evidenced-based approaches to breaking down language barriers, *Nursing* 47(9):34–40, 2017.

17. American Nurses Association Position Statement: *Nursing advocacy for LGBTQ+ populations*, 2018. https://www.nursingworld.org/~49866e/globalassets/practiceandpolicy/ethics/nursing-advocacy-for-lgbtq-populations.pdf. Accessed October 4, 2018.

18. Tanenbaum: *The medical manual for religio-cultural competence: caring for religiously diverse populations*, New York, 2009, Center for Interreligious Understanding.

19. Foronda C, Baptiste DL, Reinholdt M, Ousman K: Cultural humility: a concept analysis, *J Transcult Nurs* 27(3):210–217, 2016.

20. Kardong-Edgren S, Carson LC, Hummel F, et al: Cultural competency of graduating BSN nursing students, *Nurs Educ Perspect* 31(5):278–285, 2010.

21. McCord G, Gilchrist VJ, Grossman SD, et al: Discussing spirituality with patients: a rational and ethical approach, *Ann Fam Med* 2(4):356–361, 2004.

22. Fagan A: *The spirit catches you and you fall down: a Hmong child, her American doctors, and the collision of two cultures*, New York, 1997, Farrar, Straus and Giroua.

23. Huber L: Making community health care culturally correct, *Am Nurs Today* 4(5):13–15, 2009.

24. Borneman T, Ferrell B, Puchalski CM: Evaluation of the FICA tool for spiritual assessment, *J Pain Symptom Manage* 40(2):163–173, 2010.

25. Puchalski CH, Romer AL: Taking a spiritual history allows clinicians to understand patients, *J Palliat Med* 3:129–137, 2000.

26. Ambuel B, Weissman D: *Fast facts and Concept #19: taking a spiritual history*. http://www.mywhatever.com/cifwriter/library/eperc/fastfact/ff19.html.

CHAPTER 6: PAIN ASSESSMENT

1. Interagency Pain Research Coordinating Committee: *National pain strategy: a comprehensive population-level health strategy for pain*, 2016. https://iprcc.nih.gov/sites/default/files/HHSNational_Pain_Strategy_508C.pdf.

2. Pasero C: Challenges in pain assessment, *J PeriAnesthesia Nurs* 24(1):50–54, 2009.

3. No author: Joint Commission enhances pain assessment and management requirements for accredited hospitals, *Jt Comm Perspect* 37(7):1, 3–4, 2017. www.jointcommission.org.

4. American Nurses Association Center for Ethics and Human Rights: *The ethical responsibility to manage pain and the suffering it causes*, 2018, pp 6–7. https://www.nursingworld.org/~495e9b/globalassets/docs/ana/ethics/theethicalresponsibilitytomanagepainandthesufferingitcauses2018.pdf.

5. Merskey H, Bogduk N, et al: Pain terms: a list with definitions and note on usage (Recommended by the IASP subcommittee on taxonomy), *Pain* 6(3):247–252, 1979.

6. McCaffery M: *Nursing practice theories related to cognition, bodily pain, man-environment interactions*, Los Angles, 1968, University of California Los Angles Students' Store.

7. Hagler D: Tissue integrity. In Giddens J, editor: *Concepts for nursing practice*, ed 3, St Louis, 2021, Elsevier.

8. Starkweather A: Pain. In Giddens J, editor: *Concepts for nursing practice*, ed 3, St Louis, 2021, Elsevier.

9. Pasero C, Portenoy RK: Neurophysiology of pain and analgesia and pathophysiology of neurologic pain. In Pasero C, McCaffery M, editors: *Pain assessment and pharmacologic management*, St Louis, 2011, Elsevier.

10. Huether S, Rodway G: Pain, temperature regulation, sleep, and sensory function. In McCance K, Huether S, editors: *Pathophysiology: the biologic basis for disease in adults and children*, ed 8, St Louis, 2017, Elsevier.

11. Chapman CR, Okifuji A: Pain mechanisms and conscious experience. In Dworkin RH, Breitbart WS, editors: *Psychosocial aspects of pain: a handbook for health care providers*, Seattle, 2004, IASP Press.

12. Narayan M: Culture's effects on pain assessment and management, *Am J Nurs* 110(4):38–47, 2010.

13. Campbell L, Andrews N, Scipio C, et al: Pain coping in Latino populations, *J Pain* 10(10):1012–1019, 2009.

14. Meints S, Miller M, Hirsh A: Differences in pain coping between black and while Americans: a meta-analysis, *J Pain* 17(6):642–653, 2016.

15. Hollingshead N, Ashburn L, Stewart J, Hirsh T: The pain experience of Hispanic Americans: a critical literature review and conceptual model, *J Pain* 17(5):513–528, 2016.

16. Shavers V, Bakos A, Sheppard V: Race ethnicity, and pain among the U.S. adult population, *J Health Care Poor Underserved* 21(1):177–220, 2010.

17. Staton LJ, Panda M, Chen I, et al: When race matters: disagreement in pain perception between patients and their physicians in primary care, *J Natl Med Assoc* 99(5):532–538, 2007.

18. D'Arcy Y: Pain management survey report, *Nursing* 38(6):42–49, 2008.

19. Pasero C, McCaffery M: Assessment tools. In Pasero C, McCaffery M, editors: *Pain assessment and pharmacologic management*, St Louis, 2011, Elsevier.

20. D'Arcy Y: Managing chronic pain in acute care, *Nursing* 40(4):49–51, 2010.

21. Hicks CL, von Baeyer CL, Spafford PA, et al: The Faces Pain Scale-Revised: toward a common metric in pediatric pain measurement, *Pain* (93):173–183, 2001.

22. Ferreira-Valente MA, Pais-Ribeiro JL, Jensen MP: Validity of four pain intensity rating scales, *Pain* (152): 2399-2404, 2011.

23. Topham D, Ware D: Quality improvement project: replacing the numeric rating scale with a Clinically Aligned Pain Assessment (CAPA) tool, *Pain Manag Nurs* 18(6):363–371, 2017.

24. Herr K, Coyne PJ, Key T, et al: Pain assessment in the non-verbal patient: position statement with clinical practice recommendations, *Pain Manag Nurs* 7(2):44–52, 2006.

25. Voepel-Lewis T, Zanotti J, Dammeyer JA, Merkel S: Reliability and validity of the face, legs, activity, cry, consolability behavioral tool in accessing acute pain in critically ill patients, *Am J Crit Care* 19(1):55–61, 2010.

26. McGuire D, Kaiser K, Haisfield-Wolfe, ME, Iyamu F: Pain assessment in noncommunicative adult palliative care patients, *Nurs Clin N Am* 51(3):397–431, 2016.

CHAPTER 7: MENTAL HEALTH ASSESSMENT

1. World Health Organization: *Mental health: strengthening our response*, 2018. https://www.who.int/news-room/fact-sheets/detail/mental-health-strengthening-our-response.

2. Ball JW, Dains JE, Flynn JA, et al: *Seidel's guide to physical examination: an interprofessional approach*, ed 9, St. Louis, 2019, Elsevier.

3. Kerr LM, Huether SE, Sugarman RA: Structure and function of the nervous system. In Huether S, McCance K, editors: *Understanding pathophysiology*, ed 6, St Louis, 2017, Elsevier.

4. Murphy K: Shedding the burden of depression and anxiety, *Nursing* 38(4):34–41, 2008.

5. Halter M, Kozy M: Depressive disorders. In Halter M: *Varcarolis' foundations of psychiatric mental health nursing: a clinical approach*, ed 8, St Louis, 2018, Elsevier.

6. Sherin KM, Sinacore JM, Li XQ, et al: HITS: a short domestic violence screening tool for use in a family practice setting, *Fam Med* 30(7):508–512, 1998.

7. US Preventive Services Task Force. Screening for intimate partner violence and abuse of elderly and vulnerable adults: US Preventive Services Task Force Recommendation Statement. AHRQ Publication No 12-05167-EF-2, 2013.

http:www.uspreventiveservicestaskforce.org/uspstfl2/ipvelder/ipvelderfinalrs.htm.

8. National Institute of Mental Health: *Bipolar disorder*, 2016. www.nimh.nih.gov/health/topics/bipolar-disorder/index.shtml#part_145402.

9. McCormick U, Murray B, McNew B: Diagnostic and treatment of patient with bipolar disorder: a review for advanced practice nurses, *J Am Assoc Nurse Pract* 27(9):530–542, 2015.

10. Centers for Disease Control and Prevention: *Fast facts-suicide and self-inflicted injury*, 2017. https://www.cdc.gov/nchs/fastats/suicide.htm.

11. Curtin SC, Warner M, Hedegaard H: *Suicide rates for females and males by race and ethnicity: United States, 1999 and 2014*, 2016. https://www.cdc.gov/nchs/fastats/suicide.htm.

12. National Center for Injury Prevention and Control: *Suicide at a glance*, 2015. https://www.cdc.gov/violenceprevention/pdf/suicide-datasheet-a.pdf.

13. Spitzer RL, Kroenke K, Williams J, Lowe B: A brief measure for assessing generalized anxiety disorder: the GAD-7, *Arch Intern Med* 166(10):1092–1097, 2006.

14. Halter M: Anxiety and obsessive-compulsive disorders. In Halter M, editor: *Varcarolis' foundations of psychiatric mental health nursing: a clinical approach*, ed 8, St Louis, 2018, Elsevier.

15. National Institute on Alcohol Abuse and Alcoholism: *What is a standard drink?* 2019. https://www.niaaa.nih.gov/alcohol-health/overview-alcohol-consumption/what-standard-drink.

16. National Institutes of Health, National Institute on Alcohol Abuse and Alcoholism: *Helping patients who drink too much: a clinician's guide.* 2005.

17. Jesse S, Ferrara M, Keindl M, et al: Alcohol withdrawal syndrome: mechanisms, manifestations, and management, *Acta Neurol Scand* 135:4–16, 2017.

18. National Institute on Drug Abuse: *Drug screening and assessment resources,* 2018. https://www.drugabuse.gov/nidamed-medical-health-professionals/tool-resources-your-practice/additional-screening-resources.

19. Schirmer J, Campbell P, Cyr PR: *It never hurts to ask. You may save a life: screening, assessment, and management of domestic violence in the primary care setting*, Portland, ME, 2003, National Child Welfare Resource Center for Organizational Improvement.

20. American Medical Association diagnosis and treatment guidelines for domestic violence, 1992. In Basile KC, Hertz MF, Back SE, editors: *Intimate partner violence and sexual violence victimization assessment instruments for use in healthcare settings: Version 1*, Atlanta, GA, 2007, Centers for Disease Control and Prevention, National Center for Injury Prevention and Control, p 25.

21. Touchy T, Jett K: *Ebersole and Hess gerontological nursing and healthy aging*, ed 5, St. Louis, 2018, Elsevier.

22. The National Institute of Mental Health: *Major depression*. https://www.nimh.nih.gov/health/statistics/major-depression.shtml. Updated November 2017.

23. American Psychiatric Association: *Diagnostic and statistical manual of mental disorders*, ed 5, 2013, Washington, DC, 2013, Author.

24. Webber E, Benedict J: Postpartum depression: a multidisciplinary approach to screening, management and breastfeed support, *Arch Psychiat Nurs* 33(6):284, 2019.

25. Centers for Disease Control and Prevention: *Postpartum depression*. https://www.cdc.gov/reproductivehealth/depression/index.htm#Postpartum. Last reviewed July 24, 2019.

26. The National Institute of Mental Health: *Bipolar disorder*. https://www.nimh.nih.gov/health/topics/bipolar-disorder/index.shtml#part_145402. Revised April 2016.

27. The National Institute of Mental Health: *Bipolar disorder*. https://www.nimh.nih.gov/health/statistics/major-depression.shtml. Updated November 2017.

28. Halter M: Bipolar and related disorders. In Halter M, editor: *Varcarolis' foundations of psychiatric mental health nursing: a clinical approach*, ed 8, St Louis, 2018, Elsevier.

29. National Institute of Mental health: *Schizophrenia*. www.nimh.nih.gov/health/statistics/schizophrenia.shtml#_154880. Updated May 2018.

30. National Institute of Mental Health: *Schizophrenia*. www.nimh.nih.gov/health/topics/schizophrenia/index.shtml. Updated February 2016.

31. The National Institute of Mental Health: *Any anxiety disorder*. https://www.nimh.nih.gov/health/statistics/any-anxiety-disorder.shtml. Updated November 2017.

32. The National Institute of Mental Health: *Obsessive-compulsive disorder*. https://www.nimh.nih.gov/health/statistics/obsessive-compulsive-disorder-ocd.shtml. Updated November 2017.

33. The National Institute of Mental Health: *Obsessive-compulsive disorder*. https://www.nimh.nih.gov/health topics/obsessive-compulsive-disorder-ocd/index.shtml. Revised January 2016.

34. The National Institute of Mental Health: *Post-traumatic stress disorder*. https: www.nimh.nih.gov/health/statistics/post-traumatic-stress-disorder-ptsd.shtml#part_155467 Updated November 2017.

35. The National Institute of Mental Health: *Post-Traumatic Stress Disorder (PTSD)*. https://www.nimh.nih.gov/health/topics/post-traumatic-stress-disorder-ptsd/index.shtml. Last reviewed May 2019.

36. Humeniuk RE, Ali RA, Babor TF, et al: *The alcohol, smoking and substance involvement screening test (ASSIST)*, World Health Organization, 2010. http://apps.who.int/iris/bitstream/10665/44320/1/9789241599382_eng.pdf.

37. Governors Highway Safety Association (GHSA): *Alcohol impaired driving*, 2018. https://www.ghsa.org/state-laws/issues/alcohol%20impaired%20driving.

38. Epstein J, Halter M: Substance-related and addictive disorders. In Halter M, editor: *Varcarolis' foundations of psychiatric mental health nursing: a clinical approach*, ed 8, St Louis, 2018, Elsevier.

39. European Delirium Association, American Delirium Society: The DSM-5 criteria, level of arousal and delirium diagnosis: inclusiveness is safer, *BMC Med* 12:141, 2014. https://www.ncbi.nlm.nih.gov/pmc/articles/PMC4177077/.

40. Stein-Parbury J: Neurocognitive disorders. In Halter M, editor: *Varcarolis' foundations of psychiatric mental health nursing: a clinical approach*, ed 8, St Louis, 2018, Elsevier.

41. Dementia. *Mayo Clinic*. https://www.mayoclinic.org/diseases-conditions/dementia/symptoms-causes/syc-20352013. Updated November 2018.

CHAPTER 8: NUTRITIONAL ASSESSMENT

1. Dietary Guidelines Advisory Committee: *US Department of Health and Human Services and US Department of Agriculture: dietary guidelines for Americans, 2015–2020.* http://www.health.gov/dietaryguidelines/.

2. Fletcher J: Identifying patients at risk of malnutrition: nutrition screening and assessment, *Gastrointest Nurs* 7(5):12–17, 2009.

3. Pender N, Murdaugh C, Parsons MA: *Health promotion in nursing practice*, ed 7, Upper Saddle River, NJ, 2015, Pearson.

4. American College of Allergy, Asthma, and Immunology: *Food allergy.* https://acaai.org/allergies/types/food-allergy.

5. Laforest A: *The prevalence of food intolerance*, 2014. https://foodconnections.org/2014/02/25/food-intolerance-prevalence/.

6. American Society for Metabolic and Bariatric Surgery: *Bariatric surgery misconceptions*, n.d. https://asmbs.org/patients/bariatric-surgery-misconceptions.

7. Helder SG, Collier DA: The genetics of eating disorders, *Curr Top Behav Neurosci* 6:157–175, 2011.

8. US Department of Health and Human Services: *Physical activity guidelines for Americans*, ed 2, Washington DC, 2018, US Department of Health and Human Services.

9. Coleman-Jensen A, Rabbitt MP, Gregory CA, Singh A: *Household food security in the United States in 2017, ERR-256*, 2018, US Department of Agriculture, Economic Research Service.

10. Walton J: Dietary assessment methodology for nutritional assessment: a practical approach, *Top Clin Nutr* 30(1):33–46, 2015.

11. Freisling H, Ocke M, Cassagrande C, et al: Comparison of two food record-based dietary assessment methods for a pan-European food consumption survey among infants, toddlers, and children using data quality indicators, *Eur J Nutr* 54(3):437–45, 2015.

12. Yaroch A, Tooze J, Thompson F, et al: Evaluation of three short dietary instruments to assess fruit and vegetable intake: The National Cancer Institutes' food attitudes and behavior survey, *J Acad Nutr Diet* 112(10):1570–77, 2012.

13. US Department of Agriculture: *MyPlate.* http://www.choosemyplate.gov/.

14. Grodner M, Escott-Stump, Dorner S: *Nutritional foundations and clinical applications: a nursing approach*, ed 6, St Louis, 2016, Elsevier.

15. National Institute of Diabetes and Digestive and Kidney Diseases: *Overweight and obesity statistics, 2013–2014.* https://www.niddk.nih.gov/health-information/health-statistics/overweight-obesity.

16. National Institute of Diabetes and Digestive and Kidney Diseases: *Health risks of being overweight*, 2015. https://www.niddk.nih.gov/health-information/weight-management/health-risks-overweight.

17. Centers for Disease Control and Prevention: *High cholesterol facts*, 2019. https://www.cdc.gov/cholesterol/facts.htm.

18. Pagana KD, Pagana TJ, Pagana TN: *Mosby's diagnostic and laboratory test reference*, ed 13, St Louis, 2017, Mosby.

19. Favaro-Moreira N, Krausch-Hofmann S, Matthys C, et al: Risk factors for malnutrition in older adults: a systematic review of the literature based on longitudinal data, *Adv Nutr* 7(3):507–522, 2016.

20. National Institute of Mental Health: *Eating disorders*, 2017. https://www.nimh.nih.gov/health/statistics/eating-disorders.shtml#part_155059.

CHAPTER 9: SKIN, HAIR, AND NAILS

1. Centers for Disease Control and Prevention: *What are the risk factors for skin cancer?* 2018. https://www.cdc.gov/cancer/skin/basic_info/risk_factors.htm.

2. National Institute for Occupational Safety and Health (NIOSH): *Skin exposures and effects.* https://www.cdc.gov/niosh/topics/skin/default.html.

3. Lurati A: Occupational risk assessment and irritant contact dermatitis, *Workplace Health Saf* 63(2):81–87, 2015.

4. Anderson SE, Meade BJ: Potential health effects associated with dermal exposure to occupational chemicals, *Environ Health Insights* 8(Suppl 1):51–62, 2014.

5. Mayo Clinic: *Pruritus*, 2019. https://www.mayoclinic.org/diseases-conditions/itchy-skin/symptoms-causes/syc-20355006.

6. Centers for Disease Control and Prevention: *What are the symptoms of skin cancer?* 2018. https://www.cdc.gov/cancer/skin/basic_info/symptoms.htm.

7. Reeder S, Eggen C, Maessen-Visch B, et al: Recurrence of venous leg ulceration, *Rev Vasc Med* 1(4):63–65, 2013.

8. Sudheendra D: *Peripheral artery disease*, Medline Plus, 2019. https://medlineplus.gov/ency/article/000170.htm.

9. Safer J: Thyroid hormone action on skin, *Dermatoendocrinol* 3(3):211–215, 2011.

10. Rosen J, Yosipovitch G: *Skin manifestations of diabetes mellitus*, Endotext, 2018. https://www.ncbi.nlm.nih.gov/books/NBK481900/.

11. Drake MT: Hypothyroidism in clinical practice, *Mayo Clin Proc* 93(9):1169–1172, 2018.

12. Kumar G, Vaidyanathan M, Stead L: Koilonychia associated with iron-deficiency anemia, *Ann Emerg Med* 49(2):243–244, 2007.

13. Enamandram M, Duncan L, Kimball A: Delivering value in dermatology: insights from skin cancer detection in routine clinical visits, *J Am Acad Dermatol* 72(2):310–313, 2015.

14. National Pressure Ulcer Advisory Panel: *Prevention and treatment of pressure ulcers: quick reference guide*, Osborne Park, Western Australia, 2014, Cambridge Media.

15. Milstein A: Ending extra payment for "never events"—stronger incentives for patients' safety, *N Engl J Med* 360(23):2388–2390, 2009.

16. Centers for Disease Control and Prevention: *Lyme disease data and statistics*, 2019. https://www.cdc.gov/lyme/datasurveillance/index.html?CDC_AA_refVal=https%3A%2F%2Fwww.cdc.gov%2Flyme%2Fstats%2Findex.html.

17. American Cancer Society: *Cancer facts & figures 2020*, Atlanta, GA, 2020, American Cancer Society.

18. Child Welfare Gateway. *What is child abuse and neglect? Recognizing the signs and symptoms*, Washington, DC, 2013, US Department of Health and Human Services. https://www.childwelfare.gov/topics/systemwide/assessment/family-assess/id-can/.

19. Giardino AP, Giardino ER, Moles, RL: *Physical child abuse*, Medscape, 2015. http://emedicine.medscape.com/article/915664-overview.

20. Centers for Disease Control and Prevention: *Parasites—lice*, 2013. http://www.cdc.gov/parasites/lice/.

21. Ekback M, Wijma K, Benzein E: It is always on my mind: women's experiences of their bodies when living with hirsutism, *Health Care Women Int* 30(5):358–372, 2009.

22. Ghannoum M, Isham N: Fungal nail infections (Onychomycosis): a never-ending story? *PLoS Pathog* 10(6):e1004105, 2014.

23. Haneke E: Controversies in the treatment of ingrown nails, *Dermatol Res Pract* 2012:783924, 2012.

CHAPTER 10: HEAD, EYES, EARS, NOSE, AND THROAT

1. Rossini B, Penido N, Munhoz M, et al: Sudden sensorineural hearing loss and autoimmune systemic diseases, *Int Arch Otorhinolaryngolo* 21(3):213–223, 2017.

2. Cone B, Konrad-Martin D, Lister J, et al: *Ototoxic medications (medication effects)*, American Speech-Language-Hearing Association, n.d. https://www.asha.org/public/hearing/ototoxic-medications/.

3. Abe S, Nishio S, Yokota Y, et al: Diagnostic pitfalls for GJB2-related hearing loss: a novel deletion detected by Array-CBH analysis in a Japanese patient with congenital profound hearing loss, *Clin Care Rep* 6(11):2111–2116, 2018.

4. Occupational Safety and Health Administration: *Occupational noise exposure standards*, n.d. http://www.osha.gov/SLTC/noisehearingconservation/standards.html.

5. Nguyen-Huynh A: Evidence-based practice: management of vertigo, *Otolaryngol Clin North Am* 45(5):925–940, 2012.

6. Mueller M, Strobl R, Klaus J, et al: Burden of disability attributable to vertigo and dizziness in the aged: results from the KORA-Age study, *Eur J Public Health* 24(5):802–807, 2014.

7. Hall D, Fackrell K, Beatrice L, et al: A narrative synthesis of research evidence for tinnitus-related complaints are reported by patients and their significant others, *Health Qual Life Outcomes* 16:61, 2018. doi:10.1186/s12955-018-0888-9.

8. Akarcay M, Miman M, Erdem T, et al: Comparison of clinical differences between patients with allergic and nonallergic rhinitis, *Ear Nose Throat J* 92(9):E1–E6, 2013.

9. Centers for Disease Control and Prevention: *Sexually transmitted diseases: STD risk and oral Sex—CDC Fact Sheet*, 2016. https://www.cdc.gov/std/healthcomm/std-fact-stdriskandoralsex.htm.

10. Schmid-Schwap M, Bristela M, Kundi M, Piehslinger E: Sex-specific differences in patients with temporomandibular disorders, *J Orofac Pain* 27(1):42–50, 2013.

11. McCullagh M, Frank K: Addressing adult hearing loss in primary care, *J Adv Nurs* 69(4):896–904, 2013.

12. McGee S: *Evidence-based physical diagnosis*, ed 4, Philadelphia, 2018, Elsevier.

13. Kaminski J, Mitchell V, Drinane J: Learning the oral and cutaneous signs of micronutrient deficiencies, *J Wound Ostomy Continence Nurs* 41(2):127–135, 2014.

14. World Health Organization: *Headache Disorders*, 2016. https://www.who.int/news-room/fact-sheets/detail/headache-disorders.

15. Charles A: Migraine, *N Engl J Med* 377(6):553–560, 2017.

16. Shivang J, Rizzoli P, Loder E: The comorbidity burden of patients with cluster headaches: a population-based study, *Journal of Headaches & Pain* 18(1):1-9, 2017.

17. National Eye Institute: *Cataract data and statistics*, 2019. https://nei.nih.gov/eyedata/cataract.

18. Lieberthal AS, Carroll AE, Chonmaitree T, et al: The diagnosis and management of acute otitis media, *Pediatrics* 131(3):e964–e999, 2013.

19. National Institute on Aging: *Hearing loss: a common problem for older adults*, 2018. https://www.nia.nih.gov/health/hearing-loss-common-problem-older-adults.

20. Santos M, Corte F, Orfao T, et al: Risk factors for the occurrence of epistaxis: prospective study, *Auris Nasus Larynx* 45(3):471–475, 2018.

21. Rosenfeld RM: Acute sinusitis in adults, *N Engl J Med* 375(10):962–970, 2016.

22. American Academy of Dermatology: *Herpes simplex*, 2018. https://www.aad.org/public/diseases/contagious-skin-diseases/herpes-simplex.

23. Mayo Clinic: *Gingivitis*, 2017. https://www.mayoclinic.org/diseases-conditions/gingivitis/diagnosis-treatment/drc-20354459.

24. Mayo Clinic: *Tonsillitis*, 2018. https://www.mayoclinic.org/diseases-conditions/tonsillitis/symptoms-causes/syc-20378479.

25. Thoppay J: *Aphthous ulcers*, 2018. http://emedicine.medscape.com/article/867080-overview.

26. American Cancer Society. *Cancer facts and figures 2020*, Atlanta, GA, 2020, American Cancer Society.
27. De Leo S, Lee S, Braverman L: Hyperthyroidism, *Lancet* 388(10047):906–918, 2016.
28. McAninch EA, Bianco A: The history and future treatment of hypothyroidism, *Ann Intern Med* 164(1):50–56, 2016.

CHAPTER 11: LUNGS AND RESPIRATORY SYSTEM

1. US Preventive Services Task Force. Screening for latent tuberculosis infection in adults: US Preventive services task force recommendation statement, *JAMA*, 316(9): 962-969, 2016.
2. Social determinants of health: quality of housing, Healthy People 2020. https://www.healthypeople.gov/2020/topics-objectives/topic/social-determinants-health/interventions-resources/quality-of-housing. Updated 6/19/20.
3. Secondhand smoke, January 17, 2018. https://www.cdc.gov/tobacco/data_statistics/fact_sheets/secondhand_smoke/general_facts/index.htm.
4. US Department of Labor. Occupational Safety and Health Administration. *Respiratory protection*, 2002. https://www.osha.gov/Publications/osha3079.pdf
5. Chronic cough, August 22, 2017. https://www.mayoclinic.org/diseases-conditions/chronic-cough/symptoms-causes/syc-20351575.
6. Swartz MH: *Textbook of physical diagnosis: history and examination*, ed. 7, Philadelphia, 2014, Elsevier.
7. McGee S: *Evidence-based physical diagnosis*, ed 4, Philadelphia, 2018, Elsevier.
8. Wilson S: Gas exchange. In Giddens J, editor: *Concepts for nursing practice*, ed 2, St Louis, 2013, Elsevier.
9. Ball JW, Dains JE, Flynn JA, et al: *Seidel's guide to physical examination: an interprofessional approach*, ed 9, St. Louis, 2019, Elsevier.
10. Bohadana A, Izbicki G, Kraman SS: Fundamentals of lung auscultation, *N Engl J Med*, 370(8):744–751, 2014.
11. American Lung Association: *Acute bronchitis symptoms, causes & risk factors*, 2018. Last update March 13, 2018.
12. Centers for Disease Control: *Coronavirus Disease 2019 (COVID-19). Symptoms of Coronavirus*. https://www.cdc.gov/coronavirus/2019-ncov/symptoms-testing/symptoms.html. Last reviewed 3/20/20.
13. American Lung Association: *Pneumonia symptoms, causes & risk factors*, 2019. https://www.lung.org/lung-health-and-diseases/lung-disease-lookup/pneumonia/symptoms-and-diagnosis.html. Last updated February 14, 2019.
14. Miramontes R, Hill AN, Lambert LA, et al: Tuberculosis infection in the United States: prevalence estimates from the National Health and Nutrition Examination Survey (NHANES), 2001–2012, *PLoS One* 10(11):e0140881, 2015.
15. Parmer J, Allen L, Walton W: Tuberculosis: a new screening recommendation and an expanded approach to elimination in the United states, *AJN* 117(8):24–34, 2017.
16. Centers for Disease Control and Prevention: *Asthma numbers*. https://www.cdc.gov/asthma/archivedata/2015/2015_data.html. Last updated May 2018.
17. Centers for Disease Control and Prevention: *Chronic obstructive pulmonary disease (COPD) includes: chronic bronchitis and emphysema*. https://www.cdc.gov/nchs/fastats/copd.htm. Last updated May 3, 2017.
18. Collazo S: Obstructive pulmonary disease. In Lewis S, et al, editors: *Medical-surgical nursing: assessment and management of clinical problems*, ed 10, St Louis, 2017, Elsevier.
19. US National Library of Medicine: *Hemothorax*. https://medlineplus.gov/ency/article/000126.htm. Reviewed June 24, 2018.
20. US Cancer Statistics Working Group: *US Cancer Statistics Data Visualizations Tool, based on November 2017 submission data (1999–2015): US Department of Health and Human Services, Centers for Disease Control and Prevention and National Cancer Institute*, June 2018. www.cdc.gov/cancer/dataviz.
21. Lung cancer 101: *What is lung cancer?* https://www.lung-cancer.org/find_information/publications/163-lung_cancer_101/265-what_is_lung_cancer.

CHAPTER 12: HEART AND PERIPHERAL VASCULAR SYSTEM

1. American Heart Association: *Recommendations for physical activity in adults and kids*. https://www.heart.org/en/healthy-living/fitness/fitness-basics/aha-recs-for-physical-activity-in-adults. Last reviewed April 18, 2018.
2. US Department of Health and Human Services. *Physical activity guidelines for Americans*, ed 2, Washington, DC, 2018, US Department of Health and Human Services. https://health.gov/paguidelines/second-edition/pdf/Physical_Activity_Guidelines_2nd_edition.pdf#page=55.
3. Brown HL, Warner JJ, Gianos E, et al: Promoting risk identification and reduction of cardiovascular disease in women through collaboration with obstetricians and gynecologists, *Circulation* 137:e843–e852, 2018.
4. McGee S: *Evidenced-based physical diagnosis*, ed 4, Philadelphia, 2018, Elsevier.
5. Shaffer R, Bucher L: Coronary artery disease and acute coronary syndrome. In Lewis S, Bucher L, Heitkemper MM, et al., editors: *Medical-surgical nursing: assessment and management of clinical problems*, ed 10, St Louis, 2017, Elsevier.
6. Kalman M, Wells M: Women and cardiovascular disease, *American Nurse Today*, 13(6):22–26, 2018.
7. Wipke-Tevis D, Rich K: Vascular disorders. In Lewis S, Bucher L, Heitkemper MM, et al., editors: *Medical-surgical nursing: assessment and management of clinical problems*, ed 10, St Louis, 2017, Elsevier.

8. Swarts MH: *Textbook of physical diagnosis: history and examination*, ed 7, Philadelphia, 2014, Elsevier.

9. Bickley LS: *Bates' guide to physical examination and history taking,* ed 12, Philadelphia, 2017, Wolters Kluwer.

10. Lanier J, Mote MB, Clay EC: Evaluation and management of orthostatic hypotension, *Am Fam Physician* 84(5):527–536, 2011. https://www.aafp.org/afp/2011/0901/p527.html.

11. Simon E: Leg edema assessment and management, *Med Surg Nurs* 23(1):44, 2014.

12. Ankle-Brachial Index. *Mayo Clinic.* https://www.mayoclinic.org/tests-procedures/ankle-brachial-index/about/pac-20392934. Last updated January 10, 2018.

13. Will JC, Yuan K, Ford E: National trends in the prevalence and medical history of angina: 1988 to 2012. *Circ Cardiovasc Qual Outcomes*, March 20, 2015. https://www.ncbi.nlm.nih.gov/pmc/articles/PMC4366681/.

14. Benjamin EJ, Blaha MJ, Chiuve SE, et al: *Heart disease and stroke statistics—2017 update: a report from the American Heart Association.* 135:e1–e458, 2017. DOI: 10.1161/CIR.0000000000000485. https://www.cdc.gov/heartdisease/heart_attack.htm.

15. Heart failure. https://www.cdc.gov/dhdsp/data_statistics/fact_sheets/fs_heart_failure.htm. Last updated January 8, 2019.

16. Kupper N, Mitchell DF: Inflammatory and structural heart disorders. In Lewis S, Bucher L, Heitkemper MM, et al., editors: *Medical-surgical nursing: assessment and management of clinical problems*, ed 10, St Louis, 2017, Elsevier.

17. American Heart Association News: *More than 100 million Americans have high blood pressure*, AHA says, January 31, 2018. https://www.heart.org/en/news/2018/05/01/more-than-100-million-americans-have-high-blood-pressure-aha-says.

18. Centers for Disease Control and Prevention: *Venous thromboembolism (blood clots) Facts.* https://www.cdc.gov/ncbddd/dvt/facts.html. Last reviewed January 29, 2019.

19. Centers for Disease Control and Prevention: *Venous thromboembolism (blood clots).* https://www.cdc.gov/ncbddd/dvt/data.html. Last reviewed February 5, 2018.

20. Centers for Disease Control and Prevention: *Peripheral arterial disease (PAD) in the legs.* https://www.cdc.gov/dhdsp/data_statistics/fact_sheets/fs_pad.htm. Reviewed June 16, 2016.

21. Patel SK, Surowiec SM: *Venous insufficiency.* https://www.ncbi.nlm.nih.gov/books/NBK430975/. Last update November 18, 2018.

CHAPTER 13: ABDOMEN AND GASTROINTESTINAL SYSTEM

1. National Institute on Aging: *Urinary incontinence in older adults.* https://www.nia.nih.gov/health/urinary-incontinence-older-adults. Content Reviewed May 16, 2017.

2. Argyrou A, Legaki E, Gazouli M, et al: Risk factors for gastroesophageal reflux disease and analysis of genetic contributors, *World J Clin Cases* 6(8):76–182, 2018. https://www.ncbi.nlm.nih.gov/pmc/articles/PMC6107529/.

3. Malaty HM, Graham DY, Isaksson I, et al: Are genetic influences on peptic ulcer disease dependent or independent of genetic influences for Helicobacter pylori infection? *Arch Intern Med* 160(1):105–109, 2000. https://www.ncbi.nlm.nih.gov/pubmed/10632311.

4. Genetics Home Reference, National Library of Medicine, National Institutes of Health: *Crohn disease,* March 19, 2019. Retrieved from https://ghr.nlm.nih.gov/condition/crohn-disease#inheritance. Reviewed December 2017.

5. Genetics Home Reference, National Library of Medicine, National Institutes of Health: *Ulcerative colitis.* https://ghr.nlm.nih.gov/condition/ulcerative-colitis#inheritance.

6. American Cancer Society: *Colorectal cancer risk factors.* https://www.cancer.org/cancer/colon-rectal-cancer/causes-risks-prevention/risk-factors.html. Last reviewed February 21, 2018.

7. Genetics Home Reference, National Library of Medicine, National Institutes of Health: *Kidney stones,* March 19, 2019. Retrieved from https://ghr.nlm.nih.gov/condition/kidney-stones#inheritance.

8. American Cancer Society: *Risk factors for kidney cancer.* https://www.cancer.org/cancer/kidney-cancer/causes-risks-prevention/risk-factors.html. Last Revised August 1, 2017.

9. American Cancer Society: *Bladder cancer risk factors.* https://www.cancer.org/cancer/bladder-cancer/causes-risks-prevention/risk-factors.html. Last revised January 30, 2019.

10. Cartwright S, Knudson M: Evaluation of acute abdominal pain in adults, *Am Fam Physician* 77(7):971–978, 2008. https://www.aafp.org/afp/2008/0401/p971.html.

11. Holcomb S: Acute abdomen: what a pain, *Nursing* 38(9):26–32, 2008.

12. Swartz MH: *Textbook of physical diagnosis: history and examination*, ed 7, Philadelphia, 2014, Elsevier.

13. Madsen D, Sebolt T, Cullen L, et al: Listening to bowel sounds: an evidenced-based practice project, *Am J Nurs* 105(12):40–50, 2005.

14. Felder S, Margel D, Murrell Z, et al: Usefulness of bowel sounds auscultation: a prospective evaluation, *J Surg Educ* 71(5):768–773, 2014.

15. McGee S: *Evidenced-based physical diagnosis*, ed 4, Philadelphia, 2018, Elsevier.

16. Ball JW, Dains JE, Flynn JA, et al: *Seidel's guide to physical examination: an interprofessional approach*, ed 9, St. Louis, 2019, Elsevier.

17. Cox-North P: Upper gastrointestinal problems. In Lewis S, Bucher L, Heitkemper MM, et al., editors: *Medical-surgical nursing: assessment and management of clinical problems*, ed 10, St Louis, 2017, Elsevier.

18. US Department of Health and Human Services, Centers for Disease Control and Prevention: *Inflammatory bowel*

disease (IBD). https://www.cdc.gov/ibd/ibd-epidemiology.htm. Last Reviewed March 31, 2015.

19. Gallager DL, Harding MM: Lower gastrointestinal problems. In Lewis S, Bucher L, Heitkemper MM, et al, editors: *Medical-surgical nursing: assessment and management of clinical problems*, ed 10, St Louis, 2017, Elsevier.

20. American Cancer Society: *Cancer facts & figures 2020*, Atlanta, 2020, American Cancer Society.

21. US Department of Health and Human Services, Centers for Disease Control and Prevention: *The ABCs of hepatitis*. https://www.cdc.gov/hepatitis/resources/professionals/PDFs/ABCtable.pdf. Updated 2016.

22. Wu KH: Liver, pancreas, and biliary problems. In Lewis S, Bucher L, Heitkemper MM, et al., editors: *Medical-surgical nursing: assessment and management of clinical problems*, ed 10, St Louis, 2017, Elsevier.

23. Tapper EB, Parikh ND: Mortality due to cirrhosis and liver cancer on the United States, 1999–2016: an observational study, *BMJ* 362:k2617, 2018. https://www.bmj.com/content/362/bmj.k2817.

24. Yaday D, Lowenfels AB: The epidemiology of pancreatitis and pancreatic cancer, *Gastroenterology* 144(6):1251–1261, 2013. https://www.ncbi.nlm.nih.gov/pmc/articles/PMC3662544/.

25. Urology Care Foundation: *What is a urinary tract infection (UTI) in adults?* https://www.urologyhealth.org/urologic-conditions/urinary-tract-infections-in-adults. Updated April 2019.

26. Renal and urologic problems. In Lewis S, Bucher L, Heitkemper MM, et al., editors: *Medical-surgical nursing: assessment and management of clinical problems*, ed 10, St Louis, 2017, Elsevier.

27. Preminger GM: *Stones in the urinary tract*. https://www.merckmanuals.com/home/kidney-and-urinary-tract-disorders/stones-in-the-urinary-tract/stones-in-the-urinary-tract. Last reviewed May 2018.

28. Scales CD, Smith AC, Hanley JM, et al: Prevalence of kidney stones in the United States, *Eur Urol* 62(1):160–165, 2012. https://www.ncbi.nlm.nih.gov/pmc/articles/PMC3362665/.

29. Mayo Clinic: *Bladder stones*. https://www.mayoclinic.org/diseases-conditions/bladder-stones/symptoms-causes/syc-20354339. Updated October 27, 2016.

CHAPTER 14: MUSCULOSKELETAL SYSTEM

1. Ball JW, Dains JE, Flynn JA, et al: *Seidel's guide to physical examination: an interprofessional approach*, ed 9, St. Louis, 2019, Elsevier.

2. National Institutes of Health: *Exercise and bone health*. www.bones.nih.gov/health-info/bone/bone-health/exercise/exercise-your-bone-health. Last reviewed October 2018.

3. Smith MA, Jackson A: Tobacco use, tobacco cessation, and musculoskeletal health, *Orthop Nurs* 37(5):280–284, 2018.

4. Price MC: Musculoskeletal problems. In Lewis S, Bucher L, Heitkemper MM, et al, editors: *Medical-surgical nursing: assessment and management of clinical problems*, ed 10, St Louis, 2017, Elsevier.

5. Roberts D: Arthritis and connective tissue diseases. In Lewis S, Bucher L, Heitkemper MM, et al, editors: *Medical-surgical nursing: assessment and management of clinical problems*, ed 10, St Louis, 2017, Elsevier.

6. McGee S: *Evidenced-based physical diagnosis*, ed 4, Philadelphia, 2018, Elsevier.

7. Swartz MH: *Textbook of physical diagnosis: history and examination*, ed 7, Philadelphia, 2014, Elsevier.

8. Harris H, Crawford A: Recognizing and managing osteoarthritis, *Nursing* 45(1):37–42, 2015.

9. Bickley LS: *Bate's guide to physical examination and history taking*, ed 12, Philadelphia, 2017, Wolter Kluwer.

10. Corrarino JE: Fracture repair: mechanisms and management, *J Nurs Pract* 11(10): 960–967, 2015.

11. National Osteoporosis Foundation: *What causes osteoporosis and what causes it?* https://www.nof.org/patients/what-is-osteoporosis/. Accessed April 15, 2019.

12. Crawford A, Harris H: Understanding the effects of rheumatoid arthritis, *Nursing* 45(1):32–38, 2015.

13. Hunter TM, Boytsov NN, Zhang X, et al: Prevalence of rheumatoid arthritis in the United States adult population in healthcare claims databases, 2004–2014, *Rheumatol Int* 37(9):1551–1557, 2017. https://www.ncbi.nlm.nih.gov/pubmed/28455559.

14. Centers for Disease Control and Prevention: *Osteoarthritis*. www.cdc.gov/arthritis/basics/osteoarthritis.htm. Last reviewed January 10, 2019.

15. Mayo Clinic: *Bursitis*. https://www.mayoclinic.org/diseases-conditions/bursitis/symptoms-causes/syc-20353242. Reviewed August 12, 2017.

CHAPTER 15: NEUROLOGIC SYSTEM

1. Mozzafarian D, Benjamin EJ, Go AS, et al, on behalf of the American Heart Association Statistics Committee and Stroke Statistics Subcommittee: Heart disease and stroke statistics—2016 update: a report from the American Heart Association, *Circulation* 133(4):e38–e360, 2016. www.cdc.gov/stroke. Last reviewed April 11, 2019.

2. Epilepsy foundation: *What are the risk factors?* www.epilepsy.com/learn/about-epilepsy-basics/what-are-risk-factors. Reviewed March 2014.

3. American Brain Tumor Association: *Brain tumor education*. www.abta.org/about-brain-tumors/brain-tumor-education/. Accessed May 10, 2019.

4. Smith G, Wagner J, Edwards J: Epilepsy update part I: redefining our understanding of a complex disease, *Am J Nsg* 115(5):40–47, 2015.

5. Cummings J, Soomans D, Jodoin A, et al: Sensitivity and specificity of a nurse dysphagia screen in stroke patients, *MegSurg Nurs* 24(4):219–222, 263, 2015.

6. Morley J: Dysphagia and aspiration, *JAMDA* 16:631–634, 2015.

7. Littlejohn L: Acute intracranial problems. In Lewis S, Bucher L, Heitkemper MM, et al, editors: *Medical-surgical*

nursing: assessment and management of clinical problems, ed 10, St Louis, 2017, Elsevier.

8. McGee S: *Evidenced-based physical diagnosis,* ed 4, Philadelphia, 2018, Elsevier.

9. Ball JW, Dains JE, Flynn JA, et al: *Seidel's guide to physical examination: an interprofessional approach,* ed 9, St. Louis, 2019, Elsevier.

10. Bickley LS: *Bate's guide to physical examination and history taking,* ed 12, Philadelphia, 2017, Wolter Kluwer.

11. Sullivan CM: Spinal cord and peripheral nerve problems. In Lewis S, Bucher L, Heitkemper MM, et al, editors: *Medical-surgical nursing: assessment and management of clinical problems,* ed 10, St Louis, 2017, Elsevier.

12. Swartz MH: *Textbook of physical diagnosis: history and examination,* ed 7, Philadelphia, 2014, Elsevier.

13. Braine ME, Cook N: The Glasgow Coma Scale and evidence-informed practice: a critical review of where we are and where we need to be, *J Clin Nurs* 26:280–293, 2016.

14. Wallin MT, Culpepper WJ, Campbell JD, et al: The prevalence of MS in the United States: a population-based estimate using health claims data, *Neurology* 92(10):e1029–e1040, 2019.

15. Roberts D, Plueger M: Chronic neurologic problems. In Lewis S, Bucher L, Heitkemper MM, et al, editors: *Medical-surgical nursing: assessment and management of clinical problems,* ed 10, St Louis, 2017, Elsevier.

16. Centers for Disease Control and Prevention: *Meningococcal disease: technical and clinical information.* www.cdc.gov/meningococcal/clinical-info.html. Last reviewed May 31, 2019.

17. National Spinal Cord Injury Statistical Center: *Facts and figures at a glance,* Birmingham, AL, 2018, University of Alabama at Birmingham.

18. Centers for Disease Control and Prevention: *Traumatic brain injury & concussion: get the facts.* https://www.cdc.gov/traumaticbraininjury/get_the_facts.html. Last reviewed March 11, 2019.

19. Marras C, Beck JC, Bower JH, et al: Prevalence of Parkinson's disease across North America, *Parkinson's Dis* 4(1):1–7, 2018. https://parkinson.org/Understanding-Parkinsons/Statistics.

20. Parkinson's Foundation: *What is Parkinson's?* https://parkinson.org/understanding-parkinsons/what-is-parkinsons. Accessed June 4, 2019.

21. Zamaradi M: Stroke. In Lewis S, Bucher L, Heitkemper MM, et al, editors: *Medical-surgical nursing: assessment and management of clinical problems,* ed 10, St Louis, 2017, Elsevier.

22. National Institute of Neurological Disorders and Stroke: *Myasthenia gravis fact sheet.* https://www.ninds.nih.gov/Disorders/Patient-Caregiver-Education/Fact-Sheets/Myasthenia-Gravis-Fact-Sheet. Last modified May 14, 2019.

23. National Institutes of Health, US National Library of Medicine, Genetics Home Reference: *Myasthenia gravis.* https://ghr.nlm.nih.gov/condition/myasthenia-gravis#statistics. Last reviewed May 22, 2019.

24. *What is the incidence of Guillain Barre Syndrome (GBS) in the U.S.?* Medscape. https://www.medscape.com/answers/315632-14154/what-is-the-incidence-of-guillain-barre-syndrome-gbs-in-the-us. Updated October 6, 2017.

CHAPTER 16: BREAST AND AXILLA

1. McCance K, Huether S, Brashers VL, Rote NS: *Pathophysiology: the biologic basis for disease in adults and children,* ed 8, St Louis, 2019, Elsevier.

2. American Cancer Society (ACS): *Cancer facts and figures 2020,* Atlanta, GA, 2020, ACS.

3. de Blok C, Wiepjes C, Nota N, et al: Breast cancer risk in transgender people receiving hormone treatment: nationwide cohort study in the Netherlands, *Br Med J* 365: 1653, 2019.

4. Centers for Disease Control and Prevention: *What are the risk factors for breast cancer?* 2018. https://www.cdc.gov/cancer/breast/basic_info/risk_factors.htm.

5. US Preventive Services Task Force: *Breast cancer: screening recommendation summary,* 2016. https://www.uspreventiveservicestaskforce.org/Page/Document/UpdateSummaryFinal/breast-cancer-screening1?ds=1&s=breast%20cancer%20screening.

6. Eren T, Aslan A, Ozemir I, et al: Factors effecting mastalgia, *Breast Care* 11(3):188–193, 2016.

7. Smania MA: Evaluation of common breast complaints in primary care, *Nurse Pract* 42(10):8–15, 2017.

8. Patel BK, Falcon S, Drukteinis J: Management of nipple discharge and associated imaging findings, *Am J Med* 128(4):353–360, 2015.

9. Brents M, Hancock J: Ductal carcinoma in situ of the male breast, *Breast Care* 11(4):288–290, 2016.

10. Bryan T, Snyder E: The clinical breast exam: a skill that should not be abandoned, *J Gen Intern Med* 28(5): 719–722, 2013.

11. Saslow D, Hannon J, Osuch J, et al: Clinical breast examination: practical recommendations for optimizing performance and reporting, *CA Cancer J Clin* 54(6): 327–344, 2004.

12. Figueroa JD, Pfeiffer RM, Brinton LA, et al: Standardized measures of lobular involution and subsequent breast cancer risk among women with benign breast disease: a nested case-control study, *Breast Cancer Res Treat* 159(1):163–172, 2016.

13. Orr B, Kelley J: Benign breast diseases: evaluation and management, *Clin Obstet Gynecol* 59(4):710–726, 2016.

14. Ajmal M, Fossen, KV: Breast Fibroademoma, *StatPearls,* 2018. https://www.ncbi.nlm.nih.gov/books/NBK535345/.

15. American Cancer Society: *Fibroadenoma,* 2017. http://www.cancer.org/healthy/findcancerearly/womenshealth/non-cancerousbreastconditions/non-cancerous-breast-conditions-fibroadenomas.

16. American Cancer Society: *Duct ectasia,* 2017. http://www.cancer.org/healthy/findcancerearly/womenshealth/non-cancerousbreastconditions/non-cancerous-breast-conditions-duct-ectasia.

17. Tarallo V, Canepari E, Bortolotto C: Intraductal papilloma of the breast: a case report, *J Ultrasound* 15(2):99–101, 2012.
18. National Cancer Institute: *Breast cancer treatment for health professionals: ductal carcinoma in situ*, 2019. https://www.cancer.gov/types/breast/hp/breast-treatment-pdq.
19. Amir L, Trupin S, Kvist L: Diagnosis and treatment of mastitis in breastfeeding women, *J Hum Lact* 30(1):10–13, 2014.
20. Pena KS, Rosenfeld JA: Evaluation and treatment of galactorrhea, *Am Fam Physician* 63(9):1763–1771, 2001.
21. Huang W, Molitch M: Evaluation and management of galactorrhea, *Am Fam Physician* 85(11):1073–1080, 2012.
22. Dickson G: Gynecomastia, *Am Fam Physician* 85(7):716–722, 2012.

CHAPTER 17: REPRODUCTIVE SYSTEM AND PERINEUM

1. National Institute on Aging: *Age page: menopause*, 2017. https://www.nia.nih.gov/health/publication/menopause.
2. Momenimovahed Z, Tiznobaik A, Taheri S, Salehiniya H: Ovarian cancer in the world: epidemiology and risk factors, *Int J Womens Health* 11:287–299, 2019.
3. Johnson-Mallard V, Curry K, Chandler R, et al: Managing sexually transmitted infections: beyond the 2015 guidelines, *Nurse Pract* 43(8):28–34, 2018.
4. American Cancer Society (ACS): *Cancer facts and figures 2020*, Atlanta, GA, 2020, ACS.
5. Committee on Gynecologic Practice: Well-woman visit, *Obstet Gynecol* 132(4):e181–e186, 2018.
6. Shroff S, Spataro B, Jeong K, Rothenberger S, Rubio D: Let's talk about sex: development and evaluation of a sexual history and counseling curriculum for internal medicine interns, *Patient Educ Couns* 101:1298–1301, 2018.
7. Hill G, Aning J: Investigating the underlying cause of erectile dysfunction, *Practitioner* 263(1822):23–26, 2019.
8. Kimerling R: Sexual assault and women's health: universal screening or universal precautions? *Medical Care* 56(8):645–648, 2018.
9. Moore G: Sexual assault screening in the outpatient setting, *Am Nurse Today* 10(8), 2015.
10. Lobo RA, Gershenson DM, Lentz GM: *Comprehensive gynecology*, ed 7, St. Louis, 2016, Mosby.
11. American Society of Colon and Rectal Surgeons: *Pelvic floor dysfunction expanded version*. https://www.fascrs.org/patients/disease-condition/pelvic-floor-dysfunction-expanded-version. Accessed June 10, 2019.
12. Hill G, Aning J: Investigating the underlying cause of erectile dysfunction, *Practitioner* 263(1822):23–26, 2019.
13. Khera M: *Update on 2018 AUA testosterone and ED guidelines*. grandroundsinurology.com. Accessed September 14, 2018.
14. Unger CA: Hormone therapy for transgender patients, *Transl Androl Urol* 5(6):877–884, 2016.
15. Centers for Disease Control and Prevention: *Bacterial Vaginosis (BV) statistics*, 2015. https://www.cdc.gov/std/bv/stats.htm.
16. Yonkers KA, Simoni MK: Premenstrual disorders, *Am J Obstet Gynecol* 218(1):68–74, 2018.
17. American Urological Association: *Early detection of prostate cancer*, 2018. www.auanet.org.
18. Marsicovetere P, Ivatury JA: Anorectal evaluations: diagnosing and treating benign conditions, *Clin Rev*, November, 27(11):28-38, 2017.

CHAPTER 18: DEVELOPMENTAL ASSESSMENT THROUGH THE LIFE SPAN

1. Erickson EH: *Childhood and society*, ed 2, New York, 1963, Norton.
2. Boeree CG: *Personality theories: Erick Erickson*. http://webspace.ship.edu/cgboer/erikson.html.
3. Piaget J, Inhelder B: *The psychology of the child* (Weaver H, translator), New York, 1969, Basic Books.
4. Duvall EM, Miller BC: *Marriage and family development*, ed 6, New York, 1985, Harper & Row.
5. Wilson D: Health promotion of the infant and family. In Hockenberry MJ, Wilson D, Rodgers CC, editors: *Wong's nursing care of infants and children*, ed 11, St Louis, 2018, Elsevier.
6. Wilson D: Health promotion of the toddler and family. In Hockenberry MJ, Wilson D, Rodgers CC, editors: *Wong's nursing care of infants and children*, ed 11, St Louis, 2018, Elsevier.
7. Monroe RA: Health promotion of the preschooler and family. In Hockenberry MJ, Wilson D, Rodgers CC, editors: *Wong's nursing care of infants and children*, ed 11, St Louis, 2018, Elsevier.
8. Rodgers CC. Health promotion of the school-age child and family. In Hockenberry MJ, Wilson D, Rodgers CC, editors: *Wong's nursing care of infants and children*, ed 11, St Louis, 2018, Elsevier.
9. Kollar LM: Health promotion of the adolescent and family. In Hockenberry MJ, Wilson D, Rodgers CC, editors: *Wong's nursing care of infants and children*, ed 11, St Louis, 2018, Elsevier.
10. Leifer G, Fleck E: *Growth and development across the life span*, ed 2, St Louis, 2013, Elsevier.
11. Schaie KW: Intellectual development in adulthood. In Birren JE, Schaie KW, editors: *Handbook of the psychology of aging*, ed 2, Orlando, FL, 1996, Academic Press.
12. Cavanaugh JC, Blanchard-Fields F: *Adult development and aging*, ed 8, Boston, MA, 2019, Cengage.
13. Parker K, Patten E: *The sandwich generation: rising financial burdens for middle-aged Americans*, Pew Research Center Social & Demographic Trends; January 30, 2013. https://www.pewsocialtrends.org/2013/01/30/the-sandwich-generation/.
14. Touhy TA: Gerontological nursing in an aging society. In Touhy T, Jett K, editors: *Ebersole and Hess' toward healthy*

aging: human needs & nursing response, ed 8, St Louis, 2011, Elsevier.

15. West Midland Family Center: *Generational difference chart.* www.wmfc.org/uploads/GenerationalDifferences Chart.pdf.

16. Dimock M: *Defining generations: where millennials end and Generation Z begins,* Pew Research Center. https://www.pewresearch.org/fact-tank/2019/01/17/where-millennials-end-and-generation-z-begins/.

CHAPTER 19: ASSESSMENT OF THE INFANT, CHILD, AND ADOLESCENT

1. Alderman EM: AMA Guidelines for Adolescent Preventive Services (GAPS): Recommendations and Rationale, *JAMA* 272(12):980–981, 1994.

2. Jellinek MS, Murphy JM, Little M, et al: Use of the pediatric symptom checklist to screen for psychosocial problems in pediatric primary care: a national feasibility study, *Arch Pediatr Adolesc Med* 153:254–260, 1999.

3. Armstrong S: Instruments to identify commercially sexually exploited children: feasibility of use in an emergency department setting, *Pediatr Emerg Care* 33(12):794–799, 2017.

4. Birnie KA, Hundert AS, Lalloo C, Nruyen C, Stinson JN: Recommendations for selection of self–report pain intensity measures in children and adolescents: a systematic review and quality assessment of measurement properties, *Pain* 160:5–18, 2019.

5. Riddell A, Eppich W: Should tympanic temperature measurement be trusted? *Arch Dis Child* 85:433–434, 2001.

6. Paes BF, Vermeulen K, Brohet RM, et al: Accuracy of tympanic and infrared skin thermometers in children, *Arch Dis Child* 95(12):974–978, 2010.

7. US Department of Health and Human Services, National Institutes of Health: *The 4th report on the diagnosis, evaluation, and treatment of high blood pressure in children and adolescents,* National Institutes of Health Publication No. 05-5267, 2005. http://www.nhlbi.nih.gov/health-pro/guidelines/current/hypertension-pediatric-jnc-4/blood-pressure-tables.

8. Centers for Disease Control: *Childhood obesity facts,* 2015. https://www.cdc.gov/obesity/data/childhood.html.

9. Hockenberry MJ, Wilson D. *Wong's nursing care of infants and children,* ed 10, St. Louis, MO, 2015, Mosby.

10. Cornelissen M, Ottelander B, Rizopoulos D, et al: Increase of prevalence of craniosynostosis. *J Craniomaxillofac Surg* 44(9):1273–1279, 2016.

11. US Preventive Services Task Force: *Universal screening for hearing loss in newborns: US Preventive Services Task Force Recommendation Statement,* AHRQ Publication No. 08-05117-EF-2, 2008. http://www.infanthearing.org/resources/USPSTF_Clinical_Summary.pdf

12. Centers for Disease Control: *Congenital heart defects (CHDs).* https://www.cdc.gov/ncbddd/heartdefects/facts.html.

13. Huang W, Molitch ME: Evaluation and management of galactorrhea, *Am Fam Physician* 85:1073–1080, 2012.

14. Sphoorthi J, Livingston N, Moles R: Cutaneous sign of abuse: kids are not just little people, *Clin Dermatol* 35:504–511, 2017.

15. Oregon Evidence-based Practice Center: Screening for visual impairment in children ages 1–5 years: systematic review to update the 2004 U.S. Preventive Services Task Force Recommendation. Evidence Synthesis Number 81, 2011.

16. Arnold RW, O'Neil JW, Cooper KL, Silbert DI, Donahue SP: Evaluation of a smartphone photoscreening app to detect refractive amblyopia risk factors in children aged 1–6 years, *Clin Ophthalmol* 12:1533–1537, 2018.

17. American Academy of Pediatrics: Instrument-based pediatric vision screening policy statement, *Pediatrics* 130(5):983–986. 2012.

18. Loh AR, Chiang MF: Pediatric vision screening, *Pediatr Rev* 39(5):225–234, 2019.

19. Selway J: Case review in adolescent acne: multifactorial considerations to optimizing management, *Dermatol Nurs* 22:1, 2010.

20. Tanner JM: *Growth at adolescence,* ed 2, Oxford, UK, 1962, Blackwell Scientific Publications.

21. Harlan WR, Harlan EA, Grillo GP: Secondary sex characteristic of girls 12–17 years of age: the U.S. health examination survey, *J Pediatr* 96:1074–1078, 1980.

22. Mayo Clinic: *Impetigo,* n.d. https://www.mayoclinic.org/diseases-conditions/impetigo/symptoms-causes/syc-20352352.

23. Albert M, Rui P, Ashman JJ. *Physician office visits for attention-deficit/hyperactivity disorder in children and adolescents aged 4–17 years: United States, 2012–2013,* NCHS Data Brief Number 269, 2017.

CHAPTER 20: ASSESSMENT OF THE PREGNANT PATIENT

1. Woods SM, Melville JL, Guo Y, Fan MY, Gavin A: Psychosocial stress during pregnancy, *Am J Obstet Gynecol* 202:61.e1–e7, 2010.

2. Chambers C: Over-the-counter medications: risk and safety in pregnancy, *Semin Perinatol* 39:541–544, 2015.

3. Lynch MM, Squiers LB, Kosa KM, et al: Making decisions about medication use during pregnancy: implications for communication strategies, *Matern Child Health J* 22:92–100, 2018.

4. Garner GD: Nutrition in pregnancy. In Melin JA, editor: *UpToDate,* 2019. https://www.uptodate.com/contents/nutrition-in-pregnancy.

5. Roy A, Fuentes-Afflick E, Fernald LCH, Young SL: Pica is prevalent and strongly associated with iron deficiency among Hispanic pregnant women living in the United States, *Appetite* 120:163–170, 2017.

6. Wright TE, Terplan M, Ondersma SJ, et al: The role of screening, brief intervention, and referral to treatment in the perinatal period, *Am J Obstet Gynecol* 215:539–547, 2016.

7. Kuehn B: Vaping and pregnancy, *JAMA* 321(14):344, 2019.

8. Volkow ND, Han B, Compton WM, et al: Self-reported medical and nonmedical cannabis use among pregnant women in the United States, *JAMA* 322(2):167–169, 2019.

9. Coleman-Cowger VH, Schauer GL, Peters EN: Marijuana and tobacco co-use among a nationally representative sample of US pregnant and non-pregnant women: 2005–2014 national survey on drug use and health findings, *Drug Alcohol Depend* 177:130–135, 2017.

10. Centers for Disease Control and Prevention: *Substance use during pregnancy*, 2019. https://www.cdc.gov/reproductivehealth/maternalinfanthealth/substance-abuse/substance-abuse-during-pregnancy.htm.

11. The American College of Obstetrics and Gynecologists: *Frequently asked questions, FAQ 170 Pregnancy*, 2019. https://www.acog.org/patient-resources/faqs/pregnancy/tobacco-alcohol-drugs-and-pregnancy.

12. Centers for Disease Control and Prevention: *Parasites—toxoplasmosis (toxoplasma infection)*, 2019. https://www.cdc.gov/parasites/toxoplasmosis/gen_info/pregnant.html.

13. DeNicola N, Slatnik MG, Conry J: Toxic environmental exposures in maternal, fetal, and reproductive health, 2018. https://www.contemporaryobgyn.net/view/toxic-environmental-exposures-maternal-fetal-and-reproductive-health.

14. Poston L: Gestational weight gain. In Melin JA, editor: *UpToDate*, 2019. https://www.uptodate.com/contents/gestational-weight-gain.

15. Santos S, Voerman E, Amiano P, et al: Impact of maternal body mass index and gestational weight gain on pregnancy complications: an individual participant data meta-analysis of European, North American and Australian cohorts, *BJOG* 126(8):984–995, 2019.

16. Cunningham FG, Leveno KJ, Bloom SL, et al: *Williams obstetrics*, ed 25, New York, 2018, McGraw-Hill.

17. Voerman E, Santos S, Inskip H, et al: Association of gestational weight gain with adverse maternal and infant outcomes, *JAMA* 321(17):1702–1715, 2019.

18. World Health Organization: *Care of the preterm and low-birth-weight newborn*, 2019. https://www.who.int/maternal_child_adolescent/newborns/prematurity/en/.

19. Office of Women's Health: *Pregnancy complications*, 2019. https://www.womenshealth.gov/pregnancy/youre-pregnant-now-what/pregnancy-complications.

20. Tikkanen M: Placental abruption: epidemiology, risk factors, and consequences, *Acta Obstet Gynecol Scand* 90(2):140–149, 2011.

21. Beloosesky R, Ross MG: Polyhydraminos. In Melin JA, editor: *UpToDate*. https://www.uptodate.com/contents/polyhydraminos.

22. Bateman BT, Shaw KM, Kuklina EV, et al: Hypertension in women of reproductive age in the United States. NHANES 1999–2009. *PLoS One* 7(4):e36171, 2012. https://www.ncbi.nlm.nih.gov/pmc/articles/PMC3340351/.

23. Duff P: Preterm prelabor rupture of membranes: clinical manifestations and diagnosis. In Melin JA, editor: *UpToDate*, 2019. https://www.uptodate.com/contents/preterm-prelabor-rupture of-membranes-clinical-manifestations-and-diagnosis.

CHAPTER 21: ASSESSMENT OF THE OLDER ADULT

1. US Census Bureau: *QuickFacts*, July 1, 2018. https://www.census.gov/quickfacts/fact/table/US/PST045218.

2. Administration on Aging, Administration for Community Living: *A profile of older Americans*, Washington, DC, 2018, US Department of Health and Human Services. https://acl.gov/aging-and-disability-in-america/data-and-research/profile-older-americans.

3. Briscoe LA: Older adults. In Halter M, editor: *Varcarolis' foundations of psychiatric mental health nursing: a clinical approach*, ed 8, St Louis, 2018, Elsevier.

4. Cavanaugh JC, Blanchard-Fields F: *Adult development and aging*, ed 8, Boston, 2019, Cengage.

5. Touhy T, Jett K, editors: *Ebersole and Hess' toward healthy aging: human needs & nursing response*, ed 9, St Louis, 2015, Elsevier.

6. Jett K: Biological theories of aging and age-related physical changes. In Touhy TA, Jett K, editors: *Ebersole and Hess' gerontological nursing and healthy aging*, ed 5, St Louis, 2018, Elsevier.

7. Mangels AR: Malnutrition in older adults, *Am J Nursing* 118(3):34–41, 2018. [Mini Nutritional Assessment-Short Form (MNA-SF) https://www.mna-elderly.com/forms/mini/mna_mini_english.pdf].

8. Jett K: Assessment and documentation of optimal care. In Touhy TA, Jett K, editors: *Ebersole and Hess' gerontological nursing and healthy aging*, ed 5, St Louis, 2018, Elsevier.

9. Touhy TA: Mental health. In Touhy TA, Jett K, editors: *Ebersole and Hess' gerontological nursing and healthy aging*, ed 5, St Louis, 2018, Elsevier.

10. The National Institute of Mental Health: *Suicide*, 2019. https://www.nimh.nih.gov/health/statistics/suicide.shtml.

11. Touhy T: Rest, sleep, and activity. In Touhy T A, Jett K, editors: *Ebersole and Hess' Gerontological nursing and healthy aging*, ed 5, St Louis, 2018, Elsevier.

12. National Institute on Alcohol Abuse and Alcoholism: *Older adults*, 2019. https://www.niaaa.nih.gov/alcohol-health/special-populations-co-occurring-disorders/older-adults. Accessed July 24, 2019.

13. Jett K: Pain and comfort. In Touhy TA, Jett K, editors: *Ebersole and Hess' gerontological nursing and healthy aging*, ed 5, St Louis, 2018, Elsevier.

14. Booker S, Haedtke C: Assessing pain in verbal adults, *Nursing* 46(2):65–68, 2016.

15. National Institute on Aging: *Urinary incontinence in older adults*, May 16, 2017. https://www.nia.nih.gov/health/urinary-incontinence-older-adults.

16. Palmer MH, Willis-Gray MG: Overactive bladder in women: an evidenced review of screening, assessment, and management, *Am J Nurs* 117(4):34–41.

17. Fulmer T, Guadagno L, Bitondo Dyer C, Connolly MT: Progress in elder abuse screening and assessment instruments, *J Am Geriatr Soc* 52(2)297–304, 2004.

18. Touhy T: Hydration and oral care. In Touhy TA, Jett K, editors: *Ebersole and Hess' gerontological nursing and healthy aging*, ed 5, St Louis, 2018, Elsevier.

19. National Institutes of Health, National Institute on Aging: *Alzheimer's disease fact sheet*, May 22, 2019. https:www.nia.nih.gov/health/alzheimers-disease-fact-sheet019.